P9-CMB-631

SECOND EDITION

DRUG THERAPY IN OBSTETRICS AND GYNECOLOGY

Editors

William F. Rayburn, M.D.
Associate Professor and Director
Division of Maternal-Fetal Medicine
Department of Obstetrics and Gynecology
Associate Professor, Department of Pharmacology
University of Nebraska College of Medicine
Omaha, Nebraska

Frederick P. Zuspan, M.D.
Richard L. Meiling Professor and Chairman
Department of Obstetrics and Gynecology
The Ohio State University College of Medicine
Obstetrician-Gynecologist-in-Chief
University Hospitals
Columbus, Ohio

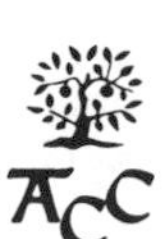

APPLETON-CENTURY-CROFTS/Norwalk, Connecticut

0-8385-1809-5

Notice: Our knowledge in clinical sciences is constantly changing. As new information becomes available, changes in treatment and in the use of drugs become necessary. The author(s) and the publisher of this volume have taken care to make certain that the doses of drugs and schedules of treatment are correct and compatible with the standards generally accepted at the time of publication. The reader is advised to consult carefully the instruction and information material included in the package insert of each drug or therapeutic agent before administration. This advice is especially important when using new or infrequently used drugs.

86 87 88 89 90 / 10 9 8 7 6 5 4 3 2 1

Prentice-Hall of Australia, Pty. Ltd., Sydney
Prentice-Hall Canada, Inc.
Prentice-Hall Hispanoamericana, S.A., Mexico
Prentice-Hall of India Private Limited, New Delhi
Prentice-Hall International (UK) Limited, London
Prentice-Hall of Japan, Inc., Tokyo
Prentice-Hall of Southeast Asia (Pte.) Ltd., Singapore
Whitehall Books Ltd., Wellington, New Zealand
Editora Prentice-Hall do Brasil Ltda., Rio de Janeiro

Library of Congress Cataloging-in-Publication Data

Drug therapy in obstetrics and gynecology.

Includes bibliographies and index.
1. Gynecological drugs. 2. Women—Drug use.
I. Rayburn, William F. II. Zuspan, Frederick P.,
1922- . [DNLM: 1. Genital Diseases, Female—drug therapy. 2. Pregnancy Complications—drug therapy.
WQ 240 D7929]
RG131.D78 1986 618 86-7987
ISBN 0-8385-1809-5

Design: Lynn Luchetti
Cover: Cindy Lee Lombardo

PRINTED IN THE UNITED STATES OF AMERICA

CONTRIBUTORS

Craig W. Anderson, M.D.
Director of Newborn Medicine
Grant Medical Center
Columbus, Ohio

Brian D. Andresen, Ph.D.
Director, Mass Spectrometry Facilities
Biomedical and Environmental Science Division
University of California
Lawrence Livermore National Laboratory
Livermore, California

Sherif G. Awadalla, M.D.
Clinical Instructor
Department of Obstetrics and Gynecology
The Ohio State University College of Medicine
Columbus, Ohio

John G. Boutselis, M.D.
Professor and Director
Division of Gynecologic Oncology
Department of Obstetrics and Gynecology
The Ohio State University College of Medicine
Columbus, Ohio

Richard C. Bump, M.D.
Assistant Professor and Director
Division of Gynecologic Urology
Department of Obstetrics and Gynecology
Medical College of Virginia
Richmond, Virginia

William E. Copeland, Jr., M.D.
Clinical Assistant Professor
Department of Obstetrics and Gynecology
The Ohio State University College of Medicine
Columbus, Ohio

Leandro Cordero, Jr., M.D.
Professor of Pediatrics and Obstetrics and Gynecology

Director of Newborn Services
The Ohio State University College of Medicine
Columbus, Ohio

James K. Crane, M.D.
Clinical Instructor
Department of Obstetrics and Gynecology
The University of Illinois College of Medicine
Peoria, Illinois

Donald M. DeDonato
Instructor and Staff Physician
Department of Obstetrics and Gynecology
Northwestern University Medical Center
Chicago, Illinois

Jeffrey M. Dicke, M.D.
Assistant Professor
Department of Obstetrics and Gynecology
The University of Texas Health Science Center
San Antonio, Texas

Nancy K. Eberhard
Clinical Assistant Professor
College of Pharmacy
The Ohio State University
Columbus, Ohio

Roger G. Faix, M.D.
Assistant Professor of Pediatrics
Section of Newborn Services
Department of Pediatrics and Communicable Diseases
The University of Michigan Medical School
Ann Arbor, Michigan

Chad I. Friedman, M.D.
Assistant Professor
Division of Reproductive Endocrinology and Infertility
Department of Obstetrics and Gynecology
The Ohio State University College of Medicine
Columbus, Ohio

Debra K. Gardner, R.Ph.
Staff Pharmacist
University Hospital
The Ohio State University
Columbus, Ohio

R. Michael Gendreau, M.D.
Research Scientist
Battelle Memorial Institute
Columbus, Ohio

Paul E. Hafner, R.Ph.
Pharmacist Coordinator
University Hospitals Clinic
The Ohio State University Hospitals
Clinical Instructor
College of Pharmacy
The Ohio State University
Columbus, Ohio

Jay D. Iams, M.D.
Associate Professor
Division of Maternal-Fetal Medicine
Department of Obstetrics and Gynecology
The Ohio State University College of Medicine
Columbus, Ohio

Melanie S. Kennedy, M.D.
Associate Professor, Department of Pathology
Director, Transfusion Medicine Program

The Ohio State University College of Medicine
Columbus, Ohio

Joseph J. Kryc, M.D.
Associate Professor of Anesthesiology
Associate Professor of Obstetrics and Gynecology
Northeastern Ohio Universities College of Medicine
Rootstown, Ohio
Aultman Hospital
Canton, Ohio

Justin P. Lavin, Jr., M.D.
Associate Professor
Northeastern Ohio Universities College of Medicine
Rootstown, Ohio
Chief of Obstetrics
Akron City Hospital
Akron, Ohio

Robert M. McNulty, Pharm.D.
Pharmacist Coordinator
University Hospital
The Ohio State University
Columbus, Ohio

Richard W. O'Shaughnessy, M.D.
Associate Professor and Director
Division of Maternal-Fetal Medicine
Department of Obstetrics and Gynecology
The Ohio State University College of Medicine
Columbus, Ohio

L. L. Penney, M.D.
Professor and Director
Division of Reproductive Endocrinology and Infertility
Department of Obstetrics and Gynecology
University of Nebraska College of Medicine
Omaha, Nebraska

William K. Rand, III, M.D.
Clinical Instructor
Department of Obstetrics and Gynecology
Eastern Virginia Graduate School of Medicine
Norfolk, Virginia

William F. Rayburn, M.D.
Associate Professor and Director
Division of Maternal-Fetal Medicine
Department of Obstetrics and Gynecology
Associate Professor
Department of Pharmacology
University of Nebraska College of Medicine
Omaha, Nebraska

James A. Roberts, M.D.
Assistant Professor and Director
Division of Gynecologic Oncology
Department of Obstetrics and Gynecology
The University of Michigan Medical School
Ann Arbor, Michigan

John S. Russ, M.D.
Clinical Assistant Professor
Department of Obstetrics and Gynecology
The Ohio State University College of Medicine
Columbus, Ohio

Randy F. Schad, M.S., P.Ph.
Director of Pharmaceutical Services
William Beaumont Hospital
Royal Oak, Michigan

Grant Schmidt, M.D., Ph.D.
Assistant Professor
Division of Reproductive Endocrinology and Infertility
Departments of Obstetrics and Gynecology and Physiologic Chemistry
The Ohio State University College of Medicine
Columbus, Ohio

Thomas C. Shope, M.D.
Associate Professor of Pediatrics
Director, Section of Infectious Disease
Department of Pediatrics and Communicable Diseases
The University of Michigan Medical School
Ann Arbor, Michigan

Laurence E. Stempel, M.D.
Clinical Assistant Professor
Department of Obstetrics and Gynecology
The Ohio State University College of Medicine
Columbus, Ohio

Sheldon A. Traeger, M.D.
Assistant Professor
Northeastern Ohio Universities College of Medicine
Rootstown, Ohio
Chief, Intensive Care Services
Akron City Hospital
Akron, Ohio

James A. Visconti, Ph.D.
Professor
College of Pharmacy
The Ohio State University
Director
Drug Information Center
The Ohio State University Hospitals
Columbus, Ohio

Nichols Vorys, M.D.
Clinical Associate Professor
Department of Obstetrics and Gynecology
The Ohio State University College of Medicine
Columbus, Ohio

Robert A. Wolk, Pharm.D.
Clinical Pharmacist
Parenteral and Enteral Nutrition Team
The University of Michigan Medical Center
Ann Arbor, Michigan

Frederick P. Zuspan, M.D.
Richard L. Meiling Professor and Chairman
Department of Obstetrics and Gynecology
The Ohio State University College of Medicine
Obstetrician-Gynecologist-in-Chief
University Hospitals
Columbus, Ohio

Kathryn J. Zuspan, M.D.
Director, Obstetric Anesthesia
Cleveland Metropolitan General Hospital
Cleveland, Ohio

CONTENTS

PREFACE

Many drugs are now being prescribed to treat women with not only a variety of obstetric and gynecologic disorders but also disorders that may affect the course of a woman's pregnancy, the health of her fetus or newborn infant, or her reproductive function. This second edition was written to provide more current information about drugs used primarily or exclusively by women. The available information reflects our expanded knowledge in such subspecialties as maternal-fetal medicine, reproductive endocrinology, gynecologic oncology, and general obstetrics and gynecology.

Several texts are now available that either discuss treatment for specific disorders in obstetrics and gynecology or describe cautions about specific drugs used during pregnancy or lactation. An effort to find in-depth information about drug therapy is time-consuming and often frustrating. This book not only provides pharmacologic knowledge about these groups of drugs but also the application of this information to disease-induced abnormalities. Current drug therapy is reviewed in a concise and comprehensive manner in each of two major sections: obstetrics and gynecology.

Each chapter introduces the nature of certain disorders along with patient concerns and then describes the characteristics and indications for the use of each drug. New chapters in this second edition include discussions of drug therapy for chronic medical disorders, drug overdose during pregnancy, immune therapy during pregnancy, and parenteral nutrition. The chapters were planned, written, and revised by the combined efforts of 37 contributors within the following disciplines: obstetrics and gynecology, pharmacology, pharmacy, neonatology, anesthesiology, and internal medicine. The tables and figures have been designed to summarize facts for quick reference, while the text discourses on treatment regimens. References at the end of each chapter have been updated to ensure more appropriate and current information. Over-the-counter drugs used primarily by women are discussed, and cost comparisons are featured when appropriate.

We hope that this text is instructive to practicing physicians, house officers, and students in all disciplines for improving patient care through the safe, accurate, and rational use of drugs in the specialties of obstetrics and gynecology, family practice, internal medicine, and pediatrics.

William F. Rayburn, M.D.
Frederick P. Zuspan, M.D.

Part I

OBSTETRICS

1

Principles of Perinatal Pharmacology

William F. Rayburn and Brian D. Andresen

Pharmacology is the science which deals with the study of drugs and the complex interaction of pathways for the absorption, distribution, metabolism, and excretion of drugs (Fig. 1–1). The absorption of a drug across a membrane (gastrointestinal, placenta, or into breast milk) is related to the following factors: the chemical properties of the drug (molecular weight, spatial configurations, degree of protein binding, ionic dissociation or pKa, lipid solubility); tissue pH; drug concentration; and exposure time. Nonionized, low molecular weight, lipid-soluble compounds are usually well absorbed. The most common mechanism of drug transport across a membrane is passive or simple diffusion from a high to low concentration. Facilitated diffusion which requires a carrier, and active transport, which requires energy transport across a concentration gradient, are less common transport mechanisms for drugs.

The distribution of absorbed drugs in the bloodstream and tissues is dependent on drug binding to proteins, local blood perfusion, capillary permeability of the unbound or "free" drug, pH of the target tissue, and membrane permeability. A drug crosses cell membranes selectively by many transport mechanisms and binds to intracellular receptors. The duration of a drug effect is related to the route of administration, dissolution rate, dose, time required to reach equilibrium, half-life of the drug, and degree of drug-receptor binding.

The metabolism of a drug is a complex event occurring primarily in the liver, and is carried out by microsomal enzymes. Representative drug metabolism reactions include oxidation, reduction, dealkylation, and synthesis. These processes transform drugs into either active or inactive compounds. Most reactions form more polar, and therefore more water-soluble, compounds which can be eliminated by the kidney.

The excretion of metabolized drugs by the kidneys is related to the volume of distribution of the drug, glomerular filtration rate, renal tubular reabsorption, urine pH, and tubular secretion. Lipid-soluble, nonionized compounds are more likely to be reabsorbed than compounds which are significantly ionized at the pH of the urine.

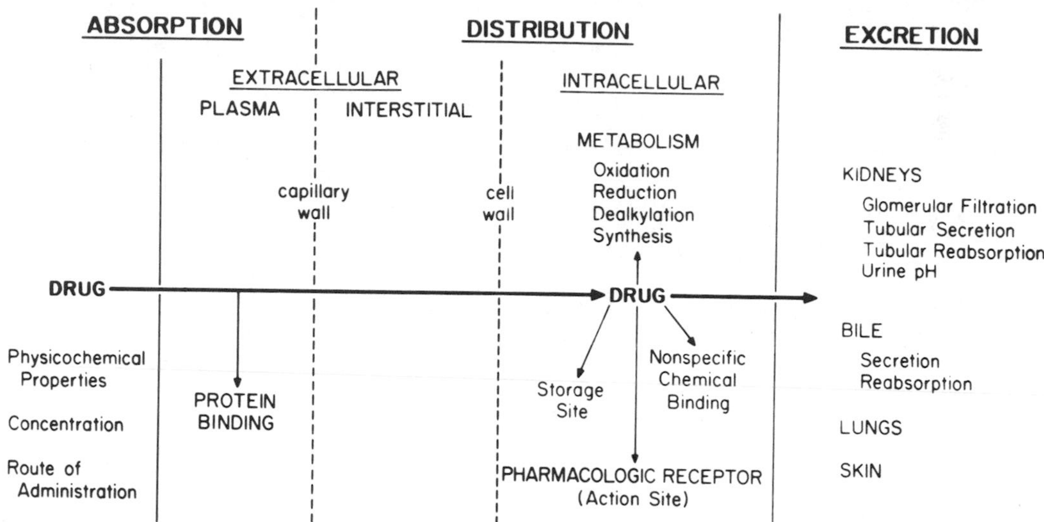

Figure 1–1. Pathways of drug metabolism.

Excretion from the intestines (in bile), lungs, and sweat glands is less common but significant for certain drugs.

Drug–drug interactions are encountered frequently and can interfere with absorption plasma and tissue protein binding, access to cell receptors, and renal excretion. Certain drugs may also induce (phenobarbital) or inhibit (disulfiram) enzymes responsible for the metabolism of other drugs or endogenous substances.[1]

The identification and quantitation of drugs and their metabolites have been accomplished primarily by the newest techniques in radioimmunoassay (RIA), combined gas chromatography and mass spectrometer (GC-MS) computer systems, and high-performance liquid chromatography (HPLC). Animal and human experiments utilizing these and other instrumental methods of analysis have revealed the potential deleterious effects and fate of drugs on the developing fetus. From these studies, new information has been gathered concerning the distribution and pharmacokinetic properties of drugs and metabolites in the maternal–fetal unit.

The study of perinatal pharmacology represents a complex interrelationship among maternal changes, placental factors, fetal development, and neonatal adaptation. These pathways are shown in Figure 1–2 and discussed in the sections that follow.

MATERNAL CHANGES

The absorption of drugs in the gastrointestinal tract during pregnancy has not been well studied but is thought to be similar to nonpregnant patients.[2] Decreased gastric tone and motility are related to progesterone effects. Hydrochloric acid secretion in the stomach is decreased during the first and second trimesters but increased during the third trimester and postpartum periods. Whether this influences the preferential absorption of certain drugs is unclear. Pregnancy has little effect on gastrointestinal secretion, digestion, or absorption.

The distribution of a drug taken during pregnancy is influenced by many factors. Before or during conception the luminal secretions and drug concentrations in the semen, fallopian tubes, and uterus are influenced by certain drugs.[3] The extracellular volume (including intravascular volume), intracellular

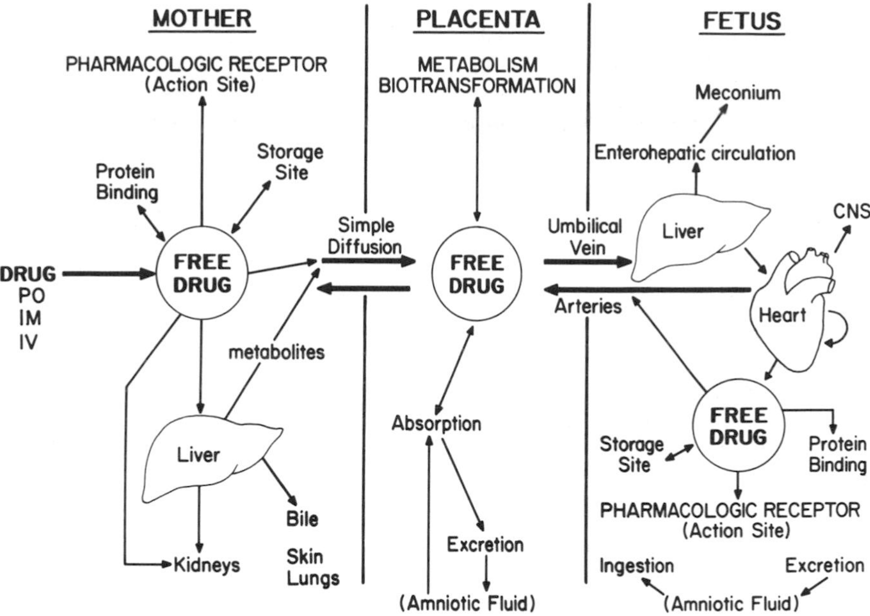

Figure 1–2. Drug pathways within the maternal, placental, and fetal units.

volume, and uterine blood flow increase gradually during pregnancy. Despite an increased production during pregnancy, serum albumin has a relatively lower concentration because of the plasma volume expansion. The albumin-binding capacity to drugs is also decreased, and more unbound or "free" drug is therefore available for placental transfer.

The metabolism of drugs in the liver during pregnancy is influenced by increasing amounts of circulating steroid hormones. Enzyme induction or inhibition by the hepatic microsomes can arise by stimulation from certain drugs. Hepatic blood flow is not increased during pregnancy, and minimal centrilobular bile stasis occurs in the liver as pregnancy progresses.[4] The excretion of drugs by the kidneys may be more rapid because of increased renal perfusion and glomerular filtration. Renal blood flow increases by 25 to 50 percent during pregnancy (550 to 800 ml/min) because of the increased cardiac output, while glomerular filtration is increased by 50 percent.[4]

The pharmacokinetics of drugs during pregnancy and delivery have been reviewed by Nöschel et al.[5] One and two compartment models were studied along with drugs delivered both intravenously and extravascularly. The concentration of a drug is diminished in the maternal circulation during late gestation, while the volume of distribution is enlarged. These changes result from an increase in extracellular fluid and inclusion of the fetoplacental unit in the distribution volume. The decrease in maternal serum drug concentration and increase in the volume of distribution depend on the physicochemical properties of the drug. Total clearance is expected to rise in late gestation, which further accentuates a reduction in serum and tissue concentrations during pregnancy. The dose of drugs prescribed during pregnancy should therefore not be reduced and the administration interval not be extended.

Most drugs are expected to have a shorter half-life in women during late pregnancy than in the nonpregnant state. This is especially true for antibiotics and barbiturates. During labor, the drug concentration may increase rather than decrease, because the clearance of a drug is thought to decrease rather than increase. For this reason, the half-life of analgesic agents, antibiotics, and hypnotics is increased during labor. Those women who have reduced renal function or are edematous may further suffer from effects of drug accumulation.

ROLE OF THE PLACENTA

The placental transfer of drugs and other substrates is complex and no method of study is ideal. Several models have been used to better understand placental transfer. Transfer of drugs across the placenta is primarily by simple diffusion and is dependent on the chemical properties and concentration gradients of the free drug.[6] Most drugs have a molecular weight of 250 to 500. An unbound and unionized drug of molecular weight less than 1000 is usually lipid-soluble and will rapidly penetrate the trophoblast, connective, and endothelial tissues which separate the fetal and maternal circulations.

Pregnant animals have been injected with drugs in varying concentrations and subsequently sacrificed at certain intervals to determine the concentration of drugs or metabolites in fetal tissues. Drug concentrations in umbilical cord or neonatal sera have also been measured and correlated with maternal serum levels. Human placentas have been cultured and exposed to drugs to determine their metabolic capabilities.

Drug transfer is greater during late gestation, and explanations[6] for this increased transfer are listed in Table 1–1. Any drug in sufficient concentration will eventually cross the placenta, especially when maternal therapeutic blood levels of a drug have been maintained for an extended period of time. Pathologic processes causing an inflammatory reaction, hypoxia, vascular degeneration, or partial separation of the placental implantation can affect uteroplacental blood flow and drug transfer. Uterine contractions, cord compression, and supine positioning of the mother can lead to transient uteroplacental hypoperfusion.

TABLE 1–1. REASONS FOR INCREASED DRUG TRANSFER ACROSS THE PLACENTA IN LATE PREGNANCY

1. Increased unbound drug available for transport
2. Increased uteroplacental blood flow (500 ml/min)
3. Increased placental surface area
4. Decreased thickness of the semipermeable lipid membranes (2 mcg at term) between the placental capillaries
5. Greater physical disruption of placental membranes
6. More acidic fetal circulation to "trap" basic drugs

Examples of drugs which readily cross the placenta within minutes after maternal administration include ampicillin, penicillin G, cephalothin, kanamycin, tetracycline, sulfonamides, streptomycin, diazepam, phenytoin, barbiturates, ethanol, meperidine, salicylate, lidocaine, mepivacaine, bupivacaine (with or without epinephrine), and propranolol.[3]

The placental metabolism of drugs is not well understood, but in vivo studies have shown the placenta to be capable of undergoing many enzymatic reactions for drug biotransformation.[7] The placenta may also act as a model for understanding drug biotransformation, since metabolized forms are often similar to those formed within the adult human liver.[8] Differences in formation of principal metabolites between adult liver and placenta may relate to differing concentrations of microsomal enzymes in the two tissues and to the tissue's specific regulation of enzymatic activity. Biochemical transformations within the placenta may be similar to those within the fetal liver. Enzymatic reactions at both sites may be necessary to explain any observed effects within the fetus.

Certain substances may cross the placenta only after transformation by any of the four possible metabolic reactions (oxidation, reduction, dealkylation, and synthesis). The synthetic capabilities of the placenta (including conjugation or oxidative metabolism) have not been well demonstrated. Certain drugs can also induce or inhibit placental enzymes necessary for the metabolic conversion of endogenous substances or for energy-requiring transport mechanisms. Furthermore, drugs may act on the fetus and placenta to reduce placental blood flow or interfere with the active transport or other nutritive functions of the placenta.[9]

DRUG EFFECTS ON THE FETUS

Drugs that cross the placental barrier usually reach fetal levels which often correspond to 50 to 100 percent of maternal serum concentrations.[3] Exceptions are diazepam and the local anesthetics that reach drug levels in the fetus at equilibria which are greater than those in the mother. The total exposure of a drug and its metabolites in the fetus is more important than the rate of transplacental transport. Chronic drug exposure, rather than single-dose therapy, may influence fetal cell growth during the early (hyperplasia stages) or later (hypertrophy stages) periods of development.[9,10] Drugs may act as teratogenic agents in many ways: abortions, malformations, altered fetal growth, functional deficits, carcinogenesis, or mutagenesis (Chap. 2).

Drugs transported in the umbilical vein travel to the fetal liver (portal vein) or are shunted through the liver to the right side of the heart (ductus venosus). Factors determining the flow direction through the ductus venosus or portal vein are not well understood. Cardiac output is proportionally greater in the fetus than in the adult, and blood is preferentially circulated to the essential organs (brain, heart, placenta) through less resistant pathways. Blood–brain permeability is greater in the fetus than in the adult. Mitochondria, the main intracellular sites for metabolism, increase in number in the fetal brain and heart and show increasing enzyme content with fetal age.[11] More than half of the cardiac output is directly returned to the placenta through the umbilical arteries. This is greater when fetal acidosis is present. The maternal–fetal concentration gradient is therefore decreased, and further transfer of drugs or metabolites is retarded.[12]

Despite preferential circulation to the heart and brain, drug distribution in the fetus eventually becomes diffuse. Total body water increases with fetal maturity but decreases proportionally with total body mass (95 percent at midgestation to 75 percent at term). The total concentration of plasma protein and the protein-binding properties are lower in the fetus than in the mother. More free drug is therefore available for tissue penetration or competitive protein binding with other drugs or endogenous compounds. Conclusions about drug deposition within the fetus obtained from maternal or fetal serum levels may therefore not accurately reflect fetal pharmacokinetics or drug distribution patterns.

Concentrations of drugs in the fetus vary but decrease when sampling from the umbilical vein, umbilical artery, and fetal tissue (fetal scalp), respectively. The rate of tissue permeability of a drug is unknown but probably increases with gestation[13] Autonomic receptors (alpha and beta) in the ileum, carotid artery, and aortic arch sinuses are present in fetal animal studies in the early second trimester and respond to catecholamine stimulation.[13,14] Response curves from drugs are considered similar throughout gestation, but the strength of receptor response increases remarkably with fetal development.[12,13] Some drugs may also have a higher affinity for specific target tissues.

Many fetal organs are capable of substantial metabolic activity, but drug metabolism occurs principally in the fetal liver. Human fetal liver microsomes have significant cytochrome P_{450} levels and NADPH–cytochrome c reductase which can be measured as early as the 14th week of gestation.[13] Oxidation and reduction reactions have been described as early as the 16th week.[15] The activity and concentration of certain hepatic microsomal enzymes and the rate of oxidative and conjugative reactions are probably less than in the adult.[15] Therefore, direct pharmacodynamic effects from drugs may be more pronounced and more prolonged in the fetus than in the mother. Certain drugs, such as phenobarbital or ethanol, which readily cross the placenta, may induce specific fetal liver enzymes.[3] Following chronic exposure, enzyme induction increases the smooth endoplasmic reticulum, and the hepatic drug metabolism capabilities of the fetus are activated. Prolonged phenobarbital, narcotic, or ethanol exposure has been shown to stimulate glucuronyl transferase to conjugate circulating bilirubin over several days and thereby diminish the amount of unconjugated hyperbilirubinemia in the neonate.[16] Furthermore, by stimulating hepatic enzymes, phenobarbital may enhance the metabolism and elimination of phenytoin.[17] An absence or excessive presence of one or more enzymes may go unrecognized if the embryo or fetus does not survive.

The excretion of most drugs is slower in the fetus than in the adult, since many systems are not fully developed. The primary routes of elimination involve the placenta and fetal urine. The placental transfer of drugs from the fetus to the mother is the primary route of drug elimination in early pregnancy and is dependent on simple diffusion, free drug chemical properties, and concentration gradients. Drug elimination in the latter half of pregnancy is determined by the immature fetal kidneys contributing to the amniotic fluid. In the absence of gastrointestinal atresia, great amounts of amniotic fluid can be swallowed by the fetus and can be recirculated into the enterohepatic circulation. The measurement of some drug and metabolite concentrations is possible by amniotic fluid sampling and by meconium analysis.

FETAL DRUG THERAPY

After crossing the placenta, pharmacologically active compounds may become localized in specific tissues or body compartments. The drugs or metabolites may then be metabolized to a limited extent by the fetal liver, eliminated into the amniotic fluid, or returned to the maternal circulation through a retrograde placental transfer. Drug uptake in specific tissues depends on the increased free drug concentration, fetal circulation, lipid solubility and specific cellular constitutents, and permeability of the specialized membranes. The drug-binding capacity to plasma proteins is less than that for the mother because of the lower albumin concentration, interfering endogenous substances, and different physicochemical properties of fetal albumin. Specialized membranes such as the blood–brain barrier within the fetus are highly permeable and may be exposed to more excessive concentrations of a drug. Specific fetal tissues may be more selective in drug uptake depending on specific cellular constituents and the lipid solubility of the drug. Examples of such tissue-specific drug uptake include teeth (tetracycline), bones (tetracycline, warfarin), middle ear (amnioglycocides), retina (quinine, chlorpromazine), Müllerian duct and vagina (diethylstebestrol), adrenal gland (corticosteroids, phenytoin), and thyroid gland (iodides, propylthiouracil). The fetal circulation is also different than the infant or adult. Much of the umbilical venous blood flow enters the liver through the portal system, while 15 to 40 percent enters through the inferior vena cava from the ductus venosus. This distribution affects drug concentrations reaching various organs.

Drug metabolism occurs primarily within the fetal liver. Hydroxylation and conjugation reactions are thought to be decreased for in vitro studies. Cytochrome P_{450} system components are present but likely specific for endogenous compounds only. Methylation, sulfation, and reduction reactions are barely mature. The renal excretion function is immature in the fetus. Elimination by the glomeruli and tubules differs for certain drugs from those in the adult.

Drug therapy for various fetal complications is another area presently under investigation. Examples of prior treatment of fetal complications are listed in Table 1–2. Drug administration can occur by the passive, transplacental route or by direct intra-amniotic instillation or intramuscular injection. The direct route has clear invasive risks, but would quickly aid the fetus if drug-transplacental transfer is slow. These risks and benefits for fetal therapy remain uncertain and require further investigation.

NEONATAL PHARMACOLOGY

Drugs absorbed transplacentally from the mother before or during labor may remain in the neonate for a variable period. Potential drug effects on the fetus may be assessed immediately at birth by Apgar scores, drug and principal metabolite concentration measurements of the umbilical blood, and a search for gross anomalies. Neurobehavioral examination of the neonate is also useful in the determination of more subtle and transient drug effects.[18] These include body tone, rooting reflex, Moro response, and response to pinprick stimulation.

Nearly all active or inactive drugs circulating within the mother can also be transferred into the breast milk or colostrum (Chap. 18). Those drugs passing into the breastfed infant may be metabolized further in the gastrointestinal tract. Absorption processes in the untested gastrointestinal tract of the neonate are similar to the adult, and lipid-soluble drugs are well absorbed. The absorption of drugs administered intramuscularly or subcutaneously is dependent on an adequate local circulation.

Distribution of drugs in the newborn is similar to that in the adult. Circulatory alterations after the umbilical cord is clamped involve more blood flow to the lungs and extremities and less to the liver and brain. Total body water and extracellular volume are proportionally higher in the infant, while adipose tissue is less than in the adult. Total serum protein is less in the infant than in the adult, and competition between drugs and endogenous substrates (sulfonamides and bilirubin) for binding sites in albumin may displace more free drugs and bilirubin into the circulation.

Metabolism in the premature and term infant occurs primarily within the liver. The four basic metabolic reactions (oxidation, reduction, dealkylation, and synthesis) for conversion or detoxification of foreign compounds are present but less active. Drugs such as salicylates, ethanol, and diazepam are therefore biotransformed much less rapidly than in the older child or adult and would contribute to any delays in neonatal adaptation.[18] Asphyxia, inadequate nutrition, hypoglycemia, insufficient body temperature control, inborn errors of metabolism, specific diseases, and toxic effects from drugs (local anesthetics, autonomic nervous system drugs,

TABLE 1–2. DRUG THERAPY FOR EVALUATION OR TREATMENT OF VARIOUS FETAL CONDITIONS

Fetal Conditions	Therapeutic Agents
Heart failure, tachycardia, bradycardia	Digoxin, verapamil
Hypothyroidism	Thyroxine
Syphilis exposure	Penicillin
Adrenal hyperplasia	Hydrocortisone, dexamethasone
Respiratory distress syndrome	Glucocorticoids
Renal insufficiency	Furosemide
Rh disease, severe	Promethazine

narcotic addiction, chronic barbiturate use) or endogenous and exogenous substrates can further retard metabolic processes.[3,20] Conversely, drugs may induce enzyme activity and accelerate the metabolism of certain drugs or other essential biochemicals. The measurement of serum bilirubin levels in the neonate can provide a better understanding of the metabolism of certain drugs (sulfonamides, diazepam, methyldopa, nitrofurantoins) since many metabolic processes are shared by other endogenous and exogenous compounds.[19]

Excretion of drugs is also delayed in the infant. Elimination processes are principally in the kidneys, while drug excretion by the lungs, bile, or sweat glands is less significant. Renal plasma flow, glomerular filtration, and tubular absorption and secretion are initially less than in the adult and become comparable only after several months of maturation. Individual drug properties, volume of drug distribution, and more basic urine pH also influence the rate of drug elimination.[20]

Toxic or serious side effects of drugs are potentially more frequent in the neonate than in the older child or adult. The reasons for this phenomenon in the neonate are similar to the fetus and include a greater concentration of free or unbound drug, greater membrane permeability, reduced hepatic capability, and delayed renal excretion capacity (Table 1–3). This observation is especially true for premature infants under these conditions. Less drug is required, and the monitoring of dosages and serum drug levels is necessary.

TABLE 1–3. REASONS FOR MORE SERIOUS SIDE EFFECTS FROM DRUGS IN THE FETUS AND NEONATE

1. More free drug available
2. Increased volume of distribution
3. Greater cell membrane and specialized membrane permeability
4. Reduced hepatic capacity
5. Delayed renal excretion

DRUGS IN BREAST MILK

Principles of drug transfer across the placenta also apply to the transfer of drugs into the breast tissues. The dose, duration of exposure, and route of administration of drugs for the mother are important considerations. Local blood flow in breast tissue is increased during lactation, and therefore drug transfer into breast milk by simple diffusion is facilitated. The chemical properties of each drug must be appreciated, but most drugs in high concentrations can be detected in breast milk. Because the breast is primarily adipose tissue, it is also a potential storage site for drugs before and after delivery. A more detailed discussion of drugs in breast milk is found in Chapter 18.

DRUG USE DURING PREGNANCY

The number of drugs taken per patient during pregnancy averages to be three (range 0 to 7).[21] Excluding iron or vitamin preparations, 75 percent of these women take one or more drugs at sometime during pregnancy and two-thirds take two or more drugs. This is not different from many of the earlier reports.[22,23] Drug use at conception is similar to that taken before gestation and often involves oral contraceptives and diet pills. Drug exposure may increase rather than decrease as gestation advances.

Iron and vitamins, mild analgesics, antiemetics, antibiotics, antacids, and decongestants are the most commonly taken medications. Almost half of all drugs taken before labor are over-the-counter rather than prescribed. Almost all analgesic agents for relief of headaches and musculoskeletal discomforts are aspirin or acetaminophen. Acetaminophen is the most commonly taken drug during pregnancy and has been reportedly used four times more frequently than aspirin.[21]

The most commonly prescribed medications during pregnancy are antibiotics, especially ampicillin, for apparent urinary tract or upper respiratory infections. Antiemetic therapy has been avoided more because of the discontinuation of Bendectin, desire to avoid any drug in general, and any concern about potential birth defects.

Illicit drug use during pregnancy depends on the social environment. Such habits are largely influenced by that person's partner or her own habits before conception. Marijuana is thought to be the most commonly used "street" drug before and during pregnancy (Chap. 4). Up to half of all women smoke cigarettes at least occasionally during pregnancy, while more than half drink caffeinated beverages such as coffee, tea, and colas on a regular basis.

Certain compounds are taken from habit instead of physical need, and are not considered medicines by patients. The initial obstetric examination should include questioning for any specific prescribed, over-the-counter, or "street" drugs. Additionally, questions concerning the mother's exposure to industrial chemicals in abnormal amounts should be included. A history of any drugs (including oral contraceptives, appetite suppressants, and alcohol) taken at conception or during the first trimester should be sought. A specific drug is to be continued during the first trimester only if the anticipated benefit is reasonable and considered to outweigh any known potential, suspected, or theoretical risk. Conversely, drugs used to treat patients with severe medical diseases (seizures, asthma, hypertension) are discontinued intentionally before advice is sought from the physician. Any indicated drug must be documented on the antepartum chart, and the pediatrician should be notified prior to the time of delivery.

The effects of a drug or its metabolites on the fetus are related to the dose, duration of administration, and developmental stage at exposure (Chap. 2). Information from case reports, epidemiologic studies, and animal studies has definite limitations. Studies with many types of animal species frequently involve the administration of large doses of a specific agent administered during early gestation. Drugs taken in high dosages and near delivery may cause more immediate and sustained neonatal effects. The effects from indiscriminate use of many drugs are not usually overtly manifested in the neonate, and less pronounced effects may be undetected.

Relief of patient symptoms and the medical welfare of the pregnant patient must not be ignored. Drugs which improve maternal health often benefit the fetus indirectly. To minimize any fetal risks or adverse side effects to the mother, a prescribed medication should be monitored closely, using a therapeutic dose for the shortest duration. Over-the-counter products used for relief of symptoms should be used sparingly with the smallest doses for the shortest time. Individual variation in patient tolerance to a certain drug must be appreciated, since recommended dosages for nonpregnant women may be inadequate or may reach toxic levels.

REFERENCES

1. Conney AH: Pharmacological implications of microsomal enzyme induction. Pharmacol Rev 19:317, 1967
2. Winship DH: Gastrointestinal diseases. In Burrow G, Ferris T (eds): Medical Complications of Pregnancy. New York, Saunders, 1975, pp 275–350
3. Mirkin BL, Singh S: Placental transfer of pharmacologically active molecules. In Mirkin BL (ed): Perinatal Pharmacology and Therapeutics. New York, Academic, 1976, pp 1–70
4. Bynum TE: Hepatic and gastrointestinal disorders in pregnancy. Med Clin North Am 61:129, 1977
5. Nöschel H, Peiker G, Müller M, et al.: Pharmacokinetics during pregnancy and delivery. Biol Res Preg 3:66, 1982
6. Juchau MR, Dyer DC: Pharmacology of the placenta. Pediatr Clin North Am 19:65, 1972
7. Rayburn W, Holsztynska E, Domino E: Phencyclidine: Biotransformation by the human placenta. Am J Obstet Gynecol 148:111, 1984
8. Rayburn W, Holsztynska E, Pohorecki R, et al.: The placenta: An active organ of drug biotransformation. Soc Gynecol Invest Abs # 198, Phoenix, Ariz, March 20–23, 1985
9. Juchau MR: Drug biotransformation reactions

in the placenta. In Mirkin BL (ed): Perinatal Pharmacology and Therapeutics. New York, Academic, 1976, p 71

10. Enesco M. Leblond CP: Increase in cell number as a factor in the growth of the organs and tissues of the young male rat. J Embryol Exp Morphol 10:530, 1962
11. Winick M. Noble A: Quantitative changes in D.N.A. and R.N.A. and protein during prenatal and postnatal growth in the rat. Dev Biol 12:451, 1965
12. Smith RJ: Mitochondria in fetal tissue. J Embryol Exp Morphol 11:424, 1964
13. Waddell WJ, Marlowe GC: Disposition of drugs in the fetus. In Mirkin M (ed): Perinatal Pharmacology and Therapeutics. New York, Academic, 1976, pp 119–269
14. Boreus LO: Pharmacology of the human fetus: Dose-effect relationship for acetylcholine during ontogenesis. Biol Neonate 11:328, 1967
15. McMurphy DM, Boreus LO: Pharmacology of the human fetus: Adrenergic receptor function in the small intestine. Biol Neonate 13:325, 1968
16. Mirkin BL: Biological maturation and drug disposition. In Perinatal Pharmacology: Mead Johnson Symposium on Perinatal and Developmental Medicine, no 5, 1974, p 31
17. Pippenger CE, Rasen TS: Phenobarbital plasma levels in neonates. Clin Perinatol 2:111, 1975
18. Seanion, JW, Alper MH: Perinatal pharmacology and evaluation of the newborn. Int Anesthesiol Clin 11:163, 1973
19. Vaisman SL, Gartner LM: Pharmacologic treatment of neonatal hyperbilirubinema. Clin Perinatol 2:37, 1975
20. Giacoia GP Gorodisher R: Pharmacologic principles in neonatal drug therapy. Clin Perinatol 2:125, 1975
21. Rayburn W, Wible-Kant J, Bledsoe P: Changing trends in drug use during pregnancy. J Reprod Med 27:569, 1982
22. Bleyer, WA, Au WY: Studies on the detection of adverse drug reactions in the newborn: Fetal exposure to maternal medication. JAMA 213:2046, 1970
23. Fofar JO, Nelson MN: Epidemiology of drugs taken by pregnant women. Clin Pharmacol Ther 14:632, 1973

2

Drug Effects on the Fetus

Jay D. Iams, William F. Rayburn, and Frederick P. Zuspan

DRUGS IN EARLY PREGNANCY

Drug use among women of childbearing age is common and does not decline during early pregnancy. Brocklebank et al. found that 15 percent of women surveyed took systemic medication in any given month during the 6 months prior to conception.[1] This figure rose to nearly 20 percent during the second and third months of pregnancy. Pregnant women may require drug therapy for an ongoing medical condition, may take drugs prior to confirmation of pregnancy, or may use over-the-counter drugs in the belief that nonprescription medications present no fetal hazard.

Drug use in early pregnancy is a problem, since there are few, if any, drugs known to be "safe" for the developing embryo. Although only a few selected drugs qualify as being definitely hazardous, most medications have unknown teratogenic potential in the human. The *Physician's Desk Reference* (PDR) and drug inserts are usually not helpful in guiding therapy during pregnancy. The inserts usually state "safety for use in pregnancy has not been established."

Drugs as Teratogenic Agents: General Principles

The role of drugs in the etiology of fetal malformation is not entirely clear. Drugs are currently believed to account for 4 to 5 percent of malformations (Table 2–1).[2] The impact of maternal medication on the incidence of spontaneous abortion, fetal growth retardation, and other adverse sequelae is more difficult to estimate.

Drugs taken by the mother may also contribute to the production of birth defects now classified as multifactorial or unknown in etiology. The general principles of teratology, outlined by Wilson and Fraser and modified here, indicate the difficulty in establishing a simple cause-and-effect relationship between a given defect and teratogen.[2] The effect of a teratogen is dependent upon:

1. The dose reaching the developing embryo or fetus. This will be affected by the maternal dose, the volume of distribution in the mother, the metabolic clearance of the drug by the mother, and the molecular weight of the drug.

TABLE 2-1. CAUSES OF HUMAN MALFORMATION (PERCENTAGE)

Known genetic transmission	20
Chromosome anomalies	5
Environmental factors	10
Irradiation— < 1%	
Infections—2–3% (rubella, cytomegalovirus, toxoplasmosis, syphilis)	
Maternal disorders—1–2% (diabetes, PKU, virilizing tumors)	
Drugs and chemicals—4–5% (see Tables 2–2 to 2–5)	
Multifactorial/unknown (e.g., most congenital heart disease, neural tube defects, facial cleft)	65

2. The gestational age at the time of exposure. Teratogenic exposure in the first 2 to 3 weeks following conception may result in spontaneous abortion. The period of organogenesis from the 3rd to 10th postconceptional week represents the critical period for major organ malformation. Physiologic deficits and growth delay are the principal effects beyond the 10th postconceptual week.
3. The duration of exposure. An agent given during the embryonic period of organogenesis and during the fetal period of growth may produce both morphologic and physiologic alterations.
4. The genotypes of the mother and fetus. Species differences in teratogenic effect abound in the literature, and illustrate the difficulty in applying animal research to predict either the safety or adverse effects on human pregnancy. Individual differences in the maternal or fetal metabolism of a given drug may produce a marked increase or decrease in the dose reaching the fetus.
5. The effect of other agents to which the embryo or fetus is simultaneously exposed. For example, drug A may be teratogenic to a given species only in the presence or absence of drug B. The addition of drug C may yield an entirely different result.
6. The difficulty to prove a drug effect unless the incidence of the effect is high. If the condition has a low natural incidence (i.e., 1 to 2/10,000), then the drug effect must be considerable for even a suspicion. Once known, randomized prospective trials should then prove cause-and-effect relationships.

The consequences of the principles cited above are several:

1. The effects of a teratogenic agent may include:
   a. No effect
   b. Abortion
   c. Malformation
   d. Altered fetal growth
   e. Functional deficit
   f. Carcinogenesis
   g. Mutagenesis
2. A given teratogenic effect may be induced by a variety of other teratogens, both pharmacologic and otherwise.
3. A single teratogen may have multiple effects, depending upon the dose, the time in gestation, as well as host and environmental factors.
4. Proof of the teratogenicity or safety of an individual drug is consequently difficult to establish. Teratogenicity may be more easily inferred if the defect produced is rare, for example, diethylstilbestrol (DES) and vaginal adenosis. Reports that a drug is associated with more common malformations such as cleft lip/palate or ventricular septal defects are much more difficult to evaluate. Conversely, the absence of reports of teratogenicity for a given drug does not imply safety. There is no drug proven to be absolutely safe for the developing fetus in human pregnancy. Data from animal studies may be either alarming or reassuring, but species differences preclude drawing definitive conclusions about drug effects on the hu-

> man fetus based on animal data alone. A drug that reliably produces defects in an animal species may not do so in humans. The converse is also true and was tragically demonstrated by the effects of thalidomide in infants, after animal studies revealed no teratogenic effects. Any drug must therefore be presumed to be a teratogen if given to a susceptible host in sufficient doses at a critical period of gestation.

The obvious conclusion is that all drugs, both prescription and over-the-counter, should be used with caution throughout pregnancy, given only for specific indication at the minimum effective dose, and for the shortest duration necessary. Pregnant women should be advised at the first prenatal care visit to consult with a physician before taking prescription or over-the-counter medications. This prospective counseling will avoid concern over the unknown effects of medication in pregnancy. Frequently, however, the physician is consulted retrospectively, after the drug has already been ingested. Before advising such a patient, the physician must first establish the exact medication, the dose and duration of the administration, and the gestational age of the pregnancy at the time of exposure.

For all but the most commonly used drugs, the next step is a careful review of the recent literature. Shepard's *Catalog of Teratogenic Agents*[3] and *The Year Book of Obstetrics and Gynecology*[4] are useful in this review. All too often these steps are ignored, and the patient is given either reassurance or alarm without adequate data collection. Tabular listings of drug effects in pregnancy must be interpreted with caution in light of the principles of teratology outlined previously.

The birth of a child with a congenital defect should prompt a review of any maternal medication during pregnancy. The same meticulous documentation of dose, duration of therapy, gestational age at exposure, and literature review are required before any causal connection between maternal medication and malformation is even implied. Failure to follow this procedure may produce unwarranted maternal guilt and anxiety.

It is clinically useful to place drugs in one of three general categories: drugs with known adverse effects, drugs with suspected adverse effects, and drugs without known adverse effects at customary dosage levels. These are listed in Tables 2–2, 2–3, and 2–4 and are described in the sections that follow and in more detail in the appropriate chapters.

Drugs with Known Adverse Effects

This category is small, and fortunately contains only one group of drugs—the anticonvulsants—where fetal risk does not conclusively exceed maternal benefit.

Anticonvulsants as teratogens are discussed extensively in Chapter 5. Trimethadione can conclusively be listed as a teratogen, producing growth retardation, microcephaly, facial dysmorphism, and other anomalies.[5] Principally used for petit mal seizures, it can frequently be avoided in pregnancy without hazard to the mother. The status of phenytoin, on the other hand, is less clear. Although the literature is inconclusive about the teratogenic effect of phenytoin, there is sufficient data to suggest that it be avoided if possible.[6] This raises the question of the relative risks of maternal seizures versus the medications used to control them.

Coumadin may be avoided in situations where anticoagulation is necessary by the substitution of self-administered heparin (Chap. 9).

The use of cancer chemotherapeutic agents in pregnancy must be considered individually. While only the folate antagonists, methotrexate and aminopterin, are listed as demonstrated teratogens, it is logical to suspect that any drug designed to kill growing malignant cells may have the same effect upon the developing embryo. Surprisingly, few cases of malformation have been reported following maternal treatment with antineoplastic drugs. Wilson and Fraser speculate that this is due to their limited use in

TABLE 2–2. DRUGS WITH KNOWN TERATOGENIC EFFECT

Drug	Effect
Anticonvulsants Trimethadione, phenytoin	Facial dysmorphogenesis, mild mental retardation, growth retardation
Anticoagulants Coumadin and congeners	Nasal hypoplasia, epiphyseal stippling, optic atrophy
Alcohol	Fetal alcohol syndrome—growth retardation, mild mental retardation, increase in anomalies
Folic acid antagonists Methotrexate, aminopterin	Abortion, multiple malformations
Hormones Diethylstilbestrol and congeners	Vaginal adenosis, carcinogenesis, uterine anomalies, epididymal anomalies, microphallus, cryptorchidism, testicular hypoplasia
Androgens	Masculinization of female fetus
Isotretinoin	CNS, cardiac anomalies, facial abnormalities, deafness, and blindness
Methyl mercury	CNS damage, growth retardation
Thalidomide	Phocomelia

pregnancy because of demonstrated teratogenicity in laboratory animals, easy justification for elective abortion under the circumstances of use, and the high rate of treatment-induced abortions and intrauterine death.[7] A recent epidemiology study has reported an association between fetal loss and occupational exposure to antineoplastic drugs during the first trimester of pregnancy. Caution should be exercised in the handling of these drugs (such as vincristine, doxorubicin, cyclophosphamide).[8]

Excessive maternal use of alcohol has now been associated with a spectrum of teratogenic effects, including growth retardation, microcephaly, shortened palpebral tissues, and mild mental retardation.[9] The frequency of other anomalies, including cardiac defects, is also slightly increased. This appears to be a dose-dependent phenome-

TABLE 2–3. DRUGS WITH SUSPECTED TERATOGENIC EFFECTS

Drug	Suspected Effect
Alkylating agents	↑ Abortion, anomalies
Hormones	
Oral contraceptives	↑ Limb and cardiac defects (?)
Progestins	↑ Limb and cardiac defects (?)
Lithium carbonate	Ebstein's anomaly
Sulfonylureas	↑ Anomalies (?)
Tranquilizers Benzodiazepines	Facial clefts (?)
Valproic acid	Neural tube defects

TABLE 2–4. DRUGS WITHOUT KNOWN TERATOGENIC EFFECT IN HUMANS AT CUSTOMARY DOSAGES*

Analgesics	Antiemetics
Acetaminophen	Phenothiazines
Narcotics-Salicylates	Corticosteroids
	Heparin
Antibiotics	
Penicillin	
Cephalosporin	
Sulfonamides	

* None of these drugs are *proven* safe. All have been associated in animal studies with malformations, but human studies have not confirmed suspected effects.

non. Several recommendations may be offered to the pregnant woman when alcohol exposure is encountered in a social setting. There is no totally safe level for drinking. Delivering an infant with the fetal alcohol syndrome increases with the average daily alcohol intake. A risk with the daily ingestion of 3 ounces of absolute alcohol (about six drinks per day) has been established, and any lesser amount is uncertain.

Isotretinoin (Accutane), a retinoic acid–vitamin A analogue, used for cystic acne and other skin conditions since 1982, is now a proven teratogen.[10,11] Reports of major human malformations and spontaneous abortions underscore the need to avoid this drug in women who are or may be pregnant. The Food and Drug Administration has received several reports of at least 16 cases of adverse pregnancy outcomes which include 9 spontaneous abortions and 7 infants with major birth defects.[11] These malformations include hydrocephalus, deformed or small external ears, completely or partially occluded external auditory canals, and cardiac abnormalities.[10,11] The half-life of isotretinoin is short, and if discontinued at least 1 month before conception, this drug should not pose any problems. Also these persons should not act as blood donors for fear of passing the potential teratogen to a recipient during early pregnancy.

The remaining drugs listed in Table 2–2 have no indication for use in pregnancy and do not ordinarily present therapeutic or counseling problems. Tetracycline is almost always a second line antibiotic; other, safer antimicrobials are available. Androgens, DES and related substances, and thalidomide are proven teratogens. Isotretinoin has now been added to the list as a proven teratogen.

Drugs with Suspected Adverse Effects

This category could conceivably include any drug that has been the subject of a case report suggesting possible teratogenicity. Such a compilation would be a book in itself, and so exhaustive as to be practically useless. Instead, a shortened list of drugs, which are likely to achieve "proven" status, is offered (Table 2–5). These medications may cause concern when inadvertent use during pregnancy is discovered. None is sufficiently studied to warrant pregnancy termination when exposure occurs.

Several of the agents in this category merit additional comment, because they illustrate some of the principles of teratogenicity. Lithium carbonate, used in the therapy of manic-depressive illness, has been associated with an increased frequency of Ebstein's anomaly, a rare congenital cardiac lesion with a reported incidence of 1 in 20,000 births. Nora et al. reported that 8 of 11 malformed infants born to mothers exposed to lithium in the first trimester had congenital heart disease.[12] Of the eight, four had the Ebstein anomaly, representing a 400-fold increase over the expected frequency. Though small, this series of patients is impressive because of the rarity of the reported defect, and the magnitude of the increase.

A large series of patients treated with progestins showed a doubling of the incidence of all forms of congenital heart disease.[13] Although the increase was statistically significant in a large population, this report must be interpreted with some care because of the relatively small increase in the incidence of a more common and less distinctive group of malformations. Since then other studies have refuted the role of progestins and oral contraceptives as teratogens.[14,15]

Studies of the sulfonylureas in the treatment of maternal diabetes present problems similar to those of the anticonvulsants. Whether the malformations observed are secondary to the maternal disorder or to the medications is not clear. Diabetic women are known to have a two- to threefold increase in the incidence of all malformations. Furthermore, it is known that if prepregnancy and first trimester blood sugars are rigidly controlled, few congenital anomalies are observed. Whether this is related to hyper- or hypoglycemia is unknown. This problem is now academic in the case of the sulfonylu-

TABLE 2–5. REPORTED EFFECTS FROM DRUG EXPOSURE ON THE HUMAN FETUS

Drugs	Reported Effect on the Human Fetus: *First Trimester Effects*	Reported Effect on the Human Fetus: *Second and Third Trimester Effects*
Analgesics (Chap. 3)		
Acetaminophen	None known	Nephrotoxicity (?)
Narcotics	None known	Depression, withdrawal
Salicylates	Frequent reports—none proven (see text)	Prolonged pregnancy and labor, hemorrhage, altered hemostasis, intracranial hemorrhage
Anesthetics (Chap. 14)		
General	Anomalies (?), abortion	Depression
Local	None known	Bradycardia, seizures
Anorexics		
Phenylpropanolamine	Eye (?), ear (?), hypospadias (?)	None known
Amphetamines	Cardiac defects (?)	Irritable, poor feeding
Phenmetrazine	None known	None known
Meclizine	Oral cleft (?)	None known
Antiasthmatics		
Theophylline	None known	Decreased respiratory distress
Terbutaline	None known	Tachycardia, hypothermia, hypocalcemia, hypo- and hyperglycemia
Anticoagulants (Chap. 9)		
Coumadin	Nasal hypoplasia, ophthalmic abnormalities, epiphyseal stippling	Hemorrhage, stillbirth
Heparin	None known	Hemorrhage, stillbirth
Anticonvulsants (Chap 5)		
Barbiturates	None known	Bleeding, withdrawal
Carbamazepine	Unknown	Bleeding, withdrawal
Clonazepam	None known	Withdrawal, depression
Ethosuximide	None known	None known
Phenytoin*	IUGR, craniofacial, abnormalities, MR, hypoplasia of phalanges	Hemorrhage } Depletion of vitamin K-dependent clotting factor
Primidone	Unknown	Hemorrhage } Depletion of vitamin K-dependent clotting factor
Trimethadione*	Mental retardation, facial dysmorphogensis	Hemorrhage } Depletion of vitamin K-dependent clotting factor; IUGR
Valproic acid	Spina bifida	None known
Anti-infection Agents		
Aminoglycosides	None known	Nephrotoxic (?), ototoxic (?)
Cephalosporins	Unknown	None known
Chloramphenicol	None known	None known
Clindamycin	None known	Unknown
Erythromycin	Unknown	None known
Ethambutol	None known	None known
Isoniazid	None known	None known
Metronidazole	None known	None known
Nitrofurantoin	None known	Hemolysis (?)

TABLE 2–5. (*Continued*)

Drugs	Reported Effect on the Human Fetus	
	First Trimester Effects	***Second and Third Trimester Effects***
Penicillins, newer synthetic	Unknown	None known
Rifampin	None known	None known
Sulfonamides	None known	Hemolytic anemia, thrombocytopenia, hyperbilirubinemia
Sulfasalazine	None known	None known
Tetracyclines	None known	Stained deciduous teeth (enamel hypoplasia)
Trimethoprim	Unknown	Hyperbilirubinemia (?)
Cancer Chemotherapy		
Alkylating agents	Abortion, anomalies	Hypoplastic gonads, growth delay
Antimetabolites		
Folic acid analogs (Methotrexate)*	Abortion, IUGR, cranial anomalies	Same as above
Pyrimidine analogs (arabinoside)	Same as above	Same as above
Purine analogs (cytosine, 5-FU)	Same as above	Same as above
Antibiotics (actinomycin)	Same as above	Same as above
Vinca alkyloids	Same as above	Same as above
Cardiovascular Drugs		
Antihypertensives		
Methyldopa	None known	Hemolytic anemia
Hydralazine	Skeletal defects (?)	Tachycardia
Propranolol	None known	Bradycardia, hypoglycemia
Reserpine	None known	Lethargy
β-Sympathomimetics	None known	Tachycardia
Digitalis	None known	Bradycardia
Cold and Cough Preparations		
Antihistamines	None known	None known
Cough suppressants	None known	None known
Decongestants	None known	None known
Expectorants	Fetal goiter (?)	None known
Dextromethorphan	None known	None known
Diuretics		
Furosemide	None known	Death from sudden hypoperfusion
Thiazides	None known	Thrombocytopenia, hypokalemia, hyperbilirubinemia, hyponatremia
Fertility Drugs		
Clomiphene	Meiotic nondisjunction (?) Neural tube defects (?)	Unknown
Hormones		
Androgens*	Masculinization of the female fetus	Adrenal suppression (?)
Corticosteroids	Cleft in animals, not in humans	None known
Estrogens	Cardiovascular anomalies	None known

(*continued*)

TABLE 2–5. (*Continued*)

Drugs	Reported Effect on the Human Fetus	
	First Trimester Effects	***Second and Third Trimester Effects***
Progestins	Limb and CV anomalies (?) "VACTERL" syndrome	None known
Danazol	Virilizing female fetus	None known
Hypoglycemics		
Insulin	Does not cross placenta	None known
Sulfonylureas	Anomalies (?)	Suppressed insulin secretion
Laxatives		
Bisacodyl	None known	None known
Docusate	None known	None known
Mineral oil	Decreased maternal vitamin absorption	Decreased maternal vitamin absorption
Milk of magnesia	None known	None known
Psychoactive Drugs		
Antidepressants tricyclics	None known	None known
Benzodiazepines	Oral clefts (?)	Depression, floppy infant
Hydroxyzine	None known	None known
Meprobamate	Cardiac anomalies (?)	None known
Phenothiazines	None known	None known
Sedatives	None known	Depression, slow learning
Thalidomide*	Phocomelia in 20 percent of cases	None known
Lithium	Facial clefts; Ebstein's anomaly	None known
Radiolabeled Diagnostic Drugs		
Albumin	Does not cross	None known
Technetium	Does not cross	None known
^{131}I (diagnostic)	None known	None known
Thyroid Drugs		
Antithyroid ^{131} therapeutic	Goiter Abortion, anomalies	Goiter, airway obstruction, hypothyroid, mental retardation
Propylthiouracil	Goiter	Same
Methimazole	Aplasia cutis, goiter	Same, aplasia cutis
Thyroid USP	Does not cross	None known
Thyroxine	Does not cross	None known
Tocolytics (Chap. 12)		
Alcohol*	Fetal alcohol syndrome	Intoxication, hypotonia; IUGR
Magnesium sulfate	None known	Hypermagnesemia, respiratory depression
β-Sympathomimetics	None known	Tachycardia, hypothermia, hypocalcemia, hypo- and hyperglycemia
Vaginal Preparations		
Antifungal agents	None known	None known
Podophyllin	Mutagenesis (?)	CNS effects (?)
Vitamins (high dose)		
A	Urogenital anomalies (?)	None known
C	None known	Scurvy after delivery
D	Supravalvular aortic stenosis (?)	None known

TABLE 2–5. *(Continued)*

Drugs	Reported Effect on the Human Fetus	
	First Trimester Effects	*Second and Third Trimester Effects*
E	None known	None known
K	None known	Hemorrhage, if deficiency
"Street" Drugs (Chap. 4)		
LSD	None known	Withdrawal
Marijuana	None known	Assoc. fetal alcohol syndrome
Methaqualone	None known	Withdrawal
Heroin	None known	Depression, withdrawal
Methadone	None known	Withdrawal
Pentazosine	None known	Withdrawal
Phencyclidine	None known	Withdrawal
Cocaine	Abortion (?)	Withdrawal
Other		
Cimetidine	None known	Liver impairment (?)
Caffeine	Anomalies (?) in high doses	Jitteriness
Azathioprine	None known	None known
Bromocriptine	None known	None known
Ibuprofen	None known	None known
Spermicides	None known	None known
Lead	Abortion, CNS disorders (?)	Stillbirth, mental retardation (?)
Isotretinoin*	CNS, cardiac, facial anomalies	Stillbirth, mental retardation (?)

*Proven teratogen.
†Unknown—No studies to investigate fetal effects. None known—No malformations reported in human studies or no consistent malformations in animal studies (when no human studies reported).
(?)Signifies conflicting information to question any increased risk of a previously reported anomaly.

reas, because oral hypoglycemics have no place in the management of glucose intolerance in pregnancy.

Recent information has implicated fetal exposure to valproic acid during the first 3 months of pregnancy and a 1 percent risk of a neural tube defect (Chap. 5). An odds ratio of approximately 20 has also been suggested for the use of this drug and neural tube defects. More information is necessary before this drug is absolutely contraindicated although its use during pregnancy is quite limited.

Drugs Without Known Adverse Effects

Some commonly used medications have not been associated with anomalies in humans despite their widespread use. The more we learn about drug effects, the smaller the list becomes. It should be assumed that all drugs cross the placenta. The real question is whether they overtly affect the fetus. Analgesic compounds including narcotics, salicylates, and acetaminophen may be used in customary doses when indicated. Salicylates are perhaps the most commonly used medication in pregnancy, taken by 80 percent of gravidas in one study.[16] Despite demonstrated embryo-toxicity in animals,[17] and retrospective analysis associating aspirin use with malformation,[18] a prospective study by Slone et al.[19] failed to identify an increase in malformation among the offspring of 5128 mothers who ingested large quantities of aspirin, or among 9736 infants exposed to episodic maternal use of aspirin in early pregnancy. Turner and Collins also found no increase in anomalies in the offspring of 144 pregnant women who used salicylates regularly.[20] Stuart et al.[21] has shown alterations in both maternal and newborn hemotasis if aspirin is ingested less than 5 days before delivery. There was no clinical significance to these observations. Both aspirin and acetaminophen have similar action on platelets but both are relatively safe for the pregnant woman to take in average doses. There has been no evidence of teratogenicity.[22]

Acetaminophen is commonly believed to have fewer side effects than aspirin, and is often used in place of salicylates during pregnancy. The paucity of data about the teratogenic potential of acetaminophen does not permit the conclusion that it is more or less safe than aspirin in pregnancy. The recent increased use of acetominophen as an over-the-counter analgesic should prompt further investigation of its risks in pregnancy.

Spermicidal contraceptives have been thought to be associated with poor pregnancy outcomes when there has been exposure around the time of conception. The first widely publicized reports linking spermicidal contraception and congenital malformations or spontaneous abortion had considerable impact on obstetric practice.[23] More recent epidemiologic studies have failed to support any early findings, and no such association has therefore been demonstrated.[24,25,26] No need for additional regulation of spermicidal contraception is thought to be necessary at this time.

Aspartame, the low-calorie sweetening agent, is broken down in the small intestine into three moieties (phenylalanine, aspartic acid, and methanol). No evidence has implicated a risk to the fetus, and aspartic acid does not cross the placenta.[27] No increases in serum formic acid, a product responsible for the acidosis and ocular toxicity in methanol poisoning, has been found in adults.[28] Phenylalanine is concentrated on the fetal side of the placenta but does not raise blood phenylalanine levels to the range generally associated with mental retardation in the offspring (even among PKU heterozygote offspring).[27] Aspartame is therefore not thought to pose a risk for use during pregnancy.

A summary of the known fetal effects from maternal medication is found in Table 2–5. Information is from human sources only. Proven teratogens are identified by an asterisk. This table should serve as a useful guideline for patient counseling. More complete information about specific reported studies may be found in Shepard's *Catalog of Teratogenic Agents*.[3]

DRUGS IN LATE PREGNANCY

Because of the possible adverse effects on fetal organ development during the first trimester, drugs are frequently avoided or not used until later in pregnancy. The fetus is not entirely spared from possible toxic effects during the latter half of pregnancy since histogenesis and functional maturation continue. Retarded growth of specific fetal organs may also occur, although malformation is unlikely after completion of organogenesis. Cells within the brain, gonads, liver, and special nervous system organs (eye, ear) continue to divide rapidly and are susceptible to drug effects. A toxic reaction within the fetus from a drug is often unpredictable and difficult to prove, because a drug may indirectly or directly act in any of the following pathways: induction or inhibition of certain enzymes, mutation of genes, changes in cell membrane integrity, competition for circulating protein-binding sites, or interactions with other drugs or teratogens.

Table 2–5 also lists specific drugs and reported effects on the human fetus during the second and third trimesters of exposure. As explained previously, these brief listings should be helpful for quick review but require more in-depth and current referencing for more definitive comments. Antibiotics, antihistamines, antihypertensives, sedatives, and mild analgesics are the most commonly prescribed drugs in the latter half of pregnancy.[1] Side effects seen in the mother may occur in the fetus with greater intensity and can interfere with normal physiologic or homeostatic processes. With the increase in uteroplacental blood flow and placental size, and with a breakdown in the placental barrier as gestation progresses, serum levels of drugs or drug metabolites in the fetus may be increased and approach or exceed maternal serum concentrations. Furthermore, the untested and immature metabolic pathways in the fetus may not adequately detoxify or degrade certain drugs. Metabolic clearance may be hindered, especially if large doses are administered over prolonged periods. Principles of drug metabolism and elimination in the fetus have been reviewed previously in Chapter 1.

REFERENCES

1. Brocklebank JC, Ray WA, Federspiel CF, et al.: Drug prescribing during pregnancy. Am J Obstet Gynecol 132:235, 1978
2. Wilson JG, Fraser FC (eds): Handbook of Teratology. New York, Plenum, 1979
3. Shepard TH: Catalog of Teratogenic Agents, ed 4. Baltimore, Johns Hopkins Univ Press, 1983
4. Pitkin RM, Zlatnik FJ (eds): The Year Book of Obstetrics and Gynecology. Chicago, Year Book Medical Publishers (whole series)
5. Feldman GL, Weaver DD, Lourien EW: The fetal trimethadione syndrome. Am J Dis Child 131:1389, Dec 1977
6. Hanson JW, Smith DW: The fetal hydantoin syndrome. J Pediatr 87:285, 1975
7. Wilson JG, Fraser FC: Handbook of Teratology, New York, Plenum, 1977, Vol 1, p 323
8. Selevan SG, Lindbohm M, Cand Pol Sci, et al.: A study of occupational exposure to antineoplastic drugs and fetal loss in nurses. N Engl J Med 313:1173, 1985
9. Clarren SK, Smith DW: The fetal alcohol syndrome. N Engl J Med 298:1063, 1978
10. Benke PJ: The isotretinoin teratogen syndrome JAMA 251:3267, 1984
11. FDA Drug Bull 14:15, 1984
12. Nora JJ, Nora AH, Toews WH: Lithium, Ebstein's anomaly, and other congenital heart defects. Lancet 2:594, 1974
13. Heinonen OP, Slone D, Monson RR, et al.: Cardiovascular birth defects and exposure to female sex hormones. N Engl J Med 296:67, 1977
14. Savolainen E, Saksela E, Saxen L: Teratogenic hazards of oral contraceptives analyzed in a national malformation register. Am J Obstet Gynecol 140:521, 1981
15. Linn S, Schoenbaum SC, Monson RR, et al.: Lack of association between contraceptive usage and congenital malformations in offspring. Am J Obstet Gynecol 147:923, 1983
16. Bodendorfer TW, Briggs GG, Gunning JE: Obtaining drug exposure histories during pregnancy. Am J Obstet Gynecol 135:490, 1979
17. Warkany J, Takacs E: Experimental production of congenital malformations in rats by salicylate poisoning. Am J Pathol 35:315, 1959
18. Nelson MM, Forton JO: Associations between drugs administered during pregnancy and congenital abnormalities of the fetus. Br Med J 1:523, 1971
19. Slone D, Siskind V, Heinonen OP, et al.: Aspirin and congenital malformations. Lancet 1:1373, 1976
20. Turner G, Collins E: Fetal effects of regular salicylate ingestion during pregnancy. Lancet 2:338, 1975
21. Stuart MJ, Gross SJ, Elrad H, et al.: Effect of acetylsalicylic acid ingestion on maternal and neonatal hemostasis. N Engl J Med 307:909, 1982
22. Rudolph A: Effects of aspirin and acetaminophen in pregnancy and in the newborn. Arch Intern Med 141:358, 1981
23. Jick H, Walker A, Rothman K, et al.: Vaginal spermicides and congenital disorders. JAMA 245:1329, 1981
24. Mills J, Reed G, Nugent R, et al.: Are there adverse effects of periconceptional spermicide use? Fertil Steril 43:442, 1985
25. Shapiro S, Slone D, Heinonen O, et al.: Birth defects and vaginal spermicides. JAMA 247:2381, 1982
26. Bracken M: Spermicidal contraceptives and poor reproductive outcomes: The epidemiologic evidence against an association. Am J Obstet Gynecol 151:552, 1985
27. Sturtevant F: Use of aspartame in pregnancy. Int J Fertil 30:85, 1985
28. Council on Scientific Affairs: Aspartame: Review of safety issues. JAMA 254:400, 1985

3

Antiemetics, Iron Preparations, Vitamins, and OTC Drugs

Randy F. Schad and William F. Rayburn

Despite growing patient awareness of the necessity to avoid drugs, many medications are commonly taken during pregnancy. Reportedly between 3.6 and 4.5 drugs have been ingested per patient during gestation, and these contain 8.7 different pharmacologic agents.[1-3] There is now a greater reluctance to take drugs during pregnancy with increased patient awareness of drug effects on the unborn infant. A more recent study at our institution has revealed that the average pregnant woman takes two drugs besides iron or vitamin supplementations before labor.[4]

Drug ingestion is most common during the first and third trimesters, exposing the fetus during organogenesis and predelivery. Approximately one-half of these drugs are over-the-counter preparations (acetaminophen, aspirin, decongestants, etc.). Many over-the-counter drugs are taken without physician knowledge and are not recognized by the pregnant patient as being potentially harmful. Furthermore, over-the-counter drugs have been reported to be taken four times more often than prescribed medications during pregnancy.[4] This chapter evaluates the drugs most commonly taken during pregnancy.

ANTIEMETICS

The "morning sickness" of early pregnancy is a frequent patient complaint. Although the etiology is unclear, increased levels of pregnancy-related hormones and certain psychologic factors have been implicated. Other conditions that may lead to persistent nausea and vomiting (urinary tract infections, influenza, appendicitis, cholecystitis, bowel obstruction, cerebral tumors) must also be considered.

Preparations

The manufacturers of Bendectin reluctantly decided to cease the production of this antiemetic in June, 1983. Despite no association being found with adverse fetal effects, significant damaging publicity undermined patient confidence. The cost of the drug with more limited patient use multiplied greatly.

Pyridoxine or vitamin B_6, formerly found in Bendectin in a 10-mg dose, has been used alone to treat nauseous pregnant women. Its mechanism of action is unknown. A 4- to 10-mg dose is found in most prenatal vitamins. A daily oral dose of 10 to 25 mg or a 100-mg injection may be moderately helpful, although no randomized prospective trials have been published. Vitamin B_6 may be purchased easily as an over-the-counter preparation in doses often larger than those recommended above.

The antihistamine doxylamine was the other component within Bendectin. Its use as an antinauseant has also not been studied, although no known teratogenic risks have been conclusively shown with antihistamine use during pregnancy. Many concentrated glucose syrups (Emetrol, Pepto Bismol) are available as over-the-counter remedies for nausea. Success with these expensive elixirs during gestation has not been reported but is unlikely.

If psychologic reassurance and frequent small dry meals of mostly carbohydrates offer no improvement, phenothiazine medications have been prescribed. The phenothiazines are thought to act by blocking the chemoreceptor trigger zone (CTZ) and the vomiting center in the brain. Promethazine (Phenergan) and prochlorperazine (Compazine) require prescription and may be dispensed as tablets, spansules, or rectal suppositories. These preparations are listed in Table 3–1, along with scopolamine and metoclopramide.

Modes of Administration

If nausea is recurrent at predictable times, the medication may be taken before its onset. The two common phenothiazine preparations may be given rectally if oral administration is not tolerated. Parenteral administration is infrequent but necessary when oral or rectal therapy is inadequate. After initial treatment, the dosage of any medication should be adjusted to the smallest amount necessary to relieve symptoms.

Precautions

No known anomalies are associated with phenothiazine usage (see Table 2–5). Phenothiazines are not approved for this use by the FDA; their liberal use as an antiemetic is therefore not encouraged. Common side ef-

TABLE 3–1. ANTIEMETICS COMMONLY USED DURING PREGNANCY*

Trade Name	Generic Name	Dose	Strength (mg, unless otherwise indicated)
Phenergan	Promethazine	25 mg repeated every 4 to 6 hr	25 mg tablet 25 mg suppository 25 mg/ml
Compazine	Prochlorperazine	5 to 10 mg every 4 to 6 hr	5 mg tablet 10 mg tablet 25 mg suppository 5 mg/ml injection
Reglan	Metoclopramide	10 mg 4 times a day 30 min before meal	10 mg capsule 5 mg/ml
Transderm Scop	Scopolamine	1 disk behind ear every 3 days	1 disk

* Experience with the use of these drugs is limited and placebo-controlled studies are lacking. Although the risk of anomalies is no greater with the use of these drugs, the benefits should outweigh any known hazards to the mother.

fects of antiemetics include drowsiness and relaxation. The concomitant use of analgesics, sedatives, and alcohol with antiemetics can further depress the central nervous system and should be avoided. Patients should be cautioned against driving automobiles or performing any actions that require coordination. Occasional side effects of phenothiazines include hypotension, extrapyramidal effects, dyskinesias, dry mouth, skin reactions, jaundice, and blood dyscrasias.

An overdose of the phenothiazines can cause central nervous system depression, coma, convulsions, fever, dry mouth, hypotension, ileus, extrapyramidal reactions, dystonic reactions, headache, vertigo, disorientation, and blurred vision. Treatment may require gastric lavage, along with symptomatic and supportive care. Emesis should be attempted cautiously, since a dystonic reaction of the head or neck may develop and lead to aspiration of vomitus. Persistent extrapyramidal signs are treated with trihexyphenidyl (Artane).

IRON

Requirements During Pregnancy

The natural course of pregnancy, due to increasing fetal and maternal needs, requires approximately twice the daily requirement of elemental iron as the nonpregnant state. A minimum of 750 mg of additional utilizable elemental iron is necessary during the course of pregnancy to meet the demands for increased maternal red blood cell volume (500 mg), fetal needs (200 mg), and placental and cord requirements (50 mg).[5] Additionally, the nursing mother loses 1 or 2 mg of iron per day via breast milk. Therefore, a total of 4 mg of absorbed elemental iron is required daily to meet the demands of normal adult losses and pregnancy or lactation needs.

The demands for iron during pregnancy are in excess of dietary sources (red meats, liver); hence, iron supplementation is recommended. Approximately 10 percent of iron contained in food and iron supplements is absorbed. Intestinal absorption of elemental iron increases further with gestational age and during iron deficiency (about 20 percent). Although no teratogenic effects have been reported in physiologic doses, iron is usually unnecessary until the second trimester, when the demand for iron increases. Iron may also be perceived by the patient as contributing to nausea of early pregnancy, which should subside by the second trimester.

Iron deficiency anemia is the most common form of anemia during pregnancy and occurs in 60 percent of gravid women if iron supplements are not given. Causes for this deficiency include inadequate dietary intake, occult hemorrhage, diminished gastrointestinal absorption, and fetal requirements. Additional iron therapy is necessary after iron deficiency anemia is confirmed. The prevention of iron deficiency anemia and the replenishment of iron stores during each pregnancy should prevent anemia in subsequent pregnancies.

Preparations

Many over-the-counter and prescription products are available that contain iron in varying dosages. Differences between oral products relate to the amount of elemental iron (10 to 33 percent) in the form of iron salt (Table 3–2). Iron-containing liquids should be taken if tablets cannot be tolerated or if intestinal absorption of iron from the tablets is questioned. Sustained release iron preparations have not proven to be more useful than other preparations, since they are relatively expensive and are transported beyond the duodenum and proximal jejunum where iron is less likely to be absorbed.

Other ingredients that are added to oral iron products include vitamin C and docusate sodium (Colace), a stool softener. Vitamin C promotes iron absorption, and docusate sodium counteracts the constipating effect of iron. The added expense for these preparations must be considered.

TABLE 3-2. IRON PRODUCTS CURRENTLY AVAILABLE

Dosage Form	Trade Name	Generic Name	Strength (mg, unless otherwise indicated)	Elemental Iron (mg)	Cost*
Liquids	Fer-In-Sol	Ferrous sulfate	90 mg/5 ml	18	7
	Feosol Elixir	Ferrous sulfate	220 mg/5 ml	44	5
	Fergon Elixir	Ferrous gluconate	300 mg/5 ml	34	6
	Mol-Iron Liquid	Ferrous sulfate	244 mg/15 ml	49	13
Tablets/capsules	Feosol	Ferrous sulfate	325	65	4
	Fergon	Ferrous gluconate	320	37	3
	Fumasorb	Ferrous fumarate	200	66	4
	Ferancee-HP	Ferrous fumarate	330	110	9
		Ascorbic acid	600	—	
	Mol-Iron with	Ferrous sulfate	195	39	4
	Vitamin C	Ascorbic acid	75	—	
Sustained release oral preparations	Ferro Sequels	Ferrous fumarate	150	50	13
		Docusate sodium	100	—	
	Feosol Spansule	Ferrous sulfate	250	50	13
	Fergon Capsules	Ferrous gluconate	435	50	13
	Fero-Gradumet	Ferrous sulfate	525	105	9
	Fero-Grad-500	Ferrous sulfate	525	105	11
		Vitamin C	500	—	
	Mol-Iron chronsule	Ferrous sulfate	390	78	9
Injection	Imferon	Iron dextran complex	50 mg/ml	50	5

* The number reflects the average wholesale cost of that dosage form rounded to the next whole dollar. It represents the cost of 100 tablets, capsules, or oral liquid doses of the indicated volume. For injections, it reflects the cost per ampule.

Injectable iron contains elemental iron (iron dextran). It is available with a preservative (0.5 percent phenol) in multiple dose vials for intramuscular injection or without a preservative in ampules for intravenous administration.

Modes of Administration and Dose

Oral iron therapy is the preferred and safest route of administration. Ferrous sulfate or gluconate, 325 mg daily, is sufficient to provide the iron requirements of pregnancy for those patients who are not iron-deficient. Patients with iron deficiency should receive 325 mg of ferrous sulfate two or three times daily. Six months of iron supplementation is necessary to replenish already depleted iron stores in the bone marrow.

Parenteral administration of iron is necessary when the response to oral iron is inadequate or not tolerated (Table 3–3) by the patient. The rate of hemoglobin production is essentially the same whether iron is administered orally, intramuscularly, or intravenously.[6–8] The total dose of parenteral iron needed to restore hemoglobin and to replen-

TABLE 3-3. REASONS FOR FAILURE OF ORAL IRON THERAPY

Inadequate patient compliance
Inability to tolerate or absorb the iron
Nonbioavailable iron preparation
Antacid therapy
Concurrent infection, inflammation, or malignancy
Undetected blood loss
Non-iron-deficient anemia

ish iron stores in the bone marrow can be calculated by the following formula:

Milligrams total
iron to be injected* =

$$\frac{0.3 \times \text{body weight in pounds} \times (100 - \text{patient hemoglobin gram·percent} \times 100)}{14.8}$$

A test dose of 0.5 ml should be administered intramuscularly or intravenously initially if parenteral therapy is necessary. If no reaction occurs within several hours, a maintenance dose of 2 ml can be given. The patient can either receive an intramuscular dose daily or twice weekly until the desired total dose is administered. The Z-track technique for intramuscular injection should be performed using a 2- or 3-in, 19- or 20-gauge needle in the upper outer quadrant of the buttock only.† Needle size is important and should be judged upon the size of the patient.

Intravenous administration of iron dextran is approved by the Food and Drug Administration, but is reserved for those patients with poor muscle mass who would require multiple injections. Intravenous injection may involve a daily bolus of 100 mg (2 ml) over 2 minutes (Table 3–4).

Precautions

Ingested iron may irritate the gastrointestinal tract. Abdominal cramps, diarrhea, constipation, and nausea are frequent patient complaints. Taking the iron preparation with a meal may improve these side effects, but iron absorption may be reduced. Antacids also impair absorption and should not be taken simultaneously with iron. Black, tarry stools are caused by the accumulated unabsorbed iron.

Local effects from intramuscular injections include pain, sterile abscess formation, hematoma formation, and skin discoloration (lasting up to 3 years). Phlebitis may occur at the intravenous administration site. Systemic reactions from parenteral administration occur in less than 1 percent of all patients and are usually manifested within 10 minutes. Systemic signs and symptoms include headache, dyspnea, myalgia, arthralgia, flushing, dizziness, nausea and vomiting, fever, and death from severe anaphylaxis.

An overdose of iron therapy may occur, particularly in children who are attracted to the candy-like appearance of the tablets. The average lethal dose of iron is 200 to 250 mg/kg body weight.[9] Death has been reported in small children who have ingested 2 gm or less of ferrous sulfate. It results from metabolic derangements, liver necrosis, extensive gastrointestinal mucosal damage, and renal failure. The treatment of iron overdose requires the immediate induction of vomiting with syrup of ipecac (15 to 30 ml). The hospitalized patient should be treated with gastric lavage using sodium phosphate, administration of intravenous deferoxamine (an iron-binding compound), and supportive care. There has been some concern about administering deferoxamine in pregnancy because of its teratogenic potential. However, there have been two successful reports of its use in combination with other therapies.[10,11]

Anemia refractory to iron therapy may result from folic acid deficiency, hemoglobinopathies, chronic disease, or infection. A cause must be sought but may not be found. Spontaneous remission may occur after delivery.

VITAMINS AND MINERALS

Requirements During Pregnancy

A balanced diet provides an adequate supply of vitamins and minerals for the pregnant patient and supplementation is usually unnecessary. The United States Recommended Daily Allowances (USRDA) for vitamins and minerals for pregnant and lactating patients

*To calculate the dose in milliliters of Imferon, divide the total milligrams by 50.

† The Z-track technique involves displacing the skin laterally prior to injection and not releasing the skin until the needle is withdrawn.

TABLE 3–4. TOTAL VOLUME OF IRON DEXTRAN INJECTION NEEDED TO TREAT IRON DEFICIENCY ANEMIA

Patient's Weight (lb)	Observed Hemoglobin (g/100 ml)				
	4.4%	*5.9%*	*7.4%*	*8.9%*	*10.4%*
100	42	36	30	24	18
110	46	39	33	26	20
120	51	43	36	29	22
130	55	47	39	31	23
140	59	50	42	34	25
150	63	54	45	36	27
160	68	57	48	38	29
170	72	61	51	41	31
180	76 ml	64 ml	54 ml	43 ml	32 ml

From Huff BB (ed): Physicians Desk Reference. Oradell, NJ, Medical Economics Co, 1985, p 1367, with permission.

have been established by the FDA and are listed in Table 3–5.[9]

Folic acid is an especially important vitamin for red blood cell production during the last trimester of pregnancy, for multifetal gestation, multiple gestations, and during lactation. A lack of folic acid affects nucleic acid metabolism. Folic acid deficiency with or without an adequate iron intake is the second leading cause of anemia during pregnancy. It is frequently seen in women of lower socioeconomic status, in adolescents with inadequate diets, and in high-risk pregnancies.

The daily adult requirement for folic acid is 0.4 mg, but increases to 0.8 mg during pregnancy.[12] A daily oral supplementation of 1 mg of folic acid should be prescribed for those patients who cannot maintain a well-balanced diet (including green vegetables) or those taking anticonvulsant medications with

TABLE 3–5. UNITED STATES RECOMMENDED DAILY ALLOWANCES (USRDA) OF VITAMINS AND IRON

Vitamin	Nonpregnant	Pregnant or Lactating
A (IU)*	5000	8000
D (IU)	400	400
E (IU)	30	30
C (mg)	60	60
Folic acid (mg)	0.4	0.8
Niacin (mg)	20	20
B_1 (mg)	1.5	1.7
B_2 (mg)	1.7	2
B_6 (mg)	2	2.5
B_{12} (mg)	0.006	0.008
Iron (mg)	18	18
Calcium (mg)	800–1200	1200

* IU = International Units.

antifolate properties. Many of the prenatal vitamin preparations contain 1 mg of folic acid.

The routine prescribing of calcium salt tablets is unnecessary during pregnancy, as the dietary requirements for calcium during pregnancy and lactation are not thought to be increased. Because of fetal and nursing demands for calcium, the maternal parathyroid glands undergo hyperplasia, and parathormone (PT) levels are greater than in the nonpregnant state. Parathormone acts to increase the calcium available by increasing intestinal absorption, reabsorption at the distal renal tubules, and bone calcium mobilization. Calcium for fetal bone deposition represents only about 2.5 percent of the total maternal calcium. It crosses the placenta by active diffusion, so that adequate fetal levels are ensured.

Even though a patient may not tolerate the gastrointestinal effects from as little as 1 cup of milk each day (30 percent of daily requirement), calcium is supplied in other dairy products (cheese, cottage cheese, yogurt, ice cream) and in the standard prenatal vitamins (125 to 600 mg of elemental calcium, 15 to 50 percent of daily requirement). Natafort has the greatest concentration of elemental calcium (350 mg, over 25 percent of daily requirement). Calcium supplementation should be considered only in treating hypoparathyroidism (Chap. 7) or prolonged malabsorption conditions.

The daily supplementation of 2.2 mg of sodium fluoride during the second and third trimesters of pregnancy has been suggested to reduce the incidence of dental caries in children.[13] This is in addition to fluoride being present in drinking water. Despite the low cost and attractive theoretic benefit, more investigation at other centers is needed to support these preliminary findings.

Preparations

Prenatal vitamin preparations are a source of folic acid, iron, and other vitamins. These products are not to be substituted for a minimum of three well-balanced meals each day. Table 3–6 lists many of the common prenatal vitamins. The cost is approximately five times greater than ferrous sulfate tablets alone. All contain varying amounts of folic acid, iron (usually the fumarate salt), and other vitamins. The amount of each ingredient either meets or exceeds the recommended daily allowances. Recently, Seligman et al. have demonstrated decreased iron absorption from some brands of prenatal vitamins. They should not be relied upon entirely as a source of iron. A periodic diet history and repeat blood count later in pregnancy are recommended.[14]

Over-the-counter vitamin preparations are also listed in Table 3–6. Not all of these preparations contain folic acid and iron. Furthermore, absolute amounts of elemental iron and folic acid may be inadequate for pregnancy needs. The risks and benefits of taking separate vitamins (C, D, A, etc.) in differing amounts are poorly understood and should be avoided. Vitamins should not be taken without the physician's knowledge.

Precautions

Although rare during pregnancy, deficiency of folic acid or vitamin B_{12} from malabsorption can lead to megaloblastic anemia and neurologic damage (paresthesia, poor muscle coordination, confusion, mental slowness). Folic acid without vitamin B_{12} given to pregnant patients with pernicious anemia may correct the anemia, but will not affect neurologic sequelae from vitamin B_{12} deficiency. A monthly injection of 0.1 mg of vitamin B_{12} is therefore necessary in addition to the folic acid.

Folic acid is nontoxic in humans, but large doses of fat-soluble vitamins A and D have been associated with a broad spectrum of congenital abnormalities and toxic reactions.[15] Vitamin A toxicity occurs both in children and adults receiving more than 100,000 units per day over several months. The com-

TABLE 3–6. COMMON PRENATAL VITAMINS AND OVER-THE-COUNTER (OTC) VITAMINS

Trade Name	Elemental Iron Content† (mg)	Folic Acid Content‡ (mg)
Prenatal Vitamins		
Filibon*	18	0.4
Filibon F.A.	45	1
Filibon Forte	45	1
Materna 1–60	60	1
Natabec*	30	0
Natabec R_x	30	1
Natabec-F.A.*	30	0.1
Natafort	65	1
Natalins*	45	0.8
Natalins R_x	60	1
Pramilet-F.A.	40	1
Stuart Prenatal*	60	0.8
Stuart Natal 1 + 1	65	1
OTC Vitamins		
Dayalets Plus Iron	18	0.4
One-A-Day	0	0.4
One-A-Day Plus Iron	18	0.4
Micebrin	15	0
Stresstabs 600 with Iron	27	0.4
Theragran-M	12	0
Theragran Hematinic	67	0.33

* OTC prenatal vitamins.
† Minimum daily requirement of absorbed elemental iron during pregnancy and lactation is 4 mg. However, approximately 10% of elemental iron is absorbed.
‡ Minimum daily requirement of absorbed folic acid during pregnancy and lactation is 0.8 mg.

mon signs and symptoms are fatigue, malaise, lethargy, abdominal upset, bone and joint pain, hair loss, brittle nails, and scaly skin. In addition to the above, infants may have increased intracranial pressure, bulging fontanels, hypoprothrombinemia, decalcification of bone, and arrest or retardation of growth. Treatment consists of discontinuing the vitamin A.

Vitamin D toxicity is seen when doses exceed 50,000 units per day for prolonged periods (Chap. 2). Toxic effects include anorexia, nausea, vomiting, weakness, weight loss, polyuria, constipation, soft tissue calcification, nephrocalcinosis, hypertension, hypercalcemia, acidosis, and renal failure. Treatment consists of a discontinuation of vitamin D, a low calcium diet, and an increased intake of fluid.

Mineral oil taken as a laxative may prevent the intestinal absorption of fat-soluble vitamins (A, D, E).

OVER-THE-COUNTER DRUGS

The basic pharmacologic principles described in Chapter 1 also apply to over-the-counter drugs used during pregnancy. The initial obstetric examination should include the questioning and documentation of any specific over-the-counter drugs taken at conception and during the first trimester. Effects from the indiscriminate use of over-the-counter drugs are not usually obvious in the neonate. Less pronounced effects can be unappreciated, even though each preparation may contain several active ingredients and preservatives.

Certain over-the-counter preparations may be taken from habit, instead of physical need, and may not be considered as medicines by the patient. Relief of patient symptoms is important, and many over-the-counter preparations are permissible during the second and third trimesters in minimal dosages and for short durations. However, all drugs should be used cautiously during pregnancy. The cost of brand name preparations containing the same basic ingredients is similar and usually higher than generic preparations.

Mild Analgesics

Aspirin is effective and should not be absolutely discouraged. Certain aspirin preparations contain magnesium or aluminum buffers (Bufferin) or caffeine (Excedrin, Anacin, Doans Pills, Vanquish).[16] However, large doses or chronic use may inhibit prostaglandin synthetase activity and thereby prolong gestation or increase the duration of labor. The effects of ibuprofen (Advil, Nuprin) in pregnancy are probably similar to aspirin, since it also inhibits prostaglandin synthetase activity. The in utero closure of the fetal ductus arteriosus is a theoretic yet unproven concern.

Excessive maternal hemorrhage can occur from aspirin effects by inhibiting platelet aggregation and inhibiting factor XII synthesis. Hemorrhage in the fetus and neonate has also been reported.[17] Even in minimal doses, aspirin can cause decreased platelet aggregation in the fetus for several days, thus avoiding aspirin late in pregnancy is probably wise.

Acetaminophen remains the most commonly taken drug during pregnancy. The effects of acetaminophen (Tylenol, Datril) in pregnancy are unknown. It does inhibit—in large doses only—prostaglandin activity (Chap. 21) and may not necessarily be a better substitute for aspirin in late gestation. Acetaminophen does not alter platelet properties but can be toxic to the liver in large doses and may be less desirable.

Decongestants, Antihistamines, Antitussives

Decongestants, antihistamines, and antitussives are frequently requested and used during early pregnancy. All "cold" preparations combine a sympathomimetic, an antihistamine, or a mild analgesic (Dristan, Co-Tylenol, Triaminicin).[16] Two antihistamine compounds, cyclizine (Marezine) and meclizine (Bonine), are available as antinauseants used to treat motion sickness. At one time these agents were required to carry a warning label against their use in pregnancy. A study by Milkovich and van den Berg found no increase in embryo deaths or malformations in children of women who used these drugs during pregnancy.[18] However, these agents are not promoted for nonprescription treatment of morning sickness and their use cannot be encouraged. Cough syrups (Robitussin D. M., Vicks Cough Syrup, Nyquil, Romilar, Halls) contain an antitussive (dextromethorphan) or an antihistamine, and alcohol.

Decongestants (Neosynephrine, Sinex, Dristan, Sudafed) should be used in the lowest concentrations, because they contain a sympathomimetic that may influence uterine perfusion in large doses. They should not be used if uteroplacental insufficiency is suspected. The teratogenic potential is unconfirmed, but withdrawal in infants born to chronic abusers of these agents can include tremulousness, agitation, irritability, and poor feeding. Sustained acting antihistamines or decongestants should be avoided during pregnancy.

Antacids

Antacids should be taken only after diet manipulation and conservative treatment for dyspepsia is unsuccessful. Patients should realize that antacids may cause diarrhea or constipation. A buffered preparation of calcium carbonate (Tums, Camalox, Chooz), a mixture of magnesium and aluminum hydroxide (Gelusil, Maalox, Riopan, Digel, Kolantyl), or magnesium hydroxide alone (Phillip's Milk of Magnesia) is recommended. Excess sodium is related to fluid retention and possibly to the onset of toxemia. Sodium is present in certain preparations (Rolaids, Alka-Seltzer, Bromo-Seltzer).[16] Patients on a low sodium diet should use a low sodium antacid such as Riopan.[16] Otherwise, the newer low sodium antacids do not seem to offer other advantages during pregnancy.

Laxatives and Stool Softeners

Laxatives and stool softeners are permitted for relief of constipation only after diet manipulation (additional fluids, fruits, bran foods) has been attempted unsuccessfully. Natural vegetable concentrates (Senokot, Metamucil, Serutan, Konsyl) are recommended bulk laxatives. Castor oil, epsom salts, or milk of magnesia may also be used occasionally. Laxatives usually contain phenolphthalein (Ex-lax, Feen-A-Mint) or docusate sodium or calcium (Correctol, Regutol, Colace, Doxidan, Dialose).[16]

Excess cathartic use may promote labor and should be taken with caution. In addition, enemas may contain high concentrations of sodium (Fleets enema). Antidiarrheals (Kaopectate, Donnagel) contain kaolin and pectin and may be used in moderation. Pepto-Bismol contains bismuth subsalicylate and significant amounts of salicylate are released with large doses. Preparation H contains no topical anesthetic and is perhaps the best hemorrhoidal preparation during pregnancy. Antihemorrhoidal suppositories with corticosteroids may be used sparingly if these steps fail.

Sedatives

Sedatives contain the antihistamine diphenhydramine (Nytol, Sominex-2, Sleep-Eze, Nervine, Compoz) or pyrilamine maleate (Quiet World). Insomnia is common during pregnancy, but these drugs should be avoided in general. Excess use may cause a worrisome decrease in fetal activity. Withdrawal symptoms in the neonate can include irritability, tremulousness, a high-pitched cry, and poor feeding.

Topical Preparations

Acne creams (Stridex, Clearasil, Phisoac, Fostex, Cuticura) and lotions contain benzoyl peroxide or sulfa, salicylate, and alcohol, and are safe in moderation.[16] First-aid ointments or lotions (Johnson & Johnson, Bacitracin, Neosporin, Betadine, Cruex, Calamine) and topical steroids (Cortaid, Lanacort) are likely safe with moderate use. Pain-relieving rubs (Mentholatum, Ben-Gay) contain methyl salicylate and menthol and should be used in moderation during pregnancy because they increase circulation to the skin which may cause an increased absorption.

Aerosols and Chemicals

Aerosol and chemical-fume exposure from hair sprays, paint, pesticides, methane, spray adhesives, household cleaners, and laboratory chemicals are frequent patient concerns. The effect on fetal cerebral development is probably negligible, but maternal exposure should be discouraged or minimized in a well-ventilated area. No fetal effects have been observed with hair dye application.

Caffeine

The structural similarity of caffeine to the DNA base pairs adenine and guanine has prompted laboratory investigation to determine any teratogenic effect. Skeletal variations have been found in fetal rats exposed to high doses of caffeine.[19] It is not known whether caffeine or its principal metabolite, paraxanthine, is teratogenic in humans. In contrast to recent large epidemiologic studies, Weathersbee et al. found excess caffeine ingestion (at least 600 mg/day) to be associated with a high incidence of abortion, stillbirth, or premature birth.[20] Caffeine in brewed coffee (125 mg), tea (65 mg), 6-oz service of cola soft drinks (50 mg), and mild analgesics (30 to 60 mg) is transferred to the fetus and breastfed infant. Stimulant tablets (NoDoz, Vivarin, Caffedrine) contain 100 to 200 mg of caffeine and are to be discouraged.[16] Drinking decaffeinated or caffeinated beverages in moderation with an adherence to a proper diet is strongly recommended.

Artificial Sweeteners

Artificial sweeteners (saccharin, sorbitol) in beverages or commercial preparations (Sucaryl, Sweeta) readily cross the placenta. However, no increase in abortion or teratogenic effects has been evident; such additives should be used in moderation during pregnancy.[21,22] Aspartame (Nutra Sweet) is hydrolyzed in the intestines to methanol and two amino acids (aspartic acid and phenylalanine). Women with phenylketonuria who wish to have children should avoid aspartame-containing foods. They should switch to a diet low in phenylalanine before conception. Otherwise, the amount of these two amino acids in a standard cola beverage is much lower than most high-protein foods. Any concern during pregnancy is strictly theoretic and unfounded by any data. Only minimal use during pregnancy would seem wise.[23,24]

Diet Pills

Diet pills (Grapefruit Diet Plan, AYD's, Appedrine, Prolamine, Dexatrim, Thinz-span) contain phenylpropanolamine alone or in combination with caffeine and other products.[16] Their effect during early, unsuspected pregnancy is unknown. Phenylpropanolamine is a stimulant that is structurally similar to epinephrine and amphetamine. No specific malformations are associated with its use, so pregnancy termination should not be offered. "Water" pills (Diurex, Tri-Aqua, Aqua-Ban) contain caffeine and potassium or ammonium chloride and are to be discouraged.[16]

Alcohol

The ingestion of alcoholic beverages (beer, wine, distilled spirits) at conception or during pregnancy is a frequent patient concern. Reports from human and animal studies have involved excessive or chronic exposure of alcohol to the fetus. A fetal alcohol syndrome has been delineated in the human and is described in Chapter 2. A 25-percent malformation rate, which includes cardiac anomalies and cleft palates, has been reported in children born to alcoholic mothers. Mills et al. reported that consuming 1 to 2 drinks daily was associated with low birth weights.[25] What effect in utero exposure to alcohol has on the child's subsequent neurobehavioral development is unclear and nearly impossible to determine before delivery. Other conditions, such as inadequate nutrition (poor protein intake, pyridoxine or other vitamin B deficiencies), contaminants in the alcohol, and genetic factors, may also play an important etiologic role.

There is no safe threshold for alcohol consumption, but no cases of fetal alcohol syndrome have been reported with the mother ingesting less than 2 oz of absolute alcohol daily. Two ounces of absolute alcohol (100 percent) is equivalent to one-half glass of distilled spirits (50 percent), two glasses of wine (12 percent), or four glasses of beer (6 percent). We recommend that a pregnant woman be discouraged from drinking alcoholic beverages during the first trimester and should avoid two or more drinks each day during the second and third trimesters.

Cigarette Smoking

Cigarette smoke contains more than 1000 chemicals, with carbon monoxide and nicotine being best known. The effects from fetal exposure to carbon monoxide and nicotine have been extensively studied in animals.[26]

Both chemicals have been associated with delayed fetal growth. The incidence of neonatal mortality and congenital defects is not increased by smoking. Preterm rupture of the amniotic membranes may occur more frequently in heavy smokers. Other possible problems associated with smoking during pregnancy include spontaneous abortion, placental abruption, placenta previa, and decreased infant length.

Whether or not cigarette smoking during pregnancy impairs the subsequent intellectual function of the exposed fetus is controversial. Davie et al. reported a 3- to 4-month delay in reading achievement, while Hardy and Mellitus could find no intellectual impairment in offspring of heavy smokers.[27,28]

Sexton and Hebel reported that an antismoking campaign results in twice the number of women discontinuing or cutting down to five cigarettes or less per day and that the intervention results in an important augmentation in birth weight and length.[29] If the patient is unable to quit smoking during pregnancy, she is to be encouraged to smoke five or less cigarettes each day, using a low tar and nicotine brand.

Nicorettes, a preparation containing 2 mg of nicotine and used to help stop smoking cigarettes, is not approved for use during pregnancy. The direct effect of nicotine to increase catecholamines and decrease uterine blood flow is undesirable in pregnancy.

REFERENCES

1. Peckham CH, King RW: A study of intercurrent conditions observed in pregnancy. Am J Obstet Gynecol 87:609, 1963
2. Bleyer WA, Au WY: Studies on the detection of adverse drug reactions in the newborn: Fetal exposure to maternal medication. JAMA 213:2046, 1970
3. Fofar JO, Nelson MM: Epidemiology of drugs taken by pregnant women: Drugs that may affect the fetus adversely. Clin Pharmacol Ther 14(pt 2):632, 1973
4. Rayburn WF, Wible-Kant J, Bledsoe P: Changing trends in drug use during pregnancy. J Reprod Med 27:569, 1982
5. Hambidge KM, Mauer AM: Trace elements, in Laboratory Indices of Nutritional Status in Pregnancy, ed 1. National Academy of Sciences, 1978, pp 157–165
6. McCurdy PR: Oral and parenteral iron therapy. JAMA 191:859, 1965
7. Olsen KS, Weinfeld A: Availability of iron dextran for hemoglobin synthesis as studied with phlebotomy. Acta Med Scand 192:543, 1972
8. Pritchard, JA: Hemoglobin regeneration in severe iron deficiency anemia. JAMA 195:97, 1966
9. Arena JM: Poisoning. Springfield, Ill, Thomas 1979, p 432
10. Rayburn WR, Donn SM, Wulf ME: Iron overdose during pregnancy: Successful therapy with deferoxamine. Am J Obstet Gynecol 146:717, 1983
11. Blanc P, Hryhorczuk D, Daniel I: Deferoxamine treatment of acute iron intoxication in pregnancy. Obstet Gynecol 64:125, 1984
12. AMA Department of Drugs: AMA Drug Evaluations. Chicago, American Medical Association, 1983, pp 1124–1125
13. Glenn FB, Glenn WD, Duncan RC: Fluoride tablet supplementation during pregnancy for caries immunity: A study of the offspring produced. Am J Obstet Gynecol 143:560, 1982
14. Seligman PA, Casken JH, Frazier JL, et al.: Measurement of iron absorption from prenatal multivitamin–mineral supplements. Obstet Gynecol 61:356, 1983
15. Gosselin RE, Hodge HC, Smith RP, et al.: Clinical Toxicology of Commercial Products. Baltimore, Williams & Wilkins, 1984, pp 264–265
16. Handbook of Nonprescription Drugs, ed 7. Washington, D.C., American Pharmaceutical Association, 1982
17. Corby DG: Aspirin in pregnancy: Maternal and fetal effects. Pediatrics 62:930, 1978
18. Milkovich L, van den Berg BJ: An evaluation of the teratogenicity of certain antinauseant drugs. Am J Obstet Gynecol 125:244, 1976
19. Collins TF, Welsh JJ, Black TN, et al.: A comprehensive study of the teratogenic potential of caffeine in rats when given by oral intubation. In Report on Caffeine. Food and Drug Administration, Sept 1980
20. Weathersbee PS, Olsen LK, Lodge JR: Caffeine and pregnancy. Postgrad Med 62:64, 1977
21. Kroes R, Peters P, Berkvens J, et al.: Longterm toxicity with cyclamate, saccharin, and cyclohexylamine. Toxicology 8:285, 1977

22. Kline J, Stern Z, Susser M et al.: Spontaneous abortion and the use of sugar substitutes. Am J Obstet Gynecol 130:708, 1978
23. Tenbrink MJ, Stroud HW: Normal infant born to mother with phenylketonuria. JAMA 247:2139, 1982
24. Lenke RR, Levy HL: Maternal phenylketonuria—Results of dietary therapy. Am J Obstet Gynecol 142:548, 1982
25. Mills JL, Graubard BI, Harley EE, et al.: Maternal alcohol consumption and birth weight. JAMA 252:1875, 1984
26. Landesman-Dwyer S, Emanuel I: Smoking during pregnancy. Teratology 19:119, 1979
27. Davie R, Butler N, Goldstein H: In From Birth to Seven: A Report of the National Child Development Study. London, Longman and the National Children's Bureau, 1972, pp 175–177
28. Hardy JB, Mellitus ED: Does maternal smoking have a long-term effect on the children? Lancet 2:1332, 1972
29. Sexton M, Hebel JR: A clinical trial of change in maternal smoking and its effect on birth weight. JAMA 251:911, 1984

4

Drug Abuse During Pregnancy

Frederick P. Zuspan and William F. Rayburn

DRUG ADDICTION

The problems of drug addiction in pregnancy are frequently unrealized and may not become apparent until the problem of newborn withdrawal is identified. Most health care practitioners think of drug addiction as involving chronic heroin or methadone dependence. Instead, marijuana and alcohol are the most commonly abused drugs, with other street drugs being used much less commonly. Other medications must also be considered, such as juveniles experimenting with different drugs and emotionally distraught individuals on psychotropic medications. Inadequate reporting is inherent without a systematic polydrug history being taken routinely, and the patients most likely to volunteer that they have a drug dependency are patients in a recognized methadone program. Most others will not admit to drug dependence and will go undetected unless a high degree of suspicion exists or a somatic problem emerges. Some of the questions that are necessary in the prenatal history concern drug dependence and usage of not just heroin or methadone but any of the psychotropic or off-street drugs, including marijuana. Information about the spouse's drug habits is often quite helpful.

Drug dependence during pregnancy involves all classes of society. The lack of awareness or inquisition about drug addiction is common in the United States. We tend to underestimate the existence of these problems because we find it socially unattractive. As a result, drug addiction creates a negative relationship between the patient and the physician. Drug-dependence studies have classically involved heroin and methadone, but reports of neonatal withdrawal have also been seen in patients receiving drugs such as phenobarbital, alcohol, pentazocaine, propoxyphene, nicotine, and caffeine.[1,2] Due to their low molecular weight, stimulants and depressants cross the placenta easily and are also excreted in breast milk. The drug reaction in the fetus is often the same as in the mother. A patient who is addicted to a narcotic, such as heroin, may be unable to sustain her habit or enter a recognized methadone maintenance program during her pregnancy.

As a result, she and the fetus will have withdrawal symptoms with increased agitation, convulsions, and often intrauterine death.[3]

Street drug use is almost impossible to study except to recognize that it does exist. The most extensive experience in drug dependency in pregnancy comes from methadone maintenance programs, which have done an exemplary job of maintaining addicted women through their pregnancies. Each major city has a methadone maintenance program for pregnant and nonpregnant individuals.[4–6]

Menstrual Dysfunction and Fertility

Menstrual abnormalities are common findings in drug-dependent women. Amenorrhea and menstrual irregularities are seen often in heroin abusers, polydrug abusers using heroin, and methadone-dependent women. Amenorrhea is the most frequently reported symptom[7,8] and it is not unusual to find a pregnant patient near term who has been amenorrheic for several years.

Fertility is difficult to assess among drug addicts. It is not uncommon to find sexually transmitted diseases with a high incidence of pelvic inflammatory disease, which may cause tubal occlusion. Coupled with the higher incidence of amenorrhea and anovulation, conception is often difficult in the drug-dependent patient. Women in methadone maintenance programs who abstain from other drugs, including alcohol, are more likely to resume normal menstrual functions.

Diagnosis of Early Pregnancy

Early diagnosis of pregnancy is important so that any desire to terminate the pregnancy can be discussed openly. At the University of Chicago, we found less than 10 percent of drug-addicted patients desired an interruption of pregnancy, which was lower or about the same as in the conventional population. An abortion against the patient's will should not be urged, because the patient's psychologic makeup is often quite fragile and may precipitate a worsening of the situation.[9] The pregnant drug addict is seldom seen early unless she is in a methadone maintenance program.

The standard techniques for diagnosing pregnancy are more difficult in the pregnant drug addict. A history of amenorrhea *may* be present in the nonpregnant methadone patient, but is usually present in the nonpregnant heroin addict. A positive pregnancy test is not always valid, because narcotics or narcotic metabolites may inhibit latex particle agglutination during the urine testing for pregnancy. Fatigue, headache, nausea and vomiting, and hot sweats or flushes can be signs and symptoms of either early pregnancy or withdrawal. Auscultation of fetal heart tones and sonographic visualization of a gestational sac are the only definitive techniques for the diagnosis of pregnancy.

Antepartum Management

The woman who is drug-dependent deserves special attention and support throughout her pregnancy. A complete and comprehensive medical and drug history is of paramount importance. Table 4–1 identifies medical and obstetric problems more commonly found among drug addicts who are pregnant. The most notable pertain to infection. These complications as reported by Finnegan[10] were similar to the University of Chicago study involving 106 patients,[9] where the incidence of specific prenatal complications included:

• Anemia	24.0%
• Syphilis	17.8%
• Urinary tract infections	15.3%
• Gonorrhea	5.1%
• Pulmonary pathology	4.2%
• Cellulitis or abscess	4.2%
• Severe edema	4.2%

A positive hepatitis history is common and was apparent in 23 percent of pregnant drug addicts in the University of Chicago study, and the use of contaminated needles may explain this high incidence. Over 12 percent of

TABLE 4–1. COMPLICATIONS ENCOUNTERED IN PREGNANT DRUG ADDICTS

MEDICAL

Alcoholism

Anemia

Bacteremia

Endocarditis (valvular heart disease)

Cellulitis

Poor dental hygiene (peridontitis)

Edema and "woody" subcutaneous tissue

Hepatitis—acute and chronic

Pelvic inflammatory disease

Phlebitis and lack of available veins

Pneumonia (may be associated with granuloma lung), pulmonary edema

Polydrug use

Septicemia

Smoking

Tetanus

Tuberculosis

Urinary tract infections (cystitis, urethritis, pyelonephritis)

Venereal infection (condyloma accuminatum, gonorrhea, *Hemophilis vaginalis*, herpes, trichomonas, syphilis)

OBSTETRIC

Intrauterine growth retardation

Stillbirth

Premature labor

Meconium

Birth asphyxia

Neonatal withdrawal

Adapted from Finnegan L et al., 1981.[10]

TABLE 4–2. RECOMMENDED PRENATAL BASELINE LABORATORY TESTS

1. Complete blood count with indices
2. Blood smear
3. Urine culture (minimum of three during pregnancy)
4. Chest x-ray
5. TB skin test
6. Hemoglobin electrophoresis
7. Folic acid level
8. Total protein—A:G ratio
9. Liver function profile
10. Rubella titer
11. Serology VDRL and FTA
12. Gonorrhea culture (cervical and rectal) initial and repeat at 36 weeks
13. Hepatitis-associated antigens (HAA)
14. Pap smear
15. Blood type, Rh and antibody screen
16. Ultrasound scan
17. Herpes culture (if positive history)
18. Urine (not amniotic fluid) for drug screen

heroin addicts and former addicts have been reported to be chronic carriers of hepatitis B-antigen.[11]

Laboratory baseline studies should be performed in case a problem develops during the antenatal course (Table 4–2).

Nutrition

A proper diet of 100 g of protein per day is beneficial in the drug-dependent patient, even though this is seldom accomplished despite nutrition counseling. Studies that we have done utilizing the urea nitrogen and creatinine ratio indicate poor protein nutrition in these women; hence, an extra effort must be made for nutrition counseling. The average protein intake proved to be less than 50 g/day.

Prenatal vitamins are essential. Iron supplementation in the form of ferrous sulfate, 300 mg, or ferrous gluconate, 300 mg, twice daily is essential to correct the nutritional anemia seen in one-fourth of these patients.

Folic acid levels were routinely screened in 106 pregnant addicts, and 64 patients had abnormally low folic acid levels of less than 2.6 mg. All patients with low serum folic acid levels were treated with additional oral folic acid throughout pregnancy. In the absence of folic acid deficiency, drug-dependent women require the routine prenatal capsule with folic acid.

Fetal Assessment

Risks to the fetus are often poorly understood. None of the illicit drugs has been shown to be associated with specific anomalies or chromosomal aberrations in humans. Any hazard to central nervous system development in humans is difficult or impossible to prove. Other accompanying obstetric and medical complications make it difficult to assess any direct adverse effects from in utero exposure to the drug or principle metabolites.

It is important to understand that detoxification during pregnancy, if too rapid, will result in undesirable side effects to the fetus. Figure 4–1 identifies the sequence of events seen with rapid detoxification of fetal withdrawal. A decreased dose of methadone, reduced by 2 mg/week, should obviate this problem.

Figure 4–2 identifies marked stimulation of the fetal adrenal and the sympathetic nervous system in response to diminishing doses of methadone. Because increased fetal activity correlates with the peak of epinephrine and norepinephrine in the amniotic fluid, fetal movement charting during one or more convenient hours each day is useful during the gradual methadone detoxification. A gradual reduction of methadone should occur in a controlled clinical atmosphere. Fetal movement charting in the hard-core drug addict need not be done as the baby is addicted and seldom moves. This would lead to spurious results.

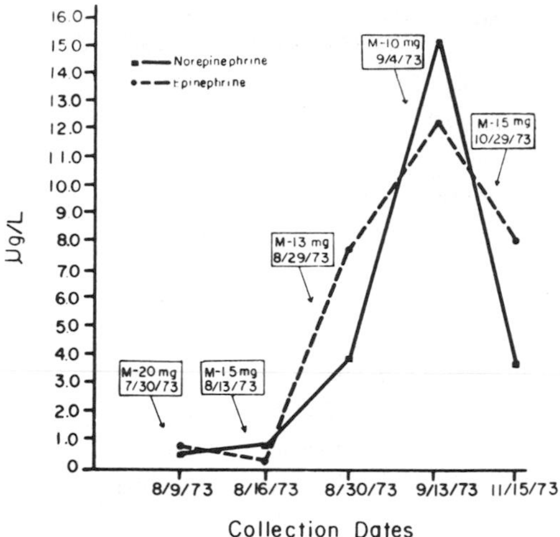

Figure 4–2. The response of the fetal adrenal and sympathetic nervous system in response to diminishing doses of methadone.

Any abnormal baseline laboratory tests should be repeated as pregnancy ensues, especially in the third trimester. At least two ultrasound examinations should be made to assess fetal growth and well-being. Of these patients, 10 percent should be anticipated to be intrauterine growth retarded. When compared to a similar group of control patients,

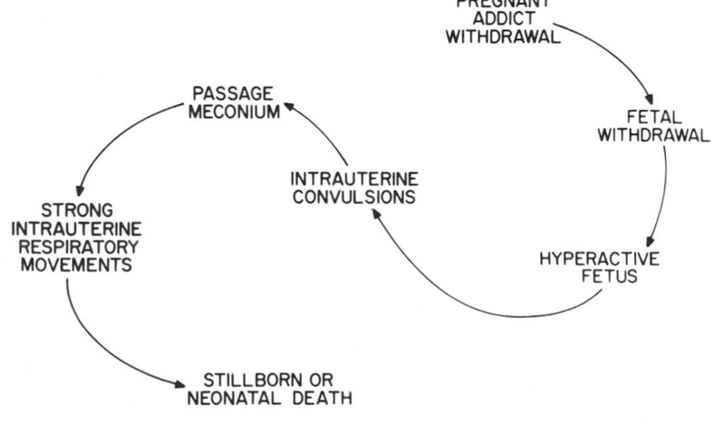

Figure 4–1. Sequence of events in fetal withdrawal of narcotics or sedatives.

this is no higher than would be expected in that general population.[5] Ultrasound is also reliable to help redetermine the expected date of confinement, provide an approximation of the weight of the fetus, and assess fetal well-being by observing limb and trunk motion and breathing movements.

Nonstress tests and contraction stress tests are not indicated routinely, as there are few drug-related problems encountered during the antenatal period except for premature rupture of membranes or premature labor. Amniocentesis prior to the 37th week may reveal a delayed maturation of the L:S ratio for comparable weeks of gestation in the methadone-dependent patient. This does not apply after the 37th week of gestation.[12]

Rehabilitation and Drug Withdrawal

The artificial sense of well-being in the patient who is a drug abuser inhibits the development of important psychologic and social skills. The emotional stresses of pregnancy are exacerbated, especially if these women attempt to abstain from drugs. Rehabilitation of the pregnant addict is often complicated by more intense fear, guilt, and shame than is seen in the nonpregnant patient. Enrollment in a drug-dependent program is likely beneficial in improving the obstetric performance by decreasing perinatal deaths and improving fetal growth.[6] Hospitalization with gradual withdrawal is appropriate.

The patient's reaction to rehabilitation may take two paths. She responds with either more profound drug use or attempts to achieve complete abstinence from drugs, which may affect the intrauterine environment and create profound physiologic changes in the fetus.[13,14] Instead of using high doses of methadone, the goal of therapy is to orient the patient to a low-dose regimen.[15-17]

The model proposed by Senay[18] and Davis[19] used methadone as a temporary support for the patients, while their basic human needs were met by psychotherapeutic and resocialization measures. During this period of approximately 6 to 8 months, the patient may gain psychologic strength by working through some of the problems that are encountered during pregnancy. This is followed by an increased emphasis on the use of medical, legal, psychologic, vocational, and social services to help readapt the patient to her environment. The pregnant patient frequently adopts an immature behavior, an inability to tolerate delayed gratification, and a poor control of her impulses. Requests for tranquilizing medication may further potentiate depressive traits in methadone patients.[20]

Patients may turn to alcohol as the most easily accessible method to handle depression and anxiety, since alcohol consumption is estimated to range from 15 to 40 percent in patients in drug abuse programs. Alcohol and tranquilizers also act as major deterrents to mental health. Fetal wastage and perinatal loss have been shown to be as much as 30 percent higher in a group of patients known to have been using central nervous system altering drugs.[19]

The following are recommendations for supportive care in the antepartum period: (1) avoid physical and emotional stresses that cause the pregnant addict to continue drug abuse, (2) emphasize prenatal classes and groups designed specifically to educate patients and help them work through issues related to drug use during pregnancy, (3) use intramural and extramural crisis intervention and counseling programs staffed by professionals and paraprofessionals (former drug addicts) to intervene in marital and family conflicts during pregnancy, and (4) collaborate frequently with the drug program staff and hospital staff to eliminate prejudicial attitudes.

Table 4–3 lists problems seen during drug withdrawal during pregnancy. The physician should be aware of how manipulative the pregnant drug addict can be and should prescribe sparingly any medicine other than

TABLE 4–3. PROBLEMS ASSOCIATED WITH DRUG WITHDRAWAL

1. The manipulative patient
2. Multiple drug regimens—not of value (use only methadone)
3. Diazepam—potentiates depressive traits
4. Alcohol—used by 15–40% of pregnant addicts
5. Multiple-abused drugs cause 30% increase in perinatal loss

methadone.[13] Eliminating the use of alcohol is difficult, but the patient should understand that alcohol potentiates the problem and increases perinatal loss.

Methadone Therapy

The ideal narcotic-dependent patient is one who is only on methadone and no other medications. Table 4–4 identifies the different philosophies of therapy of the methadone programs. Three different programs (narcotic blockade, small-dose regimen, gradual detoxification) exist in this country, and each has cared for large numbers of pregnant addicts with impressive results. Beginning methadone therapy late in pregnancy is not considered to be more acceptable than continued narcotic use.

We have been believers in utilizing the smallest dose possible to achieve control of the patient and using various supportive measures to help in this effort.[18,21] The maternal dose directly correlates with the percentage of patients having newborns exhibiting withdrawal symptoms. For example, if patients are on greater than 20 mg/day, the assumption can be made that at least 90 percent of newborns will have withdrawal symptoms of one form or another, and that half will need to have some form of therapy (methadone, diazepam, or phenobarbital) for at least 7 to 15 days.[21]

TABLE 4–4. PHILOSOPHY OF METHADONE THERAPY

1. Narcotic blockade[11,12]—large doses of methadone 80–120 mg/day
2. Small dose regimen[5,10]—controls the patient with less than 40 mg/day
3. Cold turkey or complete detoxification[7]—has no place in therapy of the pregnant patient
4. Gradual detoxification[3,8]—decreased dose (2 mg/week) only with caution, with an attempt to achieve 20 mg/day or less at delivery

If a pregnant woman is taking street heroin, the most efficacious way to switch to a methadone program is to begin between 20 and 40 mg of methadone per day. An average dose of 30 mg is acceptable. Additional 5-mg increments every 3 to 5 days can then be given based on the individual needs of the patient to prevent withdrawal. If this is insufficient, then 10 mg every 3 to 5 days may need to be given. A weekly urinalysis should be obtained to check for any illicit drug use and to help manage the noncompliant patient. When the pregnant patient is converted and stable in the methadone maintenance program, a decision must then be made as to whether or not the patient feels that she would like to have a gradual detoxification program begun at 2-mg increments per week until 20 mg/day or less is attained.

Narcotic Overdose

Whether narcotic overdose is intentional or unintentional, the route of administration determines how promptly action needs to take place. After oral dosages are taken, symptoms are most likely to appear 1 to 3 hours after ingestion, and gastric lavage is indicated. If awake, eventually the patient may not need tracheal intubation. If comatose, tracheal intubation with inflation of the tube should be performed before gastric lavage. The usual supportive measures, including maintenance of the airway and an intravenous line for medications, should be performed.

It is imperative to know the drug taken in the overdose. The drug of choice to counteract the effect from narcotics is naloxone (Narcan). Naloxone is a narcotic antagonist with almost no central nervous system depressant effects. It should be administered intravenously at doses of 0.01 mg/kg and readministered at short intervals every 5 to 10 minutes until the patient regains consciousness. Naloxone has a maximum duration of action of 2 hours, compared with most short-acting narcotics, which have a 6- to 8-hour duration of action, and methadone, which has a 12- to 48-hour duration of action.

Great care must be given to the fetus during this period of time, and monitoring of movement and heart rate is essential. Naloxone will cause precipitous withdrawal symptoms in the fetus, and it may be necessary to administer intra-amniotic medications into the fetus to control abnormal fetal activity. Observation of fetal movement can be made by utilizing an external fetal heart rate and tocodynamometer or by real-time ultrasonography.

Neither peritoneal dialysis nor hemodialysis is indicated in pregnancy overdose, nor is hemodialysis, because narcotics are extensively bound to plasma proteins and are therefore not dialyzable.

Labor and Delivery

The incidence of delivery complications in drug-dependent women varies little from normal pregnant patients. In our experience, premature rupture of the membranes was noted in 21 percent of 119 pregnant drug addicts. This is two and one-half times greater than in the normal population and underscores a need for careful attention to the microbiology of the vagina in the drug addict during pregnancy by repeated speculum examinations and appropriate cervical cultures in the early third trimester of pregnancy.

During labor, the adrenal glands in the mother excrete epinephrine, which can be measured in maternal urine to monitor maternal adrenal gland activity. Measurable norepinephrine comes principally from the sympathetic nervous system and is a reflection of the neurohormonal milieu in the mother. Urine from pregnant addicts has been assayed for epinephrine, norepinephrine, and creatinine, and these values were compared to similar urine collections from normal pregnant patients. Results revealed that the pregnant drug addict has a greater adrenal response than the nonaddict during pregnancy as evidenced by elevated urinary epinephrine levels (Fig. 4–3). There was no difference in sympathetic nervous system activity in the antepartum period.[22,23] The pregnant drug addict thus appears to have a hyperactive adrenal gland that further responds to labor, delivery, and the postpartum period by elevated epinephrine levels. The sympathetic nervous system, as indicated by urinary norepinephrine, is similar to that of nonaddicted mothers except that it lacks the ability to react to labor and delivery (Fig. 4–4), but does respond in a late fashion in the postpartum period.

The heroin addict typically consumes a "bag of heroin" prior to admission and often enters the hospital in the acceleration phase of labor, delivering a short time after arrival. This is in contrast to the methadone-dependent pregnant patient who enters the hospital at variable periods, depending on when her labor begins or if she has premature rupture of membranes. It is important that she receive her daily dose of methadone and that supplemental pain medications be used in an appropriate manner for labor. The patient requires the methadone to avoid intrauterine fetal withdrawal if her labor is protracted. The analgesic agent of choice is meperidine (Demerol) if supplemental narcotic medication is necessary, and the dosage may be larger than customary because of the addict's tolerance of narcotics.

Satisfactory analgesia may be obtained by epidural analgesia, which can also be used for delivery. A pudendal block and supplemental nitrous oxide can also be used for delivery. Barbiturates, if given to the methadone-dependent patient, may cause transient arterial hypotension and are not recommended. If the methadone maintenance dose was given that day, the pregnant addict usually does well in labor and delivery without major complications.

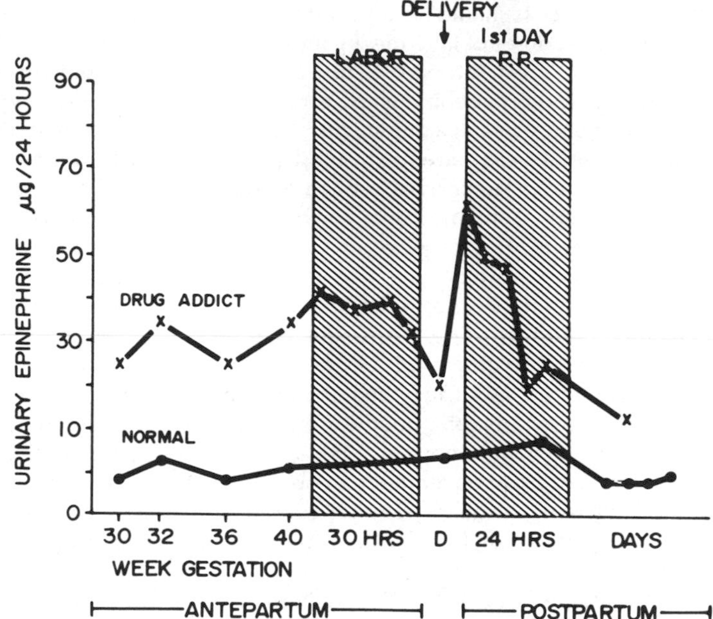

Figure 4–3. Urinary epinephrine levels in the normal pregnant patient and the pregnant drug addict.

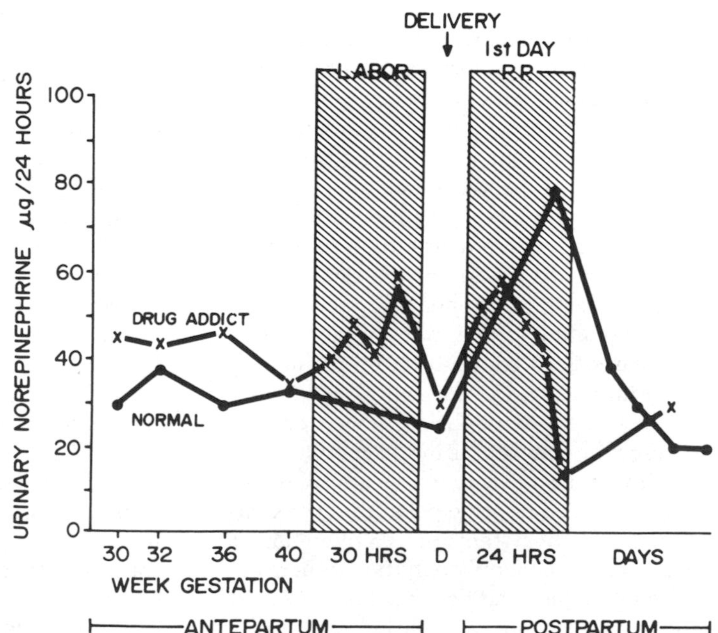

Figure 4–4. Comparison between urinary norepinephrine levels of the pregnant drug addict and the normal pregnant patient.

The Newborn

The infant of the drug-dependent mother may be smaller than those of nondependent women. In a group of 117 infants born to drug addicts from our study, the mean birth weight was 2680 g with 12.5 percent of the infants being considered small for gestational age. At birth, 88 percent had Apgar scores of 7 or above at 1 minute and 94 percent had scores of about 7 at 5 minutes. Of 117 infants, 8 had congenital malformations, of which three were minor and four major, two with talipes equinovarus and two with cardiac murmurs considered to be due to patent ductus arteriosis.[22] One infant with Potter's syndrome died because of renal agenesis.

Unless the nursery team is skilled in looking for special characteristics other than overt signs of withdrawal, these may be subtle. This is based on the daily dose, the duration of therapy, and the last dose before delivery. Table 4–5 identifies newborn withdrawal signs and symptoms, not all of which need to be present before therapy is begun. Narcotic or sedative withdrawal is accompanied by tremulousness, increased muscle tone, and hyperreflexia. Tremulousness is the first sign of withdrawal and can be evoked by startling the infant or by minimal tactile stimulation. In the severely affected infant undergoing withdrawal, tremulousness occurs without provocation. It is necessary to screen for hypocalcemia and hypoglycemia, as tremulousness is similar to both conditions.

An increase in flexor tone may accompany the tremulousness, and flexor rigidity is the most characteristic single sign of neonatal withdrawal. The attitude of flexion in the withdrawing infant increases to a point where there is marked resistance to extension. The infant becomes almost board-like, with the neck flexors sustaining the head in the same plane as the trunk for a prolonged period of time. Irritability is more pronounced than seen in normal patients, and the infant appears to be hyperalert and wakeful, with interferences being identified in the sleep cycle. The characteristic cry is shrill and high-pitched; however, this is not frequently seen as the patient is usually treated prior to this degree of withdrawal. The infant often roots and sucks on its fist. Seizures should be uncommon since the infant should be treated before this occurs. Developmental testing later in infancy and childhood would be worthwhile to assess perception and organizational skills.

Madden studied 110 newborns in a randomized blind trial utilizing methadone, phenobarbital, and diazepam with the dosage schedules outlined in Table 4–6.[3,22] Withdrawal symptoms were noted in 94 percent of patients (103 out of 110) and 45 percent required therapy. The decision to treat the neonate was based on clinical assessment of severity and whether the condition worsened. Treatment was started 2.7 days after delivery; the duration of treatment for methadone was 11.8 days; phenobarbital, 14.5 days; and diazepam, 10.2 days.

There appears to be a direct correlation between maternal methadone maintenance dose and the presence or absence of newborn withdrawal. In our experience if the maternal

TABLE 4–5. NEWBORN WITHDRAWAL

1. Tremulousness (no hypoglycemia or hypocalcemia)
2. Flexor tone increase (characteristic sign)
3. Sweating, yawning, thermal instability
4. GI disturbances (i.e., vomiting and diarrhea)
5. Tachypnea (respiratory alkalosis)
6. Irritability (hyperalert, sleep disturbance)
7. Cry—shrill and high-pitched
8. Seizures (late findings)

TABLE 4–6. NEWBORN WITHDRAWAL MEDICATIONS

Methadone	0.25 mg every 6 hr (maximum dose 0.5 MS)
Phenobarbital	5–8 mg/kg every 24 hr (given in divided doses every 8 hr)
Diazepam	0.5–2 mg every 8 hr

dose is less than 20 mg/day, only 18 percent of the infants required therapy. When the dose was greater than 20 mg/day, 62 percent of the infants required therapy.

Other Addicting Drugs

A common misconception is that fetal addiction takes place only with narcotic-like drugs. Although the narcotic group of drugs has been studied more extensively, other abused drugs affect the mother and her fetus to alter newborn behavior during withdrawal. Studies of drug abuse during pregnancy are limited to animal studies, anecdotal case reports, small sample sizes, use of other drugs, and inability to assess neurobehavioral function well in the newborn.

The drugs in Table 4–7 are grouped according to their chemical names. Signs and symptoms of an overdose, withdrawal symptoms, and any known fetal or neonatal effects are described. Abused drugs are mixed frequently and may cause different effects that may occur at lower threshold levels. Effects on the fetus are variable, difficult to predict, and may lead to an abortion or stillbirth, teratogenic effects, or developmental or growth delays later in life.

DRUG OVERDOSE DURING PREGNANCY

Suicide attempts during pregnancy are alarming events. Although rarely successful, such threats are as common during pregnancy as in the nonpregnant state.[69–71] A passive method by the ingestion of large quantities of pills is reported to occur in 95 percent of suicide attempts, regardless of pregnancy.[72] This is the first reported gesture in 83 percent of affected pregnancies.[70] They may occur at any time but especially once gestation is diagnosed or during the early third trimester.

Most suicide gestures are impulsive, and pregnancy alone is not thought to be a precipitator. Typically, the suicidal woman is emotionally immature and comes from a broken home or has an unhappy relationship with a lover or her parents.[69,72] True mental illness is infrequent, but neurotic depression is the most common psychiatric diagnosis.[69,72]

Experience at the Poison Control Center, Children's Hospital of Michigan, revealed 119 telephone calls pertaining to drug overdose in 111 pregnant patients between 1980 and 1983.[73] This represented 0.07 percent of the total 180,000 telephone calls. An attempted suicide was defined as a drug taken in excess and not intended for therapeutic benefit. This usually involved seven or more tablets (or their equivalent) at one time. A single product was ingested in 76 percent of cases, whereas two products were ingested in 22 percent of cases and three or four in 2 percent of cases. Alcoholic beverages were also consumed in 4 percent of cases. Help was usually sought within the first hour after the drug overdose.

A wide variety of prescriptions and over-the-counter products has been misused (Table 4–8).[73] Analgesic preparations are the most commonly abused drugs, especially those containing acetaminophen. The next most common medications include prenatal vitamins or iron, controlled analgesics, antianxiety agents, sedatives, antibiotics, and antihistamines or decongestants. Most of these medications are used during the second half of pregnancy and are therefore often available.[74]

Signs or symptoms from drug overdose have been found to be absent or mild in approximately half of these women.[73] Tiredness or drowsiness, nausea or vomiting, and slurred speech are the most common findings. Major signs or symptoms, such as a rapid or irregular heart rate or labored breathing, may occur. Life-threatening signs, such as coma, convulsions, or respiratory arrest, are to be anticipated although less commonly seen.

Home therapy before examination may include the ingestion of lard, mustard, or syrup of ipecac. Safe and successful therapy at home is impossible to determine, however,

TABLE 4–7. DRUG ABUSE DURING PREGNANCY

Drug Groups	Maternal Effects: *Signs and Symptoms of Overdose*	Maternal Effects: *Withdrawal Symptoms*	Fetal Effects	References
Alcohol	Unusual behavior, mostly depressant with stupor, loss of memory, hypotension	Agitation, tremors	Microcephaly, mental retardation, altered facial expressions, abortion	24–32
Anticholinergics Atropine Belladonna Scopolamine	Pupils—dilated and fixed Heart rate—increased Temperature—increased; flushed skin Sensorium—clouded, amnesia	None	None	33
Cannabis Marijuana THC Hashish Hash oil	Pupils—normal but conjunctiva injected BP—decreased in standing Heart rate—increased Sensorium—clear, dreamy, fantasy state, time and space distorted	None	Subtle behavioral alterations No anomalies or growth delay	32, 34–38
CNS Sedatives Barbiturates Chlordiazepoxide Diazepam Flurazepam Glutethimide Meprobamate Methaqualone, etc.	Pupils—unchanged BP—decreased $\pm$ shock Respiration—depressed Tendon reflexes—decreased drowsiness, coma, lateral nystagmus, ataxia, slurred speech, deliriums, convulsions	Tremulousness, insomnia, chronic blink reflex, agitation, toxic psychosis	No anomalies Withdrawal Floppy	39–47

(*continued*)

TABLE 4–7. (*Continued*)

Drug Groups	Maternal Effects: *Signs and Symptoms of Overdose*	Maternal Effects: *Withdrawal Symptoms*	Fetal Effects	References
CNS Stimulants Antiobesity drugs Amphetamines Cocaine Methylphenidate Phenmetrazine	Pupils—dilated and reactive Respiration—shallow BP—increased Tendon reflexes—hyperactive Cardiac arrhythmias Dry mouth, tremors, hyperactivity, sensorium hyperacute	Muscle aches, abdominal pain, hunger, prolonged sleep, ± suicidal	Abortion (?) Hyperactivity with increased kicks Cardiac defects (?) Depression of interactive behavior	48–53
Hallucinogens LSD Ketamine Mescaline Dimethyltryptamine Phencyclidine (PCP)	Pupils—dilated BP—elevated Heart rate—increased Tendon reflexes—increased Face flushed, euphoria, anxiety, inappropriate effect, illusions, halluciniations, realization	No withdrawal symptoms	Limited information in humans Dysmorphic face Behavioral problems	54–57
Narcotics Codeine Heroin Hydromorphone Meperidine Morphine Opium Pentazocine (and pyribenzamine)	Pupils—constricted Respiration—depressed BP—decreased Reflexes—hypoactive Sensorium—obtunded	Flu-like syndrome, agitation, dilated pupils, abdominal pain	Intrauterine withdrawal with increased fetal activity; newborn withdrawal; depressed breathing movements	58–68

TABLE 4-8. DRUGS OVERDOSED AS SUICIDAL GESTURES DURING PREGNANCY

	Percent
Analgesics, nonnarcotic	26
Vitamins or iron	12
Antianxiety agents	11
Sedatives-Hypnotics	10
Analgesics, controlled	8
Antibiotics	7
Antihistamines-Decongestants	6
Antipsychotic agents	3
Appetite suppressants	2
Hormones	2
Antidepressants	2
Anticonvulsants	2
Other	9
Total	100

From Rayburn WF et al., 1984, with permission.[73]

and the patient should be encouraged to visit her nearby emergency room. The chemical name of the drug, along with its description and pharmacokinetic properties, and the number of tablets taken, must be sought. The extent of that person's symptoms and signs must be assessed promptly. Initial blood tests should include arterial blood gases, renal function tests, and determination of any drug levels in the blood, urine, and gastric aspirate, if possible. The woman's vital signs, fluid balance, and consciousness should be monitored closely.

We assume that treatment recommendations for pregnant patients are the same as for nonpregnant women. Current information may be obtained through references at any poison control center.[75] Reassurance is often all that is necessary when mild or no symptoms exist, but symptoms may be delayed as long as 6 hours. Supportive therapy with supplemental oxygen, intravenous fluids, and vasopressors (if shock is present) is to be anticipated. Mechanical respiratory exchange may be necessary through a patent airway and with assisted or controlled ventilation. Any specific and effective antagonistic drugs or antidotes should be given.

If the abused drug was ingested and if the patient is conscious with no loss of gag reflex, emesis should be induced. Syrup of ipecac may be used, although no information exists about its safety during pregnancy. Minimal systemic absorption would be expected, and it is presumed to be safe under these circumstances. Ipecac syrup is available without prescription as 1 fl oz (30 ml). The usual dose of 1 tablespoonful (15 ml) should be followed by the ingestion of 200 to 300 ml of water. An adequate dose causes vomiting within 30 minutes in more than 90 percent of patients. Special attention should be placed on the avoidance of aspiration of vomitus and monitoring of any uterine contractions. Once emesis has occurred, 30 to 100 g of activated charcoal powder in a glass of water is then recommended.

If emesis is contraindicated, gastric lavage should be considered using a cuffed 34 Fr lavage tube and 300 to 400 ml of normal saline or tap water. The slowly instilled fluid should remain in place for 1 minute, then should be drained during a 3 to 4 minute period. Hemodialysis is seldom necessary and should be used as a last resort. The fetus should be monitored closely throughout therapy and the remainder of the hospitalization with periodic fetal heart rate determinations and ultrasound visualizations.

Specific reasons for the suicide gesture are often difficult to discern. Any mental disturbance may continue for several years in one-third of these women.[69] Although repeated suicide attempts during pregnancy are very unlikely, emotional support throughout the pregnancy and for several months after delivery is recommended to ease any interpersonal difficulties and to reduce the possibility of child abuse.[70] Adjustment difficulties and another drug overdose in the postpartum period are more likely, because the fetus is no longer in utero and that person may be less reluctant to take her own life during this complex period.

REFERENCES

1. Zelson C: Infant of the addicted mother. N Engl J Med 288:1393, 1973
2. Tyson HK: Neonatal withdrawal symptoms associated with maternal use of propoxyphene (Darvon). J Pediatr 85:684, 1974
3. Madden JD, Chappel JN, Zuspan FP, et al.: Observation and treatment of neonatal narcotic withdrawal. Am J Obstet Gynecol 127:199, 1977
4. Harper RG, Solish GI, Purrow HM, et al.: The effect of a methadone treatment program upon pregnant heroin addicts and their newborn infants. Pediatrics 54:300, 1974
5. Zuspan FP: Drug addiction in pregnancy: An invitational symposium. J Reprod Med 20:301, 1978
6. Rosner MA, Keith L, Chasnoff I: The Northwestern University drug-dependence program: The impact of intensive prenatal care on labor and delivery outcomes. Am J Obstet Gynecol 144:23, 1982
7. Gaulden EC, Littlefield DC, Putoff OE, Seivert AL: Menstrual abnormalities associated with heroin addiction. Am J Obstet Gynecol 90:155, 1964
8. Santen RJ, Sofsky J, Bilic N, Lippert R: Mechanism of action of narcotics in the production of menstrual dysfunction in women. Fertil Steril 26:538, 1975
9. Gumpel J, Mejia-Zelaya A: Prenatal management, labor and delivery care and postpartum follow-up of the drug addict. J Reprod Med 20:333, 1978
10. Finnegan L, Chappel JN, Kreek MJ, et al.: Narcotic addiction in pregnancy. In Neibyl J (Ed): Drugs in Pregnancy. Philadelphia, Lea and Febiger, 1981
11. Kreek MJ, Dodes L, Kane S, Knobler J: Long-term methadone maintenance therapy: Effects on liver function. Ann Intern Med 77:598, 1972
12. Singh EJ, Mejia A, Zuspan FP: Studies of human amniotic fluid phospholipids in normal, diabetic, and drug-abuse pregnancy. Am J Obstet Gynecol 119:623, 1974
13. Blinick G, Wallach RC, Jerez E: Pregnancy in narcotic addicts treated by medical withdrawal. Am J Obstet Gynecol 105:997, 1969
14. Zuspan FP, Gumpel JA, Mejia-Zelaya A, et al.: Fetal stress from methadone withdrawal. Am J Obstet Gynecol 122:43, 1975
15. Dole VP, Nyswander M: Methadone maintenance and its implications for theories of narcotic addiction. Res Publ Assoc Res Nerv Ment Dis 46:359, 1968
16. Dole VP, Nyswander M: The use of methadone for narcotic blockade. Br J Addict 63:55, 1968
17. Davis RC, Chappel JN: Pregnancy in the context of addiction and methadone maintenance. In Proceedings 5th National Conference on Methadone Treatment. New York, National Association for the Prevention of Addiction to Narcotics, 1973, Vol 2, p 1146
18. Senay EC, Weight M: The human need approach to the treatment of drug dependence. In Proceedings of the International Council on Alcoholism and Addiction. Amsterdam, 1972
19. Davis RC, Chappel JN, Mejia-Zelaya A, et al.: Clinical observations on methadone maintained pregnancies. Int J Addict Dis 2:101, 1975
20. Davis RC: Psycho-social care of the pregnant narcotic addict. J Reprod Med 20:316, 1978
21. Madden JD: Problems pertaining to the care of newborn infants of drug-addicted women. J Reprod Med 20:303, 1978
22. Zuspan FP: Urinary excretion of epinephrine and norepinephrine during pregnancy. J Clin Endocrinol Metab 30:357, 1970
23. Zuspan FP: Urinary amine alterations in drug addiction pregnancy. Am J Obstet Gynecol 120:955, 1976
24. Jones KL, Smith DW: Recognition of the fetal alcohol syndrome in early infancy. Lancet 2:999, 1973
25. Jones KL, Smith DW: The fetal alcohol syndrome. Teratology 12:1, 1975
26. Hanbson JW, Stressguth AP, Smith DW: The effects of moderate alcohol consumption during pregnancy on fetal growth and morphogenesis. J Pediatr 92:457, 1978
27. Landesman-Dwyer S, Keller LS, Streissguth AP: Naturalistic observations of newborns: Effects of maternal alcohol intake. Alcoholism. Clin Exper Res 2:171, 1978
28. Kline J, Shroat P, Stein Z, et al.: Drinking during pregnancy and spontaneous abortion. Lancet 2:176, 1980
29. Veghelyi PV, Osztovics J, Kardos G, et al.: The fetal alcohol syndrome: Symptoms and pathogenesis. Acta Paediatr Acad Sci Hung 19:171, 1978
30. Clarren SK, Smith DW: The fetal alcohol syndrome. N Engl J Med 298:1063, 1978

31. Hanson JW, Streissguth AP, Smith DW: The effects of moderate alcohol consumption during pregnancy on fetal growth and morphogenesis. J Pediatr 92:457, 1978
32. Gibson GT, Baghurst PA, Colley DP: Maternal alcohol, tobacco and cannabis consumption and the outcome of pregnancy. Austr NZ J Obstet Gynaecol 23:15, 1983
33. Arcuri PA, Gautieri RF: Morphine-induced fetal malformations: III. Possible mechanisms of action. J Pharm Sci 62:1616, 1973
34. Hecht F, Beals RK, Lees MHJ, et al.: Lysergic-acid–diethylamide and cannabis as possible teratogens in man. Lancet 2:1087, 1968
35. Neu RL, Powers H, Kings S, et al.: Cannabis and chromosomes. Lancet 1:675, 1969
36. Fleischman RW, Hayden DW, Rosenkrantz H, et al.: Teratologic evaluation of delta-9-tetrahydrocannabinol in mice, including a review of the literature. Teratology 12:47, 1975
37. Fried PA, Watkinson B, Willan A: Marijuana use during pregnancy and decreased length of gestation. Am J Obstet Gynecol 150:23, 1984
38. Fried PA: Marijuana use by pregnant women: Neurobehavioral effects in neonates. Drug Alcohol Depend 6:415, 1980.
39. Milkovich L, Vandenberg BJ: Effects of prenatal meprobamate and chlordiazepoxide hydrochloride on human embryonic and fetal development. N Engl J Med 291:1268, 1974
40. Shapiro S, Hartz SC, Siskind V, et al.: Anticonvulsants and prenatal epilepsy in the development of birth defects. Lancet 1:272, 1976
41. Crombie DL, Pinsent RJ, Fleming DM, et al.: Fetal effects of tranquilizers in pregnancy. N Engl J Med 293:198, 1975
42. Hartz SC, Heinonen OP, Shapiro S, et al.: Antenatal exposure to meprobamate and chlordiazepoxide in relations to malformations, mental development, and childhood mortality. N Engl J Med 292:726, 1975
43. Safra MJ, Oakley GP: An association of cleft lip with or without cleft palate and prenatal exposure to valium. Lancet 2:478, 1975
44. Saxen I: Associations between oral clefts and drugs taken during pregnancy. Int J Epidemiol 4:37, 1975
45. Saxen I, Saxen L: Association between maternal intake of diazepam and oral clefts. Lancet 2:498, 1975
46. McColl JD, Globus M, Robinson S: Drug-induced skeletal malformations in the rat. Experimentia 19:183, 1963
47. Bough RG, Gurd MR, Hall JE, et al.: Effect of methaqualone hydrochloride in pregnant rabbits and rats. Nature 200:656, 1983
48. Heinonen OP, Slone D, Shapiro S: Birth Defects and Drugs in Pregnancy. Littleton, Mass., Publishing Sciences Group, 1977
49. Nora JJ, Vargo TA, Nora AH, et al.: Dexamphetamine: A possible environmental trigger in cardiovascular malformations (letter). Lancet 1:1290, 1970
50. Milkovich L, Vandenberg BJ: Effects of antenatal exposure to anorectic drugs. Am J Obstet Gynecol 129:637, 1977
51. Larsson G: The amphetamine-addicted mother and her child. Acta Paediatr Scand (Suppl) 278:6, 1980
52. Fantel AG, MacPhail BJ: The teratogenicity of cocaine. Teratology 26:17, 1982
53. Chasnoff IJ, Burns WJ, Schnoll SH, et al.: Cocaine use in pregnancy. N Engl J Med 313:666, 1985
54. Geber WF: Congenital malformations induced by mescaline, lysergic acid diethylamide and bromolysergic acid in the hamster. Science 158:265, 1967
55. McGlothlin WH, Sparkes RS, Arnold DO: Effect of LSD on human pregnancy. JAMA 2:1483, 1970
56. Zellweger H, McDonald JS, Abbo G: Is lysergic-acid diethylamide a teratogen? Lancet 2:1066, 1967
57. El-Karim AH, Benny R: Embryotoxic and teratogenic action of ketamine hydrochloride in rats. Ain Shavis Med J 27:459, 1976
58. Wilson GS, Desmond MM, Varniann WM: Early development of infants of heroin-addicted mothers. Am J Dis Child 126:457, 1973
59. Zelson C, Lee SJ, Casalino M: Neonatal narcotic addiction. N Engl J Med 289: 1215, 1973
60. Naeye RL, Blanc W, et al.: Fetal complications of maternal heroin addiction. J Pediatr 83:1055, 1973
61. Geber WF, Schramm, LC: Congenital malformations of the central nervous system produced by narcotic analgesics in the hamster. Am J Obstet Gynecol 123:705, 1975
62. Friedler G: Pregestational administration of morphine sulfate to fetal mice: Long-term effects on development of subsequent progeny. J Pharmacol Exp Therap 205:33, 1978
63. Wilson GS, McCreary R, Kean J, Baxter JC: The development of preschool children of her-

oin-addicted mothers: A controlled study. Pediatrics 63:135, 1979
64. Richardson BS, O'Grady JP, Olsen GD: Fetal breathing movements and the response to carbon dioxide in patients on methadone maintenance. Am J Obstet Gynecol 150:400, 1984
65. Golden NL, Sokol RJ, Rubin IL: Angel dust: Possible effects on the fetus. Pediatrics 65:18, 1980
66. Nicholas JM, Lipshitz J, Schreiber EC: Phencyclidine: Its transfer across the placenta as well as into breast milk. Am J Obstet Gynecol 143:153, 1982
67. Rayburn WF, Holsztynaska EF, Domino EF: Phencyclidine: Biotransformation by the human placenta. Am J Obstet Gynecol 148:111, 1984
68. Golden ML, Kuhnert BR, Sokol RJ, et al.: Phencyclidine use during pregnancy. Am J Obstet Gynecol 148:254, 1984
69. Whitlock FA, Edwards JE: Pregnancy and attempted suicide. Compr Psychiatry 9:1, 1968
70. Gabrielson IH, Klerman LV, Currie JB, et al.: Suicide attempts in a population pregnant as teenagers. J Public Health 60:2289, 1970
71. Lewis GJ, Fay R: Suicide in pregnancy. Br J Clin Pract 35:51, 1981
72. Otto U: Suicidal attempts made by pregnant women under 21 years. Acta Paedopsychiatr 31:276, 1964
73. Rayburn W, Aronow R, DeLancy B, et al.: Drug overdose during pregnancy: An overview from a metropolitan poison control center. Obstet Gynecol 64:611, 1984
74. Rayburn W, Wible J, Bledsoe P: Changing trends in drug use during pregnancy. J Reprod Med 7:569, 1982
75. Haddad LM, Winchester JF: Clinical Management of Poisoning and Drug Overdose. Philadelphia, Saunders, 1983

5

Anticonvulsant Therapy During Pregnancy

Laurence E. Stempel and William F. Rayburn

Epilepsy is one of the most common disorders in the world with an incidence of 0.5 percent.[1,2] In most cases, the seizure disorder commences before the age of 20, making epilepsy a frequent accompaniment to the childbearing years.[2] In the past, marriage and reproduction by epileptics were limited by social stigma and public statutes. With improved social acceptance, advances in medical therapy, and decreased emphasis on the genetic transmission of epilepsy, many epileptics are now able to marry and lead nearly normal lives.

Epilepsy is now a frequent medical complication of pregnancy, with an estimated incidence of 0.3 to 0.5 percent.[3-6] Without treatment, epilepsy is a socially, psychologically, and physically disabling condition, and hence it is almost always imperative that anticonvulsant medications be continued during pregnancy. The major concern of the obstetrician caring for the pregnant epileptic should be the prevention of seizures; however, it is also important that adverse fetal effects from anticonvulsants be minimized as much as possible.

GENERAL CONSIDERATIONS

Definition and Classification

Epilepsy is not a disease, but rather a complex syndrome characterized by brief recurrent paroxysmal episodes of disturbed central nervous system (CNS) function, often with alteration in the state of consciousness. These episodes, known as seizures, may be accompanied by altered behavior, or motor or sensory activity.

The term convulsion is reserved for seizures that have a predominant motor component, such as the tonic–clonic movements of grand mal epilepsy. Seizures may vary from a momentary absence spell, as in petit mal, to the repetitive convulsions of status epilepticus, which may last for hours or days. Patients who have a single isolated seizure should not be stigmatized as having epilepsy, as this term implies a recurrent disorder. Nevertheless, anyone who experiences even one seizure should be thoroughly evaluated and treated if the seizures recur.

There are many different forms of epilepsy, and the proper therapy depends on a correct diagnosis. There are a number of different classifications of epilepsy and a wide variety of atypical forms. Most patients, however, have either grand mal, focal motor, psychomotor, or petit mal epilepsy, or a combination of these forms.

Grand Mal Epilepsy

Over 70 percent of epileptics have grand mal epilepsy, either alone or in combination with petit mal or psychomotor epilepsy.[7] Grand mal seizures are characterized by total loss of consciousness, followed by a tonic phase during which the arms are flexed, the legs are extended, and the patient is apneic. This is soon followed by the clonic phase, with alternate contraction and relaxation of skeletal muscles. The convulsion often lasts only a few minutes and the patient usually experiences a postictal depression characterized by drowsiness and confusion.

Focal Epilepsy

This form of epilepsy may be primarily motor or sensory. It is usually indicative of focal disease of the cerebral cortex, but it may also be seen with metabolic disorders such as hypoglycemia and hypocalcemia. Motor seizures often begin peripherally with twitching of the thumb, big toe, or face, which are all disproportionally represented in the cerebral cortex. The seizure may remain confined to these twitchings, or may progress to a generalized tonic–clonic convulsion. It may be followed by Todd's paralysis, a transient paralysis of that part of the body corresponding to the epileptogenic focus.

Psychomotor Epilepsy

This bizarre form of epilepsy is caused by an epileptogenic focus in the temporal lobe. Seizures may include subjective experiences, such as altered mood, repetitive disturbing thoughts, a sensation of impending disaster, and visual distortions. The patient may also experience automatisms, such as lip smacking and chewing motions, and autonomic changes including salivation, perspiration, and pupillary dilatation. Although often brief, these seizures may last for hours or days. Psychomotor seizures account for 15 percent of epilepsy.[7]

Petit Mal Epilepsy

Petit mal seizures are characterized by brief absence spells, often lasting less than 10 seconds. There is usually no major motor activity or loss of posture, although the patient may blink or roll the eyes. These seizures are not followed by postictal depression, and the patient can usually resume prior activity. Although petit mal accounts for 10 percent of all epilepsy,[7] it rarely persists past adolescence, and therefore is infrequently seen during pregnancy.

Etiology

There are many causes of seizures, some of which are listed in Table 5–1. Unfortunately, in most cases, the etiology is unknown. Correctable problems should always be diligently sought, because correction of underlying disorders is frequently as important as drug therapy.

There appears to be a familial component to epilepsy, although it is not nearly as strong as once believed. If one parent is epileptic, there is a 2.5 percent chance that the offspring will develop epilepsy[8]; this is five times the risk in the general population. The risk is even higher if both parents are epileptic.[8] Forty-one percent of epileptics have a positive family history of epilepsy, whereas the corresponding figure for control patients is only 6.3 percent.[9] Although this familial tendency is probably in part genetic it may also represent environmental influences, such as maternal seizure-related hypoxia during pregnancy.

It is important to distinguish precipitating factors from etiologic factors. Edema, hyperventilation, stress, fatigue, and fever may provoke seizures in patients with a low seizure threshold, but do not in themselves cause seizures.[8] Nevertheless, they should be avoided by susceptible individuals.

TABLE 5-1. ETIOLOGY OF EPILEPSY

Infectious	Meningitis, encephalitis, brain abscess
Metabolic	Alkalosis, hypocalcemia, hypoglycemia, hyponatremia, porphyria
Toxic	Mercury, lead, carbon monoxide, amphetamines, phenothiazine, and tricyclic antidepressant toxicity
Traumatic	Cerebral injury (especially penetrating wounds)
Vascular	Cerebrovascular accident, A-V malformation
Drug withdrawal	Alcohol, barbiturate, anticonvulsant
Degenerative disease of the CNS	
Perinatal	Trauma, asphyxia, anomalies
Neoplastic	Primary or metastatic
Genetic	

Effects of Pregnancy on Epilepsy

Pregnancy has an unpredictable effect on the frequency and severity of seizures.[10,11] Almost half of gravid epileptics will experience an exacerbation of their seizure disorder during pregnancy, while another 45 to 50 percent will show no change. The remaining 5 to 10 percent will have fewer seizures during pregnancy.[10,12] The prognosis is unrelated to maternal age, age at onset of epilepsy, and any seizure activity with a prior pregnancy.[10] Only 25 percent of patients with rare seizures, less than one every 9 months, will get worse during pregnancy, while virtually all patients who convulse at least once a month will deteriorate.[10] The course of epilepsy during previous pregnancies is not predictive either, because only half of epileptics show a similar response in subsequent pregnancies.[10] The effects of pregnancy on epilepsy are temporary, and most patients revert to their pregestational pattern after the puerperium.[10]

Many explanations have been offered for the rare improvement and frequent deterioration of epilepsy during pregnancy. Epilepsy shows natural fluctuations with time, and some of the changes may be totally unrelated to pregnancy. Improvement may also be related to better drug compliance.[12] There are numerous factors that may be responsible for the exacerbations that are so often seen during pregnancy. Many of the physiologic changes of pregnancy, such as hyperventilation, hyponatremia, hypocalcemia, and expansion of the extracellular fluid volume are well known to precipitate convulsions in susceptible individuals.[12,13] Indeed hyperventilation and hydration are frequently used in diagnostic testing to bring out electroencephalogram (EEG) abnormalities. Emotional stress and anxiety are frequent accompaniments of pregnancy, and are also known to precipitate seizures. However, the most important reason for the worsening of seizures in pregnancy may be the decrease in anticonvulsant serum levels which many patients experience.

Anticonvulsant serum levels are reduced during pregnancy for a variety of reasons. Patients may refuse to take their medications because of fears of teratogenesis, or they may fail to ingest or absorb their medication because of nausea and vomiting. Serum levels may also drop because of dilution by the expanded extracellular fluid volume, increased hepatic and renal clearance, and possibly also because of fetoplacental drug metabolism.[14]

In a retrospective study, Mygind found increased plasma clearance of phenytoin during pregnancy, with half of the patients showing more than a 100 percent increase in clearance. He also found a correlation between loss of seizure control and decreased levels of phenytoin.[15] Mirkin found that gravid mothers maintained on standard doses (300 to 400 mg/day) of phenytoin had a mean plasma level of 3.6 mcg/ml, far below the therapeutic range of 10 to 20 mcg/ml.[16] Lander et al. also found increased phenytoin requirements in 10 patients during pregnancy, with some patients needing as much as 50 percent more medication.[14] Serum levels of phenobarbital and primidone have also been shown to decrease during pregnancy, although there is considerable individual variation.[14] It is important that serum anticonvulsant levels be checked frequently during pregnancy, with appropriate adjustments made in dosage to maintain levels in the therapeutic range.

Effects of Epilepsy and Anticonvulsant Therapy on Pregnancy

Epilepsy and its therapy may have a variety of adverse effects on the pregnancy and the fetus. While some investigators have found no increase in spontaneous abortion, prematurity, toxemia, and multiple gestation,[10,17] others have found a significant increase in complications such as vaginal bleeding, toxemia, prematurity, and low birth weight infants.[18] Epileptics have a perinatal mortality twice that of the general population,[18,19] largely due to an increase in congenital malformations and neonatal hemorrhage.[19]

Because most epileptics are on chronic anticonvulsant therapy, it is often difficult to separate the effects of epilepsy from those of the therapy. Although it is sometimes helpful to compare treated and untreated epileptics, it is likely that untreated patients represent a heterogenous and quite different group, including those with mild disease, noncompliant patients, and patients resistant to prior treatment.[3] The problem is further complicated by the fact that most epileptics take multiple anticonvulsant drugs, all of which have overlapping side effects.

Several adverse effects of epilepsy and anticonvulsants that are of particular concern to the obstetrician include congenital malformations, altered maternal folate metabolism, vitamin D deficiency, neonatal coagulopathy, depression, low thyroxine levels, and drug withdrawal. While many of these problems are due to anticonvulsants or alterations in metabolism, others such as teratogenesis may relate to both anticonvulsants and epilepsy. These complications may not be of clinical significance with proper prenatal care but are discussed later with the individual anticonvulsant agents.[7] Because of the great concern that has been expressed about the teratogenicity of anticonvulsants, this subject is discussed in greater detail in the following sections.

Fetal Malformations

It has been demonstrated repeatedly that the offspring of epileptic women taking anticonvulsant medications have a two- to three-fold increase in congenital anomalies.[4,19–22] Nevertheless, the teratogenicity of most antiepileptic agents remains to be established, as there are several possible explanations for the increased incidence of malformations, including:

1. Epilepsy might in some way be linked to congenital anomalies. Dronamraju demonstrated a greater than expected number of epileptics among the first- and second-degree relatives of patients with orofacial clefts.[23] Friis found three times the expected number of epileptics among the parents of children with facial clefts.[24] In a review from the Mayo Clinic, however, Annegers et al. were unable to confirm this relationship.[3] Further evidence that epilepsy and anomalies may be linked is the finding that the children of epileptic fathers may also have an increased incidence of malformations.[25] Finally, epileptics and their relatives have a higher than expected incidence of anomalies.[26]
2. Epileptic patients as a group have a number of characteristics associated with an increased risk of malformations, including older age, lower socioeconomic class, and a higher rate of past stillbirths.[20,22] However, Monson et al. found an in-

creased incidence of anomalies in the children of mothers taking phenytoin during the first trimester, even after correcting for some of these confounding factors.[22]

3. Epileptic convulsions are often associated with hypoxia and acidosis, and these metabolic disturbances could be teratogenic during the first trimester.[1] However, Fedrick and others found no relationship between the frequency of seizures during pregnancy and congenital anomalies.[19,20]

Despite these considerations, most of the evidence supports the concept that some anticonvulsants are teratogenic, and that this teratogenicity accounts for most of the increase in anomalies in the offspring of epileptics.

Since Meadow's report in 1968 of six cases of orofacial clefts and other anomalies in fetuses exposed in utero to anticonvulsants,[27] there have been numerous epidemiologic surveys of the offspring of epileptic patients.[1,6,19–22] A variety of study designs have been used; some investigators have compared epileptics with the general population, whereas others have used matched controls. Some studies have differentiated between treated and untreated patients, whereas others have not. Furthermore, the definition of malformation, the patient follow-up, and the method of ascertainment of children with anomalies have varied widely.

Although some investigators have found no increase in malformations among the offspring of treated epileptics,[17,28,29] the vast majority of studies have shown a 1.25- to 3-fold relative increase in the incidence of anomalies in fetuses exposed to anticonvulsants.[6,19–22]

In a review of over 2000 children of epileptics taking anticonvulsants, the most commonly reported defects were orofacial clefts (3.0 percent), skeletal anomalies (1.9 percent), heart defects (1.4 percent), CNS malformations (1.2 percent), gastrointestinal malformations (1.1 percent), facial anomalies (1.0 percent), mental retardation (0.7 percent), and genitourinary anomalies (0.6 percent).[30] A recent prospective study of infants exposed in utero to anticonvulsants has shown a 10 to 20 percent incidence of major anomalies and a similar incidence of decreased mental capacity.[31] While these figures are disturbing, most authorities agree that with the exception of trimethadione, anticonvulsant medications should not be discontinued during pregnancy.

ANTICONVULSANT THERAPY DURING PREGNANCY

General Guidelines

The primary objective of anticonvulsive therapy is to reduce the frequency and severity of seizures without causing excessive adverse effects. With appropriate therapy, seizures can be completely abolished in 65 percent of epileptics, while another 20 percent will show a reduction in the frequency and severity of seizures.[8] In designing an anticonvulsant regimen for the individual patient, the following principles should be kept in mind:

1. An appropriate primary drug should be chosen. This drug should have the best possible balance between efficacy and adverse effects. The patient should undergo thorough evaluation prior to the institution of therapy, as agents that are effective for some forms of epilepsy may exacerbate others.
2. The patient should be initially treated with a *single* anticonvulsant agent. It should be started at a moderate dosage, and increased gradually until either seizures are controlled or evidence of toxicity develops. The dose should not be increased any more frequently than once every three to four half-lives, to allow serum levels to reach a steady state.
3. If toxicity develops before seizures are controlled, the dosage should be reduced and a second drug should be added. Noncompliance or sleep deprivation should

also be considered as causes before a second drug is prescribed.[7] These same principles apply to the second drug and third drugs.

4. If complete seizure control is achieved with a second drug, the initial drug should be slowly tapered and even withdrawn, if possible. A therapeutic serum drug level should be present for at least one of these drugs. This process would also apply if a third drug becomes necessary.
5. Changes in the anticonvulsant regimen should be made slowly. Rapid changes may precipitate status epilepticus.
6. When anticonvulsant therapy is being started in the previously untreated pregnant woman, one-half of the usual maintenance dose should be given. This dosage can be increased weekly until the full maintenance dosage is reached. Phenytoin is an exception to this general concept, and a single loading dose of 900 mg may be given on the first day.
7. In some cases, complete control of seizures may not be possible.
8. The most common reasons for the failure of anticonvulsants to control seizures are patient noncompliance and the use of the wrong drug or dosage.[8]
9. Seizure prophylaxis must continue during labor, delivery, and immediately postpartum. Intravenous phenytoin using a 500-mg dose should be given every 12 hours.

Monitoring Anticonvulsant Levels

The unbound concentration of the drug in plasma should equate with the unbound drug at the receptor site. A decline in the plasma level of anticonvulsant drugs is expected during pregnancy when the maintenance dose remains constant. Low serum anticonvulsant levels may also be caused by inadequate dosage, noncompliance, incomplete absorption, or abnormally rapid elimination. High serum levels may be caused by improper dosage, impaired elimination, or drug interactions.

Serum levels of anticonvulsants should be maintained within the therapeutic range, which is the concentration of drug at which most patients show the best seizure control without evidence of toxicity. It is especially important to monitor serum levels after changing drugs or dosages, and in patients with renal or hepatic disease. Serum levels should also be checked if other medications are added or withdrawn, because of the potential for drug interactions. It is also helpful to measure the serum levels in patients with signs or symptoms of toxicity, or if seizures recur. It is sometimes necessary to monitor the levels of active metabolites, for example, phenobarbital in patients taking primidone.

Phenytoin and carbamazepine are cleared more rapidly from the plasma by perhaps accelerated metabolism and by increased renal elimination.[32] There is little doubt that the availability of the plasma phenytoin assay has greatly improved the clinical use of phenytoin. Sampling of the blood in a fasting state before the next dose is desirable because a trough plasma level (the lowest in a 24-hr period) should be measured. There is nothing magic about a therapeutic range, however, and some patients will do well with subtherapeutic plasma concentrations.

Anticonvulsant drugs are also transferred across the placenta. Phenytoin concentrations at term are identical in the maternal serum and umbilical cord blood. The half-life of phenytoin in the plasma of the newborn ranges from 55 to 69 hours.[33] The elimination of the drug by the fetus is presumed to be completed by the fifth day. Phenobarbital concentrations are also virtually identical in the umbilical cord blood with those in the mother's plasma. Elimination of phenobarbital in newborns is within 2 to 7 days.[33]

Treatment of Specific Disorders

Many drugs are available for the treatment of seizure disorders. The first- and second-line drugs for the various forms of epilepsy are shown in Table 5–2. Dosage considerations and effective serum concentrations of

TABLE 5–2. ANTICONVULSANT DRUGS OF CHOICE FOR TREATING SEIZURE DISORDERS DURING PREGNANCY

Seizure Disorder	Primary Drug	Secondary Drugs
Grand mal and focal motor	Phenobarbital	Phenytoin Primidone Carbamazepine
Psychomotor	Primidone	Phenytoin Phenobarbital Carbamazepine
Petit mal	Ethosuximide	Clonazepam

these anticonvulsants are listed in Table 5–3. Adverse maternal and fetal effects of these agents are shown in Table 5–4.

Grand Mal and Focal Motor Epilepsy

Phenobarbital and phenytoin are the first-line drugs for the treatment of grand mal and focal motor epilepsy.[8] For women in the reproductive age group, phenobarbital is probably the drug of choice, as it appears to have less teratogenic potential than phenytoin.[4,5,20] However, phenytoin should be used when a second agent is required. Primidone is effective for both of these disorders, but should not be used in conjunction with phenobarbital, as this latter drug is one of the active metabolites of primidone. Other second-line drugs, which are useful for grand mal and focal motor epilepsy, are carbamazepine and occasionally, valproic acid.

Psychomotor Epilepsy

Primidone is the drug of choice for psychomotor epilepsy.[7,8] If a second agent is needed, then phenytoin may be added. Phenobarbital and carbamazepine are other useful second-line drugs. This form of epilepsy may be especially difficult to control.[8]

Petit Mal Epilepsy

This disorder rarely persists past adolescence, and is therefore an uncommon complication of pregnancy. Ethosuximide is the drug of choice for petit mal, although clonazepam occasionally may be necessary.[8] Trimethadione is highly teratogenic, and should never be

TABLE 5–3. DOSAGE CONSIDERATIONS OF ANTICONVULSANTS IN ADULTS

Drug	Starting Daily Dose (mg)	Daily Dose (mg)	Time Before Steady State (days)	Therapeutic Level* (mcg/ml)	Serum Half-Life† (hr)	Protein Binding %
Phenytoin	900 (loading dose)	300–500	5–10	10–20	22–40	88–92
Phenobarbital	30–60	120–250	16–21	10–35	96	50
Valproic acid	250	1000–3000	2–4	50–120	7–17	90–95
Ethosuximide	250	750–2000	12	40–100	50–60	0
Primidone	50–125	750–1500	1–5	4–12	15.6	0–20
Carbamazepine	100–200	600–1200	3–6	4–12	Single dose: 40–50 Long-term dose: 8–18.7	67–81

* Therapeutic level may change with multiple drugs.

† Half-life may change with multiple drugs; steady state reached in five half-lives.

TABLE 5–4. ADVERSE MATERNAL AND FETAL EFFECTS FROM ANTICONVULSANT USE

Anticonvulsant	Maternal	Fetal/Neonatal
Phenytoin (Dilantin)	Cardiovascular collapse after rapid IV injection, ataxia, nystagmus, GI upset, increased incidence of seizures, gingival hyperplasia, behavioral changes, osteomalacia, megaloblastic anemia, hirsutism, lymphadenopathy, skin rashes, Stevens-Johnson syndrome, lupus syndrome, and hepatic necrosis	Probable teratogenicity, possible carcinogenicity, neonatal coagulopathy, and neonatal hypocalcemia and tetany
Phenobarbital	Drowsiness (transient), ataxia, respiratory depression, sleep abnormalities, hypotension, allergic reaction, megaloblastic anemia, agranulocytosis, thrombocytopenia	Possible low-level teratogenicity, neonatal coagulopathy, neonatal depression, neonatal withdrawal
Primidone (Mysoline)	Ataxia, vertigo, headache, nausea, morbilliform rash, edema, nystagmus, impotence, leukopenia, and megaloblastic anemia	Possible teratogenicity, neonatal coagulopathy, neonatal depression
Carbamazepine (Tegretol)	Diplopia, drowsiness, leukopenia, transient blurred vision, rash, disturbance of equilibrium, transient paresthesias, proteinuria, neutropenia, systemic lupus erythematosus, left ventricular failure, hypertension, hypotension, syncope and collapse, edema	None known
Ethosuximide (Zarontin)	Hematopoietic complications, including aplastic anemia, pancytopenia, agranulocytosis, and eosinophilia. Morphologic and functional changes in the liver, GI upset, nausea, vomiting, diarrhea Hyperactivity, hypoactivity, behavioral changes, paranoid and suicidal ideations Stevens-Johnson syndrome, systemic lupus erythematosus, and pruritic erythematous rash	Possible low-level teratogenicity
Valproic acid (Depakene)	GI upset, sedation, ataxia and incoordination, hepatotoxicity, and thrombocytopenia	Hyperglycinemia, teratogenic in animals; neural tube defects(?)
Diazepam	Drowsiness, ataxia	
Clonazepam (Clonopin)	Depressed respiration, bradycardia, hypotension, cardiovascular collapse, and paradoxical hyperexcitability. Caution should be exercised not to use small veins or the dorsum of the hand or wrist to administer diazepam. Extreme care should also be taken to avoid intra-arterial administration or extravasation because of the irritating properties of the drug	Decreased fetal heart rate variability, possible low-level teratogenicity, neonatal depression, neonatal hypotension, neonatal withdrawal, impaired neonatal thermoregulation

used in fertile women during the reproductive years.[34–36]

Status Epilepticus

Status epilepticus is the occurrence of repetitive grand mal seizures between which the patient does not regain consciousness. Without adequate therapy, the seizures may continue for hours or even days, frequently resulting in death or anoxic brain damage. Even with prompt treatment, mortality is still high, making status epilepticus a serious medical emergency. The patient's prognosis depends on the underlying cause of the seizures, the general condition of the patient, and the interval between the onset of seizures and the institution of therapy.[37] Although status epilepticus may be triggered by a variety of insults, the most common precipitating factor is the abrupt cessation of anticonvulsant medications.[38] Although status epilepticus is no more common during pregnancy, it can be disastrous for both the mother and the fetus, though normal infants have been born after an episode of status epilepticus.[10]

Patients with status epilepticus should be hospitalized immediately, preferably in an intensive care unit. Supportive care includes an intravenous line, padded side rails, and maintenance of a patent airway. The underlying cause of the seizures should be sought diligently and treated promptly. Initial laboratory tests should include serum levels of anticonvulsants, glucose, urea nitrogen, and electrolytes and arterial blood gases. A bolus injection of 50 ml of a 50 percent glucose solution should be infused.

The mainstay of treatment is the use of large doses of intravenous anticonvulsant medications. There is no evidence that this has any adverse effect on the fetus, especially when one considers the alternative injurious effects on the fetus of continuous inadequate oxygenation. Table 5–5 lists drugs of choice to be prescribed. The intermittent infusion of diazepam is the first drug to be used. If seizures persist, other options include intravenous phenobarbital or phenytoin or a diazepam intravenous drip. Experience with intravenous magnesium sulfate for this condition is limited and not recommended. General anesthesia with halothane and neuromuscular-junction blockade should be instituted if seizures persist.

Because of its rapid effect on the CNS, intravenous diazepam is the drug of choice for status epilepticus.[38] The benefits of prompt seizure control far outweigh the risks of hypotension and respiratory depression.[37] Diazepam is administered intravenously in a dose of 5 to 10 mg over a 2- to 4-minute period. It should not be given any faster than 2 mg/min. If there is no response to the initial dose, then it may be repeated several times at 10-minute intervals, or until a total 20-mg dose is given; however, this may necessitate the use of artificial ventilation. The anticonvulsant action of intravenous diazepam lasts for only 15 to 20 minutes, and therefore treatment with long-acting agents, such as phenytoin or phenobarbital, must begin as soon as seizures have been stopped.[38]

Phenytoin is not often used as the primary therapy of status epilepticus, because it is effective in stopping seizures in only about half of the cases.[37] As soon as seizures are controlled with diazepam, the patient should receive an intravenous loading dose of phenytoin. This drug has a rapid onset of action, and unlike phenobarbital, it does not potentiate the depressant actions of diazepam. Even if the patient receives a modest overdose, the symptoms of nystagmus and ataxia are not dangerous.[39] Phenytoin should be given in a loading dose of 1000 to 1500 mg (18 mg/kg), at a rate not to exceed 50 mg/min. When given any faster, phenytoin may cause hypotension, arrhythmias, and cardiac arrest.[37–39] The blood pressure and electrocardiogram (ECG) should be monitored care-

TABLE 5–5. DRUGS OF CHOICE FOR TREATING ADULTS WITH STATUS EPILEPTICIES

Drugs of Choice	Usual Initial Dose	Usual Rate (mg/min)	Repeat Doses PRN every 20–30 min	Maximum /24 hr
Diazepam, IV	5–10 mg	1–2	5–10 mg	100 mg
Phenytoin, IV	15 mg/kg	30–50	100–150 mg	1.5 g
Phenobarbital, IV	300–800 mg	25–50	120–240 mg	1–2 g

fully while the loading dose is being given. After the patient has received her loading dose, daily maintenance therapy should be started.

Intravenous phenobarbital has been used to treat status epilepticus, but its slow onset of action (15 to 30 minutes) makes it less useful than diazepam.[38] When administered in conjunction with diazepam, the hypotensive and respiratory depressant actions of the two drugs are additive.[38] Phenobarbital may be used to treat status epilepticus caused by barbiturate withdrawal. In these cases, it should be given intravenously in a dose of 250 mg administered over 3 to 5 minutes (no more than 100 mg/min). This dose may be repeated once after 30 minutes. It should be noted that it may be necessary to artificially support respiration when large doses of intravenous phenobarbital are given.

Paraldehyde and general anesthesia have been used rarely when the seizures continue.

Special Considerations in Pregnancy

Phenytoin

Phenytoin requirements generally increase during pregnancy, although there is considerable individual variation[14-16,33] and dosage changes should be dictated by serum levels. Phenytoin crosses the human placenta rapidly, so that with chronic usage, maternal and fetal serum levels are identical.[40] This drug is eliminated quite slowly by the neonate, with a half-life of approximately 60 hours, compared to only 24 hours in the adult.[16] Although phenytoin may have a number of adverse effects on the fetus and neonate, including teratogenesis, coagulopathy, and vitamin deficiency, it differs from some of the other anticonvulsants in that it is not associated with neonatal depression or withdrawal.[16]

TERATOGENICITY. Phenytoin is known to be teratogenic in some laboratory animals.[2,41,42] In mice, the severity of malformation is related to both the dosage and the stage of gestation at which it is administered.[42] The numerous difficulties involved in defining the teratogenic potential of an anticonvulsant drug in humans have already been discussed. Nevertheless, there is considerable evidence that phenytoin is teratogenic in humans. In a retrospective study, Monson et al. found that infants exposed to phenytoin on a daily basis early in pregnancy had a 6.1 percent incidence of selected malformations, including orofacial clefts, neural tube defects, congenital heart lesions, and limb defects. Even after correcting for confounding variables such as age, race, and socioeconomic status, this incidence of malformations was 2.4 times higher than that of nonepileptics, and also considerably higher than the rate among fetuses exposed to phenytoin sporadically or later in pregnancy. There was no evidence that the risk of anomalies was dose-related.[22] Fedrick also found that phenytoin was much more likely to produce defects than phenobarbital, although the combination was additive. Infants exposed in utero to phenytoin had a 15.2 percent incidence of malformations, compared with 4.9 percent with phenobarbital alone and 22.0 percent when both agents were used. Of the control patients, 5.6 percent gave birth to anomalous infants. Fedrick also was unable to find a relationship between phenytoin dosage and the risk of malformations.[20]

Hanson has described a fetal hydantoin syndrome (FHS) consisting of pre- and postnatal growth deficiency, microcephaly, mental retardation, developmental delay, and a wide variety of dysmorphic features (Table 5–6). These infants may manifest a variety of limb abnormalities, including distal phalangeal and nail hypoplasia and finger-like thumbs.[43,44] Other frequently reported lesions include congenital heart defects and diaphragmatic hernias. In a retrospective review of data from the Collaborative Perinatal Study, Hanson and co-workers found that 11 of 104 infants exposed in utero to phenytoin had FHS.[43] In a companion prospective study of 35 infants exposed to phenytoin during pregnancy, he found that 11 percent mani-

TABLE 5–6. FEATURES OF THE FETAL HYDANTOIN SYNDROME

- Intrauterine growth retardation
- Postnatal growth retardation
- Microcephaly
- Mental or motor deficiency
- Ridging of metopic suture
- Facial dysmorphisms
  - Low-set or abnormal ears
  - Broad, depressed nasal bridge
  - Short nose
  - Anteverted nostrils
  - Wide mouth
  - Prominent upper lip
  - Inner epicanthal folds
  - Ptosis
  - Strabismus
  - Cleft lip and/or palate
  - Hypertelorism
- Limb anomalies
  - Hypoplastic nails
  - Hypoplastic distal phalanges
  - Finger-like thumbs
- Congenital heart defects
- Hernias
  - Diaphragmatic
  - Inguinal
- Genitourinary anomalies
- Abnormal genitalia

fested FHS, whereas an additional 31 percent showed some of the features of the syndrome. None of the infants exposed only to phenobarbital had features of FHS.[43] The permanent impairment of neurologic function in some of these infants has caused greater concern than the structural defects, most of which are readily correctable.[30] It should be noted, however, that some investigators have questioned Hanson's figures.[4,17,25,26,45] Several types of anomalies have been reported in infants whose mothers were treated with either no anticonvulsant or a drug other than phenytoin. The FHS may represent an aggregation of unfavorable findings for which any epileptic pregnant woman is at risk.[7]

The current feeling is that infants exposed to phenytoin in utero have a somewhat increased risk of mental retardation, and a two- to threefold increased incidence of congenital malformations. These risks appear to be unrelated to dosage, although this has never been studied prospectively. Phenytoin is probably more teratogenic than phenobarbital, and several authorities have recommended that when possible, women in the reproductive age group should be treated with phenobarbital alone.[4,5,32] However, when needed to control seizures, the benefits of phenytoin far outweigh the risks.

CARCINOGENICITY. There have been four reported cases of neuroblastoma in children with FHS. Because of the rarity of these two conditions it has been calculated that it should take approximately 60 years to produce three cases of FHS with neuroblastoma if the two conditions are not related.[46] The fact that these four cases were reported over only a 3-year period suggests that phenytoin may be carcinogenic.

NEONATAL COAGULOPATHY. Another serious complication of maternal anticonvulsant use (especially phenytoin and phenobarbital) is neonatal hemorrhage, which contributes significantly to the high perinatal mortality in the offspring of epileptics. First reported in 1957, it was a number of years before the nature of this problem became clear. It is now known that almost half of all infants exposed in utero to anticonvulsants will exhibit a severe coagulopathy, and half of these children will experience significant bleeding if they are not given vitamin K at birth.[47] These infants tend to bleed soon after birth, often during the first 24 hours of life.[48,49] This is in contrast to hemorrhagic disease of the newborn (HDN), in which the infants usually bleed during the second to fifth day. This syndrome also differs from HDN in that these infants may bleed in unusual places, such as into the pleural, pericardial, or peritoneal cavities, or into the retroperitoneal space. Intracranial bleeding may also occur.[9,19,48,49] This bleeding appears to be unrelated to prematurity, hypoxia, or birth trauma.

Anticonvulsant-associated coagulopathy is characterized by a deficiency of the vitamin K-dependent coagulation factors, that is numbers II, VII, IX and X.[47,49] It can usually be prevented by treating the infant at birth with 1 mg of intramuscular vitamin K.[47–50] As this vitamin is used prophylactically in many hospitals in the United States, most of the reports of neonatal bleeding have come from Europe. Because infants may occasionally bleed despite treatment with vitamin K at birth,[9] it has been recommended that epileptics be treated with vitamin K prophylactically during the final months of pregnancy.[47–49] Clotting studies should be obtained on the cord blood from all newborns exposed in utero to anticonvulsant agents; if these studies are severely abnormal, the infant should be treated with additional doses of vitamin K and with fresh frozen plasma, as some infants will die if treatment is delayed until there is clinical evidence of bleeding.[47,48]

Anticonvulsant-associated coagulopathy is usually seen only after treatment with barbiturates or primidone,[47,48] but it may occasionally be seen with phenytoin alone.[48] In fact, phenytoin has been shown to depress vitamin K-dependent clotting factors in animals in a dose-dependent fashion, and this drop can be prevented by the administration of vitamin K.[49] Other anticonvulsants besides phenytoin, phenobarbital and primidone have not been reported to cause this syndrome.

FOLATE DEFICIENCY. Folate deficiency is a frequent complication of several anticonvulsant agents, including phenytoin, phenobarbital and primidone.[50,51] Because of the increased metabolic demands of pregnancy, this problem can be especially severe in the pregnant epileptic. Between 33 and 91 percent of patients taking anticonvulsants are folate-deficient, depending on the population being studied, the definition of normal, and the particular test which is used.[52] Only a small fraction of these patients demonstrate macrocytosis, and fewer yet have megaloblastic anemia.[51–53] All of these changes respond readily to folic acid supplementation.[51]

Anticonvulsants may cause folate deficiency through several mechanisms. By inducing hepatic microsomal enzymes, these drugs increase the demand for folates, which act as cofactors in the hepatic reactions responsible for drug hydroxylation.[54] In addition, phenytoin has been shown to interfere with intestinal absorption of folates.[55,56]

The only complication of pregnancy that has been definitely linked to folate deficiency is megaloblastic anemia.[57] However, folate antagonists, such as aminopterin, are well known to be potent teratogens,[58] and folate deficiency has been shown to induce malformations in some animals.[52] Although several retrospective studies have suggested a relationship between folate deficiency and malformations in humans,[59,60] other studies have failed to confirm this.[61,62] Furthermore, a prospective study of approximately 3000 patients showed no relationship between serum folate levels during early pregnancy and fetal anomalies.[63] At the present time, the relationship between folate and congenital malformations (especially neural tube defects) remains controversial.[7,52]

Some authorities have recommended that all pregnant epileptics be given prophylactic folic acid. However, correction of folate deficiency may increase hepatic drug hydroxylation, with a resultant decrease in serum phenytoin levels.[54] This drop is usually small, and rarely results in the loss of seizure control.[52,53] Nevertheless, patients receiving supplemental folic acid should have their anticonvulsant levels monitored carefully. The monitoring of maternal serum folate levels does not seem worthwhile and low levels do not relate to the finding of anomalies.[64]

ALTERED CALCIUM METABOLISM. Another complication of chronic phenytoin therapy is abnormal calcium metabolism. Phenytoin is thought to induce the enzymes that increase the metabolism of cholecalciferol to inactive compounds.[65] Phenytoin may also interfere with intestinal absorption of calcium.[66] These changes may cause hypocalcemia, rickets, or osteomalacia. In addition, cases have been described of severe, prolonged neonatal hypocalcemia and tetany refractory to calcium therapy in infants exposed to phenytoin and phenobarbital during pregnancy.[67] This has led some investigators to suggest that pregnant epileptics be given supplemental vitamin D.[50,67]

BREASTFEEDING. Phenytoin crosses poorly into the breast milk, attaining levels that are only one-fourth to one-third of those in the maternal serum.[16] These low levels have not been shown to be harmful, despite slow elimination by the neonate.[16] Hence, breastfeeding is not contraindicated in patients taking phenytoin.

Phenobarbital

Phenobarbital levels frequently decrease during pregnancy, often necessitating increases in the daily dosage.[14] Barbiturates cross the placenta without difficulty, rapidly reaching an equilibrium between mother and fetus.[68] At birth, levels in the cord blood are approximately 95 percent of those in the maternal serum.[69] After delivery, the neonate excretes phenobarbital slowly, clearing only 1 to 20 percent every 24 hours.[69] Although phenobarbital is probably less teratogenic than phenytoin, it has some of the same adverse effects. For example, phenobarbital often contributes to folate deficiency in the mother, and coagulation defects in the neonate. In addition, phenobarbital has several adverse effects that are not seen with phenytoin, such as neonatal depression and withdrawal. Nonetheless, it remains the drug of choice for the young epileptic woman with grand mal or focal motor epilepsy.[5,32]

TERATOGENICITY. Phenobarbital appears to have much less teratogenic potential than phenytoin.[4,5,20,32] However, several retrospective studies have shown a significant association between maternal phenobarbital ingestion and congenital anomalies, even among nonepileptic patients.[70–72] There is also recent evidence that a fetal barbiturate syndrome may exist.[73] These findings have been contradicted by other studies. Shapiro et al. found no evidence of fetal damage in approximately 8000 nonepileptic patients who took phenobarbital during pregnancy.[25] Thus, the question of phenobarbital's teratogenicity remains controversial. Most authorities are convinced, however, that even if phenobarbital is teratogenic, it is probably much less so than phenytoin.

NEONATAL COAGULOPATHY. Phenobarbital and primidone, which is partially metabolized to phenobarbital, are the anticonvulsants most commonly associated with neonatal coagulopathy. The diagnosis, prevention, and therapy of this disorder are discussed in the section on phenytoin.

FOLATE DEFICIENCY. Like phenytoin, phenobarbital and primidone may cause maternal folate deficiency, and occasionally megaloblastic anemia. This problem is discussed in a previous section.

NEONATAL DEPRESSION. Maternal ingestion of barbiturates during the last few days of pregnancy may cause neonatal depression, manifested by decreased alertness, respiratory depression, and hypotonia.[74] In addition, barbiturates may cause a 48-hour lag in the neonate's ability to adapt to breastfeeding.[75]

NEONATAL WITHDRAWAL. Barbiturates are well known to posses addictive potential in adults, and recently a neonatal withdrawal syndrome has been described.[74] Between 10 and 20 percent of neonates exposed to as little as 60 mg/day of phenobarbital during the third trimester will exhibit symptoms of withdrawal.[74] These symptoms frequently commence after the infant has left the hospital, usually between the fourth and seventh days of life. The neonatal phenobarbital withdrawal syndrome is characterized by generalized neuromuscular excitability, with hyperactivity, tremulousness, hyperreflexia, excessive crying, sleep disturbances, vomiting, diarrhea, hyperphagia, and occasionally seizures. Some of these symptoms may persist for 2 to 6 months. This syndrome differs from neonatal heroin withdrawal in that the onset is much later and the infant is usually appropriately grown. Phenobarbital withdrawal is treated by minimizing stimulation of the newborn and, when necessary, sedation with phenobarbital, phenothiazines, or paregoric.

BREASTFEEDING. As noted above, barbiturates may cause a 2-day lag in the newborn's ability to nurse.[75] Barbiturates enter the breast milk, attaining levels of 10 to 30 percent of those in the maternal serum.[76] This level, combined with the slow rate of elimination of the drug by the neonate, may lead to continued depression in a small percentage of newborns.[69,77] Breastfeeding is not contraindicated in mothers taking phenobarbital unless the neonate manifests signs or symptoms of generalized depression.

Primidone

Primidone crosses the placenta to a variable degree. Nine out of 10 patients given a single 250-mg tablet during labor had detectable primidone in the cord blood.[78] Because phenobarbital is one of its major active metabolites, patients taking primidone during pregnancy can expect all of the same problems that are seen with phenobarbital, including folate deficiency, and neonatal coagulopathy, depression, and withdrawal. There is one report that suggests the possibility of a primidone embryopathy, consisting of craniofacial and cardiac malformations.[79] In addition, Shapiro et al. found an 8 percent (2 of 26) malformation rate in the fetuses of epileptics taking primidone alone.[25] Primidone crosses poorly into breast milk,[80] and nursing should be avoided only in those infants showing signs of generalized depression.

Carbamazepine

Carbamazepine is now being used more often as a primary drug for clonic seizures. Although some investigators have found that serum levels of carbamazepine decrease during pregnancy,[80,81] others have not found this to be true.[14] Carbamazepine readily crosses the placenta in humans, with drug levels in the cord blood approximating those in the maternal circulation.[80] Carbamazepine is eliminated by the neonate at approximately the same rate as adults, with a half-life of 8 to 28 hours.[82]

The teratogenicity of carbamazepine in humans has not been fully investigated, as relatively few pregnant epileptics have received this agent and of those who have, most have been taking other anticonvulsants as well. Of the 94 reported cases of infants exposed to carbamazepine, only five took this agent alone. Four of these 94 patients delivered anomalous infants.[80] Although this incidence is no greater than expected in the general population, there is not yet enough data to recommend switching pregnant patients from other potentially more harmful drugs to carbamazepine. Conversely, carbamazepine should not be discontinued when the epileptic patient becomes pregnant.

Carbamazepine crosses poorly into breast milk, with levels less than 40 percent of those in the maternal serum.[80] Because chronically exposed neonates are able to metabolize this drug as efficiently as adults, nursing is not contraindicated in epileptic patients taking this drug.

Ethosuximide

Like most other anticonvulsants, ethosuximide crosses the placenta.[83] It appears to be far less teratogenic in humans than trimethadione, the other first-line drug used for petit mal epilepsy.[84] Because petit mal is rare after adolescence, there is little data on the effects of ethosuximide on the fetus; however, one estimate puts the risk of malformations at approximately 6 percent, somewhat higher than the general population.[84]

Ethosuximide is eliminated slowly by the neonate, with a half-life of 41 hours.[83] Levels in the breast milk are only slightly lower than those in the maternal serum.[83] However, toxicity has not been observed in nursing infants, and there is therefore no contraindication to breastfeeeding in mothers who must take this drug.

Valproic Acid

Valproic acid readily crosses the placenta, with fetal and maternal serum levels being about equal or slightly higher in the fetus.[85,86] This drug produces a transient neonatal hyperglycinemia; while serum levels of glycine are not high enough to impair neuronal development, they may cause a false-positive screen for aminoacidemia.[85] Valproic acid has been shown to have a dose-related teratogenic effect in mice, rats, and rabbits.

New information provided by the Centers for Disease Control (CDC) has indicated that valproic acid prescribed during pregnancy is associated with a 1 percent risk of bearing a child with a neural tube defect.[7] This risk is similar for a woman who has had a prior child with a neural tube defect. The greater danger to the fetus occurs during the first 3 months of pregnancy.[87,88] Robert and Guibaud found that among 72 women giving birth to offspring with caudal neural tube defects, 9 were taking valproic acid.[89] The doses were usually over 1 g daily, giving an odds ratio of approximately 20 for the defect to occur among valproic acid users.[89] International studies are in progress, and the CDC has established a registry of women who have taken valproic acid during pregnancy. Dalens et al. reported a severely malformed infant who was born to a woman who took valproic acid throughout her pregnancy.[90] There is not enough evidence to warrant changing anticonvulsant therapy from valproic acid during pregnancy; instead this agent should be discontinued and changed to phenobarbital if it is necessary to maintain adequate seizure control. An ultrasonic imaging of the fetal spine and either a maternal serum or amniotic fluid α-fetoprotein determination is recommended if the drug was used in early gestation.

Valproic acid crosses poorly into the breast milk, with levels less than 2 percent of those in the maternal serum.[87] Therefore, there is no contraindication to nursing in mothers taking this drug.

Trimethadione

Trimethadione is the most potent teratogen among the anticonvulsants. The fetal trimethadione syndrome, described in Table 5–7, includes a variety of congenital defects, many of which are also seen with FHS.[7,34,36,91] When used during pregnancy, trimethadione is associated with an 83 percent incidence of major fetal malformations among live-born infants, and a high rate of spontaneous abortion. In one review of exposed patients, 87 percent of pregnancies were complicated by either fetal anomalies or first trimester loss.[34]

TABLE 5–7. FEATURES OF THE FETAL TRIMETHADIONE SYNDROME

Intrauterine growth retardation
Postnatal growth deficiency
Microcephaly
Mild to moderate mental retardation
Developmental delay
Speech difficulties
Facial dysmorphisms
- V-shaped eyebrows
- Hypertelorism
- Strabismus
- Inner epicanthal folds
- Visual impairment
- Low-set ears with anterior folded helix
- Hearing loss
- Broad, depressed nasal bridge
- High, arch palate
- Orofacial clefts
- Irregular teeth

Congenital heart defects
Tracheoesophageal anomalies
Hypospadias
Inguinal hernias
Assorted gastrointestinal and genitourinary defects

Several families have been reported in which numerous consecutive pregnancies resulted in spontaneous abortion or fetal malformations while the mother was taking the drug, followed by several consecutive normal children after the drug was discontinued.[34,35] Trimethadione is useful only for the treatment of petit mal epilepsy, a relatively benign disorder which is rarely seen after adolescence. This drug should be avoided by women during the reproductive years, since ethosuximide and clonazepam may be used more effectively.

Diazepam

Diazepam crosses the human placenta within seconds, with fetal levels of the parent drug and its active metabolites exceeding maternal levels for the first 4 to 6 hours.[91–94] The neonate metabolizes diazepam very slowly, and it frequently takes more than a week for drug elimination.[95]

Diazepam is used only for the control of status epilepticus. This disorder is so life-threatening for both the mother and the fetus that almost any adverse fetal effect is acceptable. Diazepam administered during labor may cause numerous neonatal problems, including low Apgar scores, apneic spells, hypotonia, poor suckling, reluctance to feed, impaired metabolic response to cold stress, and hypothermia. These effects are most pronounced when the mother has received more than 30 mg of the drug during the 15 hours preceding delivery.[95,96] When used during labor, diazepam depresses short-term, beat-to-beat variability of the fetal heart rate.[94] A syndrome resembling narcotic withdrawal has been observed in neonates after prolonged intrauterine exposure to diazepam,[97] but this is rarely a problem in the epileptic patient.

Diazepam crosses the placenta as early as the first trimester.[98] In rats, benzodiazepines are not teratogenic, even in high doses.[99] In a study in humans, there was no increase in the incidence of malformations when diazepam was used in cases of threatened abortion.[32] One group found that a related compound, chlordiazepoxide, was associated with a fourfold increase in congenital malformations when used in early pregnancy,[100] but this was not confirmed in a larger study.[101] However, four retrospective case control studies in three countries have shown an association between oral clefts and first trimester exposure to diazepam.[102] The risk was increased by three to four times, but the absolute risk for any fetus was quite small. Therefore diazepam should not be withheld in cases of status epilepticus during pregnancy because of fears of teratogenesis.

Diazepam crosses into the breast milk and may cause lethargy and impaired suckling.[103] Because neonates eliminate diazepam slowly, it is best avoided in nursing mothers. This is rarely a problem, as it is unlikely that a woman who has recently been treated for status epilepticus will be in any condition to breastfeed.

GUIDELINES FOR MANAGEMENT OF EPILEPSY IN PREGNANCY

1. Epileptic women should not be discouraged from becoming pregnant unless seizures are difficult to control, making the patient incapable of responsible parenthood.
2. If the mother has idiopathic epilepsy, she should be advised that the risk of her child developing epilepsy is approximately 2 to 3 percent, or five times higher than the general population.
3. If the patient is not pregnant when first seen, has been seizure-free for several years, and has a normal EEG, an attempt should be made to withdraw anticonvulsants over a period of several months prior to the patient attempting pregnancy.
4. If the patient is not pregnant, and is taking a combination of anticonvulsants, an attempt should be made to see if she can be controlled with only one agent, preferably phenobarbital. However, the patient should be maintained on as many medications as are necessary to control her seizures, because seizure control is of more concern than teratogenesis. The only exception to this rule is that trimethadione should never be used in young women during the reproductive years.
5. If the patient is first seen during pregnancy and is well controlled on her current regimen, anticonvulsant agents should not be withdrawn, as this may put the patient into status epilepticus.
6. Status epilepticus should be treated vigorously, without regard for the pregnancy.
7. Patients should be advised that the risk of fetal anomalies is increased two- to

threefold in patients taking anticonvulsants, and that there is a somewhat increased risk of mental retardation with certain agents.

8. Pregnant epileptics should be warned that excessive weight gain and sudden fluid retention may increase the risk of seizures.
9. Patients should be advised that there is a 50 percent risk that epilepsy will worsen during pregnancy, and that this risk is even higher if she has frequent seizures.
10. Anticonvulsant serum levels should be measured monthly during pregnancy and the puerperium, with adjustments in dosage to keep levels in the therapeutic range.
11. Pregnant epileptics receiving phenytoin, phenobarbital, or primidone should be given prophylactic folic acid, with careful monitoring of serum anticonvulsant levels.
12. Pregnant epileptics taking phenytoin, phenobarbital, or primidone should be given vitamin K, 5 to 10 mg/d by mouth during the last 1 or 2 months of pregnancy to prevent neonatal coagulopathy. Coagulation studies should be obtained on the cord blood, and the infants should be given 1 mg of vitamin K intramuscularly at birth.
13. During labor, anticonvulsants should be administered parenterally whenever possible to prevent intrapartum or postpartum seizures.
14. The infants of mothers receiving phenobarbital or primidone should be carefully observed for evidence of generalized depression or neonatal withdrawal symptoms.
15. There is no contraindication to breastfeeding in mothers taking anticonvulsants, as long as the infant shows no signs of generalized depression. Early weaning may be considered if the infant suckles poorly or is somnolent.

REFERENCES

1. Speidel BD, Meadow SR: Epilepsy, anticonvulsants and congenital malformations. Drugs 8:354, 1974
2. Mercier-Parot L, Tuchmann-Duplessis H: The dysmorphogenic potential of phenytoin: Experimental observations. Drugs 8:340, 1974
3. Annegers JF, Elveback, LR, Hauser WA, et al.: Do anticonvulsants have a teratogenic effect? Arch Neurol 31:364, 1974
4. Committee on Drugs, American Academy of Pediatrics: Anticonvulsants and pregnancy. Pediatrics 63:331, 1979
5. Golbus MS: Teratology for the obstetrician: Current status. Obstet Gynecol 55:269, 1980
6. Janz D: The teratogenic risk of antiepileptic drugs. Epilepsia 16:159, 1975
7. Dalessio DJ: Seizure disorders during pregnancy. N Engl J Med 312:559, 1985
8. Parker WA: Epilepsy. In Herfindal ET, Hirschmann JL (eds): Clinical Pharmacy and Therapeutics, ed 2. Baltimore, Williams & Wilkins, 1979, pp 569–580
9. Hill RM, Verniaud WM, Horning MG: Infants exposed in utero to antiepileptic drugs. Am J Dis Child 127:645, 1974
10. Knight AH, Rhind EG: Epilepsy and pregnancy: A study of 153 pregnancies in 59 patients. Epilepsia 16:99, 1975
11. Schmidt D, Canger R, Avanzini G, et al.: Changes of seizure frequency in pregnant epileptic women. J Neurol Neurosurg Psychiatry 46:751, 1983
12. Suter C, Klingman WO: Seizure states and pregnancy. Neurology 7:105, 1957
13. Niswander KR, Gordon M: The women and their pregnancies. [DHEW publication no. (NIH) 73] Washington, D.C.: Government Printing Office, 1972
14. Lander CM, Edwards VE, Eadie MJ, et al.: Plasma anticonvulsant concentrations during pregnancy. Neurology 27:128, 1977
15. Mygind KI, Dam M, Christiansen J: Phenytoin and phenobarbitone plasma clearance during pregnancy. Acta Neurol Scand 54:160, 1976
16. Mirkin BL: Diphenylhydantoin: Placental transport, fetal localization, neonatal metabolism, and possible teratogenic effects. J Pediatr 78:329, 1971
17. Janz D: On major malformations and minor anomalies in the offspring of parents with epi-

lepsy: Review of the literature. In Janz D, Bossi L, Dam M et al. (eds): Epilepsy, Pregnancy, and the Child. New York, Raven Press, 1982, p 211
18. Bjerkedal T, Egenaes J: Outcome of pregnancy in women with epilepsy: Norway 1967–1978. Description of material. In Janz D, Bossi L, Dam M, et al. (eds): Epilepsy, Pregnancy, and the Child. New York, Raven Press, 1982, p 75
19. Speidel BD, Meadow SR: Maternal epilepsy and abnormalities of the fetus and newborn. Lancet 2:839, 1972
20. Fedrick J: Epilepsy and pregnancy: A report from the Oxford record linkage study. Br Med J 2:442, 1973
21. Nakane Y, Okuma T, Takahashi R, et al.: Multi-institutional study on the teratogenicity and fetal toxicity of antiepileptic drugs: A report of a collaborative study group in Japan. Epilepsia 21:663, 1980
22. Monson RR, Rosenberg L, Hartz SC, et al.: Diphenylhydantoin and selected congenital malformations. N Engl J Med 289:1049, 1973
23. Dronamraju KR: Epilepsy and cleft lip and palate. Lancet 2:876, 1970
24. Friis ML: Epilepsy among parents of children with facial clefts. Epilepsia 20:69, 1979
25. Shapiro S, Hartz SC, Siskind V, et al.: Anticonvulsants and parental epilepsy in the development of birth defects. Lancet 1:272, 1976
26. Stumpf DA, Frost M: Seizures, anticonvulsants, and pregnancy. Am J Dis Child 132:746, 1978
27. Meadow SR: Anticonvulsant drugs and congenital abnormalities. Lancet 2:1296, 1968
28. Bird AV: Anticonvulsant drugs and congenital anomalies. Lancet 1:311, 1969
29. Livingston S, Berman W, Pauli LL: Maternal epilepsy and abnormalities of the fetus and newborn. Lancet 2:1265, 1973
30. Hill RM: Teratogenesis and antiepileptic drugs. N Engl J Med 289:1089, 1973
31. Hill RM: Anticonvulsant medication. Am J Dis Child 133:449, 1979
32. Hooper WD, Bochner F, Eadie MJ, Tyrer JF: Plasma protein binding of diphenylhydantoin: Effects of sex hormones, renal and hepatic disease. Clin Pharmacol Ther 15:276, 1974
33. Mygind KI, Dam M, Christiansen J: Phenytoin and phenobarbitone plasma clearance during pregnancy. Acta Neurol Scand 54:160, 1976
34. Feldman GL, Weaver DD, Lovrien EW: The fetal trimethadione syndrome. Am J Dis Child 131:1389, 1977
35. German J, Ehlers KH, Kowal A, et al.: Possible teratogenicity of trimethadione and paramethadione. Lancet 2:261, 1970
36. Zackai EH, Mellman WJ, Neiderer B, et al.: The fetal trimethadione syndrome. J Pediatr 87:280, 1975
37. Sodha NB: Neurologic emergencies. In Costrini NV, Thomson WM (eds): Manual of Medical Therapeutics, ed 22. Boston, Little Brown, 1977, pp 363–378
38. Cloyd JC, Gumnit RJ, McLain, W: Status epilepticus: The role of intravenous phenytoin. JAMA 244:1479, 1980
39. Easton JD: Diphenylhydantoin and epilepsy management. Ann Int Med 77:421, 1972
40. Mirkin BL: Placental transfer and neonatal elimination of diphenylhydantoin. Am J Obstet Gynecol 109:930, 1971
41. Gibson JE, Becker BA: Teratogenic effects of diphenylhydantoin in Swiss-Webster and A/J mice. Proc Soc Exp Biol Med 128:905, 1968
42. Harbison RD, Becker BA: Relation of dosage and time of administration of diphenylhydantoin to its teratogenic effect in mice. Teratology 2:305, 1969
43. Hanson JW, Myrianthopoulos NC, Sedgwick MA, et al.: Risks to the offspring of women treated with hydantoin anticonvulsants, with emphasis on the fetal hydantoin syndrome. J Pediatr 89:662, 1976
44. Hanson JW, Smith DW: The fetal hydantoin syndrome. J Pediatr 87:285, 1975
45. Shapiro S, Slone D, Hartz SC, et al.: Are hydantoins (phenytoins) human teratogens? J Pediat 90:673, 1977
46. Allen RW, Ogden B, Bentley FL, et al.: Fetal hydantoin syndrome, neuroblastoma, and hemorrhagic disease in a neonate. JAMA 244:1464, 1980
47. Mountain KR, Hirsh J, Gallus AS: Neonatal coagulation defect due to anticonvulsant drug treatment in pregnancy. Lancet 1:265, 1970
48. Bleyer WA, Skinner A: Fatal neonatal hemorrhage after maternal anticonvulsant therapy. JAMA 235:626, 1976
49. Solomon GE, Hilgartner MW, Kutt H: Coagulation defects caused by diphenylhydan-

toin. Neurology 22:1165, 1972
50. Seip M: Effects of antiepileptic drugs in pregnancy on the fetus and newborn infants. Ann Clin Res 5:205, 1973
51. Reynolds EH: Anticonvulsants, folic acid, and epilepsy. Lancet 1:1376, 1973
52. Norris JW, Pratt RF: Folic acid deficiency and epilepsy. Drugs 8:366, 1974
53. Grant RHE, Stores OPR: Folic acid in folate-deficient patients with epilepsy. Br Med J 4:644, 1970
54. Maxwell JD, Hunter J, Stewart DA, et al.: Folate deficiency after anticonvulsant drugs: An effect of hepatic enzyme induction. Br Med J 1:297, 1972
55. Gerson CD, Hepner GW, Brown N. et al.: Inhibition by diphenylhydantoin of folic acid absorption in man. Gastroenterology 63:246, 1972
56. Dahlke MB, Mertens-Roesler E: Malabsorption of folic acid due to diphenylhydantoin. Blood 30:341, 1967
57. Strauss RG, Ramsay RE, Willmore LJ, et al.: Hematologic effects of phenytoin therapy during pregnancy. Obstet Gynecol 51:682, 1978
58. Milunsky A, Graef JW, Gaynor MF: Methotrexate-induced congenital malformations. J Pediatr 72:790, 1968
59. Fraser JL, Watt HJ: Megaloblastic anemia in pregnancy and the puerperium. Am J Obstet Gynecol 89:532, 1964
60. Hibbard ED, Smithells RW: Folic acid metabolism and human embryopathy. Lancet 1:1254, 1965
61. Pritchard JA, Scott DE, Whalley PJ, et al.: Infants of mothers with megaloblastic anemia due to folate deficiency. JAMA 211:1982, 1970
62. Scott DE, Whalley PJ, Pritchard JA: Maternal folate deficiency and pregnancy wastage. Obstet Gynecol 36:26, 1970
63. Hall MH: Folic acid deficiency and congenital malformation. J Obstet Gynaecol Br Commonw 79:159, 1972
64. Hiilesmaa V, Teramo K, Granstrom J-L, et al.: Serum folate concentrations during pregnancy in women with epilepsy: Relation to antiepileptic drug concentrations, number of seizures, and fetal outcome. Br Med J 287:577, 1983
65. Stamp TCB, Round JM, Rowe DJF, et al.: Plasma levels and therapeutic effect of 25-hydroxycholecalciferol in epileptic patients taking anticonvulsant drugs. Br Med J 4:9, 1972
66. Goldberg MA: Anticonvulsant drugs. In Bevan JA (ed): Essentials of Pharmacology, ed 2. Hagerstown, Harper & Row, 1976, pp 239–247
67. Friis B, Sardemann H: Neonatal hypocalcaemia after intrauterine exposure to anticonvulsant drugs. Arch Dis Child 52:239, 1977
68. Flowers CE: The placental transmission of barbiturates and thiobarbiturates and their pharmacological action on the mother and the infant. Am J Obstet Gynecol 78:730, 1959
69. Melchior JC, Svensmark O, Trolle D: Placental transfer of phenobarbitone in epileptic women, and elimination in newborns. Lancet 2:860, 1967
70. Crombie DL, Pinsent RJFH, Slater BC, et al.: Teratogenic drugs—R.C.G.P. survey. Br Med J 4:178, 1970
71. Greenberg G, Inman WHW, Weatherall JAC, et al.: Maternal drug histories and congenital abnormalities. Br Med J 2:853, 1977
72. Nelson AM, Forfar JO: Associations between drugs administered during pregnancy and congenital abnormalities of the fetus. Br Med J 1:523, 1971
73. Smith DW: Teratogenicity of anticonvulsive medications. Am J Dis Child 131:1337, 1977
74. Desmond MM, Schwanecke RP, Wilson GS, et al.: Maternal barbiturate utilization and neonatal withdrawal symptomatology. J Pediatr 80:190, 1972
75. Brazelton TB: Psychophysiologic reactions in the neonate. J Pediatr 58:513, 1961
76. Donaldson JO: Neurology of Pregnancy. Philadelphia, Saunders, 1978, pp 190–210
77. Tyson RM, Shrader EA, Perlman HH: Drugs transmitted through breast milk. J Pediatr 13:86, 1938
78. Martinez G, Snyder R: Transplacental passage of primidone. Neurology 23:381, 1973
79. Rudd NL, Freedom RM: A possible primidone embryopathy. J Pediatr 94:835, 1979
80. Niebyl JR, Blake DA, Freeman JM, et al.: Carbamazepine levels in pregnancy and lactation. Obstet Gynecol 53:139, 1979
81. Montouris GD, Fenichel GM, McLain WL: The pregnant epileptic: A review and recommendations. Arch Neurol 36:601, 1979
82. Rane A, Bertilsson L, Palmer L: Disposition

of placentally transferred carbamazepine in the newborn. Eur J Clin Pharmacol 8:283, 1975

83. Koup JR, Rose JQ, Cohen ME: Ethosuximide pharmacokinetics in a pregnant patient and her newborn. Epilepsia 19:535, 1978
84. Fabro S, Brown NA: Teratogenic potential of anticonvulsants. N Engl J Med 300:1280, 1979
85. Simila S, von Wendt L, Hartikainen-Sorri A-L: Sodium valproate, pregnancy, and neonatal hyperglycinemia. Arch Dis Child 54:985, 1979
86. Dickinson RG, Harland RC, Lynn RK, et al.: Transmission of valproic acid (Depakene) across the placenta: Half-life of the drug in mother and baby. J Pediatr 94:832, 1979
87. Hiilesmaa VK, Bardy AH, Granstrom M-L, et al.: Valproic acid during pregnancy. Lancet 1:883, 1980
88. Gomez, MR: Possible teratogenicity of valproic acid. J Pediatr 98:508, 1981
89. Robert E, Guiband P: Maternal valproic acid and congenital neural tube defects. Lancet 2:937, 1982
90. Dalens B, Raynaud EJ, Gaulme J: Teratogenicity of valproic acid. J Pediatr 97:332, 1980
91. Zackai EH, Mellman WJ, Neiderer B, Hanson JW: The fetal trimethadione syndrome. J Pediatr 87:280, 1975
92. Idanpaan-Heikkila JE, Jouppila PI, Puolakka JO, et al.: Placental transfer and fetal metabolism of diazepam in early human pregnancy. Am J Obstet Gynecol 109:1011, 1971
93. McAllister CB: Placental transfer and neonatal effects of diazepam when administered to women just before delivery. Br J Anaesth 52:423, 1980
94. Scher J, Hailey DM, Beard RW: The effects of diazepam on the fetus. J Obstet Gynecol Br Commonw 79:635, 1972
95. Cree JE, Meyer J, Hailey DM: Diazepam in labour: Its metabolism and effect on the clinical condition and thermogenesis of the newborn. Br Med J 4:251, 1973
96. Gillberg C: "Floppy infant syndrome" and maternal diazepam. Lancet 2:244, 1977
97. Rementeria JL, Bhatt K: Withdrawal symptoms in neonates from intrauterine exposure to diazepam. J Pediatr 90:123, 1977
98. Erkkola R, Kanto J, Sellman R: Diazepam in early human pregnancy. Acta Obstet Gynecol Scand 53:135, 1974
99. Beall JR: Study of the teratogenic potential of diazepam and SCH 12041. CMA Journal 106:1061, 1972
100. Milkovich L, Van den Berg BJ: Effects of prenatal meprobamate and chlordiazepoxide hydrochloride on human embryonic and fetal development. N Engl J Med 291:1268, 1974
101. Hartz SC, Heinonen OP, Shapiro S, et al.: Antenatal exposure to meprobamate and chlordiazepoxide in relation to malformations, mental development, and childhood mortality. N Engl J Med 292:726, 1975
102. Safra MJ, Oakley, GP: Valium: An oral cleft teratogen? Cleft Palate J 13:198, 1976
103. Patrick MJ, Tilstone WJ, Reavey P: Diazepam and breast-feeding. Lancet 1:542, 1972

6

Acute and Chronic Hypertension During Pregnancy

Frederick P. Zuspan and Kathryn J. Zuspan

Hypertension in pregnancy is best understood if divided into four different types of pregnancy-related elevations of blood pressure. Such a classification follows: (1) acute hypertension in pregnancy, preeclampsia–eclampsia, and pregnancy-induced hypertension (PIH); (2) chronic hypertension during pregnancy; (3) chronic hypertension during pregnancy with superimposed acute hypertension (preeclampsia); and (4) transient hypertension in pregnancy which occurs during labor or immediately postpartum, then subsides.

The first two categories, acute and chronic hypertension, are well described and treated with specific drugs and regimens. Chronic hypertension with a superimposed acute component is managed using the drug regimens for chronic hypertension along with those drugs used to control the acute hypertensive (preeclampsia) episode. Finally, transient hypertension in the absence of signs of preeclampsia is treated with intravenous hydralazine as needed, just as in regimens which follow. Most likely, transient hypertension is a form of preeclampsia.

Acute Hypertension of Pregnancy

Acute hypertension during pregnancy is a condition that is synonymous with the terms toxemia of pregnancy, preeclampsia–eclampsia, and pregnancy-induced hypertension. Conditions often associated with this form of hypertension are listed in Figure 6–1. Patients who have these conditions deserve special attention as they are potentially high risk for hypertension.

The description of the patient with mild preeclampsia is an individual who, after the 20th week of gestation, develops, in sequential fashion: overt edema of the face or hands; hypertension, that is, blood pressure greater than 140/90, or an incremental increase in the diastolic of greater than 15, or in the systolic greater than 30; and the development of proteinuria noted in clean-catch specimen. Usually there are no other clinical signs. It is important to understand that in more than 90 percent of patients, this will be a sequential development of edema, hypertension, and proteinuria. If other signs or symptoms are seen in a different sequence then a sus-

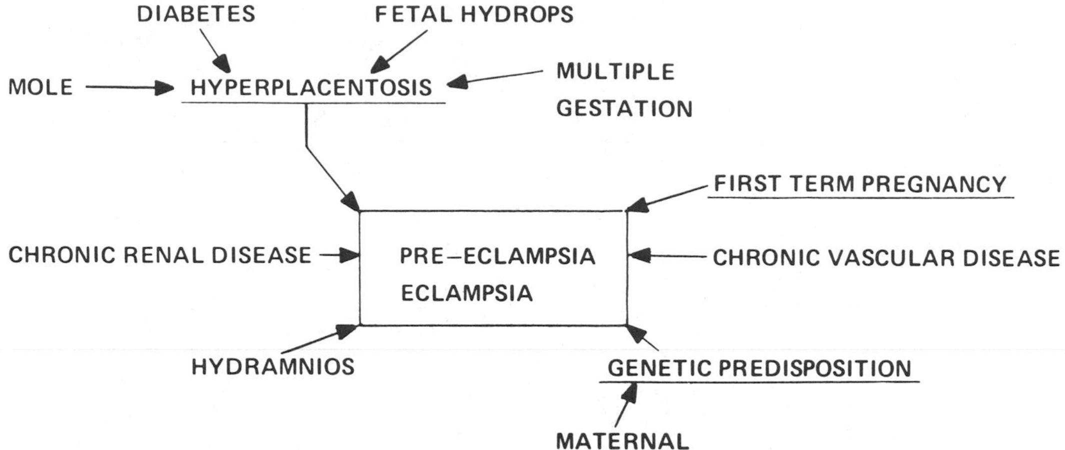

Figure 6–1. The cause of preeclampsia–eclampsia is multifaceted. Many different maternal and fetal conditions can act as catalytic agents in its development. When these conditions are present, meticulous prenatal care and diagnosis are essential for prevention and early diagnosis.

picion should be entered that perhaps other conditions also exist. The patient with preeclampsia is usually a primigravida, less than 25 years old, with proteinuric hypertension that subsides after delivery. The mild forms of preeclampsia are treatable but not preventable. With proper identification and management of the mild forms, their complications may be preventable and should not occur. These severe forms, i.e., eclampsia, have a maternal mortality of more than 10 percent in developing countries and less than 1 percent in the United States. The perinatal mortality should be less than 10 percent in developed countries if the protocol outlined in this chapter is used.

The common denominator of therapy is a pharmacologic amount of magnesium sulfate and the relative absence of other medications, except for antihypertensive medications to prevent stroke.

The key to treatment is prevention or early diagnosis. Patients who are prone to develop preeclampsia must be identified early and seen at weekly intervals. The development of preeclampsia consists of mild preeclampsia progressing on to severe preeclampsia and then to eclampsia. The rapidity in which one stage passes to another is variable and dependent upon many factors, including the individual variations of patients. It would be most unusual for a patient to present first with eclampsia without progressing through the milder forms of the disease.

Once the diagnosis of mild preeclampsia is made, the patient should be hospitalized on complete bedrest (lying on her side) with a nutritious diet. The only medication given is a sedative, such as phenobarbital 30 mg three times daily to improve comfort during bedrest. Diuresis may be expected in 48 hours, with associated weight loss and symptoms abating in 3 to 5 days. If the patient is at or near term, oxytocin induction of labor should be considered.

The diagnosis of the severe form of preeclampsia is based on one or more of the following criteria:

1. Systolic pressure of 160 or diastolic pressure of 100 taken two times, recorded 6 hours apart, with the patient at bed rest.
2. Proteinuria of greater than 5 g in 24 hours or a 3 to 4+ protein on dipstick.

3. Oliguria, defined as urinary output of less than 400 ml in 24 hours.
4. Cerebral or visual disturbances, including eye-ground changes.
5. Pulmonary edema or cyanosis.

The patient with severe preeclampsia is seriously ill and must be hospitalized on bedrest, with frequent blood pressure recordings and evaluation of deep tendon reflexes. The major therapy is administration of magnesium sulfate either intravenously (IV) or intramuscularly. The IV route is both more appropriate for the disturbed pathophysiology and less painful. Magnesium sulfate is given via a controlled administration system such as an infusion pump, with 4 to 6 g magnesium sulfate being given slowly IV over 5 to 10 minutes as a loading dose, then 1 to 2 g thereafter. The patient is monitored by examination of (1) deep tendon reflexes which should be hypoactive but present, (2) urine output which should be greater than 25 ml/hour, and (3) respirations that are in excess of 10 per minute. Loss of reflexes, decrease in urine output, and depressed respirations are signs of magnesium overdose. Magnesium toxicity is managed by decreasing the rate of magnesium infusion or, in severe toxicity, by IV administration of 1 g of IV calcium chloride. It is usually not necessary to obtain plasma magnesium levels as long as clinical evidence is satisfactory.

If the diastolic blood pressure is consistently greater than 100 mm Hg, hydralazine is given to prevent a cerebrovascular accident. A 5-mg IV bolus is infused and followed by administration using an infusion pump, with the hydralazine placed in an IV solution of 100 mg hydralazine in 200 ml saline. The diastolic blood pressure should be maintained between 80 and 90 mm Hg.

Most patients with severe preeclampsia should be delivered. Labor is easily induced with small doses of oxytocin given by infusion pump (Chap. 13). Electronic fetal heart rate surveillance is essential during this process. Table 6–1 provides a listing of the relative risk of fetal mortality with an increase of maternal blood pressure.

TABLE 6–1. RELATIVE RISK OF FETAL MORTALITY WITH INCREASED MATERNAL BLOOD PRESSURE

Diastolic Pressure Maximum (mm Hg)	Proteinuria	Relative Fetal Risk*
94	≥1+	20×
94	None	4×
85	≥2+	10×
85	≥1+	7×
75–84	≥1+	4×

* Compared with a diastolic pressure maximum of 75 to 84 mm Hg with no proteinuria.

The drug of choice to control an eclamptic convulsion is IV magnesium sulfate (4 to 6 g slowly over at least 5 minutes). Following a generalized clonic convulsion, the patient may be obtunded, and the possibility always exists of aspiration during the seizure. An aggressive action-oriented program that is the same as the one outlined for severe preeclampsia should be instituted. This does not infer emergency cesarean section. With the eclamptic seizure there is an associated maternal apnea that resolves as the seizure abates. The fetus responds with bradycardia that resolves as oxygen flow returns to the fetus. The temptation to perform an emergency cesarean section for "fetal distress" is a poor one. This places the mother in maximum anesthetic jeopardy for several reasons. As noted, aspiration may have occurred. Secondly the patient is obtunded and general anesthesia may further complicate evaluation of her neurologic status. Most importantly, these patients are at a significant risk for cerebral hemorrhage and cerebral edema. The usual general anesthetic techniques for emergency cesarean may increase the intracerebral pressure and thus increase the brain damage. Once the patient is under good control (a process requiring no more than 4 hours), a decision must be made concerning delivery. Delivery cures the problem of preeclampsia–eclampsia. Convulsions are controlled with 4 to 6 g of magnesium sulfate IV, and not with other drugs. Diuretics are not used, and antihypertensive therapy should be instituted to prevent stroke, as described previously using hydralazine (Figs. 6–2 and 6–3).

Chronic Hypertension of Pregnancy

Chronic hypertension during pregnancy is defined as hypertension usually antedating pregnancy or seen prior to the 20th week of gestation. Pregnancy tends to provoke the unmasking of chronic hypertension, which is seen more commonly in the multigravida. Fetal wastage in patients with mild hypertension may be as high as 16 percent, whereas in those with severe hypertension (blood pressure greater than 160/100), fetal wastage is as high as 40 percent.

Chronic hypertension is subdivided into primary and secondary. Primary hypertension is that which is not related to any specific disease and comprises 95 percent of chronic hypertensive patients. Secondary hypertension is hypertension related to a known disease process. A specific diagnosis is mandatory, because some forms are treatable, such as some neurohumoral disorders, endocrine factors, renal pressor mechanisms, and cardiovascular factors.

Initial management involves electrocardiogram (ECG), chest x-ray, and laboratory studies. The patient is maintained on the antihypertensive medications used prior to pregnancy, but those on diuretics should be discontinued after 20 weeks' gestation. It is important that the patient be taught self-blood pressure determinations with a two-headed stethoscope. The morning blood pressure and again the noon blood pressure are important at least three times a week. It is known that the office blood pressure agrees with the home blood pressure but one-third of the time. The home blood pressure is considered more accurate in deciding antihypertension medications.[1,2] The blood pressure should always be taken with patient lying on her side.

A second trimester decline in blood pressure is not observed if the blood pressure is taken on the side. If the blood pressure increases it should be considered significant. When the blood pressure no longer responds to 2 hours a day of bedrest, antihypertensive medications are used (Table 6–2). Methyldopa (Aldomet) is the preferred initial drug with doses started at 250 mg four times daily and increased to 500 mg four times daily, if necessary. Diuretics are not used. If the patient's blood pressure shows minimal or no response to this therapy, the amount of bedrest is further increased. Once maximum therapy with methyldopa is achieved (2 to 3 g/day), a second antihypertensive drug is chosen. Either a direct acting drug, such as hydralazine (20 mg qid), or a β-blocker is used, such as propranolol (20 mg qid), atenolol (25 mg qd), or labetalol (100 mg bid). If an acute hypertensive episode intervenes, treatment is with IV hydralazine. A bolus injection of 5 mg IV gives an indication of response. The 100 mg of hydralazine are then

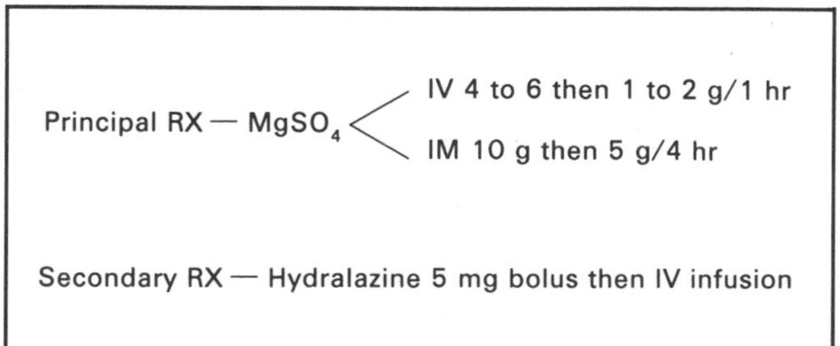

Principal RX — $MgSO_4$ < IV 4 to 6 then 1 to 2 g/1 hr; IM 10 g then 5 g/4 hr

Secondary RX — Hydralazine 5 mg bolus then IV infusion

Figure 6–2. The major therapy for preeclampsia–eclampsia in the United States is the use of parenteral magnesium sulfate. An antihypertensive (hydralazine) is used to prevent a stroke in the mother. (*Note*: The IV route is preferred to avoid pain and assure accurate drug delivery.)

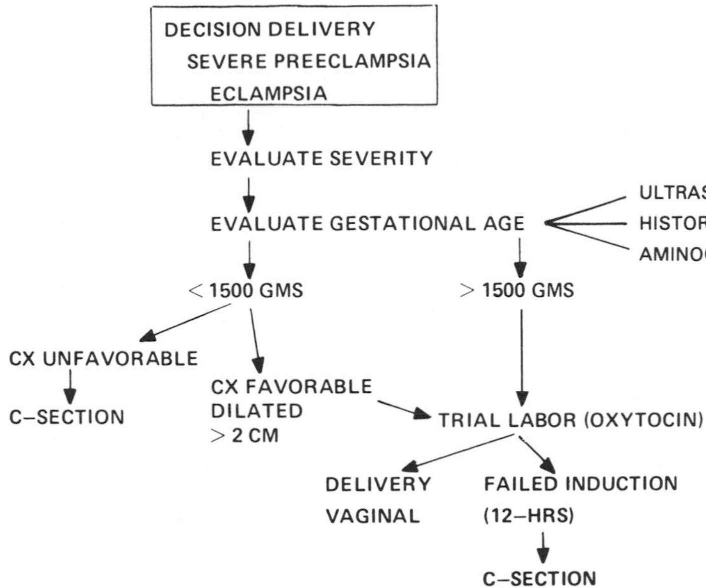

Figure 6–3. The decision for delivery is outlined in this flowchart. It must be stressed that the decision should be made early in the affected patient. Delivery mode depends upon the condition of the cervix, fetal size, and gestational age.

added to an IV bag of 200 ml saline and infused via infusion pump at a rate adequate to control the diastolic blood pressure between 80 and 90 mm Hg. If preeclampsia superimposes on the chronic hypertension, the preeclampsia is treated with IV magnesium sulfate (4 to 6 g loading dose and then 1 to 2 g/hr maintenance dose).[1]

In cases of severe preeclampsia, the option of pregnancy termination should be con-

TABLE 6–2. ANTIHYPERTENSIVE DRUGS USED IN CHRONIC HYPERTENSION

Drug	Action	Standard Oral Dose
Methyldopa (Aldomet)	Inhibition of vasoconstricting impulses from vasoregulating center in medulla oblongata Inhibition of impulses from hypothalamus	500 mg tid
Propranalol (Inderal)	β-Adrenergic blockade Usually associated with decreased cardiac output	100 mg tid
Hydralazine (Apresoline)	Direct relaxation of arterioles Action on vascular smooth muscle	20–40 mg qd
Atenolol (Tenormin)	Cardioselective (β-adrenoreceptors) in low doses (less selective in high doses)	25 mg qd
Labetalol (Trandate, Normodyne)	Nonselective β-blocker with α-adrenergic blocking properties	100 mg bid
Captopril (Capoten)	Angiotensin-converting enzyme inhibitor Not to be used in pregnancy but may be used postpartum	100 mg qd

sidered. Evaluation of fetal pulmonary maturity is carried out by amniocentesis. If less than 34 weeks' gestation and pulmonary immaturity, 12 mg of betamethasone is given for two doses 12 hours apart if the pregnancy termination can wait 36 hours. We have found no increase in blood pressure using corticosteriods.[3] Delivery is then induced, using oxytocin or, in cases of an unfavorable cervix and small baby (<1250 g), abdominal delivery is indicated.

ANESTHESIA CONSIDERATIONS

Anesthesia for women with acute and chronic hypertension during pregnancy has gained much attention recently. Spinal and epidural conduction anesthesia was once contraindicated because of severe hypotension that commonly accompanied their use. Now, with appropriate evaluation, monitoring, hydration, and use of epidurals, conduction anesthesia is often the technique of choice.[4,5] Spinal anesthesia is contraindicated. Laboratory data should include serum electrolytes, hematocrit, prothrombin time, partial thromboplastin time, and platelet count. Severe acute hypertensive patients also need a bleeding time, because platelet dysfunction may exist despite a normal platelet count.[6]

Invasive cardiovascular monitoring is usually unnecessary for mild hypertensives when urine output is adequate. Women with severe hypertension may need a central venous pressure (CVP) catheter placed to assess and correct fluid status. In the event of pulmonary disease or pulmonary edema, a Swan-Ganz catheter would more accurately reflect pulmonary circulation and left-sided cardiac function than the CVP. An arterial line is useful in women with uncontrolled hypertension or on continuous infusion of antihypertensive medications.[7] It is imperative that a clotting defect is not present if this is to be used.

Despite their edematous appearance, many acutely hypertensive pregnant persons have contracted intravascular volumes and their CVP or pulmonary capillary wedge pressure (PCWP) measurements are usually below normal.[8] This should be corrected to a normal CVP of 6 to 8 cm H_2O or PCWP of 10 to 15 torr before induction of any form of anesthesia. This is best achieved with the infusion of albumin alone or in combination with a crystalloid.[9]

Epidural anesthesia offers many advantages to the hypertensive pregnant patient. Unlike spinals, the onset of analgesia is slower, so precipitous falls in blood pressures are avoided more easily. Epidural anesthesia can be used throughout labor and during a vaginal delivery or cesarean section. Because of the pain relief provided, the calmer patient is more likely to release fewer endogenous catecholamines. The average blood pressures and the risk of a seizure are thought to decrease with epidural anesthesia, while urine output and uteroplacental blood flow improve.

Patients with a corrected fluid status and a normal coagulation profile qualify for epidural anesthesia, which should be given early in labor and maintained through delivery. Any evidence for a coagulopathy increases the risk of an epidural hematoma and potential for paralysis. Use of epinephrine in the epidural should be avoided due to the patient's increased sensitivity to catecholamines.[10] Intravenous ephedrine is the drug of choice for hypotension refractory to further fluid administration or Trendelenberg positioning. Patellar reflexes may be dulled by the epidural, but arm reflexes remain intact and can be used to check effects from magnesium sulfate.

Hypertensive persons requiring cesarean section need preoperative prophylaxis with sodium citrate or ranitidine for aspiration pneumonitis. Magnesium sulfate must be continued intraoperatively, and left lateral uterine displacement is essential to avoid vena caval compression. Anesthetic options are epidural or general anesthesia. Epidural anesthesia is preferred for patients with a controlled blood pressure, corrected fluid status, and normal coagulation profile. Supplemental oxygen by mask should be used until delivery of the neonate. General anesthesia is the better choice for patients with either an uncontrolled blood pressure, hypovolemia, abnormal coagulation profile, or obtundation. The endotracheal tube helps protect the patient's airway (which may be more edematous), and anesthetic agents may be used to better control blood pressure fluctuations. Rehydration to attain a normal fluid status is still necessary using urine output, CVP, or PCWP measurement as a guide.

Perioperative magnesium sulfate obviates the need for precurarization and potentiates muscle relaxants especially the nondepolarizing type such as pancuronium. Succinylcholine, a depolarizing relaxant, is potentiated less, and its use may reduce the need for possible postoperataive mechanical ventilation. Intubation and extubation are periods of precipitous increases in blood pressure. If needed, this can be managed with continuous infusion of nitroglycerine or nitropruside.

POSTPARTUM HYPERTENSION

Once delivery has been achieved, it is important to protect the mother from sequelae of hypertension such as coma, heart failure, and intracerebral hemorrhage. The best way to treat the hypertension is with suspected anticipation by assuming that there will be an increased liberation of more epinephrine in the immediate postpartum period. Recommendations for drug therapy during a hypertensive crisis are outlined in Table 6–3. If a patient is receiving hydralazine prior to delivery, the controlled infusion source should be brought to the delivery room and continued. If hydralazine is insufficient in controlling the hypertension, sodium nitroprusside, which acts in 1 to 3 minutes, should be considered. An IV bolus of 300 mg of diazoxide may be used if sodium nitroprusside is unavailable but concern for hypotension and uterine tocolysis may occur.

The use of methyldopa, atenolol, and labetalol are not as rapid acting as the drugs already mentioned but can be instituted for long-term care and taken upon discharge from the hospital. We try to avoid oral antihypertensive medication until approximately 3 days after delivery to see what happens to the blood pressure. The pregnancy-induced vasoconstrictive changes should have subsided, and the dynamics which affect blood pressure changes may be better appreciated. Restarting the patient on the same medication and dose as before pregnancy seems appropriate before the end of the first postpartum week if blood pressure remains elevated with diastolic values above 100 mm Hg. Education on self-blood pressure monitoring is important.

TABLE 6–3. DRUG TREATMENT DURING A HYPERTENSIVE CRISIS

1. Hydralazine (Apresoline)
   - 5 mg push and evaluate
   - If no effect in 20 minutes give IV infusion of 100 mg hydralazine in 200 ml saline
   - Drug of choice if fetus present
2. Diazoxide (Hyperstat)
   - 20 ml ampule with 300 mg
   - 300 mg IV push (binds to plasma proteins)
   - Not drug of choice with fetus present as hypotension unpredictable
   - Excellent drug for postpartum hypertension
3. Sodium nitroprusside*
   - 50 mg of sodium nitroprusside into 250 ml D5W and use as a constant infusion
4. Nitroglycerin*
   - 50 mg into 250 ml 250 D5W infusion

* Needs arterial monitoring due to rapid onset and profound hypotension.

Summary

In summary, the drugs used in the treatment regimen described for acute hypertension include magnesium sulfate to prevent or control convulsions, hydralazine as an antihypertensive agent, phenobarbital for sedation, calcium chloride as an antidote for magnesium toxicity, and oxytocin for induction of labor. The drugs used in chronic hypertension therapy as outlined include α-methyldopa as an antihypertensive, with propranolol; atenolol, labetalol, and intravenous hydralazine added if needed; a diuretic such as hydrochlorthiazide or diazide is usually not used periodically; phenobarbital for sedation; hydrocortisone or betamethasone[3] to mature fetal lungs; and oxytocin for induction.

The challenge for the obstetrician in chronic hypertension is to choose the appropriate drug with maximum safety for the fetus and therapeutic response in the mother. Over the past several years many drugs have been used, but until recently randomized clinical trials had not been undertaken. The objectives of therapy include delivery of a viable baby with no morbidity, and prevention of maternal cardiac decompensation, stroke, and morbidity.

A number of drugs are employed in different treatment regimens. Lindheimer and Katz have recently reviewed current therapy for hypertension in pregnancy.[11] Blood pressure control is sought using sympatholytics such as α-methyldopa; β-adrenergic agents such as propranolol, atenolol, and labetalol; vasodilators such as prazosin, hydralazine, minoxidil, diazoxide, and sodium nitroprusside; and diuretics such as thiazide, furosemide, ethacrynic acid, chlorthalidone, and spironolactone. Each of these agents is discussed in this chapter and is listed in Table 6–4.

DIURETICS

The use of diuretics, particularly the thiazides, in the treatment of hypertension is well established in the nonpregnant patient.[11] Although recommended as the primary drug in the stepped-care approach to the treatment of hypertension they are not indicated during pregnancy.[12–18] Diuretics do not alter the incidence of preeclampsia and eclampsia, and do not influence perinatal mortality or birth weight.[15,18] The use of diuretics may induce maternal hypovolemia and a decrease in placental and uterine perfusion.[19–22] Studies utilizing diuretics in chronic hypertensive patients have shown a decrease in blood volume and an increase in fetal loss when compared to control patients.

Maternal side effects include those seen in nonpregnant patients; hypokalemia, hypovolemia, pancreatitis, decreased carbohydrate tolerance, and hyperuricemia.[23] In addition, there have been case reports of hypokalemia and metabolic alkalosis,[24] hemorrhagic pancreatitis,[25] and maternal death[26] when thiazide diuretics are administered to the pregnant patient.

Reported fetal side effects include hyponatremia,[12,27] thrombocytopenia,[28,29] jaundice,[17] and the possibility of hypertension at maturity.[30] Chlorthiazide appears to freely cross the placenta, with essentially equal maternal and neonatal levels being found at birth.[31] Fetal heart rate abnormalities have been reported in a pregnant patient with hypokalemia secondary to diuretics.[32] Lethargy and poor Apgar scores secondary to hyponatremia were found in two infants whose mothers received thiazide diuretics antepartum.[27] However, the rarity of these complications in practice is pointed out by several large studies which reported no adverse fetal or neonatal effects.[18,33,34]

It has been suggested by several authors[12,35,36] that the use of furosemide should be limited to patients with pulmonary edema or heart failure. Furosemide has been reported to freely cross the placenta, leading to equal maternal and fetal blood levels.[37] Ethacrynic acid is similar in mechanism of action and clinical effects to furosemide. The use of ethacrynic acid during pregnancy should be avoided because of the potential for ototoxicity and nephrotoxicity.[13,35]

The use of chlorthalidone[38,39] and spironolactone[14] in pregnant patients has been reported, but their routine use cannot be recommended because of a paucity of data.

SYMPATHOLYTICS

Reserpine exerts its hypotensive effect via depletion of catecholamines from peripheral nerve endings. Adverse effects reported in adults include depression, nasal congestion, and galactorrhea. Fetal and neonatal adverse effects reported are: bradycardia, lethargy, alteration of thermal equilibrium, congenital anomalies, and mucous membrane engorgement.[40-42] Because of these problems, the use of reserpine during pregnancy should be avoided. Reserpine is seldom used in current times, except in developing countries.

α-Methyldopa is currently the most widely used hypotensive agent in pregnancy. Side effects in nonpregnant adults include drowsiness, fatigue, and rarely Coomb's positive hemolytic anemia and hepatic disorders. Methlydopa is the most extensively studied hypotensive drug used in pregnancy. Fetal and neonatal adverse effects have not been reported up to the present time.[43-48] Leather et al.[46] and Redmon et al.[44,45] showed increases in fetal survival rates, decreases in maternal blood pressure, and an increase in the length of gestation of approximately 2 weeks when compared with an untreated control group. The major difference that made these studies statistically significant was the decrease in midtrimester fetal loss. Doses of methyldopa in both trials ranged from 0.5 to 2 g daily, and allowed the addition of hydralazine or a diuretic if indicated by less than optimal response. Other authors have noted similar results,[43,47,49] but the work of Leather and Redmon were the first randomized trials published in the literature. There are now more randomized trials published.

The transfer of methyldopa across the "placental barrier" has been noted.[47,49] Samples of amniotic fluid contained higher total levels of drug, but with a greater percentage of conjugated drug than in the maternal or fetal circulation. Free or unconjugated drug appears to cross the placenta where it is conjugated and excreted by the fetus. The specific effect of methyldopa on fetal amines has yet to be studied.[50]

To summarize, methyldopa's effectiveness and apparent safety make it an agent of choice for the treatment of chronic hypertension in pregnancy in the United States.

β-ADRENERGIC BLOCKING AGENTS

β-Adrenergic blocking agents form a large part of antihypertensive therapy today. They have been found to be useful alone[51] or in combination with a diuretic[52] in the treatment of hypertension in the nonpregnant patient. Potential maternal adverse effects are the same as those found in nonpregnant patients: interference with diabetic control, bradycardia, drowsiness, aggravation or precipitation of heart failure, or bronchoconstrictive disease.[53] Propranolol constitutes the greatest portion of β-adrenergic blocking agents used in the United States. Propranolol appears to cross the placenta freely, leading to essentially equal maternal and fetal concentrations.[54] Reported fetal complications include neonatal hypoglycemia, intrauterine growth retardation, and neonatal respiratory depression and bradycardia.[54-66] Caution must be used in interpreting the incidence of these side effects, as all of these reports are anecdotal. No teratogenic effects have been reported for propranolol, and there is a paucity of data for other newer agents. Some side effects of β-blockers may be dose-related,[58] and can possibly be prevented by using lower doses or by discontinuing the drug 1 to 2 weeks prior to the expected delivery date. The inability to accurately predict the date of delivery and the increase in maternal pressure, which follows drug discontinuation, probably preclude the use of propranolol during pregnancy. In the only random double-blind study of the effects of propranolol on the fetus, a 5- to 6-minute delay occurred in the onset of spontaneous respiration, possibly requiring intubation in babies born to mothers receiving 1 mg of propranolol IV prior to cesarean section.[65]

Propranolol is not routinely indicated for antihypertensive use during pregnancy, because there are insufficient clinical data to evaluate their role in the management of maternal hypertension.[66] The effects on the fetus and neonate have been discussed in Chapter 2. We have followed many pregnant

TABLE 6–4. ADVERSE EFFECTS ON THE MOTHER AND FETUS OF DRUGS USED TO TREAT HYPERTENSION DURING PREGNANCY

Drug	Placental Transfer	Maternal Adverse Effects	Fetal Adverse Effects	References
Diuretics				
Thiazides	Yes, chlorothiazide–fetal levels equal to maternal[30]	Hypokalemia, hyperglycemia, hyperuremia, hypercalcemia, skin rashes, pancreatitis, hypovolemia	Hyponatremia, thrombocytopenia, jaundice, increased risk of hypertension at maturity	101–108
Furosemide	Unknown	Hypokalemia, hyperuricemia, hyperglycemia, gastrointestinal upset, hypovolemia	None reported	101, 109
Ethacrynic acid	Unknown	Same effects as furosemide plus hearing loss	Deafness	110, 111
Spironolactone	Unknown	Hyperkalemia, gynecomastia, amenorrhea	Unknown	
Triamterene	Unknown	Leg cramps, dizziness, hyperkalemia	No available data	
Chlorthalidone	Unknown	Same effects as furosemide	Unknown	112, 113
Sympatholytics				
Reserpine	Yes—not quantified	Depression, sedation, bizarre dreams, nasal congestion, galactorrhea, increased gastric acid secretion, abdominal cramps, diarrhea, breast cancer (?)	Bradycardia, lethargy, nasal congestion, altered thermoequilibrium, stillbirth and congenital anomalies, anorexia, death	
α-Methyldopa	Unknown	Sedation, decreased mental acuity, fatigue, sodium retention, hepatitis, drug fever, positive Coombs test, hemolytic anemia, galactorrhea, postural hypotension	None reported	114–120

β-Adrenergic Agents				
Propranolol	Yes—fetal levels similar to maternal	Sodium retention, aggravation of heart failure, bradycardia, depression, aggravation of bronchoconstrictive disease, vivid dreams, interference of diabetic control, CNS disturbances	Intrauterine growth retardation, hypoglycemia, respiratory depression, bradycardia	101, 121–123
Metoprolol, Atenolol, Timolol Labetalol	Unknown	Similar to propranolol	No available data	
Vasodilator				
Clonidine	Unknown	Sedation, dry mouth, sodium retention, orthostatic hypotension, constipation, CNS disturbances, rebound hypertension when stopped	Embryotoxic in animals; none reported in humans	114, 120
Guanethidine	Unknown	Postural hypotension, diarrhea, depression, sodium retention, aggravation of heart failure	No available data	101
Hydralazine	Unknown	Tachycardia, palpitations, flushing, headache, sodium retention, aggravation of angina, Lupus syndrome, neuropathy, dizziness	None reported in long-term use; fetal heart rate changes when given acutely at term	101, 124, 125
Prazosin	Unknown	Sodium retention, sudden hypotension, palpitations, tachycardia	No available data	126
Minoxidil	Unknown	Tachycardia, hypotension, palpitations, hypertrichosis	No available data	
Magnesium Sulfate	Yes—fetal levels similar to maternal	Overdose—decreased respirations, absent reflexes Increased urine calcium loss, increased parathyroid hormone secretion	Excess level excreted in 4 to 24 hr; rare bladder atony and myotonia	
Calcium Gluconate (Magnesium overdose)	Yes	Give to mother when magnesium overdose suspected by no reflexes, decreased respiration, or cardiac arrest	No fetal effects	

patients with cardiac disease (notably mitral valve prolapse) and symptomatic hyperthyroidism who were on propranolol, and all delivered without event to either mother or baby. The lowest necessary dose of propranolol should be taken for the shortest time.

Other β-blocker drugs have been used with satisfactory results. The agents used have been oxprenolol and atenolol under double-blind conditions and both have proven satisfactory.[67-69] Labetalol has been studied in Europe and Australia and appears safe to use.

VASODILATORS

Prazosin, hydralazine, minoxidil, diazoxide, and sodium nitroprusside reduce blood pressure through direct effects on arterioles. They are useful when added to previously ineffective therapy with maximal doses of other antihypertensive agents or for the latter three, when used acutely to treat hypertensive exacerbations. Treatment with these agents is limited by a reflex increase in sympathetic activity and heart rate, an increase in plasma renin activity, and the corresponding retention of sodium, fluid, and circulation plasma volume. Combination therapy with a diuretic and β-blocker or sympatholytic obviates these problems in chronic use.

Hydralazine, when used *parenterally*, is the drug of choice in pregnancy, and is an effective agent when used acutely to control exacerbations of maternal blood pressure.[70] Adverse effects in pregnant and nonpregnant patients include tachycardia and palpitations, flushing, and headaches. The use of hydralazine in combination with methyldopa in two large studies found no adverse effects in the fetus and neonate.[69,71-73] There are conflicting reports of the effects of hydralazine on uteroplacental blood flow, though the possibility of decreased flow must be considered. Fetal heart rate changes occur when hydralazine is administered acutely[74] and the blood pressure drops precipitously. Although fetal adverse effects have rarely been reported, the possibility of neonatal thermoregulatory problems and hypothermia exist.[75] Due to the amount of experience with hydralazine, and inexperience with other agents, hydralazine can therefore be recommended for use in pregnancy as the drug of choice for parenteral use. The use of oral hydralazine is only minimally effective and is not used routinely.

Diazoxide is a thiazide congener available for IV use only. Major problems with its use include sodium and fluid retention and reflex sympathetic stimulation. Diazoxide is usually successful in lowering blood pressure, even after failures with other indirectly acting agents. Its use in pregnancy is, however, not without controversy. Diazoxide has a powerful relaxant effect on uterine smooth muscle and may stop labor (Chap. 12), necessitating the use of oxytocins to reestablish it.[76,77] Diazoxide crosses the placenta[77] and can cause neonatal hyperglycemia, as well as hyperbilirubinemia by displacement from protein-binding sites. Maternal side effects include hyperglycemia through a direct effect on pancreatic β cells and hyperuricemia. Both of these effects are mild and rarely present problems with short-term use. Headache, flushing, tachycardia, and palpitations may be seen acutely as with other vasodilators.[78]

The most distressing problem associated with the use of diazoxide is the unpredictability of the initial response. Reports of systolic and diastolic pressures decreasing to below 60 mm Hg are distressing and cause acute fetal distress and hypoxia. The implications for uteroplacental perfusion of this drop in pressure are grave. Fetal heart rate decelerations immediately following the use of diazoxide have been reported. This, along with hyperbilirubinemia and problems with fetal maternal carbohydrate metabolism, make diazoxide a poor choice in pregnancy, and it should only be used if the blood pressure cannot be controlled with hydralazine. However, diazoxide is a good agent for use in the immediate postpartum state to control acute exacerbations of high blood pressure.

Sodium nitroprusside has not been used widely or studied because of potential fetal cyanide poisoning. Because of this problem, it cannot currently be recommended except in acute transient hypertension where other medications fail. Its only use may be to control an acute blood pressure rise during anesthesia for cesarean section, when the fetus is to be extracted in a short time.

MAGNESIUM SULFATE

The most important agent used in the United States in the treatment of severe preeclampsia and eclampsia is parenteral magnesium sulfate. Of a group of academic obstetricians and gynecologists recently surveyed, 100 percent utilize this drug for severe preeclampsia and eclampsia. Similarly, 98 percent of practicing obstetricians and gynecologists in the United States use magnesium sulfate, as contrasted to 2 percent of practicing obstetricians and gynecologists in the United Kingdom.[79] This discrepancy between the two countries is felt to be due to the American promotion of the drug by academic obstetricians and gynecologists, especially by the teachings and writings of Pritchard[80,81] and Zuspan who demonstrated improved outcome.[82] The use and role of magnesium sulfate in acute hypertension in pregnancy follows.

Magnesium Metabolism

Magnesium is the fourth most common cation in the body and the second most plentiful intracellular cation. The human body contains approximately 2000 mEq of magnesium. The majority, at least 50 percent, is found in bone, and the remainder is equally distributed in muscle and nonmuscular tissue.[83-85] Magnesium is absorbed mainly in the small intestine, and disorders or alterations of the intestine, such as jejunoileal bypass, can result in magnesium deficiency. The excretion of magnesium, when it is administered IV, is principally in the urine, as only 1 to 2 percent is recovered in the feces.[86]

Magnesium is an activator of a host of enzyme systems which are critical to cellular metabolism. In addition, it is a required cofactor for oxidative metabolism in vitro. Because it is the most abundant divalent intracellular cation, it is used in many metabolic pathways.

Magnesium and calcium have a complex interdependent influence on the excitability of the components of the neuromuscular junction. There are no known studies showing that magnesium deficiency is the cause of toxemia of pregnancy or that its use in toxemia provides a correction of such a deficiency. Magnesium and calcium depletion do not lead to increased neurohormonal excitability or enhance neuromuscular transmission. Some of the effects of calcium and magnesium, however, are antagonistic to neurohormonal transmission. Magnesium in pharmacologic doses has a curariform action on the neuromuscular junction, presumably interfering with the release of acetylcholine from motor–nerve terminals. Another hypothesis is that there is a change in membrane potential by replacement of calcium with magnesium, thus altering neuromuscular transmission and excitability of the motor–nerve terminal which prevents eclamptic convulsions.

Magnesium Excess

The studies on magnesium excess in the human have resulted from clinical pharmacologic studies, most notably those in toxemia of pregnancy. It is known that infusions to animals and humans lead to an impairment of neuromuscular transmission. The sequential clinical development suggestive of magnesium excess can be noted first when deep tendon reflexes become hypoactive at serum magnesium concentrations between 8 and 10 mEq/L, followed by respiratory paralysis developing when concentrations exceed 13 to 15 mEq/L. Finally, cardiac conduction is affected with serum concentrations greater than 15 mEq/L. Cardiac arrest does not occur until extremely high concentrations take place, usually in excess of 25 mEq/L, with cardiac arrest occurring in diastole.

Use of Magnesium in Preeclampsia and Eclampsia

Since 1906 magnesium sulfate has been used for the treatment of preeclampsia and eclampsia.[87] Administration has been parenteral, with a very few clinicians in the world using intrathecal magnesium to control eclamptic convulsions. Lazard, in 1925, was the first to use IV magnesium sulfate to treat eclampsia. He gave hourly doses of 20 ml of 10 percent solution of magnesium sulfate until the convulsions ceased. The following year, Dorsett used intramuscular magnesium sulfate to treat toxemia of pregnancy. Eastman is credited with establishing the current acceptable intramuscular regimen for magnesium sulfate by giving an initial dose of 10 g (20 ml of 50 percent solution), followed by 5 g at 6-hour intervals.[88] He regarded magnesium therapy as the single most valuable agent in the treatment of severe preeclampsia, and this has not changed to this day in the United States. Pritchard popularized a regimen similar to Eastman's, except that the initial dose is 4 g of magnesium sulfate IV and thereafter, intramuscular injections.[80,81,89] Zuspan popularized the use of IV magnesium sulfate using 4 to 6 g initially, then 1 to 2 g/hour thereafter, depending on the clinical condition of the patient.[90,91] The reports of Pritchard and Zuspan in the literature identify the use of parenteral magnesium sulfate as the most efficacious means of reducing eclampsia-related perinatal mortality to 10 percent and maternal mortality to zero. Their reports, published more than 20 years ago, represent the best fetal salvage rates for this severe disease reported in the literature (Fig. 6–4).

Magnesium Sulfate Regimens

All doses of magnesium sulfate refer to the hydrated form $MgSO_4 \cdot 7\,H_2O$. The anhydrous salt contains twice as much magnesium as the hydrated salt. Various methods are available to monitor the therapeutic administration of magnesium. Flowers proposed monitoring the urine magnesium as well as the plasma levels at periodic intervals using formula calculations, thus allowing appropriate adjustment of magnesium dosage.[92] Periodic monitoring of plasma magnesium is advisable, and the ideal level is 6 to 8 mEq/L. The difficulty stems from the protracted amount of time

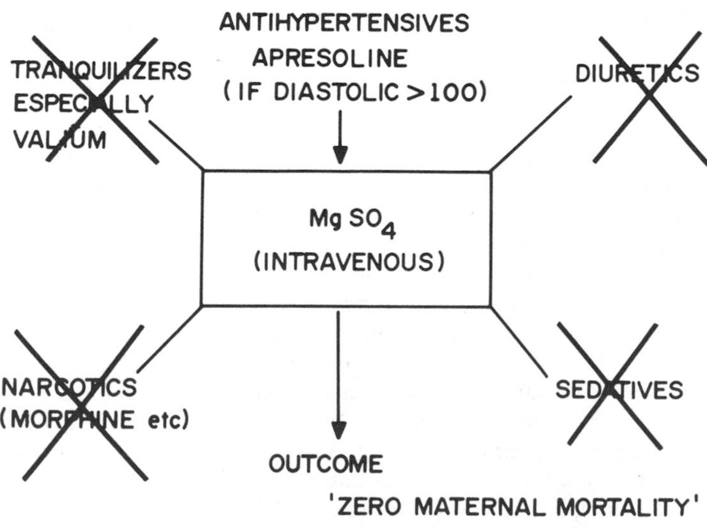

Figure 6–4. The major therapy used in preeclampsia–eclampsia is intravenous magnesium sulfate in pharmacologic doses.

required to obtain the magnesium level, thus rendering this method of little value except to monitor a trend of therapy.

Most clinicians monitor the patient using reflexes, respiration, and urine output as parameters. Reflexes should be present, respirations adequate, and urine output should be more than 100 ml every 4 hours. To assure this (1) deep tendon reflexes should be checked on an hourly basis and, if absent, the dosage should be lowered (reflexes should be hypoactive and present); (2) respirations should be counted at hourly intervals and should remain above 12 per minute; and (3) urine output should exceed 100 ml every 4 hours because magnesium is only excreted in the urine. In the event of oliguria, a plasma magnesium level should be obtained and the amount of magnesium gradually diminished; an antidote to combat a hypermagnesium state is calcium gluconate or calcium chloride in a 10 percent solution; 10 ml or 1 g is injected IV for magnesium overdose.

Pritchard demonstrated in toxemia therapy involving parenteral $MgSO_4$ that plasma levels average 6 mEq/L and often approach 8 to 10 mEq/L. The concentration of magnesium in the cerebral spinal fluid is only slightly increased and is considered essentially normal. Cerebral spinal fluid magnesium thus does not correlate with plasma magnesium.

Several investigators in the past used intrathecal magnesium to control convulsions and, despite previous information, this was an effective method, although it is not generally accepted at the present time.[93]

A major misconception concerning magnesium sulfate centers around its hypotensive qualities. Magnesium is not a hypotensive agent even though it decreases intrinsic resistance in the uterine vessels. Occasionally a transient decline in blood pressure occurs within the first hour of administration of IV magnesium; however, it returns to baseline levels following this brief period. If blood pressure needs to be controlled, an antihypertensive drug should be used. Therapeutic levels of magnesium seem to blunt the vasospastic fluctuations of the blood pressure often seen in the severe preeclamptic patient with an elevated blood pressure. It is hypothesized that magnesium may also protect the fetus by increasing uterine blood flow, a finding in experimental animals not yet documented in humans.[94] Magnesium has no direct general anesthetic property, and changes at serum concentrations above 12 mEq/L do not indicate suppressed EEG activity.[95]

Adverse Effects on the Neonate and Uterine Activity

There is divided opinion concerning the effect of magnesium sulfate on uterine activity. Zuspan was not able to show a lengthening of eclamptic labor or inductions in spite of doses of magnesium as high as 3 g/hour.[96] This is in contrast to Hall et al., who were able to demonstrate in muscle tissue excised from the gravid human uterus at the time of cesarean section that increasing concentrations of magnesium in the muscle-bath solution caused a diminution in spontaneous uterine activity.[97] Their conclusions were that magnesium inhibits the contractility of isolated muscle tissue excised from the gravid human uterus and that additionally, the magnesium ion may have a depressant action on uterine motility in vivo. These workers substantiate their latter statements by looking at the length of labor of 300 patients who, in toxemia of pregnancy, received either no magnesium, low magnesium, or high magnesium. The high magnesium patients had labor of approximately 18 hours, versus 14-hour labor in the low magnesium patients and 9-hour labor in patients without magnesium.

Pritchard also was not able to document a causal relationship of magnesium and alterations in uterine contractions by direct transabdominal percutaneous recordings of uterine pressure. There were no changes in frequency, duration, or intensity of uterine contractions following the parenteral injection of magnesium.[89]

The effect of magnesium on the fetus is

such that amniotic fluid levels are roughly 25 to 30 percent of plasma levels. Cruikshank and Pitkin sampled in a sequential manner the maternal and cord levels of magnesium with a follow-up of newborn blood levels revealing that it takes 24 to 48 hours for magnesium levels to return to normal after therapeutic doses are present in the mother.[98] Over a 14-year period, Stone and Pritchard studied some 7000 infants whose mothers had received parenteral magnesium and found no problem in its use with relation to newborns.[99] They found that the serum level of magnesium in the fetus rapidly approached that of the mother but could not be correlated with any ill effects on the newborn. Lipsitz has noted that when magnesium sulfate is given intramuscularly to the mother, the newborn is usually not compromised by excess magnesium but may be affected. However, when continuous infusion of magnesium sulfate is used and given for more than 24 hours, anticipation of the newborn manifesting signs of hypermagnesemia may be present.[100]

This is in contrast to the experience of Zuspan, who has utilized therapeutic doses of magnesium sulfate since 1960. Excessive magnesium levels present in the newborn are cleared by renal excretion if the newborn did not suffer hypoxia during labor or the birth process. Only two exceptions are notable in 26 years, and both involved urinary retention most likely due to magnesium effects on the detrussor muscle of the newborn. The point at issue is that magnesium remains the best drug for the toxemic patient, and although it may affect the fetus, it has the lowest number of side effects.

REFERENCES

1. Zuspan FP: Chronic hypertension in pregnancy. Clin Obstet Gynecol 27 (4):854, 1984
2. Rayburn WF, Zuspan FP, Piehl EJ: Self blood pressure monitoring during pregnancy. Am J Obstet Gynecol 148:159, 1984
3. Iams JD, Semchyshyn S, O'Shaughnessy RW, et al.: Blood pressure response in hypertensive pregnancies treated with cortisol. Clin Exp Hypertens 2:923, 1980
4. Shnider SM, Levinson G: Anesthesia for obstetrics, Baltimore, William & Wilkins, 1979
5. Ostheimer GW: Manual of obstetric anesthesia. New York, Churchill Livingston, 1984
6. Kelton JG, Hunter DJS, Neame PB: A platelet function defect in preeclampsia. Obstet Gynecol 65:107, 1985
7. Benedetti TJ, Kates R, Williams V: Hemodynamic observations in severe preeclampsia complicated by pulmonary edema. Am J Obstet Gynecol 152:330, 1985
8. Heller PJ, Schneider EP, Marx GF: Phoryngolaryngeal edema as a presenting symptom in preeclampsia. Obstet Gynecol 62:523, 1983
9. Berkowitz RL: Critical Care of the Obstetric Patient. New York, Churchill Livingston, 1983
10. Talledo OE, Chesley LC, Zuspan FP: Renin–angiotensin system in normal and toxemic pregnancies. Am J Obstet Gynecol 100:218, 1968
11. Lindheimer M, Katz A: Current concepts: Hypertension in pregnancy. N Engl J Med 313:675, 1985
12. Kelly JV: Drugs used in the management of toxemia of pregnancy. Clin Obstet Gynecol 20:395, 1977
13. Welt SI, Crenshaw MC: Concurrent hypertension and pregnancy. Clin Obstet Gynecol 21:619, 1978
14. Campbell DM, MacGillivary I: The effect of a low caloric diet or a thiazide diuretic on the incidence of preeclampsia and on birthweight. Br J Obstet Gynecol 82:572, 1975
15. Kraus GW, Marchese HR, Yen SSC: Prophylactic use of hydrochlorothiazide in pregnancy. JAMA 198:1150, 1966
16. Gray J: Use and abuse of thiazides in pregnancy. Clin Obstet Gynecol 11:568, 1968
17. Limited usefulness of diuretics in pregnancy. FDA Drug Bull. Sept 1977
18. Lindheimer MD, Katz AI: Sodium and diuretics in pregnancy. JAMA 198:1150, 1966
19. Gant NF, Madden JD, Siiteri PK, MacDonald PK: The metabolic clearance rate of dehydroisoandrosterone sulfate: III. The effect of thiazide diuretics in normal and preeclamptic pregnancies. Am J Obstet Gynecol 123:159, 1975
20. Gant NF, Madden JD, Siiteri PK, MacDonald PK: The metabolic clearance rate of dehydroisoandrosterone sulfate: IV. Acute effects of induced hypotension and natriuresis in normal and hypertensive pregnancies. Am J Obstet Gynecol 124:143, 1976

21. Arias F: Expansion of intramuscular volume and fetal outcome in patients with chronic hypertension and pregnancy. Am J Obstet Gynecol 123:610, 1975
22. Soffronoff EC, Kaulman RM, Connaughton JF: Intravascular volume determination and fetal outcome in hypertensive disease of pregnancy. Am J Obstet Gynecol 127:4, 1977
23. Riddiough MA: Preventing, detecting and managing adverse reactions of antihypertensive agents in the ambulant patient with hypertension. Am J Hosp Pharm 34:465, 1977
24. Pritchard JA, Walley PJ: Severe hypolkalemia due to prolonged administration of chlorothiazide during pregnancy. Am J Obstet Gynecol 81:1241, 1961
25. Minkowitz S. Soloway HB, Hall JE, Yermakov V: Fatal hemorrhagic pancreatitis following chlorothiazide administration in pregnancy. Obstet Gynecol 24:337, 1964
26. Schifrin BS, Spellacy WN, Little WA: Maternal death associated with excessive ingestion of a chlorothiazide diuretic. Obstet Gynecol 34:215, 1969
27. Alstatt LB: Transplacental hyponatremia in the newborn infant. J Pediatr 66:785, 1965
28. Merenstein GB, O'Laughlin EP, Plunkett DC: Effects of maternal thiazides on platelet counts of newborn infants. J Pediatr 76:766, 1970
29. Rodriguez SU, Leikin SL, Hiller MC: Neonatal thrombocytopenia associated with antepartum administration of thiazide drugs. N Engl J Med 270:881, 1964
30. Grollman A, Grollman EF: The teratogenic induction of hypertension. J Clin Invest 41:710, 1962
31. Garnet JD: Placental transfer of chlorothiazide. Obstet Gynecol 21:123, 1963
32. Anderson GG, Hanson TM: Chronic fetal bradycardia. Obstet Gynecol 44:896, 1974
33. Jerner K, Kutti J, Victorin LA: Platelet counts in mothers and their newborn infants with respect to antepartum administration of oral diuretics. Acta Med Scand 194:473, 1973
34. Anderson JB: The effect of diuretics in late pregnancy on the newborn infant. Acta Paediatr Scand 59:659, 1970
35. Finnerty FA: Hypertension in pregnancy. Clin Obstet Gynecol 18:145, 1975
36. Berkowitz RL: Antihypertensive drugs in the pregnant patient. Obstet Gynecol Surv 35:191, 1980
37. Riva E, Farina P, Togoni G, et al.: Pharmacokinetics of furosemide in gestosis of pregnancy. Eur J Clin Pharmacol 14:361, 1978
38. Sanders JG, Gillis OS III, Marketo DL Jr, Gready TG Jr: Chlorthalidone in edema of pregnancy. NY State J Med 65:762, 1965
39. Tenvila L, Vartainen E: The effects and side effects of diuretics in the prophylaxis of toxemia of pregnancy. Acta Obstet Gynecol Scand 50:351, 1971
40. Stirrat GM: Prescribing problems in the second half of pregnancy and during lactation. Obstet Gynecol Surv 31:1, 1976
41. Desmond MM, Rogers SE, Lindley JE, et al.: Management of toxemia of pregnancy with reserpine: II. The newborn infant. Obstet Gynecol 10:140, 1957
42. Budnich IS, Leikth S, Hoek LE: Effect in the newborn infant of reserpine administered antepartum. Am J Dis Child 90:286, 1955
43. Kincaid-Smith P, Bullen M, Mills J: Prolonged use of methyldopa in severe hypertension of pregnancy. Br Med J 1:275, 1966
44. Redmon CWG, Beitin LJ, Bonnar J. Ounsted MK: Fetal outcome in trial of antihypertensive treatment in pregnancy. Lancet 1:753, 1976
45. Redmon CWG, Beitin LJ, Bonnar J: Treatment of hypertension in pregnancy with methyldopa: Blood pressure control and side effects. Br J Obstet Gynecol 84:419, 1977
46. Leather HM, Humphreys DM, Baker P, Chadd MA: A controlled trial of hypotensive agents in hypertension in pregnancy. Lancet 2:488, 1968
47. Jones HMR, Cummings AJ: A study of the transfer of alpha-methyldopa to the human fetus and newborn infant. Br J Clin Pharmacol 6:432, 1964
48. Hans SF, Kopelman H: Methyldopa in the treatment of severe hypertension of pregnancy. Br Med J 1:736, 1964
49. Jones HMR, Cummings AJ, Sebchell KDR, Lawson AM: A study of the disposition of alpha-methyldopa in newborn infants following its administration to the mother for the treatment of hypertension during pregnancy. Br J Clin Pharmacol 8:833, 1979
50. Zuspan FP, O'Shaughnessy R: Chronic hypertension in pregnancy. In Pitkin RM, Zlatnik FL (eds): Yearbook of Obstetrics-Gynecology. Chicago, Yearbook Medical Publishers, 1979, pp 11–36
51. Zacharias FJ, Kowen KJ, Presst J, et al.: Propranolol in hypertension: A study of long-term therapy. Am Heart J 83:755, 1972

52. Joint National Committee on Detection, Evaluation, and Treatment of High Blood Pressure: Report. JAMA 237:255, 1977
53. Riddiough MA: Preventing, detecting, and managing adverse reactions of antihypertensive agents in the ambulant patient with hypertension. Am J Hosp Pharm 34:465, 1977
54. Sabom MB, Curry C, Wise DE: Propranolol therapy during pregnancy in a patient with idiopathic hypertrophic subaortic stenosis: Is it safe? South Med J 71:328, 1978
55. Levitan AA, Manion JC: Propranolol therapy during pregnancy and lactation. Am J Cardiol 32:247, 1973
56. Fiddler GI: Propranolol and pregnancy. Lancet 2:722, 1974
57. Read RL, Cheney CB, Fearon RE, et al.: Propranolol throughout pregnancy: A case report. Anesth Analg 53:224, 1974
58. Cottrill CM, McAllister RG, Genes L, et al.: Propranolol therapy during pregnancy, labor and delivery: Evidence for transplacental drug transfer and impaired neonatal drug disposition. J Pediatr 91:872, 1977
59. Tcherdekoff PH, Colliard M, Berrard E, et al.: Propranolol in hypertension during pregnancy. Br Med J 2:670, 1978
60. Eliahou HE, Silverberg DE, Reisin E, et al.: Propranolol for the treatment of hypertension during pregnancy. Br J Obstet Gynecol 85:431, 1978
61. Lieberman BA, Stirrat GM, Cohen SL, et al.: The possible adverse effects of propranolol on the fetus in pregnancies complicated by severe hypertension. Br J Obstet Gynecol 85:678, 1978
62. Habib A, McCarthy JS: Effects on the neonate of propranolol administered during pregnancy. J Pediatr 91:808, 1977
63. Gladstone GE, Hordof A, Gersony WM: Propranolol administration during pregnancy: Effects on the fetus. J Pediatr 86:962, 1975
64. Barnes AB: Chronic propranolol during pregnancy. J Reprod Med 5:179, 1970
65. Tunstall ME: The effect of propranolol on the onset of breathing at birth. Br J Anaesth 51:792, 1969
66. Pruyn SC, Phelan JP, Buchanan GC: Long-term propranolol therapy in pregnancy: Maternal and fetal outcome. Am J Obstet Gynecol 135:485, 1979
67. Rubin PE, Butters L, Clark D, et al.: Obstetric aspects of the use in pregnancy-associated hyhypertension of the β-adrenoceptor antogonist atenolol. Am J Obstet Gynecol 150:389, 1984
68. Fidler J, Smith V, Fayers P, DeSwiet M: Randomized controlled comparative study of methyldopa and oxprenolol in treatment of hypertension in pregnancy. Br Med J 286:1927, 1983
69. Fidler J, Smith V, DeSwiet M: A randomized study comparing timoloc and methyldopa in hospital treatment of puerperal hypertension. Br J Obstet Gynecol 89:1031, 1982
70. Kelly JV: Drugs used in the management of toxemia of pregnancy. Clin Obstet Gynecol 20:395, 1977
71. Redmon CWG, Beilin LJ, Bonnar J, Ounsted MK: Fetal outcome in trial of antihypertensive treatment in pregnancy. Lancet 1:753–756, 1976
72. Redmon CWG, Beilin LJ, Bonner J: Treatment of hypertension in pregnancy with methyldopa: Blood pressure control and side effects. Br J Obstet Gynecol 84:419–426, 1977
73. Leather HM, Humphreys DM, Baker P, Chadd MA: A controlled trial of hypotensive agents in hypertension in pregnancy. Lancet 2:488–490, 1968
74. Vink GJ, Moodley J, Philpott RH: Effect of dihydralazine on the fetus in the treatment of maternal hypertension. Obstet Gynecol 55:519–522, 1980
75. Gordon II: Toxemia of pregnancy. In Hawkins DF (ed): Obstetric Therapeutics. Baltimore, Williams & Wilkins, 1974, pp 274–276
76. Koch-Weser J: Diazoxide. N Engl J Med 294:1271–1274, 1976
77. Boulos BM, Davis LE, Almond CH, et al.: Placental transfer of diazoxide and its hazardous effect on the newborn. J Clin Pharmacol 11:206–210, 1971
78. Morris JA, Arce JJ, Hamilton CJ, et al.: The management of severe preeclampsia and eclampsia with intravenous diazoxide. Obstet Gynecol 49:675, 1977
79. Lewis PJ, Bulpitt CJ, Zuspan FP: A comparison of current British and American practice in the management of hypertension in pregnancy. J Obstet Gynaecol Br Commonw 1:78–82, 1980
80. Pritchard JA, Stone SR: Clinical and laboratory observations on eclampsia. Am J Obstet Gynecol 99:754, 1967
81. Pritchard JA, Cunningham FG, Pritchard SA: The Parkland Memorial Hospital protocol for

treatment of eclampsia. Am J Obstet Gynecol 148:951, 1984
82. Zuspan FP, Ward MC: Improved fetal salvage in eclampsia. Obstet Gynecol 26:893, 1965
83. Widdowson EM, McCance RA, Spray CM: Chemical composition of human body. Clin Sci 10:113, 1951
84. Wacker WEC, Parisi AF: Magnesium metabolism. N Engl J Med 278:658, 1968
85. Wacker WEC, Parisi AF: Magnesium metabolism. N Engl J Med 278:712, 1968
86. Silver L, Robertson JS, Dahl LK: Magnesium turnover in human studied with Mg^{28}. J Clin Invest 39:420, 1960
87. Chesley LE, Tepper I: Plasma levels of magnesium attained in magnesium sulfate therapy for preeclampsia and eclampsia. Surg Clin North Am April: 353–367, 1957
88. Eastman NJ: Williams Obstetrics. New York, Appleton-Century-Crofts, 1950
89. Pritchard JA: The use of the magnesium ion in the management of eclamptogenic toxemias. Surg Gynecol Obstet 100:131, 1955
90. Zuspan FP, Ward MC: Improved fetal salvage in eclampsia. Obstet Gynecol 26:893, 1965
91. Zuspan FP: Problems encountered in the treatment of pregnancy induced hypertension. Am J Obstet Gynecol 131:591, 1978
92. Flowers CE Jr: Magnesium sulfate in obstetrics: A study of magnesium in plasma, urine and muscle. Am J Obstet Gynecol 91:763, 1965
93. Watehorn E, McCance RA: Inorganic constituents of cerebralspinal fluid. Biochem J Lond 26:54, 1932
94. Harbert G: Personal communication, 1980
95. Aldrete JA, Barnes DR, Aikawa JK: Does magnesium produce anesthesia? Anesthesia and analgesia. Curr Res 47:428, 1968
96. Zuspan FP, Talledo OE, Rhodes K: Factors affecting delivery in eclampsia: The condition of the cervix and uterine activity. Am J Obstet Gynecol 100:672, 1968
97. Hall DG, McGaughey HS Jr, Corey EL, Thornton WN: The effects of magnesium therapy on the duration of labor. Am J Obstet Gynecol 78:27, 1959
98. Cruikshank D, Pitkin R: Personal communication, 1981
99. Stone SR, Pritchard JA: Effect of maternally administered magnesium sulfate on the neonate. Obstet Gynecol 35:574, 1970
100. Lipsitz PJ: The clinical and biochemical effects of excess magnesium in the newborn. Pediatrics 47:501, 1971
101. Kelly JV: Drugs used in the management of toxemia of pregnancy. Clin Obstet Gynecol 20:395–420, 1977
102. Limited usefulness of diuretics in pregnancy, FDA Drug Bull, Sept 1977
103. Gant NF, Madden JD, Siiteri PK, MacDonald PK: The metabolic clearance rate of dehydroisoandrosterone sulfate: III. The effect of thiazide diuretics in normal and preeclamptic pregnancies. Am J Obstet Gynecol 123:159–163, 1975
104. Gant NF, Madden JD, Siiteri PK, MacDonald PK: The metabolic clearance rate of dehydroisoandrosterone sulfate: IV. Acute effects of induced hypotension and natriuresis in normal and hypertensive pregnancies. Am J Obstet Gynecol 124:143–148, 1976
105. Alstatt LB: Transplacental hypoatremia in the newborn infant. J Pediatr 66:785–788, 1965
106. Rodriguez SU, Leikin SL, Hiller MC: Neonatal thrombocytopenia associated with antepartum administration of thiazide drugs. N Engl J Med 270:881–884, 1967
107. Grollman A, Grollman EF: The teratogenic induction of hypertension. J Clin Invest 41:710–714, 1962
108. Garnet JD: Placental transfer of chlorothiazide. Obstet Gynecol 21:123–125, 1963
109. Riva E, Farina P, Togoni G, et al.: Pharmacokinetics of furosemide in gestosis of pregnancy. Eur J Clin Pharmacol 14:361–366, 1978
110. Welt SI, Crenshaw MC: Concurrent hypertension and pregnancy. Clin Obstet Gynecol 21:619–648, 1978
111. Finnerty FA: Hypertension in pregnancy. Clin Obstet Gynecol 18:145–154, 1975
112. Sanders JG, Gillis OS III, Marketto DL Jr, Gready TG Jr: Chlorthalidone in edema of pregnancy. NY State J Med 65:762–764, 1965
113. Tervila L, Vartainen E: The effects and side effects of diuretics in the prophylaxis of toxaemia of pregnancy. Acta Obstet Gynecol Scand 50:351–356, 1971
114. Stirrat GM: Prescribing problems in the second half of pregnancy and during lactation. Obstet Gynecol Surv 31:1–6, 1976
115. Budnick IS, Leikin S, Hoek LE: Effect in the newborn infant of reserpine administered antepartum. Amer J Dis Child 90:286–289, 1955
116. Kincaid-Smith P, Bullen M, Mills J: Prolonged use of methyldopa in severe hypertension of pregnancy. Br Med J 1:275, 1966

117. Redmon CWG, Beilin LJ, Bonnar J, Ounsted MK: Fetal outcome in trial of antihypertensive treatment in pregnancy. Lancet 1:753–756, 1976
118. Redmon CWG, Beilin LJ, Bonnar J: Treatment of hypertension in pregnancy with methyldopa: Blood pressure control and side effects. Br J Obstet Gynecol 84:419–426, 1977
119. Leather HM, Humphreys DM, Baker P, Chadd MA: A controlled trial of hypertensive agents in hypertension in pregnancy. Lancet 1:488–490, 1968
120. Jones HMR, Cummings AJ: A study of the transfer of alpha-methyldopa to the human fetus and newborn infant. Br J Clin Pharmacol 6:432–434, 1978
121. Sabom MB, Curry C, Wise DE: Propranolol therapy during pregnancy in a patient with idiopathic hypertrophic subaortic stenosis: Is it safe? South Med J 71:328–329, 1978
122. Gladstone GR, Hordof A, Gersony WM: Propranolol administration during pregnancy: Effects on the fetus. J Pediatr 86:962–964, 1975
123. Pruyn SC, Phelan JP, Buchanan GC: Long-term propranolol therapy in pregnancy: Maternal and fetal outcome. Am J Obstet Gynecol 135:485–489, 1979
124. Soffronoff BC, Kaufman RM, Connaughton JF: Intravascular volume determination and fetal outcome in hypertensive diseases of pregnancy. Am J Obstet Gynecol 127:4–9, 1977
125. Vink GJ, Moodley J, Philpott RH: Effect of dihydralazine on the fetus in the treatment of maternal hypertension. Obstet Gynecol 55:519–522, 1980
126. Brogden RN, Heel RC, Speight TM, et al.: Prazosin: A review of its pharmacological properties and therapeutic efficacy in hypertension. Drugs 14:163–197, 1977

7

Endocrine Disorders During Pregnancy

William F. Rayburn, Robert M. McNulty, and Richard W. O'Shaughnessy

With improved medical, obstetric, and neonatal care, remarkable progress has been made in treating pregnancies complicated by endocrine disorders. Today, many more patients with endocrinopathies are able to conceive and successfully maintain their pregnancies as compared to several decades ago. Diabetes mellitus and thyroid diseases are the most common endocrine disorders seen during pregnancy, and these conditions, along with all endocrinopathies, require careful monitoring during the antepartum, intrapartum, and postpartum periods. Derangements in parathyroid, adrenal, or pituitary glands are quite uncommon but may be amenable to drug therapy. This chapter provides detailed information on the use of insulin, thyroid, and antithyroid medications during pregnancy. In addition, drugs proposed for treating other endocrine conditions are listed and briefly discussed.

DIABETES MELLITUS

The reported incidence of diabetes mellitus during pregnancy is approximately 2 to 3 percent.[1] Diabetes is due to faulty pancreatic activity with the subsequent disturbance of normal insulin release and carbohydrate metabolism, resulting in hyperglycemia, glycosuria and polyuria, and symptoms of thirst, hunger, and weakness.

An increased number of patients with diabetes are now becoming pregnant and seeking early prenatal care. A diabetic pregnancy is considered high risk, because maternal morbidity and unfavorable perinatal outcomes are significantly increased when compared to nondiabetic pregnancies. Maternal complications may arise from metabolic, vascular, and infectious derangements. Fetal complications include premature delivery, congenital anomalies, metabolic alterations, and respiratory distress. Specific fetal metabolic derangements include hypoglycemia, hypocalcemia, hypomagnesemia, hyperkalemia, and hyperbilirubinemia. Not all complications can be avoided completely during pregnancy, but maternal and fetal complications may be minimized with early screening and careful medical management.[1-6]

Pregnancy is associated with many physiologic alterations in metabolism which are hormonally influenced. Glucose intolerance may not become apparent until the onset of pregnancy. To adequately diagnose and treat diabetes during pregnancy, it is necessary to understand the metabolic changes of pregnancy and appreciate the pathophysiologic principles of diabetes.

Carbohydrate Metabolism During Pregnancy

During pregnancy, many energy-producing metabolic pathways are modified through hormonal influence. These modifications are necessary to provide essential nutrients to the fetus while maintaining normal circulating glucose levels in the mother. As the primary regulator of carbohydrate metabolism, insulin at increased levels results in increased glycogen synthesis, protein synthesis, and the conversion of carbohydrates to fat with an increased uptake of free fatty acids. Basal levels of insulin are lower or unchanged in early pregnancy, but higher levels are secreted in the second half of pregnancy from the hyperplastic β cells in the islets of Langerhans.[7,8] Insulin secretion is noted to increase rapidly after eating during pregnancy and reaches levels that are approximately twice those that would be expected in a nonpregnant patient (Fig. 7–1).

Despite this hyperinsulinemic state during the second half of pregnancy, glucose tolerance is impaired. Compared to nonpregnant values, basal glucose values after an overnight fast are lower in the first trimester and decrease progressively during gestation. This tendency toward fasting hypoglycemia, termed as "accelerated starvation" by Freinkel, is related to the following conditions: (1) increasing insulin levels, (2) increasing placental and fetal uptake of glucose, (3) subnormal hepatic production of glucose, and (4) less renal reabsorption of glucose at all levels of the filtered load.[9] After an oral glucose challenge, peak values of glucose are higher and occur later when compared to values in the early or nonpregnant state (Fig. 7–1). As pregnancy continues, serum glucose levels show decreasing fasting levels, increasing 1-hour levels, and essentially unchanged 2-hour levels after a glucose challenge. Glucose tolerance test (GTT) standards must be adjusted upward to correct for this physiologic response. The standards of O'Sullivan and Mahan for the 3-hour, 100-g oral test have been accepted widely and are listed in Table 7–1.[10]

Postprandial glucose intolerance is a diabetogenic phenomenon explained by the insulin-antagonistic effects of cortisol, progesterone, and placental lactogen (hPL). Insulin-sensitive tissues are exposed to increas-

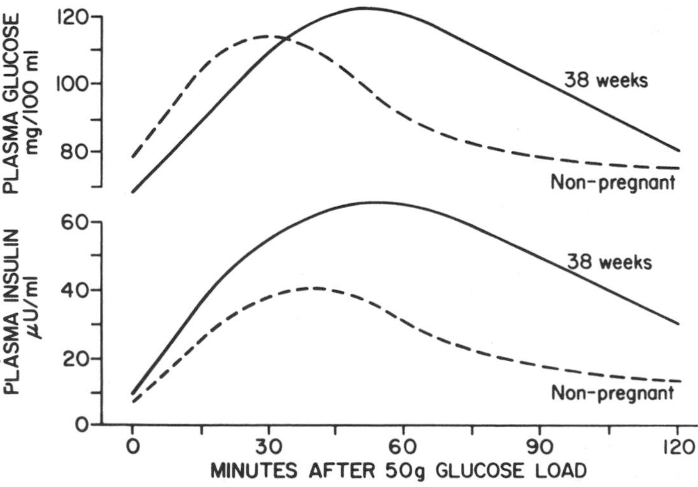

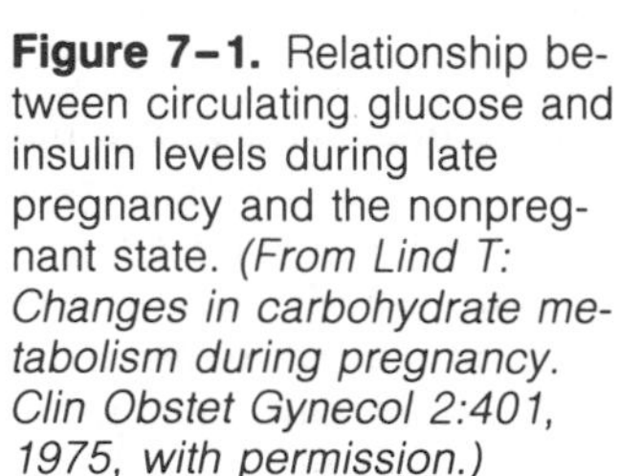

Figure 7–1. Relationship between circulating glucose and insulin levels during late pregnancy and the nonpregnant state. *(From Lind T: Changes in carbohydrate metabolism during pregnancy. Clin Obstet Gynecol 2:401, 1975, with permission.)*

TABLE 7–1. GTT VALUES DURING PREGNANCY*

	Whole Blood (mg/100 ml)	Serum (mg/100 ml)
Fasting (hr)	≤ 90	≤ 105
1	165	190
2	145	165
3	125	145

* 100-g glucose challenge.

ing levels of prolactin, which has been suggested as a possible insulin antagonist at target cell receptor sites, as well as increasing concentrations of free cortisol during pregnancy. The role of catecholamines in the metabolic changes of pregnancy is uncertain. Although the secretion of glucagon from the pancreas increases during pregnancy, its counterinsulin effects are offset by the relatively increased secretion of insulin.[11] In addition, the placenta is capable of synthesizing and secreting increasing levels of progesterone and hPL which are antagonists to insulin at the cellular level.

The kinetics of endogenous and exogenous insulin is unchanged during pregnancy.[12] Although influenced by the increased extracellular volume, placental metabolism, and lowered renal clearance, the half-life of insulin is considered to be the same in pregnancy as in nonpregnant controls or in women in the late puerperium.[12,13]

The fetus and placenta constantly drain nutrients such as glucose and amino acids from the mother. Although the placenta is impermeable to maternal or fetal insulin, glucose is known to cross the placenta by facilitated diffusion. There is a direct relationship between glucose intolerance in the mother and glucose utilization by the fetus and neonate.[14] The worse the maternal tolerance, the more rapidly glucose is assimilated by the fetus. Although fetal insulin and glucagon concentrations within the pancreas are greater than in the adult as early as the first trimester, secretory mechanisms are immature.[15] Carbohydrate metabolism is apparently independent of these hormones until the third trimester, when insulin takes over the dominant role (Fig. 7–2). An elevated maternal blood glucose level causes fetal hyperglycemia, and whether the fetus is protected from severe hyperglycemia is presently unclear. Fetal hyperinsulinemia with hyperplasia of the islets of Langerhans may occur in response to high fetal glucose concentrations secondary to persistent maternal hypergly-

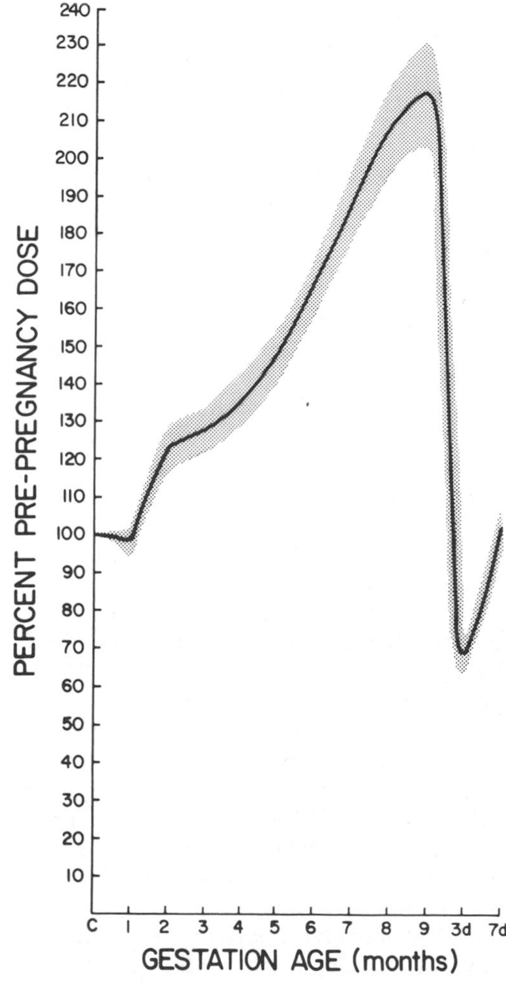

Figure 7–2. Changes in maternal insulin requirements during pregnancy and the first postpartum week. (*From Rayburn W et al., 1985, with permission.*[28])

cemia. With prolonged hyperglycemia and resultant hyperinsulinemia, macrosomia and delayed lung maturation are possible. Fetal macrosomia results from the insulin-induced deposition of fat and glycogen. Delayed fetal lung maturity can occur from the antagonism of insulin to the maturing effects of cortisol, or from a decrease in the precursors for phospholipid synthesis.

Guidelines for Therapy

Most pregnant patients tolerate well the increased demands on carbohydrate metabolism. However, when metabolic requirements at the cellular level are not met by an adequate secretion of insulin, maternal hyperglycemia may persist. A positive relationship has been shown between maternal hyperglycemia with fluctuating maternal glucose levels and subsequent perinatal morbidity and mortality. The goal of diabetic management during pregnancy is to control serum glucose values while treating any medical complications and carefully planning the delivery.[3,16-18] Strict control of blood glucose levels requires the periodic sampling of blood for glucose determination, a proper diet, and the administration of insulin if necessary.

An adequate diet may be sufficient to control glucose intolerance. Most approved diabetic diets involve a daily intake of 30 to 35 kcal/kg body weight. The calories are to be distributed more in favor of the carbohydrates (45 percent carbohydrate, 30 to 35 percent fat, 20 to 25 percent protein) and to be taken evenly throughout the day (20 percent at breakfast, 30 percent at lunch, 35 percent at dinner, and 15 percent as a late snack). Adjustments in this schedule are dependent on individual patient desires and corresponding glucose values. Prolonged periods of fasting are to be avoided.

Oral hypoglycemic agents (chlorpropamide, tolazamide, tolbutamide, acetohexamide) are contraindicated during pregnancy. Although maternal glucose levels may be decreased with these agents, they can cross the placenta to stimulate the fetal pancreas. No teratogenic effect on the major organs has been reported in human studies using oral hypoglycemic agents, but pancreatic hyperplasia and fetal hyperinsulinemia can result from persistent sulfonylurea-agent stimulation.[19] Neonatal macrosomia and profound hypoglycemia may be apparent.[19] These drugs are to be discontinued when pregnancy is being planned or at least immediately after pregnancy is confirmed.

Insulin should be continued in all insulin-dependent diabetics during pregnancy. In addition, many patients who have abnormally high glucose values on screening tests will require insulin, despite an initial attempt at diet control. It is usually recommended that the patient be admitted to the hospital for instruction on the management of her condition, to obtain the appropriate baseline tests and consultations, and either to begin or adjust insulin therapy according to serum glucose levels.

Insulin

Insulin is a protein composed of two chains of amino acids linked by two disulfide bridges. It acts to lower serum glucose levels by inhibiting glucose production and by promoting the peripheral utilization of glucose in the liver and peripheral tissues. At low concentrations, the hypoglycemic effect from insulin is primarily from a decrease in either glycogenolysis and/or gluconeogenesis within the liver. At higher physiologic concentrations, (100 mU/L or more), insulin also contributes to the peripheral utilization of glucose to decrease circulating glucose concentrations. In normal subjects, endogenous insulin probably acts primarily in the liver to block glucose production, while peripheral concentrations of insulin remain low. In insulin-dependent diabetics, however, portal vein concentrations of insulin are equal to or lower than peripheral concentrations of insulin. Because of this relative increase in peripheral insulin concentration, glucose utilization contributes more to the lowering of serum glucose.

The actions of insulin are many. Insulin is thought to bind to specific receptors on membranes of skeletal muscle and adipose cells to facilitate the transmembranous passage of glucose. Glucose metabolism for the production of energy in skeletal muscle and for triglyceride synthesis in adipose tissue is also stimulated by insulin. Insulin favors protein synthesis, nucleic acid (DNA, RNA) synthesis, glycolysis, and glycogenesis, and it inhibits glycogenolysis, gluconeogenesis, lipolysis, and proteolysis.

Following injection, insulin is rapidly degraded in the peripheral tissues by the cleavage of the disulfide bridges by the enzyme insulinase, which is found in all tissues, especially the liver and kidney. Protease enzymes further degrade the two insulin chains into individual amino acids. Placental insulinase can also degrade insulin to prevent maternal insulin from reaching the fetal circulation.[20] Its effect on insulin resistance during pregnancy is negligible.[13]

Preparations and Routes of Administration

Insulin is digested after oral intake, so subcutaneous or intravenous administration is necessary. The properties of the various insulin preparations (onset of action, duration of action) serve only as a guide, and insulin regimens must be adjusted according to individual responses after an adequate period of surveillance. Because circulating insulin is degraded rapidly, the duration of action is dependent on absorption from the injection site. The available preparations are grouped as being either fast acting, intermediate acting, or long acting (Table 7–2). Only fast acting (regular, Semilente insulin) and intermediate acting (NPH, Lente) preparations are used during pregnancy. Being a charged protamine protein, NPH should mix better with regular insulin and not affect absorption kinetics of soluble insulin. The onset of action is delayed when Lente and regular insulins are mixed, even when administered immediately after mixing.[21] Long-acting preparations are not used during pregnancy because of their variable onsets of action and prolonged duration.

Progress in purification of beef and pork insulin products has resulted from gel-filtration chromatography and ion-exchange chromatography techniques. As a result, concentrations of contaminants such as proinsulin, glucagon, somatostatin, and pancreatic polypeptides are decreased. Enhanced purification has led to a decreased risk of lipodystrophy, antibody formation, and local or systemic allergic reactions. In addition, dosage requirements of insulin may decrease when changing to a more purified insulin product.

Several purified beef or pork preparations of insulin have become available recently. Physicians must decide whether to prescribe either of these relatively expensive products or the less purified but less expensive preparations, which are usually mixtures of beef or pork. Purification removes potential antigens, such as proinsulin and pancreatic hormones, that may cause reactions and insulin resistance. Although this seems preferable in theory, no evidence exists that antibodies induced by giving the older insulins or impurities in the products (proinsulin, glucagon, or somatostatin) are harmful to the fetus.

Human insulin of recombinant DNA origin (biosynthetic human insulin, BHI), became commercially available in 1983 as a highly purified insulin, which is both chemically and structurally identical to endogenous human insulin. Pork insulin differs from human insulin by a single amino acid, whereas beef insulin contains three different amino acids. Both regular and intermediate-acting human insulin, (Humulin R, and Humulin N) have been manufactured by removing the terminal alanine from pork insulin and replacing it with threonine or using two strains of bacteria produced by gene-splicing techniques to synthesize the α-chain and the β-chain of insulin. In the future, commercially available insulin will probably be in the form of purified preparations.

As a general rule, standard beef–pork in-

TABLE 7-2. PROPERTIES OF VARIOUS INSULIN PREPARATIONS

Type	Preparation	Route	Onset (hr)	Peak (hr)	Duration (hr)	Compatible Mixed with
Fast acting	Regular	SQ	$\frac{1}{2}$–1	2–6	5–8	All preparations
		IM	$\frac{1}{4}$–$\frac{1}{2}$	1–3	2–4	
		IV	$\frac{1}{12}$	$\frac{1}{12}$	$\frac{1}{4}$	
	Prompt zinc (Semilente)	SQ	$\frac{1}{2}$–1	3–9	12–16	Lente
Intermediate	Isophane (NPH)	SQ	1–2	7–12	24–30	Regular insulin
	Insulin zinc suspension (Lente)	SQ	1–3	7–12	24–30	Regular, Semilente
	Globin insulin	SQ	1–4	6–16	16–24	—
Long acting	Protamine zinc	SQ	1–8	12–24	30–36	Regular
	Extended insulin zinc, suspension (Ultralente)	SQ	4–8	10–30	34–46	Regular, Semilente
Mixtures	Regular 30 percent Isophane 70 percent	SQ	See individual components			—

sulin preparations are to be continued during pregnancy, whereas purified preparations are usually prescribed when insulin is required for the first time and when lipoatrophy is found at injection sites. A change to a highly purified preparation may require an initial decrease of up to 20 percent of the original dose. Individual variability in adjustment to a purified insulin preparation is to be expected, especially for those with longstanding diabetes who may have developed appreciable insulin antibodies.[20]

The various insulin products may be safely stored for long periods. Cost differences between the various fast-acting and intermediate-acting preparations are negligible, although purified preparations are more expensive.

Dosing

A rigid control of serum glucose levels ($\leq$ 105 mg percent) and the avoidance of ketoacidosis are desired throughout pregnancy,[16–19,22–25] although this may be difficult to obtain.[26] The dosing of insulin is dependent on periodic glucose determinations using serum glucose determinations by venipuncture or capillary glucose determinations by finger stick using an optical reflectometer (Dextrostix-Eyetone) or enzymatic method (Chemstip, Accuchek bG).[27] These methods offer the advantage of patient participation in a relatively inexpensive manner at home. Urine glucose determinations are less reliable and predictable, because the renal threshold for glucose is decreased during pregnancy.

Regardless of the metabolic control and duration of diabetes, averaged daily insulin requirements are expected to increase twofold from early in pregnancy.[28] Fluctuation in daily insulin requirements are to be expected during the first trimester. The daily dose may remain the same or decrease slightly because of a lower caloric intake before proper instruction or anorexia from nausea of early pregnancy. Following initial hospitalization, insulin requirements often decrease before increasing almost linearly between the second and ninth month of gestation (see Fig. 7–2). This gradual rise in insulin requirements is found to be unaffected by the duration of diabetes and extent of glucose control. The third trimester is characterized by the greatest fluctuation in averaged daily insulin requirements. The doses may increase, plateau, or decrease slightly. This finding may be explained by changes in placental function and alterations in maternal activity and diet.

Split-dose insulin regimens and the mixing of regular with NPH insulin are usually necessary. Ideally, two-thirds of the total dose is usually given in the morning in a ratio of 2:1 NPH to regular insulin. The evening dose is a 1:1 mixture of NPH and regular insulin and given 1 hour before the meal. If control remains inadequate, a three-dose daily schedule (morning–regular, noon–regular, evening–regular with NPH) may be prescribed.[29] The addition of regular insulin with the NPH insulin is often used to control the rapid increase in glucose levels after a meal. The mixing of regular with NPH insulin in a syringe does not appreciably alter their respective onsets and durations of action.

Many factors should be considered when insulin requirements are increased or decreased during pregnancy. Increased insulin requirements may also result from acute infection, drugs (thyroid supplementation, glucocorticoids, diuretics), and certain endocrine disorders (hyperthyroidism, hyperadrenocorticism, hyperparathyroidism). Decreased insulin requirements may result from a degenerating placenta or uteroplacental insufficiency, inactivity, renal disease, inadequate caloric intake, or certain endocrine disorders (hypothyroidism, hypoadrenocorticism). Wide fluctuations in glucose levels may result from errors in management (diet, exercise, insulin administration, glucose determinations) or emotional disturbances.

The management of the diabetic during the intrapartum period is similar to the diabetic about to undergo surgery. Monitoring of the blood glucose level by finger stick or venipuncture every hour is essential, because strict glucose control (80 to 140 mg/dl) is necessary to avoid ketoacidosis from marked hyperglycemia or marked hypoglycemia.[24]

Insulin requirements during labor are expected to decrease during the first stage and increase slightly during the second stage.[30] Glucose control during labor and delivery is achieved by balancing the intravenous infusion of dextrose solutions with minimal or no insulin therapy. The usual dose of NPH insulin is prescribed the evening before induction. Intermittent or continuous regular insulin may then be prescribed the day of induction. Regular insulin may be given intermittently by subcutaneous administration every 4 hours, depending on the capillary or venous glucose values. Disadvantages of this method are the variability and delay in absorption of insulin. Continuous intravenous infusion of regular insulin (25 units regular insulin/250 ml of normal saline or 5 percent dextrose in water) is an alternate method, wherein the onset of action is more rapid and the duration of action is shorter.[31,32] Table 7–3 offers guidelines for adjusting the amount of insulin infused during labor.

The dose of insulin is not dependent on insulin requirements during the antepartum period.[32] Hypoglycemia, detected from blood determinations or maternal complaints of nausea, weakness, or light-headedness, can be reversed quickly by stopping the insulin infusion and maintaining a dextrose infusion.

TABLE 7–3. CONTINUOUS INSULIN INFUSION DURING LABOR

Blood Glucose (mg/100 ml)	Insulin Dosage (U/hr)*	Fluids (125 ml/hr)
<100	0.5	D5/Ringer lactate
100–140	1.0	D5/Ringer lactate
141–180	1.5	Normal saline
181–220	2.0	Normal saline
>220	2.5	Normal saline

* As 25 units of regular insulin in 250 ml normal saline with intravenous line flushed before IVAC administration.

Because insulin infusion must be carefully titrated, a constant infusion pump should be used, beginning at 0.5 to 1 unit "rations" of regular insulin per hour. Irrespective of the use of low-dose insulin, normoglycemia during labor does not necessarily prevent infant morbidity.[32]

When insulin is infused intravenously, it may adhere to the walls of glass or plastic containers and tubing to reduce the actual amount of insulin administered to the patient. Reports of 10 to 80 percent of insulin adhering to the delivery system make it difficult to predict the actual dose being infused, and it is recommended that the tubing and container be primed with an insulin solution.[33]

Following delivery of the placenta, insulin requirements are negligible.[27] Regular insulin is usually administered on a "sliding scale" every 6 hours. The dose is dependent on the glucose concentration (e.g., if 200 to 250 mg percent, give 5 to 10 units, or if 250 to 300 mg percent, give 10 to 15 units). A decrease to two-thirds the average prepregnancy insulin dose or one-third the average dose at 9 months gestation is expected by the third postpartum day.[28] Following the first postpartum week, the mean daily insulin dose should be approximately the same as the prepregnancy dose. It is not until the mother is able to eat solid foods for a full day that intermediate-acting insulin can be prescribed with confidence. Breastfeeding and the route of delivery are not thought to affect insulin requirements with proper nutritional support.

Gestational-onset Diabetes

After gestational-onset diabetes is confirmed by an abnormal GTT, insulin is started when diet alone has failed to properly regulate glucose levels or when a large for gestational age fetus is possible.[34] Monitoring glucose levels is necessary on a daily basis. A purified preparation of intermediate-acting insulin (NPH, Lente) is begun in low doses (10 or 20 units) each morning. A 20-unit dose may be safely prescribed on an outpatient basis if the mother is obese.

Although some patients may be well controlled with a single early morning dose of NPH, most are better controlled with both early morning (two-thirds total daily dose) and early evening doses (one-third total daily dose) one-half hour before meals. This "split-dose" regimen may result in improved glucose control throughout a 24-hour period without an increased risk of hypoglycemia. When converting a patient from one injection to two injections per day, less total daily insulin may be required, resulting in a decreased risk of significant hypoglycemia, particularly in the late afternoon. An additional advantage to the split-dose regimen is that the time of the evening meal can be varied without risk of hypoglycemia. The success of any insulin regimen is dependent upon adherence to a prescribed diet.

Insulin Pumps

Insulin pumps have been used recently during the antepartum period to administer regular insulin continuously.[35–37] This equipment has been used in women who have had great difficulties in adequately controlling glucose levels despite their perseverance and diligence. Continuous subcutaneous insulin infusion has been reported during the fifth through the tenth week to achieve improved diabetic control.[35] Complications with this new therapy declined as experience was gained in teaching the system. The widespread use of subcutaneous insulin pumps most probably will not occur in the near future, and this means for drug delivery will remain primarily a research procedure in specialized centers. Excellent control by intensive conventional therapy with multiple subcutaneous injections is probably as effective. The large size of the pump is a problem, and dislodging of the needle is a frequent concern. Any person on pump therapy needs to be properly motivated and capable of avoiding overinsulinization.

Hypoglycemia

Insulin administered in excess can cause iatrogenic hypoglycemia with a resultant stimulation in endogenous catecholamines (primarily epinephrine), cortisol, glucagon, and growth hormone secretion to raise circulating glucose levels. This rebound hyperglycemic effect (Somogyi phenomenon) usually develops in the morning and may lead to the erroneous administration of more insulin to compound the problem. It is diagnosed by the demonstration of wide fluctuations in serum glucose levels which are unrelated to food intake.

In striving for such metabolic control during pregnancy, insulin-dependent women are at increased risk for developing hypoglycemia.[38] Severe hypoglycemia may result from a failure to release glucagon or lack of warning signs from catecholamine release.[39] Maternal symptoms from severe hypoglycemia include headaches, loss of concentratin, confusion, visual disturbance, stupor, and unconsciousness.[40] Convulsions, coma, and even death may supervene when the unrecognized severe hypoglycemia persists. An infusion of glucose using 25 to 50 ml of a 50 percent glucose solution is used most often to reverse hypoglycemia-induced unconsciousness.

Another accepted therapy in the nonpregnant diabetic person is the injection of glucagon which offers the advantages of ease of administration, rapid action, and potential to avoid hospitalization. It appears that any pregnant woman with a history of altered neurologic states shortly before or during gestation or with repeated capillary blood glucose measurements less than 40 mg percent without any warning adenergic symptoms would benefit from instruction on the use of this medication. Preliminary information at our institution has revealed that reversal of unconciousness has been successful by the subcutaneous or intramuscular injection of a standard 1-ml (1-mg) dose of glucagon by a friend or family member. This reversal of unconciousness should occur within 5 to 20 minutes, and persons should snack to prevent hypoglycemia from recurring.

Antibodies to Insulin

Antibodies to insulin are rarely responsible for glucose intolerance. Insulin resistance is apparent when exogenous insulin demand exceeds 200 units per day and anti-insulin antibodies of IgG type exceed 30 mU/ml. Therapy for this condition usually requires a change in insulin to a monospecies (pork) preparation and may require glucocorticoids in large doses (prednisone 80 mg/day) or a change to Lente, which does not contain protamine.

Diabetic Keto-acidosis

Keto-acidosis is fortunately uncommon in closely regulated patients but may result from profound hyperglycemia and ketosis. Maternal dehydration, acidosis, and potassium depletion and the theoretic adverse effect on fetal CNS development are particular concerns.[41] Along with the appropriate replacement of fluids and electrolytes and the infusion of bicarbonate, insulin administration is necessary.

A protocol used for lowering very elevated serum glucose initially and during a recovery phase is shown in Table 7–4. The desired goal is a serum glucose level of less than 300 mg/100 ml with no urinary ketone bodies. Should there be little or no decline in serum glucose values, a double dose of IV regular insulin (up to 200 units or more) may be necessary within the next 2 hours. Once satisfactory control is achieved, only subcutaneous regular insulin is required using a sliding scale dose regimen. Intermediate-acting insulin may be added the next morning.

Allergic Reactions

Local allergic reactions are found in less than 5 percent of persons using an unpurified beef or pork preparation and usually occur within 1 month after initiation of insulin treatment. Edema, induration, urticaria, and pruritis are presenting signs.[42] Treatment is usually unnecessary, because insulin is destroyed rapidly in the tissues; however, a change in preparation may be necessary and could require a pure preparation. Signs of systematic reactions are rare but include anaphylaxis and generalized urticaria. Therapy requires supportive care.

Lipoatrophy with a loss of subcutaneous

TABLE 7-4. TREATMENT OF DIABETIC KETOACIDOSIS DURING THE INITIAL AND RECOVERY PHASES

	Initial	Recovery
General measures	If patient is comatose, insert nasogastric tube and bladder catheter Identify and treat any precipitating illness such as infection Consider low-dosage heparin Draw arterial blood gases periodically	Remove catheter as soon as possible Continue to search for precipitating or complicating illnesses
Fluids	Begin 0.9% NaCl at 1000 ml/hr Replace sodium deficit in 4–6 hr (average 500 mEq)	When BP is stable, urine output satisfactory, and serum glucose falling, decrease to 0.45% NaCl at 250–500 ml/hr When serum glucose <250 mg/100 ml, add 5% glucose to IV fluids Replace H_2O deficit (average 5–10 liters) over 12–24 hr
Insulin	10–20 U regular insulin IV bolus plus 0.15U/kg/hr constant IV infusion Increase hourly dose if serum glucose does not fall despite adequate fluid therapy	As acidosis is reversed, decrease to 5–10 U every 2–4 hr When patient is eating, restart intermediate acting insulin
Bicarbonate	If pH>7.2, give no bicarbonate If pH 7.0–7.2, ± small amounts (usually 44 mEq and not >88 mEq) If pH>7.0, give as needed to raise pH to 7.0	Give no bicarbonate
Potassium	Measure serum K^+ every 2–4 hr; monitor ECG Begin KCl at 20 mEq/hr	Adjust dose of KCL according to serum K^+ measurements Continue oral KCL replacement for 1 week to correct total deficit
Phosphorus	Measure serum phosphorus and calcium frequently If patient not oliguric, potassium phosphate may be given at 10 mEq/hr (decrease dosage of KCl accordingly)	Give no phosphorus

fat may be minimized by using a purified preparation and rotating the sites of injection. Lipohypertrophy will disappear gradually by avoiding the same injection site.

HYPERTHYROIDISM

Changes in thyroid metabolism during pregnancy relate to increased circulating levels of steroid hormones. The synthesis and release of carrier proteins by the liver are increased during pregnancy from estrogen stimulation. In particular, the serum concentration of thyroid-binding globulin (TBG) increases gradually to twice the nonpregnant value and provides an increased number of sites for thyroid hormone-binding. Although concentrations of total thyroxine (T_4) and tri-iodothyronine (T_3) are increased as early as the second trimester, circulating levels of free T_3 and T_4 are not increased throughout pregnancy because of their 99 percent protein-binding property. The measurement of resin T_3 uptake (RT_3U) is inversely proportional to the number of binding sites on TBG and is therefore found to be decreased during pregnancy. The pituitary glycoprotein required for thyroid stimulation, TSH, is unchanged during pregnancy. Placental transfer is negligible for T_4 and TSH and is poor for T_3.

Fetal thyroid function has been described as early as the end of the first trimester, with circulating levels of T_4 and TBG increasing gradually during the second half of pregnancy.[43] Production of T_3 is primarily by peripheral conversion from T_4 and increases gradually after 30 weeks of fetal life. With the development of neuroendocrine control during the latter half of pregnancy, the negative feedback by thyroid hormones on the fetal pituitary gland is found to eventually mature.

Hyperthyroidism is another common endocrine disorder during pregnancy. Graves' disease is the most common form and is characterized by a diffuse goiter. Toxic nodular goiter and thyroid hyperfunction from excess pituitary TSH secretion are very uncommon. A search for trophoblastic disease (hydatidiform mole, choriocarcinoma) is necessary when biochemical signs of hyperthyroidism are apparent during pregnancy. The signs and symptoms of thyroid hyperfunction include tachycardia, weakness, increased appetite, and shortness of breath and may be difficult to distinguish from the usual patient complaints during pregnancy.

Therapy is necessary to avoid serious maternal and fetal complications. Many patients may become more symptomatic and may develop thyrotoxicosis, which is a medical emergency, especially during labor and delivery. A goiter and hyperthyroidism in the fetus may occur when stimulated by LATS, a long-acting thyroid stimulator of IgG type, which crosses the placenta from the maternal circulation. If maternal hyperthyroidism is untreated, stillbirth rates have been reported to increase to 8 to 15 percent, and premature delivery is considered to be increased to 11 to 25 percent.[44,45]

Guidelines for Therapy

Treatment of hyperthyroidism in the nonpregnant state includes radioactive iodine, medical therapy, and surgical correction. Radioiodine (^{131}I) in therapeutic doses is contraindicated during pregnancy because of its damaging effect in the fetal thyroid after placental transfer. Hypothyroidism in the fetus is also possible, even with a brief course of radioactive iodide.

A subtotal thyroidectomy is reserved for patients who fail on medical management because of poor compliance, severe disease, or need for excessive antithyroid medication. Postoperative complications may include hypothyroidism, hypoparathyroidism, airway obstruction, recurrent laryngeal nerve paralysis, and infection.

Medical therapy of hyperthyroidism is the primary form of treatment during pregnancy. Prescribed medications are intended to decrease the amount of circulating thyroid hormones (antithyroid drugs) and to relieve severely bothersome maternal symptoms (β-adrenergic blocking agents). Hyperthyroidism may be treated effectively during pregnancy using the minimal effective doses. A relative excess of infants with a birth weight less than the 25th centile, goiter, and premature delivery is to be anticipated.[46]

Antithyroid Drugs

Two principal antithyroid preparations have been used to inhibit excess hormone production within the thyroid gland. Propylthiouracil (PTU) and methimazole (Tapazole) are thiourea derivatives that prevent the iodination of tyrosine by inhibiting the oxidation of iodide to iodine (Fig. 7–3). Prophylthiouracil also acts by blocking the conversion of thyroxine to tri-iodothyronine in peripheral tissues. Within the first 24 to 48 hours of therapy, propylthiouracil may also produce a 25 to 40 percent reduction in the peripheral conversion of T_4 to T_3 (which is three to four times more metabolically active than T_4).[47]

Oral absorption is rapid, and the duration of action is moderately short (2 to 3 hours for PTU). The drugs and their metabolites are

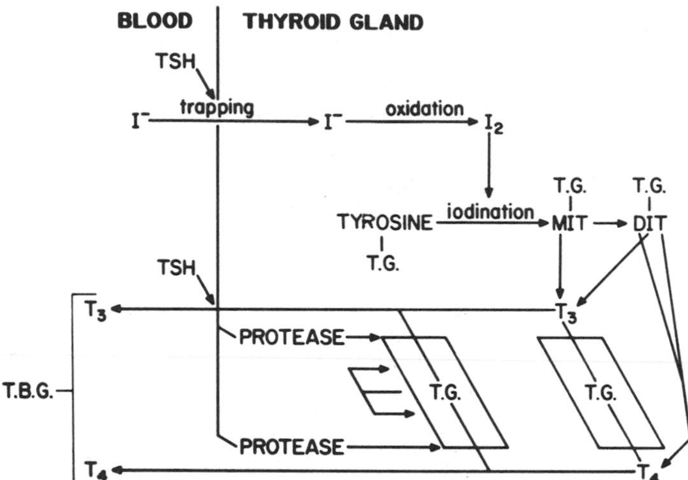

Figure 7–3. Synthetic pathways for hormone production in the thyroid. *(From Gibson M, Tulchinsky D, 1980, with permission.* [50]*)*

eliminated primarily via the kidneys. The placenta is permeable to each drug, but PTU is preferred over methimazole during pregnancy because transfer is less rapid.

Propylthiouracil

Propylthiouracil is available as 50-mg tablets, which are usually prescribed in 100- to 400-mg daily doses (100 mg each day or every 6 hours). Because of the relatively short duration of action, frequent use each day may be necessary. The response of hyperthyroidism to therapy is governed by the long time needed to deplete thyroid stores that may persist until 3 to 6 weeks after the beginning of therapy. The adjustment in daily dosage is begun after this initial period and is dependent on relief of patient symptoms and circulating levels of free T_4. It is preferred that a hyperthyroid woman requiring PTU therapy avoid pregnancy until therapy is unnecessary or only low doses are necessary. To avoid hypothyroidism and to minimize the effective dose necessary, serum-free T_4 levels should be maintained within an upper normal or slightly elevated range during pregnancy. Tapering the dose and even discontinuing the drug are possible and desirable especially late during pregnancy. Daily doses exceeding 300 mg should be avoided because of potential fetal effects.

Side effects, such as nausea, headaches, or jaundice, in the mother from PTU are uncommon and are usually well tolerated. Agranulocytosis is reported to occur in 1 in 500 cases, so a leukocyte count should be determined before therapy and periodically thereafter.[48] Allergic reactions or a mild, sometimes purpuric rash may resolve spontaneously without discontinuing the drug. Arthralgias, especially of the hands and wrist, are very uncommon.

Because of placental transfer, antithyroid substances may impair fetal thyroid function and cause an increase in fetal TSH levels. Goiter formation has been reported in up to 10 percent of all infants and is dependent on the dose and duration of in utero exposure. Neonatal hypothyroidism is short-lived, lasting only a few days.[49] The minimum effective dose to the mother is therefore recommended. Administering the usual 200 to 300 mg/day dose of PTU does not apparently pose a hazard to the fetus. However, the risks to the fetus do not appear to be reduced with low-dose thyroid supplementation to the mother although this has been challenged by Ramsey et al.[50,51]

No other anomaly has been consistently found with antithyroid use, and the perinatal outcome is usually favorable in 70 to 95 percent of the pregnancies. These infants are usually free of clinical evidence for thyroid dysfunction. Thyroxine and TSH usually revert to normal in 5 days.[44,52] In a study involving 28 children with in utero exposure to antithyroid drugs, Burrow found that long-term intellectual development was not impaired when compared to their siblings.[53] The ages of the offspring ranged from 2 to 28 years. Six were born with goiters, four with hypothyroidism, and two with hyperthyroidism.[53,54] If ablative doses of radioactive iodine are inadvertently given during early pregnancy, PTU and saturated solutions of potassium iodine have been given to blunt the fetal uptake of the radioactive isotope.

Most physicians are reluctant to encourage breastfeeding for the mother requiring PTU therapy. This is despite the findings that only 0.025 percent of the dose of propylthiouracil taken by the mother is found in breast milk. No changes in the infant's serum T_4, T_3, TSH, or T_3 uptake levels is to be anticipated.[55] Concentrations are less in breast milk than maternal serum and minimal and presumably insignificant amounts reach the suckling infants.

Methimazole

Methimazole offers no advantage over PTU during pregnancy and may have more adverse effects to the fetus. In comparable doses, methimazole lacks the ability to inhibit peripheral monodeiodination of T_4 to T_3. It is metabolized more slowly and transferred more rapidly across the placenta than PTU. A maldevelopment of the fetal scalp, aplasia cutis, has also been described with methimazole use.[56]

β-Adrenergic Blocking Agents

Tachycardia, tremors, hyperreflexia, and palpitations are frequent findings in hyperthyroidism which relate to enhanced sympathomimetic activity and increased responsiveness to β-adrenergic stimulation (Chap. 12). β-Adrenergic blocking agents are used when these findings are severe. Clinical experience with β-blocking agents has been greatest with propranolol hydrochloride (Inderal). Although not intended to correct the altered metabolism, propranolol may also inhibit the peripheral conversion of T_4 to T_3, thus decreasing the elevated circulating levels of the more metabolically active thyroid hormones.

Propranolol is a naphthyloxy propanolamine derivative, which is absorbed well after any route of administration. Following absorption from the gastrointestinal tract, propranolol is metabolized in the liver. Only a fraction of the original drug remains in the circulation and at least eight metabolites have been detected in the urine. Oral doses of 10 to 30 mg three or four times daily are usually adequate for symptomatic relief. An IV dose of 1 to 3 mg may be given slowly, either during thyrotoxicosis or to avoid thyrotoxicosis before or during an operation. Prolonged use of propranolol is to be avoided, and the dose should be titrated to maintain a maternal pulse of 80 beats/min and to control tremors and nervousness.

Maternal side effects from propranolol use in otherwise healthy women are uncommon and are dose-dependent. Toxic effects may be seen in a variety of tissues but most commonly in the heart. Bradycardia, hypotension, and congestive failure may result from the decrease inotropic, chronotropic, and metabolic effects. These adverse effects are more apparent if a preexisting heart disorder is present. In select cases, propranolol has been used as an antihypertensive agent (Chap. 6), but hypotension is an undesired effect in treating symptoms of hyperthyroidism. Because bronchial spasm is possible, propranolol should be given with caution in any patient with a history of asthma. Propranolol may compete with β_2-adrenergic agents used to inhibit premature labor (Chap. 12) and may increase uterine muscle tone.

Propranolol does cross the placenta, but no congenital anomalies have been linked with its use. The increased incidence of growth-retarded fetuses may be attributable to the underlying medical condition. A mild bradycardia of the fetal heart rate may be observed during the antepartum and intrapartum periods.[57] Propanolol concentrations in the neonate are reported to be 20 percent of the maternal concentrations. Although neonatal glucose, calcium, and electrolyte balance are usually not impaired, hypoglycemia should be suspected. Furthermore, transient neonatal respiratory depression has been associated with intravenous propranolol use prior to anesthesia for cesarean section.[58] The propranolol should be discontinued within 24 hours before delivery to minimize the risk of neonatal metabolic or respiratory complications.

HYPOTHYROIDISM

Thyroid hypofunction is more common than hyperthyroidism in reproductive-age women. It is most apparent following subtotal thyroidectomy; hypothyroidism from iodine deficiency is very unusual. Symptoms of hypothyroidism (myxedema) include increased fatigability, cold intolerance, hyporeflexia, and lethargy. Many patient complaints during pregnancy may overlap with these classical symptoms. Documented hypothyroidism by low free-T_4 levels has been reported to be associated with an increased risk of infertility and an unfavorable perinatal outcome.[59] Whether an impaired intellectual development of the offspring or an increased incidence of spontaneous abortion is more common in hypothyroid pregnant patients remains controversial.[59,60] It is recommended that thyroid supplementation be continued during pregnancy only if laboratory evidence exists and patient symptoms persist.

Thyroid Supplements

Thyroid preparations are used to supplement low serum concentrations of free thyroid hormones. The metabolic rate is increased by several mechanisms to enhance energy-requiring oxidation processes in tissues and to stimulate protein synthesis. Table 7–5 lists thyroid supplements currently available. All products are taken orally and are inexpensive. The two most commonly used preparations, thyroid extract and synthetic levothyroxine sodium, contain thyroxine (T_4). In addition, thyroid extract contains levotriiodothyronine (T_3) in variable concentrations.

Levothyroxine is the preferred drug during pregnancy, as patients seem to tolerate this therapy better than thyroid extract. There are many advantages of ingesting a thyroid supplement with T_4 alone, instead of a combination T_3:T_4 preparation. Thyroxine mimics normal thyroid physiology more closely, and 80 percent of T_3 produced is by peripheral monodeiodination from T_4.[61,62] Serum T_3 levels with combination preparations may fluctuate more, and nonphysiologic concentrations of T_3 are more common.

Fifty to eighty percent of an oral dose of levothyroxine is absorbed. Absorption is decreased by meals, intestinal flora, plasma protein in the gut, and other substances to which thyroxine may bind. Levothyroxine is 99 percent bound to plasma proteins (thyroid-binding globulin, thyroid-binding prealbumin, albumin). Each day, approximately 85 percent of T_4 is converted peripherally to T_3 at many sites, including the liver and kidney. Thyroxine may also be monodeiodinated to form reverse thyronine (RT_3) under such conditions as surgical stress, renal failure, acute or chronic starvation, cirrhosis, or chronic illness. Reverse T_3 is biologically inactive, and patients may remain clinically euthyroid despite low T_3 levels. Thyroxine may also be conjugated in the liver and undergo recirculation in the enterohepatic pathways.

Thyroid supplements do not pass the placental barrier in any appreciable amounts and should have no effect on the autonomous fetal thyroid–pituitary function. Direct administration of levothyroxine into the fetal buttock by the transabdominal route has led to the successful treatment of one fetus thought to be hypothyroid.[63] The only major complication with thyroxine therapy is overdosage, and signs of hyperthyroidism may range from subclinical to overt. Cardiovascular disease is less likely to be exacerbated by thyroxine than by thyroid hormone combinations.

TABLE 7–5. THYROID SUPPLEMENTATION PREPARATIONS

Preparation	Trade Name	Equivalent Dose	T_3 Content	T_4 Content	Comments
Levothyroxine	Synthroid Letter Levoid Levothroid	0.05–0.1 mg	0	100 mcg	Converted to thyronine peripherally. Most physiologic replacement. Long half-life duration
Thyroid extract	Various	60 mg	Variable	Variable	Reputable company standardizes thyroid content. Cheapest, but all products inexpensive. Inactive iodinated protein contamination. Variable potency
Thyroglobulin extract	Proloid	60 mg	Variable	Variable	Inactive iodinated protein removed. Variable potency
Liotrix	Thyrolar	#1 tablet	12.5 mcg	50 mcg	No advantage. Nonphysiologic replacement
	Euthyroid	#1 tablet	15 mcg	60 mcg	
Liothyronine	Cytomel	25 mcg	25 mcg	0	Absorption and onset rapid. Hormone content standardized. Physiologic fluctations with thyrotoxic levels. Expensive. Drug of choice in emergency, such as myxedema coma

The response to thyroid supplementation should therefore be determined by the standard thyroid tests. The dosage of levothyroxine should be such that the TSH level is less than 10 mU/ml. Serum thyroxine levels tend to be high when receiving maintenance thyroxine therapy. This may be explained by differences in potencies between old and new tablets and by the time relation after the tablet was ingested. The pregnant hypothyroid patient may require a higher dose of thyroxine (up to 0.4 mg/day) although 0.1 to 0.2 mg/day remain the standard doses.

OTHER ENDOCRINE DISORDERS

Pregnancies complicated by disorders of the parathyroid, pituitary, or adrenal gland are rare. Medical treatment should be continued during pregnancy, using either the same or lesser doses unless the condition worsens. Disorders involving hormone deficiency or hypofunctional states (hypoparathyroid, hypophysectomy, diabetes insipidus, Addison's disease) require appropriate hormone replacement. Surgery is often the treatment of choice with glandular hyperfunction (Cushing's syndrome, hyperparathyroid, pituitary tumor, insulinoma). Hormonal replacement therapy may be necessary postoperatively. Because of the sparsity of reported cases and the possible adverse fetal effects from drug use, controlled clinical trials comparing different drug regimens are lacking. Literature on the medical management of these rare conditions is therefore limited. Medications used to treat specific endocrinopathies and appropriate references for further reading are listed in Table 7–6.

TABLE 7–6. DRUGS USED IN THE MANAGEMENT OF ENDOCRINE DISORDERS DURING PREGNANCY

Gland	Disorder	Drug	References
Pancreas	Insulinoma	Corticosteroids	64
	Diabetes mellitus	Insulin, glucagon	
Parathyroid	Hypoparathyroidism	Calcium salts	65–67
		Vitamin D	
		Calcitriol	
		Parathormone	
		Phosphate-binding antacids	
	Hyperparathyroidism	Oral phosphates	68,69
Thyroid	Hyperthyroid	Propylthiouracil	
	Hypothyroid	Levothyroxine	
Pituitary	Hypophysectomy	Vasopressin	71
	and	Levothyroxine	70,71
	Sheehan's syndrome	Corticosteroids	70
		Mineralocorticoids	
		Estrogen-progestin	
		Human menopausal gonadotropin	
		Human chorionic gonadotropin	
	Diabetes insipidus	Vasopressin	72
		Diuretics (i.e., ethacrynic acid)	
	Pituitary tumors	Bromocriptine	73–78
		Corticosteroids	
	Acute adrenal failure	Corticosteroids	
Adrenal	Addison's disease	Corticosteroids	79–81
		Mineralocorticoids	
	Cushing's syndrome	None	82–84

REFERENCES

1. Beard RW, Oakley NW: The fetus of the diabetic. In Beard RW, Nathanietz PW (eds): Fetal Physiology and Medicine. London, Saunders, 1976, p 137
2. Pedersen J, Pedersen L, Andersen B: Assessors of fetal perinatal mortality in diabetic pregnancy. Diabetes 23:302, 1974
3. Gabbe S: Diabetes mellitus in pregnancy. In Quilligan E, Kretchmer N (eds): Fetal and Maternal Medicine. New York, Wiley, 1980, pp 587–608
4. Jonanovic L, Peterson M, Saxema B, et al.: Feasibility of maintaining normal glucose profiles in insulin dependent pregnant women. Am J Med 68:105, 1980
5. Karlsson K, Kjellmer I: The outcome of diabetic pregnancies in relation to the mother's blood sugar level. Am J Obstet Gynecol 112:213, 1972
6. Lavin J, Lovelace R, Miodovnik M, et al.: Clinical experience with 107 diabetic pregnancies. Am J Obstet Gynecol 147:742, 1983
7. Aerts L, Assche FA: Ultrastructural changes of the endocrine pancreas in pregnant rats. Diabetologia 11:284, 1975
8. Van Assche FA, Hoeb JJ, Jack PM: The endocrine pancreas of the pregnant mother, fetus, and newborn. In Beard RW, Nathanietz PW (eds): Fetal Physiology and Medicine. Philadelphia, Saunders, 1976, pp 121–136
9. Freinkel N, Metzger BE, Nitzan M, et al.: "Accelerated starvation" and mechanisms for the conservation of maternal nitrogen during pregnancy. Isr J Med Sci 8:426, 1972
10. O'Sullivan JB, Mahan CM: Criteria for the oral glucose tolerance test in pregnancy. Diabetes 13:278, 1964
11. Kitzmiller JL: The endocrine pancreas and maternal metabolism. In Tulchinsky D, Ryan KJ (eds): Maternal–Fetal Endocrinology. Philadelphia, Saunders, 1980, p 58
12. Burt RL, Davidson IW: Insulin half-life and

utilization in normal pregnancy. Obstet Gynecol 43:161, 1974

13. Bellmann O, Hartman E: Influence of pregnancy on the kinetics of insulin. Am J Obstet Gynecol 122:829, 1975
14. Wood GP, Sherline DM: Amniotic fluid glucose: A maternal, fetal, and neonatal correlation. Am J Obstet Gynecol 122:151, 1975
15. Schaeffer LD, Wilder ML, Williams RH: Secretion and contents of insulin and glucagon in human fetal pancreas slices in vitro. Proc Soc Exp Biol Med 143:314, 1973
16. Coustan DR: Recent advances in the management of diabetic pregnant women. Clin Perinatol 7:299, 1980
17. Gugliucci CL, O'Sullivan MJ, Apperman W, et al.: Intensive care of the pregnant diabetic. Am J Obstet Gynecol 125:435, 1976
18. Gyves MT, Rodman HM, Little AB, et al.: A modern approach to management of pregnant diabetics: A two-year analysis of perinatal outcomes. Am J Obstet Gynecol 128:606, 1977
19. Adam PA, Schwartz R: Diagnosis and treatment: Should oral hypoglycemic agents be used in pediatric and pregnant patients? Pediatrics 42:819, 1968
20. Heine RJ, Bilo HJG, Fonk T, et al.: Absorption kinetics and action profiles of mixtures of short- and intermediate-acting insulins. Diabetologia 27:558, 1984
21. Bressler R, Galloway JA: Insulin treatment of diabetes mellitus. Med Clin North Am 55:861, 1971
22. Jonanovic L, Peterson CM: Management of the pregnant, insulin-dependent diabetic woman. Diabetes Care 3:63, 1980
23. Weiss P, Hofmann H: Intensified conventional insulin therapy for the pregnant diabetic patient. Obstet Gynecol 64:629, 1984
24. Frienkel N, Dooley S, Metzger B: Care of the pregnant woman with insulin-dependent diabetes mellitus. N Engl J Med 313:96, 1985
25. Coustan DR, Berkowitz RL, Hobbins JC: Tight metabolic control of overt diabetes in pregnancy. Am J Med 68:845, 1980
26. Leveno J, Hauth JC, Gilstrap LC, et al.: Appraisal of "rigid" blood glucose control during pregnancy in the overtly diabetic woman. Am J Obstet Gynecol 135:853, 1979
27. Sonksen PH, Judd SL, Lowy C: Home monitoring of blood-glucose. Lancet 1:729, 1978
28. Rayburn W, Lewis R, Piehl E: Changes in insulin requirements during pregnancy. Am J Perinatol 2:271, 1985
29. Jovanovic L, Peterson M, Saxema B, et al.: Feasibility of maintaining normal glucose profiles in insulin dependent pregnant women. Am J Med 68:105, 1980
30. Peterson CM, Jovanovic L: Insulin and glucose requirements during the first stage of labor in insulin-dependent diabetic women. Am J Med 75:607, 1983
31. Yeast JD, Porreco RP, Ginsberg HN: The use of continuous insulin infusion for the peripartum management of pregnant diabetic women. Am J Obstet Gynecol 131:861, 1978
32. Golde SH, Good-Anderson B, Montoro M, et al.: Insulin requirements during labor: A reappraisal. Am J Obstet Gynecol 144:556, 1982
33. Whalen FJ, LeCain WK, Latiolais CJ: Availability of insulin from continuous low-dose infusion of insulin. Am J Hosp Pharm 36:330, 1979
34. Coustan DR, Imarah J: Prophylactic insulin treatment of gestational diabetes reduces the incidence of macrosomia, operative delivery, and birth trauma. Am J Obstet Gynecol 150:836, 1984
35. Kitzmiller J, Younger D, Hare J, et al.: Continuous subcutaneous insulin therapy during early pregnancy. Obstet Gynecol 66:606, 1985
36. Rudolf M, Coustan D, Sherwin R, et al.: Efficacy of the insulin pump in the home treatment of pregnant diabetics. Diabetes 30:891, 1981
37. Hertz RH, King KC, Kalhan SC: Management of third-trimester diabetic pregnancies with the use of continuous subcutaneous insulin infusion therapy: A pilot study. Am J Obstet Gynecol 149:256, 1984
38. Unger RH: Meticulous control of diabetes: Benefits, risks, and precautions. Diabetes 31:479, 1982
39. Santiago V, White N, Skor D, et al.: Defective glucose counter-regulation limits intensive therapy of diabetes mellitus. Am J Physiol 246:E 215, 1984
40. Goldwicht C, Stama G, Papoe L, et al.: Hypoglycemia reactions in 172 type I (insulin-dependent) diabetic patients. Diabetologia 24:95, 1985
41. Churchill JA, Berendes HW: Intelligence of children whose mothers had ketonusic during pregnancy. In Perinatal Factors Affecting Human Development (scientific publication no 185). New York, Pan American Health Organization, 1969, p 30
42. Galloway JA, deShazo R: The clinical use of insulin and the complications of insulin ther-

apy. In Ellenberg M and Rifkin H (eds): Diabetes Mellitus, Theory and Practice (3rd ed.). New York, Medical Examination, 1983, pp 519–538
43. Fesher DA, Dussault JH, Sack J, et al.: Ontogenesis of hypothalamic-pituitary-thyroid function and metabolism in man, sheep, and rat. Recent Progr Horm Res 33:59, 1977
44. Talbert LM, Thomas CG, Holt WA, et al.: Hyperthyroidism during pregnancy. Obstet Gynecol 36:779, 1970
45. Worley RJ, Crosby WM: Hyperthyroidism during pregnancy. Am J Obstet Gynecol 119:150, 1974
46. Sugrue D, Drury MI: Hyperthyroidism complicating pregnancy: Results of treatment by antithyroid drugs in 77 pregnancies. Br J Obstet Gynaecol 87:970, 1980
47. Saberi M, Sterling FH, Utiger RD: Reduction in extrathyroidal triiodothyronine production by propylthiouracil in man. J Clin Invest 55:218, 1975
48. Gilman AG, Goodman LS, Gilman A (eds): The Pharmacological Basis of Therapeutics, ed 6. New York, Macmillan, 1980, p 1410
49. Refetoff S, Ochi Y, Selenkow HA, et al.: Neonatal hyperthyroidism and goiter in one infant of each of two sets of twins due to maternal therapy with antithyroid drugs. J Pediatr 85:240, 1974
50. Gibson M, Tulchinsky D: The maternal thyroid. In Tulchinsky D, Ryan KA (eds): Maternal–Fetal Endocrinology. Philadelphia, Saunders, 1980, p 115
51. Ramsay I, Kaur S, Krassas, G: Thyrotoxicosis in pregnancy: Results of treatment by antithyroid drugs combined with T4. Clin Endocrinol 18:73, 1983
52. Mujtaba Q, Burrow GN: Treatment of hyperthyroidism in pregnancy with propylthiouracil and methimazole. Obstet Gynecol 46:282, 1975
53. Burrow GN: Hyperthyroidism during pregnancy. N Engl J Med 298:150, 1978
54. Burrow GN: Thyroid diseases. In Burrow GN, Ferris TF (eds): Medical Complications During Pregnancy. Philadelphia, Saunders, 1975, pp 196–241
55. Kampman J, Hansen P, Johansen J, et al.: Propylthiouracil in human milk. Lancet 1:736, 1980
56. Milharn S, Elledge W: Maternal methimazole and congenital defects in children. Teratology 5:125, 1972
57. Gladstone GR, Harelof A, Gersony WM: Propranolol administration during pregnancy: Effects on the fetus. J Pediatr 86:962, 1975
58. Turnstall ME: The effect of propranolol on the onset of breathing at birth. Br J Anaesth 41:792, 1969
59. Lachelin GC: Myxedema and pregnancy. J Obstet Gynaecol Br Commonw 77:77, 1970
60. Greenman GW, Gabrielson MO, Howard-Flanders J, et al. Thyroid dysfuretion in pregnancy: Fetal loss and follow-up evaluation of surviving infants. N Engl J Med 267:426, 1962
61. Brennan MD: Thyroid hormones. Mayo Clin Proc 55:33, 1980
62. Dong Betty J: Diseases of the thyroid. In Koda-Kimble MA, Katcher BS, Yound LY (eds): Applied Therapeutics for Clinical Pharmacists, ed 2. San Francisco, Applied Therapeutics, Inc., 1978, pp 494–529
63. Van Herle AJ, Young RT, Fisher DA, et al.: Intra-uterine treatment of a hypothyroid fetus. J Clin Endocrinol Metab 40:474, 1975
64. Rubens R, Carlier A, Thiery M, et al.: Pregnancy complicated by insulinoma. Br J Obstet Gynecol 84:543, 1977
65. Goodenday LS, Gordon GS: No risk from vitamin D in pregnancy. Ann Intern Med 75:807, 1971
66. O'Leary JA, Klainer LM, Newwirth RS: The management of hypoparathyroidism in pregnancy. Am J Obstet Gynecol 94:1103, 1966
67. Bolen JW: Hypoparathyroidism in pregnancy. Am J Obstet Gynecol 117:178, 1973
68. Salem R, Taylor S: Hyperparathyroidism in pregnancy. Br J Surg 66:648, 1979
69. Dorey LG, Gell JW: Primary hyperparathyroidism during the third trimester of pregnancy. Obstet Gynecol 45:469, 1975
70. Grimes HG, Brooks MH: Pregnancy in Sheehan's syndrome: Report of a case and review. Obstet Gynecol Surv 35:481, 1980
71. Corral J, Calderon J, Goldzieher JW: Induction of ovulation and term pregnancy in a hypophysectomized woman. Obstet Gynecol 39:397, 1972
72. Pico I, Greenblatt RB: Endocrinopathies and infertility: IV. Diabetes insipidus and pregnancy. Fertil Steril 20:384, 1969
73. Husami N, Jewelewicz R, Vande Wiele RL: Pregnancy in patients with pituitary tumors. Fertil Steril 28:920, 1977
74. Bigazzi M, Ronga R, Lancranjan I, et al.: A pregnancy in an acromegalic woman during bromocriptine treatment: Effects on growth

hormone and prolactin in the maternal fetal and amniotic compartments. J Clin Endocrinol Metab 48:9, 1979

75. Magyar DM, Marshall JR: Pituitary tumors and pregnancy, Am J Obstet Gynecol 132:739, 1978
76. deWit W, Bennik C, Gerards LJ: Prophylactic bromocriptine treatment during pregnancy in women with macroprolactinomas: Report of 13 pregnancies. Br J Obstet Gynaecol 91:1059, 1984
77. Bergh T, Nillius SJ, Wide L: Clinical course and outcome of pregnancies in amenorrhocic women with hyperprolactinaemia and pituitary tumors. Br Med J 1:875, 1978
78. Griffith RW, Turkalj I, Braun P: Pituitary tumours during pregnancy in mothers with bromocriptine. Br J Clin Pharmacol 7:393, 1979
79. Khunda S: Pregnancy and Addison's disease. Obstet Gynecol 39:431, 1972
80. Barber HRK, Graber EA, O'Rourke JJ: Pregnancy and delivery after previous bilateral total adrenolectomy. Obstet Gynecol 27:414, 1966
81. Poorai A, Jelercic F, Pop-Lazic B: Pregnancy with diabetes mellitus, Addison's disease and hypothyroidism. Obstet Gynecol 49(Suppl 86S):865, 1977
82. Grimes EM, Gayez JA, Miller GL: Cushing's syndrome and pregnancy. Obstet Gynecol 42:550, 1973
83. Reschini E, Giustina G, Crosignani PG, et al.: Spontaneous remission of Cushing syndrome after termination of pregnancy. Obstet Gynecol 51:598, 1978
84. Check JH, Caro JF, Kendall B, et al.: Cushing's syndrome in pregnancy: Effect of associated diabetes on fetal and neonatal complications. Am J Obstet Gynecol 133:846, 1979

8

Cardiac Drugs During Pregnancy

Justin P. Lavin, Jr. and Sheldon A. Traeger

Heart disease has been found in 0.9 to 3.7 percent of pregnancies and remains the fourth leading cause of maternal death in the United States.[1,2] Therefore, physicians caring for pregnant women will frequently be called upon to manage persons with cardiac problems during the perinatal period. While an exhaustive review of the cardiovascular changes engendered by pregnancy and cardiac disease complicating pregnancy is beyond the scope of this chapter, a basic understanding of the potential complications resulting from various cardiac lesions is central to the understanding of pharmacologic therapy.

Intravascular volume, heart rate, and stroke volume rise begin early in the pregnancy and reach a peak in the second to early third trimesters. These changes remain relatively stable until term[3–8] and are magnified further during labor, delivery, and immediately postpartum.[7,8] As a result of these physiologic alterations, there is a marked increase in cardiac work and the pregnant cardiac patient is subjected to significantly increased stress. Her prognosis depends on the functional capacity of her heart, the presence or absence of any associated disorders, the quality of her medical care and her social resources.[9]

SPECIFIC CARDIAC DISEASES

Mitral stenosis usually occurs as a result of rheumatic heart disease. The obstructed mitral valve restricts left atrial outflow and subsequently leads to left atrial and left ventricular distention. Physiologic changes of pregnancy may further tax this previously compromised cardiac function, occasioning heart failure and pulmonary congestion.[9–11] Initial therapy consists of bedrest. If this treatment does not suffice, judicious use of diuretics and digoxin may be required.[9] Additionally, distention of the myocardium during pregnancy may predispose to cardiac arrhythmia.[10,11] Atrial arrhythmias are most common[9] and usually treated with a cardiac glycoside.

Mitral insufficiency may result from rheumatic fever, endocarditis, a congenitally abnormal mitral valve, mitral valve prolapse, cardiomyopathy, and rarely from rupture of the chordae tendineae.[9] Congestive changes tend to occur at later ages than with mitral stenosis. Therefore, most women of childbearing age are asymptomatic and tolerate pregnancy well.[9,12] When congestive changes are present, acute deterioration and atrial fibrillation may occur as a result of the additional stress imposed by pregnancy.[13] Women with such changes are usually treated in a similar fashion to that outlined above for mitral stenosis.

Aortic stenosis results in obstruction of left ventricular outflow. This in turn causes increased cardiac work, left ventricular hypertrophy, and increased myocardial oxygen consumption. High maternal and fetal mortality rates have been reported in the association with this lesion.[14] Pregnant women with aortic stenosis rarely develop congestive failure, but angina may occur frequently.[9,13] Labor and delivery are particularly worrisome periods, in that these patients have difficulty in maintaining adequate cardiac output in the face of acute increases in afterload or acute decreases in preload.[9,12,13] Hypertension, fluid overload, or hypotension secondary to blood loss or regional anesthesia must be avoided.

Aortic insufficiency usually results from rheumatic fever, although endocarditis vasculitis, associated collagen vascular disease, and Marfan's syndrome may also lead to this condition. Most patients with aortic insufficiency tolerate pregnancy without difficulty.[9,12,13] However, pulmonary congestion may occur requiring rest, diuretics, and digitalis therapy.

Triscupid and pulmonic valvular disorders are rare during pregnancy and are usually well tolerated.[9,12,13] Severe pulmonary stenosis may result in chest pain, dyspnea, or fatigue.[9] The physiologic changes of pregnancy may exacerbate these symptoms.

All patients with valvular heart disease are at increased risk for bacterial endocarditis if bacteremia should occur at the time of labor and delivery. Patients with a history of rheumatic fever (particularly those with a history of rheumatic heart disease) are at risk for recurrence of this problem during pregnancy.[9,13,15,16]

Congenital cardiac abnormalities occur in 0.8 percent of newborns in the United States.[17,18] Many of these young women are now reaching childbearing age, and presenting for obstetrical care. An atrial septal defect, ventricular septal defect, and patent ductus arteriosus constitute some of the most common congenital cardiac lesions. They are characterized by communications between the left and right sides of the heart. Because of the differential in pressures between the two sides of the cardiac circulation, left-to-right shunting usually occurs. Most lesions are now recognized and repaired in childhood, and most women with these lesions do not experience deterioration during pregnancy.[9,12,13] However, pulmonary congestion, arrhythmia, and emboli may occur.[9] Patients with a ventricular septal defect and patent ductus arteriosus are at increased risk for bacterial endocarditis. This is not true for patients with atrial septal defects.[9,13,15,19] Pulmonary vascular resistance may exceed peripheral vascular resistance as a result of pulmonary vascular disease or pulmonary outflow obstruction and lead to a reversal in the direction of shunt flow with right-to-left shunting (Eisenmenger's syndrome). Patients with this syndrome are at extreme risk with reported maternal mortalities of 30 to 70 percent,[20-22] as are women with primary pulmonary hypertension.[23,24] These women should be counseled to avoid pregnancy, and if pregnancy occurs therapeutic abortion should be recommended.[9]

Coarctation of the aorta involves a narrowing of the aorta at the level of the left subclavian artery. There is usually hypertension in the right arm with normal blood pressure in the left arm and legs. Chest pain and leg fatigue may occur.[9,12,13] Patients with this lesion can be separated into complicated and uncomplicated on the basis of additional associated cardiac valvular lesions.[25] Uncomplicated pregnancies generally progress without difficulty.[12] Complicated patients are at higher risk due to potential rupture of associated intracranial aneurysms and/or aortic dissection.[9,12,25,26] Therapy for the latter group consists of control of hypertension, rest, and β-sympathetic blockers to prophylax against dissection.[9,12] Patients with coarctation of the aorta are at increased risk for endocarditis.[19]

Marfan's syndrome is an autosomal dominant disease characterized by a weakness of connective tissue, and manifested by dislocation of the ocular lens, joint deformities, and dilation of the aortic root.[27] Many patients also have associated abnormalities of the aortic and mitral valves. The major risk associated with pregnancy involves rupture of the aorta. Patients can be segregated into high- and low-risk groups on the basis of associated symptoms, additional valvular lesions, and dilation of the aortic root to greater than 4 cm. Women without these problems are at relatively low risk, and generally tolerate pregnancy without maternal mortality. Patients in the high-risk group have reported maternal mortalities from 30 to 50 percent.[27,28] Therapy for the latter group consists of rest and β-sympathetic blockers.[25,27,28] There appears to be an increased risk of bacterial endocarditis in this disease.

Idiopathic hypertrophic subaortic stenosis is a genetic cardiac disease transmitted in an autosomal dominant fashion. The lesion is associated with dyspnea, chest pain, and an increased risk of sudden death.[9] The hemodynamic changes associated with pregnancy often result in a decrease in outflow obstruction and improvement in symptoms.[9,12] Catecholamines released due to pain or anxiety or hypotension due to venal caval obstruction or blood loss, however, may aggravate outflow obstruction and increase symptomatology.[9] Propranolol may be helpful for the control of symptoms.[9]

Mitral valve prolapse is a very common congenital cardiac abnormality characterized by weakness or redundancy of the mitral valve leaflets with ballooning of the valve into the atrium during ventricular systole.[28] Most patients are asymptomatic, but occasional patients develop chest pain, arrhythmia, and light-headedness. Propranolol is useful for the control of these symptoms.[28,29] Pregnancy does not appear to markedly increase symptomatology nor does mitral valve prolapse appear to exert a deleterious effect on pregnancy.[28,29]

Peripartum cardiomyopathy is an uncommon syndrome in the absence of another etiology for heart failure or underlying heart disease[9,12,30] and is characterized by heart failure in the month before or the 5 months following delivery. The lesion is more common in black women and older women whose pregnancy is complicated by either hypertension or twins.[30] The disease is characterized by cardiomegaly, congestive failure, and thromboembolic phenomenon. Therapy consists of bedrest, diuretics, digoxin, and anticoagulation for patients with thromboembolic phenomenon.

CARDIAC GLYCOSIDES

The cardiac glycosides are steroid or steroid glycoside structures commonly employed for their positive inotropic and antiarrhythmic properties.[31] These and other cardiac drugs are shown in Table 8–1. The physiologic mechanism involved in their positive inotropic activity is not completely understood. Current theories suggest that these drugs increase the availability of calcium[31] and affect Na^+, N^+-activated adenosine triphosphatase (ATPase) inhibition.[32] Their antiarrhythmic properties relate to slowing of conduction through the atrial ventricular node, suppression of ectopic atrial pacemakers, and alterations in reenterant pathways in the atrium.[31,33]

Digoxin is the most commonly used cardiac glycoside. It is available in both oral and parenteral forms. It is intermediate in its duration of action with a half-life of 21 hours.[34,35] The oral form is absorbed in the small intestine.[34] Absorption may be hampered by the concomitant use of cholestyramine, nonabsorbable antacids, or malabsorption syndromes.[31] Drug excretion is primarily renal, and the dosage needs to be decreased in the presence of abnormal renal function.[34] Unless a loading dose is employed, several days of oral therapy are required to reach a steady-state blood level.[31] The usual "digitalizing" dose is 0.75 to 1.25 mg intravenously in divided 0.25 mg increments at 4- to 6-hour intervals. Alternately 1.25 to 2 mg may be administered orally in divided doses. The maintenance dose is 0.25 to 0.50 mg daily.[31] Caution must be employed in patients receiving quinidine or verapamil because of an associated increase in plasma levels,[31,36] so monitoring serum digoxin levels may be useful in patients receiving quinidine or verapamil or in patients with compromised renal function.

Digitoxin is a second cardiac glycoside with a longer duration of action and half-life of 4 to 6 days.[31] It is primarily excreted by the liver and therefore is particularly useful in patients with impaired renal function.[31] The usual "digitalizing" dose is from 0.70 to 1.20 mg orally or 1 mg intravenously in divided doses over 24 hours. The usual maintenance dose is 0.10 to 0.20 mg daily.[31]

Ouabain is poorly absorbed, but possesses a rapid onset of action (5 to 10 minutes) after intravenous administration. It is particularly useful in emergency situations when rapid action to control cardiac arrhythmias is required.[31] Its half-life is similar to that of digoxin. The excretion of ouabain occurs in both genitourinary and gastrointestinal tracts.[31] The usual "digitalizing" dose is 0.30 to 0.50 mg, and the usual maintenance dose is approximately 0.10 mg every 4 hours.[31]

Toxicity occurs frequently with all the cardiac glycosides. Manifestations include cardiac rhythm disturbances, nausea, vomiting, headache, and neurologic disturbances.[35-37] Toxicity is more common in the presence of hypoxia, as electrolyte (especially hypokalemia) and acid-base disturbances, so particular caution is warranted in these clinical situations.[31]

The primary uses of the cardiac glycosides during pregnancy are for treatment of pulmonary congestion unresponsive to rest and diuretics. These agents are most useful for the treatment of supraventricular tachycardias and rate control in atrial fibrillation and atrial flutter.[38] There have also been occasional reports of successful transplacental fetal cardioversion employing the cardiac glycosides,[38-40] although other attempts have been unsuccessful.[39,41] A limiting factor appears to be the occurrence of maternal toxicity before the establishment of a fetal therapeutic level.

The cardiac glycosides have been clearly demonstrated to cross the placenta.[42-46] With the exception of rare reports,[47,48] no adverse fetal effects have been noted.[31] Digoxin has been demonstrated to be secreted in the breast milk, but the concentration is low and the clinical effects on the infant are probably minimal.[31]

By reducing the impedance to left ventricular ejection and/or by reducing venous return, vasodilators can dramatically reverse signs and symptoms of heart failure such as peripheral and pulmonary edema and exercise intolerance.[49] Nitrates, prazosin hydrolazine, captopril, or nitroprusside can be used to treat severe heart failure refractory to more conventional therapy. There has been little experience with their use in pregnancy, however, and there are theoretical concerns that their effects on arterial and venous tone might compromise uterine and placental blood flow.[50]

ANTIARRHYTHMIA DRUGS

β-Adrenergic Blockers

Arrhythmias may occur during pregnancy in patients with pre-existing valvular, congenital, or ischemic cardiac lesions. They may also occur in patients who develop myocarditis and in patients with underlying endocrinopathies.[38,51] The cardiac glycosides and β-sympathetic blockers are the agents most widely used to combat these abnormal rhythms.[9,12,31,38,51] Several other antiarrhy-

TABLE 8–1. CARDIAC DRUGS UTILIZED DURING PREGNANCY

Drug	Primary Use	Loading Dose	Maintenance Dose	Excretions
Digoxin	Paroxysmal supraventricular tachyarrhythmia; rate control in atrial fibrillation	0.75–1.25 mg intravenously in 0.25-mg increments at 4–6 hr intervals 1.25–2.0 mg orally in increments at 4-6 hr intervals	0.25–0.50 mg daily, orally	Renal
Digitoxin	Same as digoxin	1.0 mg intravenously *or* 0.7–1.2 mg orally in divided doses over 24 hr	0.1 mg–0.2 mg daily, orally	Hepatic
Ouabain	Rapid control in severe arrhythmias similar to other cardiac glyco	0.3–0.5 mg intravenously	0.1 mg intravenously every 4 hr	Renal Gastrointestinal
Propanolol	Atrial and ventricular premature beats; reentrant ventricular and supraventricular tachyarrhythmia; rate control in atrial flutter and fibrillation	0.05 mg–0.15 mg/kg intravenously by slow infusion; no more than 0.15 mg/kg should be administered in a 6 hr period	40–160 mg daily in 3–4 divided doses, orally	Hepatic renal
Disopyramide	Similar to quinidine	200–300 mg orally	400–800 mg daily, divided dose	Hepatic
Phenytoin	Supraventricular and ventricular arrhythmia due to digitalis toxicity	100 mg intravenously every 5 min until arrhythmia controlled or adverse effects occur; total dose should not exceed 1,000 mg/24 hr 1,000 mg in divided doses orally over 24 hr	500 mg orally in divided dose	Hepatic
Verapamil	Paroxysmal supraventricular tachyarrhythmia; rate control in atrial fibrillation	5–10 mg over 2–3 min; intravenous dose; may be repeated in 30 min if arrhythmia remains unchanged	80–120 mg 3–4 times daily, orally	Hepatic

Half-life	Potential Maternal Side Effects	Potential Fetal Side Effects	Secreted in Breast Milk
36–38 hr	Cardiac rhythm disturbance, nausea, vomiting, headache, neurologic disturbance	None noted	Yes In low concentration; no adverse effects noted
4–6 days	Same as digoxin	None noted	Unknown
21 hr	Same as digoxin	None noted	Unknown
3–4 hr	Cardiac depression, bradycardia, drowsiness, interference with diabetic control, aggravation of bronchoconstrictor disease	No teratogenic bradycardia, hypoglycemia, respiratory depression, possible IUGR	Minimal
6–7 hr	Cardiac depression, arrhythmia, hypotension	Few reports uncertain, possible premature labor	Yes Little information available
Varies with patient's hepatic metabolism	Hypotension, bradycardia, nystagmus, lethargy, ataxia, hepatic injury, megoblast anemia, peripheralic neuropathy	Hydantoin syndrome; depression of vitamin K-dependent coagulation factors	In low concentration Neonatal usually no effect Enzyme induction possible
3–7 hr	Hypotension bradycardia, cardiac failure, asystole nausea, constipation, headache, dizziness	Uncertain; no adverse effects in the few patients reported, hypoxia and acidosis have been reported in animals treated with other calcium channel blockers	Unknown

(continued)

TABLE 8-1. (*Continued*)

Drug	Primary Use	Loading Dose	Maintenance Dose	Excretions
Lidocaine	Ventricular tachyarrhythmias, arrhythmias due to digitalis toxicity	1-1.4 mg/kg intravenously If arrhythmia not resolved in 10-20 min, ½ original loading dose may be repeated	1-4 mg/min intravenously	Hepatic
Quinidine	Paroxysmal atrial tachyarrhythmias, prophylaxis for atrial and ventricular arrhythmias	Not appropriate	1-2 g per day in twice daily dosage	Hepatic Renal
Procainamide	Treatment of prophylaxis and for atrial and ventricular tachyarrhythmias	100 mg intravenously over 4-5 min; may be repeated at 10 min intervals until arrhythmia controlled or total dose of 1000 mg given	2-6 mg/min intravenously, *or* 2-6 g daily orally by divided dose at 3-4 hr intervals	

thmic agents, however, may be required and are discussed here.

The pharmacology and maternal-fetal side effects of the β-adrenergic blockers have been described in Chapter 6 dealing with hypertension. While there is theoretical advantage to the use of metaprolol because of its selective β-1 blockade, only the use of propanolol has been reported in pregnant cardiac patients. The major indications for the use of this medication in such patients include control of coexistant hypertension,[9] control of cardiac arrhythmias including premature atrial and premature ventricular beats, supraventricular and ventricular tachycardias, and reduction of ventricular response in patients with atrial fibrillation and atrial flutter.[38] Propanolol is also useful for the reduction of cardiac output and pulse pressure to prevent aortic dissection in patients with coarctation of the aorta and Marfan's syndrome,[9,12,27] and to reduce outflow obstruction and control of symptoms in patients with idiopathic hypertropic subaortic stenosis.[9,12]

Lidocaine

Lidocaine, an amide-linked local anesthetic, is the drug of choice for the control of acute ventricular tachycardia and arrhythmias from digitalis toxicity.[38] Administration must be parenteral because of poor oral absorption.[38] The onset of action is nearly immediate. Drug elimination occurs by hepatic metabolism. A decrease in concentration usually begins within 10 to 20 minutes, and half-life is usually 100 minutes.[38,52]

To achieve rapid antiarrhythmic effect, lidocaine is usually administered with a loading dose from 1 to 1.4 mg/kg intravenously. If the arrhythmia is not terminated in 10 minutes, administration of one-half the loading

Half-life	Potential Maternal Side Effects	Potential Fetal Side Effects	Secreted in Breast Milk
100 min	Anxiety, confusion, myocardial depression, hypotension, seizure, respiratory arrest	No teratogenic; mild transient neurobehavioral depression, if fetus acidotic may cause neonatal depression	Yes No adverse effects noted
4–8 hr	Nausea, vomiting, dizziness, vertigo, depressed synthesis of vitamin K-dependent vitamins	No teratogenic; rare cases of premature labor	Yes Hepatic accumulation in premature infants
Varies with patients rate of acetylation	Liver injury, psychosis (+) ANA titers lupus-like syndrome	Uncertain	Unknown

dose may be repeated. The loading dose should be followed by a maintenance dose between 1 and 4 mg/min with subsequent infusion rates titrated to plasma levels. The appropriate therapeutic range is from 2 to 4 mcg/ml.[53] Maternal side effects due to lidocaine are rare,[38] at therapeutic concentrations. If toxic levels are reached, a typical local anesthetic toxicity reaction consisting of anxiety, confusion, myocardial depression, hypotension, respiratory arrest, and seizures may occur.[54]

Potential fetal side effects from lidocaine have been well studied and reported in the obstetrical anesthesia literature (Chap. 14). At unusually high maternal plasma concentrations, this agent may cause uterine artery constriction. However, this effect has not been noted at therapeutic concentrations.[59] Lidocaine crosses the placenta,[55–57] and fetal concentrations are usually half simultaneously obtained maternal concentrations.[58,59] The drug half-life in the fetus is usually 3 hours.[59] Lidocaine is a weak base and if the fetus is acidotic, ion trapping may occur with higher fetal concentrations.[60–62] There is no known teratogenic effect from lidocaine exposure in early pregnancy.[38] Subtle neurobehavior changes, however, have been noted among infants whose mothers have received this drug as a regional anesthetic agent (Chap. 14).[38]

Quinidine

Quinidine is the d-isomer of quinine. Its use as an antiarrhythmic agent was based on the fortuitous observation that it occasionally relieved atrial fibrillation in patients treated for malaria.[63] Quinidine is employed chiefly to control paroxysmal atrial tachycardia, atrial fibrillation, and atrial flutter. It is useful for the long-term prophylaxis against recurrence of these arrhythmias and ventricular tachycardias due to Wolfe-Parkinson-White syndrome.[38] Quinidine is well absorbed orally. Quinidine's onset of action is within 30 minutes.[38] The maintenance dose varies from 1 to 2 g per day.[38] The half-life ranges from 4 to 8 hours. Therefore, sustained released preparations and twice daily dosage are usually employed for long-term therapy.[38] Blood drug levels are helpful in determining proper dosage. Plasma levels of 2 to 5 mcg/ml are adequate for prophylaxis,[38] and levels of 4 to 9 mcg/ml may be required to affect conversion of atrial fibrillation.[64] It is metabolized primarily in the liver, although significant renal metabolism occurs.[38]

Maternal side effects are quite common. Nausea, vomiting, dizziness, and vertigo necessitate the cessation of therapy in up to one-fourth of patients receiving quinidine.[38] Hypersensitivity reactions may occur,[65,66] and toxic levels are associated with cardiac arrhythmias.[38] The synthesis of K-dependent vitamins is suppressed, and any simultaneous use of anticoagulants may cause severe clotting deficiencies.[67] Concomitant use of cardiac glycosides may result in elevated levels of the latter drugs and subsequent digitalis toxicity.[68,69]

Quinidine crosses the placenta easily, and maternal and neonatal plasma concentrations are nearly identical.[70,71] Infants of mothers taking this drug have been reported to have congenital anomalies. Given the widespread use of quinine compounds in the treatment of malaria and the low incidence of anomalies, however, it is quite unlikely that there is a significant teratogenic risk.[72] Quinidine has also been reported to exert a mild oxytocic effect, and rare cases of premature labor have been reported in association with quinidine administration.[73] Despite the aforementioned potential problems, evidence would suggest overwhelmingly that this drug can be employed with relative safety during pregnancy.[38] Quinidine is secreted in breast milk, and prolonged exposure has been reported to result in hepatic accumulation in the premature neonate.[70]

Procainamide

Procainamide is a second antiarrhythmic agent considered by most investigators to be very similar in clinical activity to quinidine.[38] Its greatest benefit is in the treatment and prevention of ventricular arrhythmias.[38] This drug may be administered either intravenously or orally. A 100-mg bolus may be given intravenously over 4 minutes for rapid control of the arrhythmia. The dose may be repeated every 5 minutes until the arrhythmia resolves or a 1000-mg total dose is reached.[74] Once the arrhythmia is corrected, intravenous infusion of 2 to 6 mg per minute should maintain therapeutic levels (3 to 10 mcg/ml).[75] Blood pressure, electrocardiographic monitoring, and measurement of blood drug levels are appropriate during intravenous administration. Oral maintenance requires a total daily dose of 2 to 6 g at dosing intervals of 3 to 4 hours. Longer dosing intervals may be appropriate in patients with serious cardiac disease in which there is a longer half-life of elimination.[76] A sustained release preparation is available for every 6-hour administration in those patients with normal elimination of procainamide.[76]

Very little information has been published regarding the placental and fetal metabolism of procainamide or the drug's effects on fetus and neonate.[77] Given the known adverse effects of lupus on pregnancy and the high incidence of positive ANA titers and a clinical lupus-like syndrome with the long-term use, procainamide is probably best avoided during pregnancy unless therapy with other safer and more commonly used antiarrhythmic drugs fails.[78-79]

Disopyramide

Disopyramide is a new antiarrhythmic agent with similar electrophysiologic properties and clinical indications to quinidine.[38] Only a few patients have been reported to have been treated with this drug during pregnancy.[80,81] Therefore, it would seem appropriate to restrict the use of this agent in pregnancy to those cases where more traditional compounds have been unsuccessful.

Phenytoin

The pharmacology and potential teratogenesis of phenytoin has been discussed in Chapter 9 dealing with antiseizure medications. Because of the teratogenic risk, this agent is usually best avoided during pregnancy, but may be required occasionally for arrhythmias caused by digitalis toxicity that do not respond to lidocaine.

Verapamil

Verapamil is papaverine derivative, calcium channel blocker developed originally as an antianginal agent, but also found to be effective in the control of superventricular arrhythmias.[38] Verapamil is well absorbed orally, although it may also be administered intravenously. It is metabolized in the liver and its half-life ranges from 3 to 4 hours.[38,82] For the rapid treatment of supraventricular arrhythmias, 5 to 10 mg is administered intravenously over 2 to 3 minutes and may be repeated in 30 minutes if the first dose is unsuccessful.[83] Blood pressure and electrocardiographic monitoring is required during intravenous administration. Oral doses of 80 to 120 mg, three to four times per day are employed for long-term prophylaxis.[38]

Potential maternal side effects include hypotension, bradycardia, cardiac failure, asystole, and occasional nausea, vomiting, constipation, and dizziness.[38] Little information has been published relating to the use of this drug for the treatment of maternal cardiac disease.[84,85] Some information is available relating to the use of calcium channel blockers as tocolytic agents. Some investigators have suggested relative fetal safety using other calcium channel blockers,[86] while others have observed declining oxygen and pH levels with prolonged administration in an animal model.[87] As with the other newer antiarrhythmic agents, it would seem appropriate to confine the use of this drug to patients who do not respond to more traditional medications.

If pharmacologic cardioversion fails or if a woman is severely hemodynamically unstable and requires rapid therapy, electrocardioversion has been employed in several instances with apparent safety.[9,12,38]

TREATMENT OF ISCHEMIC HEART DISEASE

Coronary artery disease is rare in women of childbearing age. Hankins and coinvestigators have recently reviewed the literature and found 70 cases of myocardial infarction during pregnancy.[88] The occurrence of ischemic heart disease may become more common with the current tendency to delay pregnancy until more advanced maternal ages. Additionally, the incidence of angina complicating pregnancy is much higher than that of acute myocardial infarction.[89,90]

Medical treatment of patients with coronary artery disease consists of a change in life style and an avoidance of precipitating factors.[88] If angina still persists the most commonly employed therapy involves the use of organic nitrates.[89] These agents exert their beneficial effect by relaxing smooth muscle. This in turn leads to a reduction of ventricular filling, reduction in ventricular wall tone, and decrease in myocardial oxygen consumption.[89] These compounds may also cause coronary artery dilation with increased blood flow and oxygen delivery.[83]

Nitroglycerin administered sublingually in a dose of 0.20 to 0.40 mg is the drug of choice for an acute anginal attack. This dose may be repeated at 5-minute intervals until the attack has subsided or three doses have been given. Longer acting preparations with durations of action of 2 to 4 hours are available for prolonged therapy. Side effects include headache, flushing, postural hypertension, and tachycardia.[89]

β-adrenergic blockers may also be useful for patients with coronary artery disease. They decrease oxygen consumption by decreasing the heart rate, blood pressure, and myocardial contractility.[89]

Calcium channel blockers have also been proven to be effective in the control of angina.[89] Their mode of action results from a decrease in the transport of calcium in vascular smooth muscles leading to relaxation of coronary smooth muscles and subsequent vasodilation.[89] These agents also exert a negative inotropic effect on the myocardium.[89] As noted in the previous section, there has been little published information regarding the use of calcium channel blockers during pregnancy, and their use is probably best avoided unless more traditional medications fail.

ANTICOAGULANTS AND PROSTHETIC CARDIAC VALVES

The introduction of prosthetic valves in 1952 revolutionized the treatment of many forms of cardiac disease. Young women who have undergone valve replacement are now becoming pregnant, and over 150 such pregnancies have been reported.[90] Thromboembolic phenomena represent the most important late complication, and most authorities believe that long-term anticoagulant therapy is required,[91] except for those patients with porcine valves. Two forms of anticoagulation, warfarin-like compounds or heparin are available. Only heparin is recommended preconceptually and during pregnancy because of fetal concerns with warfarin use.

Warfarin crosses the placenta easily.[92,93] First trimester exposure results in a well-recognized syndrome including nasal hypoplasia, chondrodysplasia punctata, and mental retardation in up to 10 percent of exposed fetuses.[72] Exposure during the second and third trimesters has been associated with intracranial hemorrhage and other neurologic disorders.[94] Warfarin is secreted in breast milk, but concentrations do not appear to cause a significant anticoagulation effect in the neonate.[93]

Heparin is highly negatively charged and has a large molecular weight. Because of these properties, it does not cross the placenta.[92,93] There is no oral heparin preparation and intramuscular administration is painful and poorly absorbed. Administration must be given intravenously or subcutaneously. The drug exerts its anticoagulant effect by accelerating the action of plasma antithrombin Factor III and inhibiting the intrinsic coagulation pathway.[93] Metabolism occurs in both the kidneys and liver.[92,93]

The most common maternal complication is bleeding which occurs in from 5 to 10 percent of patients.[93,94] Significant heparin-induced hemorrhage can be reversed by the use of protamine sulfate. The latter drug is given by intravenous push over approximately 30 minutes. A 1-mg dose will reverse 100 units of heparin immediately after the latter drug's administration. The dose should be reduced by 50 and 75 percent, respectively, if 1 or 2 hours have transpired since heparin administration.[93] Thrombocytopenia is also a relatively frequent side effect of heparin administration occurring in 5 to 30 percent of patients.[93-97] The mechanism by which this complication occurs is poorly understood, but it is felt to be immunologic.[93,94] Osteoporosis can also occur with long-term subcutaneous administration.[92,93] It was thought to be unlikely in pregnant women,[98] but recently this phenomenon has been reported to occur during pregnancy.[99]

While heparin does not cross the placenta, Hall et al. have described a 12 percent prevalence of stillbirth and 20 percent frequency of prematurity among 135 reported cases of infants whose mothers were treated with this medication during gestation.[94] Since there was no control group of similar patients who were not treated, it was unclear whether these adverse fetal and neonatal outcomes related to the drug or the underlying maternal diseases for which the drug was administered.

Heparin is usually administered subcutaneously in a dose of 150 to 250 U/kg every 12 hours.[100] With the onset of labor the omission of one or two doses prior to delivery or the administration of minidoses (5000 U q 12 h) usually allows adequate hemostasis. In emergency situations or while administering regional anesthetics, Saka and Marx have suggested that protamine reversal be employed.[101] Heparin therapy may be reinstituted 6 hours after delivery and continued for 48 to 72 hours. For long-term effect, warfarin therapy may be reinstituted on the 3rd or 4th postpartum day.

ANTIBIOTIC PROPHYLAXIS

Bacterial Endocarditis

Patients with valvular or severe forms of congenital heart disease are at increased risk to develop bacterial endocarditis if they experience bacteremia (Table 8–2).[9–12,15,19] The American Heart Association suggests that such patients receive antibiotic prophylaxis to prevent bacterial endocarditis before certain diagnostic and surgical procedures.[16] The incidence of bacteremia following parturition has been reported to vary from 0 to 5 percent.[102,103] No controlled study has proved that such prophylaxis has effectively reduced the incidence of bacterial endocarditis at the time of parturition.[19] Women with artificial prosthetic valves are at very high risk for the development of bacterial endocarditis, which may be devastating, and most investigators suggest that such women should receive antibiotic prophylaxis at the time of labor and delivery.[9,12,13,15,16] Opinion regarding routine prophylaxis for uncomplicated vaginal delivery in other patients at risk remains controversial. Some investigators favor this approach,[9,12,13,16,104,105] while others suggest it may be unnecessary and lead to unwarranted fetal drug exposure or predispose to the development of bacterial endocarditis due to resistant organisms.[106–108] If special risks occur, however, e.g., chorioamnionitis or cesarean section, most authors suggest antibiotic prophylaxis be employed.[19] When antibiotic prophylaxis is utilized the recommendations of the American Heart Association (Table 8–3) should be followed.[16]

TABLE 8–2. CARDIAC DISORDERS ASSOCIATED WITH INCREASED RISK OF BACTERIAL ENDOCARDITIS

Prosthetic valves
Valvular disease
Ventricular septal defect
Patent ductus arteriosus
Idiopathic subaortic hypertrophic stenosis
Mitral valve prolapse
Marfan's syndrome
Coarctation of the aorta

TABLE 8–3. DRUG REGIMEN FOR BACTERIAL ENDOCARDITIS PROPHYLAXIS

Aqueous penicillin (2 million units or ampicllin 1g, both IV or IM) plus gentamicin (1.5 mg/kg IM or IV) or streptomycin (1 g IM) 0.5–1 hr prior to the procedure.

If gentamicin is used, repeat the dose of penicillin or ampicillin and gentamicin every 8 hr for 2 additional doses.

If streptomycin is used, give penicillin or ampicillin with streptomycin every 12 hr for 2 additional doses after the procedure.

If the patient is allergic to penicillin, vancomycin (1 g IV infused over 30 min) about 1 hr prior to the procedure and gentamicin or streptomycin as above can be used. The same dose of these agents may be repeated in 8–12 hr for 2 more doses.

Rheumatic Fever

Most authorities recommend that patients with prior rheumatic fever, especially those with a history of rheumatic heart disease, should continue to receive prophylaxis during pregnancy to prevent recurrence.[9,12,13,19] The American Heart Association recommendations are the most widely accepted.[16] The most effective prophylaxis involves a monthly injection of 1.2 units of benzathene penicillin.

If this treatment is unacceptable due to pain or difficulty with patient compliance, oral penicillin G 200,000 units twice daily or penicillin V 250 mg twice daily or sulfadiazine, 1 g daily may be employed. There is a theoretical risk of competition for bilirubin-binding sites and neonatal hyperbilirubinemia with the latter medication, so penicillin is the most appropriate medication for those not allergic. In rare patients allergic to both penicillin and sulfadiazine, erythromycin 250 mg twice daily may be used.[9-15,19]

ADVERSE DRUG INTERACTIONS DURING PREGNANCY

β-adrenergic drugs including ritodrine, terbutaline, and isoxsuprine are commonly used to inhibit premature labor. These agents exert powerful inotropic effects of the myocardium.[109] Their use is associated with tachycardia, widened pulse pressure, and chest pain.[110] Rare cases of pulmonary edema have been recorded.[111] Because of the side effects, β-adrenergic drugs are relatively contraindicated in patients with cardiac disease. Magnesium sulfate may provide a more appropriate tocolytic agent in selected cases.

Oxytocin is used to induce and augment labor and to decrease blood loss at the time of delivery. While gradual infusion is usually safe, acute bolus injection may cause transient hypotension and should be avoided.[112] Ergonovine and methylergonovine maleate may cause acute hypertension imposing increased afterload and significant stress on the compromised myocardial function. It should therefore be avoided in patients with cardiac disorders.[112]

Intravenous fluids during labor and delivery must be carefully regulated to avoid both fluid overload and hypotension. In patients with mild to moderate disease, a solution such as D5 0.45 NaCl at 100 to 150 ml/hr is usually appropriate. Invasive monitoring with a Swan–Ganz catheter may facilitate management for women with more severe disease or cardiac failure.[113,114]

A full discussion of the various anesthetic techniques appropriate for the pregnant cardiac is beyond the scope of this chapter. Significant care, however, must be exercised in selecting the appropriate agent. The interested reader is referred to Joyce's excellent review.[115]

REFERENCES

1. Payne D, Fishburne J, Ruffy A, et al.: Bacterial endocarditis in pregnancy. Obstet Gynecol 60:247, 1982
2. Sullivan J, Ramanthan K: Management of medical problems: Severe cardiac disease. N Engl J Med 313:304, 1985
3. Hytten F, Paintin D: Increases in plasma volume during normal pregnancy. J Obstet Gynaecol Br Commonw 70:422, 1963
4. Pritchard J: Changes in the blood volume during pregnancy and delivery. Anesthesiology 26:293, 1965
5. Rovinsky J, Jaffin H: Cardiovascular hemodynamics in pregnancy. I. Blood and plasma volumes in multiple pregnancy. Am J Obstet Gynecol 93:1, 1965
6. Metcalfe J, Ueland K: Maternal cardiovascular adjustments to pregnancy. Prog Cardiovasc Dis 16:363, 1974
7. Ueland K, Gillis R, Hansen J: Maternal cardiovascular dynamics, I. Cesarean section under subarachnoid anesthesia. Am J Obstet Gynecol 100:42, 1968
8. Ueland K, Hansen J: Maternal cardiovascular dynamics, III. Labor and delivery under local and caudal analgesia. Am J Obstet Gynecol 103:8, 1969
9. McAnulty J, Metcalfe J, Ueland K: Cardiovascular disease. In Burrow G, Ferris T (eds): Medical Complications During Pregnancy, ed. 2. Philadelphia, Saunders, pp 145–168, 1982
10. Szekely P, Snaith L: Heart Disease and Pregnancy. Edinburgh, Churchill Livingstone, 1974
11. Szekely P, Turner R, Snaith L: Pregnancy and the changing pattern of rheumatic heart disease. Br Heart J 35:1293, 1973
12. Sullivan J, Ranathan K: Cardiovascular disorders. In Brundenell M, Wilds P (eds): Medical and Surgical Problems in Obstetrics. Bristol, John Wright, pp 11–28, 1984
13. Ueland K: Rheumatic heart disease and pregnancy. In Elkayam V, Gleicher N (eds): Cardiac Problems in Pregnancy Diagnosis and Management of Maternal and Fetal Disease. New York, Alan R Liss, pp 79–96, 1982
14. Arias F, Pineda J: Aortic stenosis and pregnancy. J Reprod Med 20:229, 1978
15. Johnstone W, Elkayam V: Infection endocarditis on pregnancy. In Elkayam V, Gleicher N (eds): Cardiac Problems in Pregnancy Diagnosis and Management of Maternal and Fe-

tal Disease. New York, Alan R Liss, pp 131–140, 1982
16. Kaplan E, Anthony B, Durack D, et al.: Prevention of bacterial endocarditis. Circulation 56:139A, 1977
17. Mitchell S, Korones S, Berendes H: Congenital heart disease in 56,109 births: Incidence and natural history. Circulation 43:323, 1971
18. Nora J, Nora A: The evolution of specific genetic and environmental counseling in congenital heart diseases. Circulation 57:205, 1978
19. Cesario T: Antibiotic therapy in pregnancy. In Elkayam V, Gleicher N (eds): Cardiac Problems in Pregnancy Diagnosis and Management of Maternal and Fetal Disease. New York, Alan R Liss, pp 289–304, 1982
20. Jones A, Howitt G: Eisenmenger syndrome in pregnancy. Br Med J 1:1627, 1965
21. Neilson G, Galea E, Blunt A: Eisenmenger's syndrome and pregnancy. Med J Aust 1:1086, 1970
22. Pelletier L Jr, Petersdorf R: Infective endocarditis: A review of 125 cases from the University of Washington Hospital, 1963–1972. Medicine 56:287, 1977
23. McCaffrey R, Dunn L: Primary pulmonary hypertension in pregnancy. Obstet Gynecol Surv 19:567, 1964
24. Neilson J, Fabricius J: Primary pulmonary hypertension with special reference to prognosis. Acta Med Scand 170:731, 1961
25. Cobb T, Gleicher N, Elkayam V: Congenital heart disease in pregnancy. In Elkayam V, Gleicher N (eds): Cardiac Problems in Pregnancy Diagnosis and Management of Maternal and Fetal Disease. New York, Alan R Liss, pp 61–68, 1982
26. Pyeritz R: Maternal and fetal complications of pregnancy in the Marfan syndrome. Am J Med 71:784, 1981
27. Ferguson J, Ueland K, Stinson E, et al.: Marfan's syndrome: Acute aortic dissection during labor, resulting in fetal distress and cesarean section followed by successful surgical repair. Am J Obstet Gynecol 147:759, 1983
28. Rayburn W: Mitral valve prolapse and pregnancy. In Elkayam V, Gleicher N (eds): Cardiac Problems in Pregnancy Diagnosis and Management of Maternal and Fetal Disease. New York, Alan R Liss, pp 191–198, 1982
29. Rayburn W, Fontana MB: Mitral valve prolapse and pregnancy. Am J Obstet Gynecol 141:9, 1981
30. Silverman R, Ribner H: Peripartal cardiomyopathy. In Elkayam V, Gleicher N (eds): Cardiac Problems in Pregnancy Diagnosis and Management of Maternal and Fetal Disease. New York, Alan R Liss, pp 93–104, 1982
31. Johnston W, Elkayam V: Cardiac glycosides and pregnancy. In Elkayam V, Gleicher N (eds): Cardiac Problems in Pregnancy Diagnosis and Management of Maternal and Fetal Disease. New York, Alan R Liss, pp 281–288, 1982
32. Lee K, Klaus W: The subcellular basis for the mechanism of inotropic action of cardiac glycosides. Pharmacol Rev 23:193, 1971
33. Rosen M, Wit A, Hoffman B: Electrophysiology and pharmacology of cardiac arrhythmias, IV. Cardiac arrhythmias and toxic effects of digitalis. Am Heart J 89:391, 1975
34. Lisalo E: Clinical pharmacokinetics of digoxin. Clin Pharmacokinet 2:1, 1977
35. Aronson J: Clinical pharmacokinetics of digoxin. Clin Pharmacokinet 5:137, 1980
36. Klein H, Lang R, Weis E, et al.: Influence of verapamil on serum digoxin concentration. Circulation 65:998, 1982
37. Smith T: Digitalis-glycosides. N Engl J Med 288:719, 1973
38. Rotemensch H, Lessing J, Dorchin Y: Clinical pharmacology of antiarrhythmic drugs in the pregnant patient. In Elkayam V, Gleicher N (eds): Cardiac Problems in Pregnancy Diagnosis and Management of Maternal and Fetal Disease. New York, Alan R Liss, pp 227–244, 1982
39. Kerenyi T, Gleicher N, Meller J, et al.: Transplacental cardioversion of intrauterine supraventricular tachycardia with digitalis. Lancet 2:393, 1980
40. Harrigan J, Kangos J, Sikka A: Successful treatment of fetal congestive heart failure secondary to tachycardia. N Engl J Med 304:1527, 1981
41. Newburger J, Keane J: Intrauterine supraventricular tachycardia. J Pediatr 95:780, 1979
42. Okita G, Plotz E, David N: Placenta transfer of radioactive digitoxin in pregnant women and its fetal distribution. Circ Res 4:376, 1956
43. Rogers M, Willerson J, Goldblatt A, et al.: Serum digoxin concentrations in the human fetus, neonate and infant. N Engl J Med 287:1010, 1982
44. Saarikosh S: Placental transfer and fetal update of ^{3}H-digoxin in humans. Br J Obstet Gynaecol 83:879, 1976
45. Allonen H, Kanto J, Iisalo E: The foeto-maternal distribution of digoxin in early human

pregnancy. Acta Pharmacol Toxicol 39:477, 1976
46. Saarikoski S: Placental transmission of foetal distribution of ^{3}H-ouabain. Acta Pharmacol Toxicol 46:272, 1980
47. Potondi A: Congenital rhabdomyoma of the heart and intrauterine digitalis poisoning. J Forensic Sci 11:81, 1966
48. Sherman J, Locke R: Transplacental neonate digitalis intoxication. Am J Cardiol 6:834, 1960
49. Levine T: Role of vasodilators in the treatment of congestive heart failure. Am J Cardiol 55:32, 1985
50. McAnulty J, Metcalfe J, Ueland K: General guidelines in the management of cardiac disease. Clin Obstet Gynecol 24:773, 1981
51. Meller J, Goldman M: Rhythm disorder and pregnancy. In Elkayam V, Gleicher N (eds): Cardiac Problems in Pregnancy Diagnosis and Management of Maternal and Fetal Disease. New York, Alan R Liss, pp 191–198, 1982
52. Benowitz N: Clinical applications of the pharmacokinetics of lidocaine. Cardiovasc Clin 6:77, 1974
53. Benowitz N, Meister W: Clinical pharmacokinetics of lidocaine. Clin Pharmacokinet 3:177, 1978
54. Rubinstein A, Rothmensch HH: A case of asystole following lidocaine administration. Harefuah J Isr Med Assoc 94:478, 1970
55. Tucker G, Boyes R, Bridenbaugh P, et al.: Binding of anilide-type local anesthetics in human plasma, II. Implications in vivo, with special reference to transplacental distribution. Anesthesiology 33:304, 1970
56. Reynolds F, Taylor G: Maternal and neonatal blood concentrations of bupivacaine: A comparison with lidocaine drug continuous extradual analgesia. Anesthesia 25:14, 1970
57. Biehl D, Shnider SM, Levinson S, et al.: Placental transfer of lidocaine. Anesthesiology 48:409, 1978
58. Blankenbaker W, DiFazio C, Barry F: Lidocaine and its metabolites in the newborn. Anesthesiology 42:325, 1975
59. Brown W, Bell G, Lurie A, et al.: Newborn blood levels of lidocaine and mepivacaine in the first postnatal day following maternal epidural anesthesia. Anesthesiology 42:698, 1975
60. Brown W, Bell G, Alper M: Acidosis, local anesthesia and newborn. Obstet Gynecol 48:23, 1976
61. Scanlon J, Estheimer G, Lurie A: Neurobehavioral responses and drug concentrations in newborn after maternal epidural anesthesia with bupivacaine. Anesthesiology 45:400, 1976
62. Brackbill Y: Obstetrical medication and infant behavior. In Osofsky JD (ed): The Handbook of Infant Development. New York, Wiley, pp 76–125, 1979
63. Moe G, Abildskov J: Antiarrhythmic Drugs, Pharmacology Basis of Therapeutics, ed 4. New York, Macmillan, pp 711–719, 1970
64. Sokolow M, Edgar A: Blood quinidine concentrations as a guide in the treatment of cardiac arrhythmias. Circulation 1:576, 1950
65. Cohen I, Fick H, Cohen S: Adverse reactions to quinidine in hospitalized patients: Findings based on data from the Boston Collaborative Drug Surveillance Program. Prog Cardiovasc Dis 20:150, 1977
66. Rotmensch H, Rubinstein A, Levni E: Quinidine-induced subclinical hepatitis. Harefuah J Isr Med Assoc 98:211, 1968
67. Koch-Weser J: Quinidine-induced hypoprothrominemic hemorrhage in patients chronic warfarin therapy. Ann Intern Med 68:511, 1968
68. Doering W: Quinidine-digoxin interaction: Pharmacokinetics, underlying mechanism and clinical implications. N Engl J Med 401:400, 1979
69. Chen T, Friedman H: Alteration of digoxin pharmacokinetics by a single dose of quinidine. JAMA 244:669, 1980
70. Hill L, Malkasian G: The use of quinidine sulfate throughout pregnancy. Obstet Gynecol 54:366, 1979
71. Conradson T, Werko L: Management of heart disease in pregnancy. Prog Cardiovasc Dis 16:407, 1974
72. Globus, M: Teratology for the obstetrician: Current status. Obstet Gynecol 55:269, 1980
73. Meyer J, Lackner JE, Schochet SS: Paroxysmal tachycardia in pregnancy. JAMA 94:1901, 1930
74. Giardina EG, Heissenbuttel RH, Guttel R, Bigger J: Intermittent intravenous procainamide to treat ventricular arrhythmias: Correlation of plasma concentrations with effects on arrhythmias, electrocardiogram and blood pressure. Ann Int Med 78:183, 1973
75. Bigger J: Management of arrhythmias. In Braunwald E (ed): Heart Disease: A Textbook of Cardiovascular Medicine. Philadelphia, Saunders, pp 691–743, 1984

76. Giardinia E, Fenster P, Paul E, et al.: Efficacy and plasma concentrations and adverse effects of a new sustained release procainamide preparation. Am J Cardiol 46:855, 1980
77. Witter F, King T, Blake D: Adverse effects of cardiovascular drug therapy on the fetus and neonate. Obstet Gynecol 58:1005, 1981
78. Gardinia E, Dreyfuss J, Bigger J: Metabolism of procainamide in normal and cardiac subject. Clin Pharmcol Ther 19:339, 1976
79. Condemi J, Blongren S, Vaughan J: The procainamide-induced lupus syndrome. Bull Rheum Dis 20:604, 1970
80. Shaxted E, Mitton P: Disopyramide in pregnancy: A case report. Curr Med Res Opin 6:70, 1979
81. Leonard R, Braun T, Levy A: Initiation of uterine contractions by disopyramide during pregnancy. N Engl J Med 299:84, 1978
82. Spiegelhalder B, Eichelbaum M: Determination of verapamil in human plasma by mass fragmentography using stable isotope labeled verapamil as internal standard. Arznemin Forsch 27:1, 1974
83. Zipes D: Management of cardiac arrhythmias. In Braunwalk E (ed): A Textbook of Cardiovascular Medicine. Philadelphia, Saunders, pp 648–682, 1984
84. Barrillon A, Grand A, Bergaux A: Treatment of the heart disease pregnancy. Ann Med Int 125:437, 1974
85. Klein V, Repke J: Supraventricular tachycardia in pregnancy cardioversion with verapramil. Obstet Gynecol 63:165, 1984
86. D'Allon M, Jillson A, Hou S, et al.: Treatment of premature labor with the calcium antagonist nifedipine. Abstract of the Society of Perinatal Obstetricians Annual Meeting, p 77, 1985
87. Ducsay C, Cook M, Ueille J, et al.: Nifedipine tocolysis in pregnant rhesus monkeys: Maternal and fetal cardiorespiratory effects. Abstracts of the Society of Perinatal Obstetricians Annual Meeting, p 295, 1985
88. Hankins G, Wendel G, Leveno K, et al.: Myocardial infarction during pregnancy: A review. Obstet Gynecol 65:139, 1985
89. Goldman M, Meller J: Coronary artery disease in pregnancy. In Elkayam V, Gleicher N (eds): Cardiac Problems in Pregnancy Diagnosis and Management of Maternal and Fetal Disease. New York, Alan R Liss, pp 141–152, 1982
90. Lutz D, Noller K, Spittell J, et al.: Pregnancy and its complications following cardiac valve prosthesis. Am J Obstet Gynecol 131:460, 1978
91. Noller K: Pregnancy after cardiac surgery. In Elkayam V, Gleicher N (eds): Cardiac Problems in Pregnancy Diagnosis and Management of Maternal and Fetal Disease. New York, Alan R Liss, pp 207–220, 1982
92. Berman L, Aledort L: Anticoagulation in pregnancy. In Elkayam V, Gleicher N (eds): Cardiac Problems in Pregnancy Diagnosis and Management of Maternal and Fetal Disease. New York, Alan R Liss, pp 261–270, 1982
93. Knuppel R, Hoffman M, O'Brien W: Precautions in OB anticoagulant use. Cont Ob-Gyn 25:53, 1985
94. Hall J, Pauli R, Wilson K: Maternal and fetal sequelae of anticoagulation during pregnancy. Am J Med 68:122, 1980
95. Bell W, Tomasulo P, Alving B, et al.: Thrombocytopenia occurring during the administration of heparin: A prospective study in 52 patients. Ann Int Med 85:155, 1976
96. Powers P, Cuthbert D, Hirsch J: Thrombocytopenia found uncommonly during heparin therapy. JAMA 241:2396, 1979
97. Kapch D, Adelstein E, Rhodes R, et al.: Heparin-induced thrombocytopenia, thrombosis and hemorrhage. Surgery 86:148, 1979
98. Griffith G, Nichols G, Asher J, et al.: Heparin osteoporosis. JAMA 193:85, 1965
99. DeSwiet M, Dorrington W, Fidler J, et al.: Prolonged heparin therapy in pregnancy causes bone demineralization. Br J Obstet Gynecol 90:1129, 1983
100. Laros R: Discussion of paper by Lutz J, et al.: Am J Obstet Gynecol 131:460, 1978
101. Saka D, Marx G: Management of a patient with cardiac valve prosthesis. Anesth Anal 55:214, 1976
102. Ramsey L, Swartwout J: Cited in Burwell CS, Metcalf JM (eds): Heart Disease in Pregnancy: Physiology and Management. Boston, Little Brown, p 277, 1959
103. Redleaf P, Fadell E: Bacteremia during parturition. JAMA 169:1284, 1979
104. Baker T, Hubbell R: Reappraisal of a symptomatic puerperal bacteremia. Am J Obstet Gynecol 97:575, 1967
105. McCormack W, Rosner B, Lee Y, et al.: Isolation of genital mycoplasmas from blood obtained shortly after delivery. Lancet 1:596, 1975
106. Sugrue D, Blake S, MacDonald D: Pregnancy complicated by maternal heart disease: The

National Maternity Hospital, Dublin, Ireland, 1969 to 1978. Am J Obstet Gynecol 139:1, 1981

107. Sugrue D, Blake S, Troy P, et al.: Antibiotic prophylaxis against infective endocarditis after normal delivery: Is it necessary? Br Heart J 44:499, 1980
108. Marquis R: Bacterial endocarditis following delivery in women with heart disease. In Anguissola, Puddu, and Turin (eds): Cardiologia D'Oggi. Rome Edizioni Mediche Scientifiche p 278, 1975
109. Hosen J, Morton M, O'Grady J: Cardiac stimulation during ritodrine hydrochloride tocolytic therapy. Obstet Gynecol 62:52, 1983
110. Barden T, Peter J, Merkatz I: Ritodrine hydrochloride: A beta mimetic agent for use in preterm labor, I. Obstet Gynecol 56:1, 1980
111. Bendetti T: Maternal complications of parenteral beta sympathamimetic therapy for premature labor. Am J Obstet Gynecol 145:1, 1983
112. Hendricks C, Brenner W: Cardiovascular effects of oxytonic drugs used postpartum. Am J Obstet Gynecol 108:751, 1970
113. Cotton D, Benedetti T: Use of Swan-Ganz catheter in obstetrics and gynecology. Obstet Gynecol 56:641, 1980
114. Berkowitz R, Rafferty T: Pulmonary artery flow directed catheter use in obstetrics patients. Obstet Gynecol 55:507, 1980
115. Joyce T: Cardiac disease. In James F, Wheeler A (eds): Obstetrical Anesthesia. Philadelphia, Davis, pp 97–101, 1982

9

Pharmacologic Therapy for Chronic Medical Disorders During Pregnancy

Justin P. Lavin, Jr.

Gravid women are generally susceptible to the same medical disorders as when nonpregnant. In many instances, treatment during pregnancy differs little from that utilized in nonpregnant women. In other disorders, pregnancy-induced physiologic changes and/or potential fetal or neonatal side effects require alterations in the usual therapeutic approach. This chapter discusses pharmacologic therapy for women with certain chronic medical disorders during pregnancy.

ASTHMA

Asthma is one of the more common disorders complicating pregnancy. The reported prevalence during the gestational period varies from 0.4 to 1.3 percent,[1] with an average frequency of about 1 percent.[2] Approximately, 10 percent of gravidas with asthma require hospitalization for acute attacks.[3] The literature contains conflicting reports regarding the effect of pregnancy on the severity of asthma.[4] Gluck and Gluck combined 9 previous series for a total of over 1000 patients, and determined that 48 percent of the patients' clinical symptoms remained unchanged, 29 percent improved, and 23 percent deteriorated.[5] However, the prognosis for any given patient was unpredictable.[1-5] There is also conflict regarding the effect of asthma on pregnancy. Gordon et al. described a twofold increase in perinatal mortality in comparison to controls[6] Other authors have not noted such marked increases, but have observed minimally increased frequencies of prematurity, low birthweight, stillbirth, and neonatal neurologic abnormalities.[1-3,7-9] Our experience has shown that women with asthma generally do well during pregnancy with cautious surveillance and proper medical treatment.

Long-term Therapy

A large number of pharmacologic agents are available for the control of asthma, and therapy in pregnancy differs little from that in the nonpregnant state. Many patients can be managed with intermittent administration of the β-sympathetic agonists, metaproterenol or albuterol, administered by inhalation. During short periods of wheezing, two inhalations every 4 to 6 hours should be employed.[7–9] To obtain an optimal effect, the patient should exhale completely beforehand, breathe in the drug to complete inhalation, and hold her breath for several seconds.

If intermittent inhalation therapy does not suffice, oral methylxanthine therapy should be initiated. Methylxanthines exert their beneficial effect by inhibiting the action of phosphodiesterase. This enzyme is involved in the metabolism of cyclic adenosine monophosphate (AMP). With its inhibition, the concentrations of the latter compound increase leading to activation of kinases and increased sequestration of intracellular calcium, which in turn leads to smooth muscle relaxation.[10] Several preparations of methylxanthines are available (Table 9–1). Aminophylline in a dose betwen 200 and 300 mg, 4 times daily may be used for short-term therapy.[3,9] Sustained-release theophylline preparations such as Theo-Dur at a dose of 300 mg daily may be employed instead for more prolonged therapy.[3,7,9] For optimal effect, the dosage should be adjusted to blood theophylline levels with serum values of 10 to 20 mcg/ml being considered therapeutic. Potential maternal side effects include nausea, vomiting, anorexia, anxiety, and tremor. At toxic levels, cardiac arrhythmias and seizures may occur.[1,3,7–9]

The methylxanthines inhibit the force but not the frequency of uterine contractions,[11] and therefore their use is associated with a theoretical risk of prolonged gestation or abnormally long labor. These medications cross the placenta, and maternal and fetal cord blood levels are nearly identical.[12] While there are no known teratogenic effects attributed to these agents,[13] it has been suggested that the methylxanthines may accelerate the development of fetal pulmonary maturity.[10]

If patients still experience respiratory symptoms after adequate xanthine therapy, oral β-mimetic agents should be employed. Several preparations are available. Oral terbutaline at a dose of 2.5 to 5.0 mg two to three times daily,[3–9] or oral metroproterenol at a dose of 10 to 20 mg three to four times daily[3,7,9] may be employed. These agents exert their bronchodilating effect by stimulat-

TABLE 9–1. SELECTED METHYLXANTHINE PREPARATIONS

	Theophylline %	Theophylline mg
Nonsustained-release tablets		
Aminophylline 100 mg	80	80
Aminophylline 200 mg	80	80
Slophylline 100 mg	100	100
Theolair 125 mg	100	125
Theolair 250 mg	100	250
Sustained-released preparations		
Slophylline Gyrocap 125 mg	100	125
Slophylline Gyrocap 250 mg	100	250
Theo-Dur 100 mg	100	100
Theo-Dur 200 mg	100	200
Theo-Dur 300 mg	100	300
Liquid preparations		
Theophylline Elixir 80 mg/15 ml	100	80
Theophylline Elixir 160 mg/30 ml	100	160
Somophylline Solution 105 mg aminophylline 5 ml	85.7	90

ing the β-2 receptors in bronchial smooth muscle leading to increased production of cyclic AMP. This increases the activity of the kinases promoting the uptake and sequestration of intracellular calcium.[14] Common maternal side effects include tremor and tachycardia.[1,3,7-9] While unlikely with an oral dosage, high-dose intravenous β-mimetic therapy for the treatment of premature labor has been associated with hyperglycemia, hypokalemia, and pulmonary edema.[14-16] Therefore adjustment of glucose control may be required in pregnant diabetics, and fluid balance must be monitored carefully. β-mimetics are widely used to treat premature labor.[14-17] Therefore, there is a theoretical risk of prolonged gestation and/or desultory labor. No teratogenic effects have been attributed to the β-mimetics.[14] High-dose therapy for the treatment of premature labor has not been associated with any excess in neonatal complications.[18]

A select group of patients may continue to have refractory symptoms, and therapy with corticosteroids is warranted.[1,3,4,7,9,10] Varying dosages from 60 to 100 mg of prednisone as a single daily oral dose have been recommended.[3,7,9] Clinical improvement is usually noted after approximately 6 hours. The dosage should usually be tapered over 5 days to 2 weeks.[3,7,9] However, occasional patients may require prolonged corticosteroid therapy. In this situation, every other day therapy should be employed to minimize side effects.[19] All patients receiving oral corticosteroid therapy for more than a few days should receive intravenous hydrocortisone, in a dose of 100 mg every 8 hours during labor, delivery, and the immediate postpartum period to prevent acute adrenal insufficiency.

As an alternate to oral steroid therapy, the aerolized corticosteroid, beclomethasone dipropione, administered by inhalation may be utilized. The usual dosage is two inhalations (100 mg), three to four times daily.[3-9,19,20] This approach may provide the advantage of avoiding systemic absorption.[3,8,9,20] However, caution must be employed in switching from oral to inhalation therapy as the occurence of acute adrenal insufficiency has been reported.

Although early animal studies suggested an increased risk of oral clefts in association with maternal consumption of corticosteroids,[21] several human studies have failed to demonstrate a teratogenic risk.[22-24] Additionally, Shatz and associates have reported that the use of these preparations in pregnant asthmatics was not associated with increased maternal, fetal, or neonatal complications.[22] Rare cases of fetal adrenal suppression after maternal ingestion of corticosteroids have been reported,[25] and all infants should be carefully monitored.

In patients not responsive to the above maneuvers, a trial of cromolyn sodium may be considered.[3,8,9] This medication is available as a powder for inhalation. The usual dosage is 20 mg four times daily.[3,7] The drug exerts its effect by inhibiting the release of chemical mediators from the pulmonary mast cells.[3,9] There have been only limited reports of the use of cromolyn sodium during pregnancy, but to date no adverse effects have been detected.[1,3,7-9]

Because of the risk of precipitating acute attacks, aspirin-containing compounds and prostaglandin F_2-α should be avoided in pregnant asthmatics.[7] Iodine-containing cough suppressants should also be avoided because of the associated risk of congenital goiter with prolonged use.[24] However, allergy desensitization may be continued without increased fetal risk.[7]

Acute Asthma Attack

Acute asthma attacks are quite frequent in gravid women. Rapid and definitive action is required to prevent maternal deterioration, status asthmaticus, and potential adverse effects due to maternal and secondary fetal hypoxia. After a rapid history, physical examination, arterial blood gas determination, gram stain of the sputum, and chest x-ray to rule out pneumonia, intravenous fluid should be administered at a rate of 100 to 200 ml/

hr, and oxygen should be provided by nasal prongs at a rate of 5 to 6 L/min. Any suspected pulmonary infection should be treated aggressively with a broad-spectrum antibiotic.

The β-adrenergic agonists, epinephrine or terbutaline, may be injected subcutaneously in doses of 0.30 to 0.50 ml of a 1:1000 solution and 0.25 to 0.50 mg, respectively.[3,7-9] The latter preparation may be preferable because of possible decreased uterine blood flow in association with the use of epinephrine.[3,7] This action will suffice in several patients. If it is unsuccessful, however, an intravenous loading dose of 4.5 to 6 mg/kg of aminophylline should be administered over 20 to 30 minutes.[3,7,9,10] To prevent maternal toxicity, this dose should be reduced to 4.5 mg/kg or omitted in patients receiving prior oral therapy. Infusion should then be continued at a rate 0.5 to 0.9 mg/kg per hour,[3,7,9,10] and adjusted to achieve therapeutic theophylline levels. The infusion should be continued until significant clinical improvement has occurred, and the patient can tolerate oral therapy. Occasionally patients will require intravenous corticosteroids in addition to the above medications to abort acute attacks. Intravenous hydrocortisone should be initiated at a dose of 7.0 mg/kg.[3,10] This medication should be continued at a dose of 100 mg intravenously every 6 hours until significant clinical improvement has occurred.[3,7,10] Thereafter, the patient can be switched to oral corticosteroid therapy and rapidly tapered from these medications as described above.

Breastfeeding should be encouraged as newborn infants inherit a tendency toward asthma and allergies. The exclusive use of breastfeeding for at least 6 months may delay the onset of these allergic problems in the child.[7] Less than 4 percent of ingested theophylline appears in breast milk. Inhaled bronchodilators have minimal systemic absorption and therefore probably no secretion in breast milk, and only small quantities of orally ingested corticosteroids reach the breast milk. Therefore, the use of these drugs is not contraindicated in the nursing mother.[7]

INFLAMMATORY BOWEL DISEASE

Inflammatory bowel disease usually begins in adolescence or early adulthood, so the prevalence of this disorder during the gestational period is high.[26-31] While some recent authors have suggested that the various manifestations of inflammatory bowel disease simply represent different presentations of the same disease process,[29] the literature dealing with this subject has tended to consider ulcerative colitis and Crohn's disease separately.

Ulcerative colitis exerts no effect on fertility.[26] In contrast, Crohn's disease is associated with decreased fertility.[28] With modern management techniques, neither ulcerative colitis or Crohn's disease appears to be associated with increased maternal–fetal or neonatal complications.[26,27,29] The older literature would suggest that pregnancy exerts a deleterious effect on the course of inflammatory bowel disease. When the incidence of exacerbations among pregnant women is compared with that among women of similar age, however, recent reports suggest that there is no increase in the frequency of exacerbation.[26,27,29]

Therapy for inflammatory bowel disease begins with modification of the diet to avoid lactulose, some fruits, and vegetables.[29] Because this dietary alteration results in decreased calcium intake due to decreased consumption of dairy products and because there is an increased requirement for calcium during pregnancy, calcium intake should be supplemented with such over-the-counter products as Os-Cal at a dose of one or two tablets three times daily.[29] Initial therapy also involves the use of constipating agents. Codeine, lomotil, or immodium are probably not associated with any increased fetal risk, and may be used judiciously during pregnancy.[29] However, other constipating agents that are poorly absorbed such as Pepto-Bismol, Amphojel, or Metamucil may be preferable during the gestational period (Chap. 3).[29]

Corticosteroids

Corticosteroids are usually employed for those patients who fail to respond to the above measures. These medications exert their beneficial effect by accumulating in the inflamed bowel tissue, exerting a dose-related inhibition of the inflammatory process.[32] In controlled studies, corticosteroids have been demonstrated to be effective for the treatment of acute flairs of both ulcerative colitis and Crohn's disease.[33] In contrast, results from studies evaluating the efficacy of corticosteroids for prevention of recurrence in quiescent ulcerative colitis have yielded conflicting results, and at present this form of therapy is highly controversial.[33] Studies examining the same issue in patients with Crohn's disease have demonstrated no beneficial effect to the use of these medications.[33]

Corticosteroids may be administered either orally or, for distal colitis, as retention enemas. Prednisone in a single daily dose of 40 mg is utilized initially.[29,31,33] This dose has been demonstrated to be more effective than 20 mg and equally effective as 60 mg for the treatment of acute disease.[32] Since corticosteroids preferentially accumulate in inflamed tissue, and single-dose administration leads to less prolonged blood levels (less adrenal suppression), a single daily dose is preferable to multiple-dose therapy.[31,33] Most patients experience a therapeutic response in 1 to 2 weeks. The dosage is then generally reduced gradually to allow for 4 to 8 weeks of total therapy.[29,31,33] If the patient does not respond within 2 weeks of therapy at a given dose, it is very unlikely that she will respond to that dose and consideration should be given to increasing the dose.[33]

Corticosteroid enemas are administered as 100 mg of hydrocortisone, 5 mg of betamethasone, or 20 mg prednisone-21-phosphate in 100 ml of saline.[33] Betamethasone offers similar therapeutic effects to that of prednisone with less systemic absorption.[33] However, both hydrocortisone and betamethasone readily cross the placenta whereas prednisone crosses poorly.[29] Therefore, there may be a theoretical advantage to using prednisone during pregnancy. It is currently unclear whether corticosteroid enemas exert their therapeutic effect through a topical anti-inflammatory action or through systemic absorption.[33]

Requirements to prevent acute maternal adrenal insufficiency, and general comments regarding the potential fetal and neonatal complications associated with maternal corticosteroid ingestion have been discussed in the preceding section. In separate publications, Willoughby and Truelove,[26] and Mogadam and associates[27] have investigated the potential fetal and neonatal side effects of corticosteroids for the treatment of inflammatory bowel disease. Neither group of investigators found any excess in fetal or neonatal complications attributable to corticosteroid therapy.[26,27]

Sulfasalazine

Sulfasalazine is also frequently used alone or in combination with corticosteroids for the treatment of patients with inflammatory bowel disease.[26–33] This medication is split by the gut bacteria to form 5-aminosalicylate and sulfapyridine.[31,33] The former compound inhibits prostaglandin synthetase activity and is responsible for the beneficial effect of this medication on inflammatory bowel syndrome.[33] Sulfasalazine has been proven to be effective for the treatment of both acute ulcerative colitis and acute Crohn's disease.[33] While there is some controversy, the body of evidence suggests that prolonged therapy for the prevention of recurrences is of little benefit.[33] For acute attacks, sulfasalazine may be administered in a dose of 2 to 6 grams orally.[29,31,33] Maintenance doses of 2 grams daily are used for long-term therapy.[33] Potential maternal side effects include nausea, anorexia, vomiting, diarrhea, and dizziness.[33] Rare idiosyncratic reactions occur. Sulfasalazine inhibits the absorption of folate in the small bowel and therefore folate supplementation is required during pregnancy.[33]

Sulfasalazine crosses the placenta.[32,33] Cord blood concentrations have been reported to have been approximately one-half those of simultaneously obtained maternal plasma concentrations.[33] Maternal and cord blood concentrations of sulfapyridine are nearly identical and cord blood concentrations of 5-aminosalicylate appear to be very low.[32] No teratogenic effect has been attributed to this medication.[27] Since sulfasalazine is a sulfur preparation, there is a theoretical risk of displacement of bilirubin from binding sites and neonatal jaundice. However, the incidence of this complication is very low. Among 102 pregnancies during which sulfasalazine was employed, Mogadam and associates reported only 1 case of severe neonatal jaundice.[27] Other potential fetal and neonatal side effects of sulfasalazine therapy have been evaluated by Willoughby and Truelove and Mogadam and associates.[26,27] Neither group detected a significant increase in any particular complication or overall complications.[26,27] Both groups have suggested that the benefits of this medication during pregnancy far outweigh the potential dangers.[26,27]

Sulfasalazine is secreted in breast milk with concentrations about 30 percent of those of simultaneous maternal serum concentrations.[33] No adverse neonatal effects have been reported, and it is permissible for women to breastfeed while taking this medication.[27,29]

Azathioprine

Azathioprine is an immune antagonist sometimes employed in patients with inflammatory bowel disease for its anit-inflammatory action.[33] Most studies have not demonstrated a significant beneficial effect of this medication upon acute ulcerative colitis or Crohn's disease.[33] Azathioprine may be beneficial for the prevention of recurrences in both patients with quiescent ulcerative colitis and Crohn's disease. However, there is considerable controversy regarding this issue.[33]

Very little information has been published regarding the use of azathioprine for the treatment of inflammatory bowel disease during pregnancy. Several gravidas with renal transplants have been treated with a combination of corticosteroids and azathioprine. Several fetal complications have been reported including lymphopenia, thymic hypoplasia, immunoglobulin deficiency, low cortisol levels, and transient chromosomal abnormalities.[34–36] Given these reported complications and the questionable efficacy of azathioprine for the treatment of inflammatory bowel disease, this medication should not be utilized during pregnancy except under very unusual circumstances.

AUTOIMMUNE THROMBOCYTOPENIA PURPURA

Idiopathic or autoimmune thrombocytopenia purpura (ATP) is a chronic autoimmune disease characterized by the production of abnormal IgG, which attaches to circulating platelets and leads to their sequestration and destruction in the reticuloendothelial system.[37,38] The degree of thrombocytopenia varies but tends to follow a course of remissions punctuated by exacerbations.[37,38] Maternal mortality is exceptionally rare, although significant maternal morbidity may occur due to hemorrhage associated with genital tract injury or operative incisions.[37–39]

The maternal IgG antibody attaches to the placental Fc receptor and traverses the human placenta.[37,38] Spontaneous abortion rates of up to 33 percent have been reported.[40,41] Perinatal mortality has ranged from as high as 15 to 25 percent, but has declined recently to less than 5 percent in expertly managed populations.[42–45] Prematurity and intracranial hemorrhage constitute the chief causes of neonatal death.[37–39] The incidence of intracranial hemorrhage is related to the degree of neonatal thrombocytopenia.[37,38,45,46] However, the degree of neonatal thrombocytopenia is poorly correlated with the maternal platelet count.[37,38,45–47] Cines and associates have recently demonstrated a correlation between the incidence of neonatal thrombocytopenia and the level of circulating antibodies as determined by indirect assay.[48] The inability to accurately predict which neonates will be thrombocytopenic, as well as the relatively low incidence of neonatal intracranial hemorrhage, has engendered considerable controversy regarding the proper mode of delivery. Some investigators favor cesarean delivery for all such women,[42,49] others advocate vaginal delivery,[39,45] and still others favor a selective approach based on the platelet level as determined by fetal scalp sampling.[46,47]

Corticosteroids

Corticosteroids represent the primary pharmacologic therapy to treat ATP. Several mechanisms of action have been proposed to explain their therapeutic effect on this disorder:[37]

1. Decreased antiplatelet antibody production by the reticuloendothelial system.
2. Interference with the interaction between antiplatelet antibody and platelet surfaces, resulting in a decrease in platelet bound antibody and an increase in circulating unbound antibody.
3. Decreased clearance of antibody or complement-bound platelets by the reticuloendothelial system, resulting in prolonged platelet survival and elevated platelet counts.
4. Decreased capillary fragility.

There is also controversy regarding the appropriate clinical criteria for initiating corticosteroid therapy during pregnancy. Some authorities believe that, as in the nonpregnant state, the platelet count itself should not be treated, but rather therapy should be reserved for those patients with clinical evidence of hemorrhagic complications.[50] Other authors have suggested the initiation of therapy when the maternal platelet count decreases to below 50,000.[37] The latter group advocates their position in hope of maintaining a "safe" fetal platelet count throughout gestation. Therapy is initiated at daily doses from 60 to 100 mg of prednisone.[37,50] Divided dose administration appears to be more effective than the use of a single daily dose.[50] A therapeutic response will occur in most patients over a period of 1 to 3 weeks.[37,50] Therapy is continued at the initial dose for this period of time, then gradually tapered to the lowest dose compatible with an adequate platelet count,[37] or the absence of hemorrhagic complications.[50] As in the previously described disorders, patients receiving prolonged corticosteroids require intravenous corticosteroid supplementation at the time of labor and delivery.

Several groups of investigators have noted higher platelet counts among the neonates of mothers who have received corticosteroids for the treatment of ATP than among the neonates of mothers who did not undergo such therapy.[44,46,51,52] This observation has led Karpatkin and associates to advocate steroid treatment during the last several weeks of pregnancy for all gravidas with ATP to enhance fetal safety during vaginal delivery.[52] Other investigators have noted a less uniform success in maintaining normal neonatal platelet counts with similar treatment plans,[51,53,54] and thus the recommendation of Karpatkin and associates remains highly controversial. Levin has suggested that the use of steroid preparations, such as dexamethasone or betamethasone, which cross the placenta with greater ease than prednisone may lead to a more optimal fetal response.[50]

Corticosteroids will engender a permanent remission in approximately 14 to 38 percent of patients treated for ATP.[55] Further therapy will be required in the remaining patients. Splenectomy is usually the next form of therapy, and this operative procedure can be utilized with relative safety in pregnant women with ATP.[37,50] Platelet transfusion may be utilized in life-threatening hemorrhagic emergencies or to prepare patients for surgery.[37,50] Immunosuppressants such as azathioprine, cyclophosphamide, vincristine, and vinblastine have been employed in selected patients unresponsive to the above measures.[50,56] Reported results have not been overwhelmingly successful, however, and these agents possess significant potential for fetal injury.[50,56] Therefore, the use of these agents should be avoided in pregnant women with ATP except in very unusual situations.[50]

Immune Globulin Therapy

Recently, several groups of investigators have reported that the intravenous infusion of high-dose human immunoglobulin has resulted in increased circulating platelet counts in approximately one-third of patients with chronic ATP refractory to corticosteroid therapy.[57-61] This preparation is administered intravenously in a dose of 400 mg/kg/day, for 5 days. When a favorable response takes place, it usually occurs within a few days.[59,60] An example of favorable responses in two cases is illustrated in Figure 9-1. Most responses have been of relatively short duration, unless immunoglobulin therapy has been continued.[37] The mechanism leading to the observed improvement in platelet counts is not clear at present. Various investigators have proposed that a decreased clearance of platelets by the reticuloendothelial system[58] or an interference with the antiplatelet antibody-platelet interaction takes place.[60] While this preparation would appear to pose minimal risk to the fetus, only a few patients have been treated during pregnancy,[61] and further research is required to clarify the

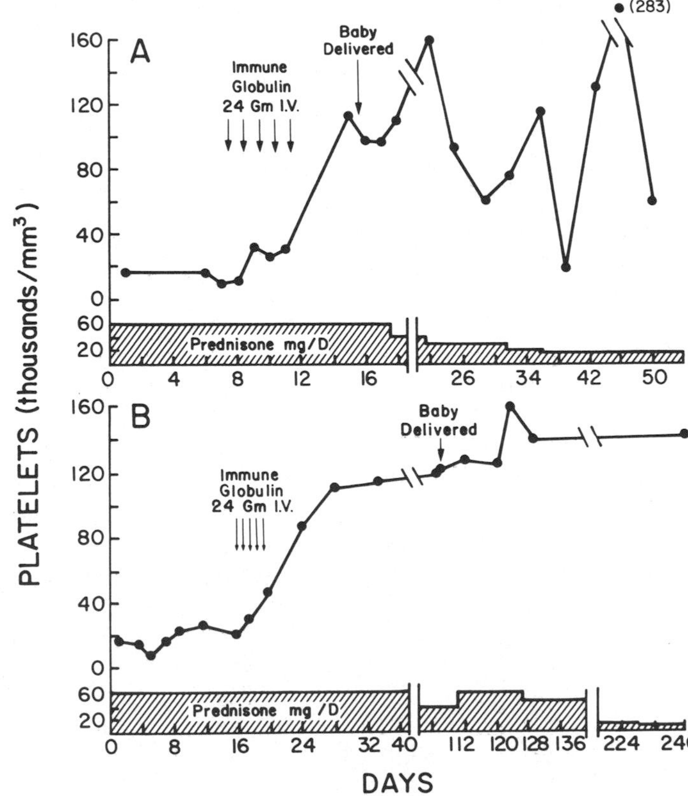

Figure 9-1. Maternal platelet response to intravenous immune globulin therapy in two cases (**A** and **B**).

proper role of immunoglobulin in the treatment of ATP during the perinatal period.[37]

THROMBOEMBOLIC DISEASE

Thromboembolic disorders have long concerned obstetricians because of the risk of maternal death due to pulmonary embolism. This anxiety has perhaps been heightened by the difficulties related to the diagnosis of these disorders during the peripartum period. Physiologic changes of pregnancy increase a gravid woman's probability of experiencing Virchow's classic triad of factors predisposing to thrombosis: alteration in the composition of the blood, venous stasis, and vessel wall injury.[62] Despite these changes, the incidence of clinically apparent deep venous thrombophlebitis during the antepartum period is similar to that observed in nonpregnant women and has been reported to range from 0.021 to 0.035 percent.[63] In contrast, the frequency of thrombophlebitis during labor, delivery, and the puerperium has been reported to be four- to sixfold that experienced in the nonpregnant state.[63] This has ranged from 0.27 to 1.2 percent on clinical grounds, to as high as 3 percent, when the diagnosis has been made on the basis of I^{125} scanning.[64] Additionally, the incidence of pulmonary embolus formation during pregnancy has been reported to range from 0.5 to 12 per 1000 deliveries.[62] Patients with superficial thrombophlebitis respond well to heat, elevation, and analgesics, and are not at increased risk to experience a pulmonary embolus.[65]

Heparin

Untreated patients with deep venous thrombophlebitis do not fare well. Finnerty and Mackay[66] reviewed the literature dealing with this subject in 1962, and reported that of 135 such women, 32 (34 percent) experienced a pulmonary embolus, and 16 (11 percent) died during pregnancy. In contrast, among 73 women with deep vein thrombophlebitis who were treated with anticoagulants, 4 (10 percent) experienced a pulmonary embolus, and none died.[66] This and similar observations[66-68] provide the rationale for anticoagulant therapy in pregnant patients with deep vein thrombophlebitis and pulmonary embolus.

Because of the potential teratogenic and late fetal complications associated with warfarin therapy (Chaps. 2 and 8), most authors recommend heparin for anticoagulation during the antepartum period.[62,69,70] (For a discussion of the pharmacokinetics, modes of action, and potential maternal and fetal side effects of heparin and warfarin, please refer to the discussion of anticoagulant therapy for patients with prosthetic cardiac valves in Chapter 8.) A variety of regimens have been proposed for initial intravenous heparin therapy. Kelton and Hirsch[62] have suggested an initial bolus of 70 U/kg, followed by an infusion of 300 to 400 U/kg over a 24-hour period. The dosage should be regulated to provide a therapeutic heparin level of 0.2 to 0.4 units per ml.[62] These authors believe that the measurement of heparin levels, as opposed to partial thromboplastin times, prevents unnecessarily high heparin dosage due to shortening of the partial thromboplastin time by pregnancy-induced alterations in coagulation Factor VIII.[62] Bolan has recommended a loading dose of 5000 units, followed by a maintenance dose of approximately 1000 units per hour regulated to achieve a partial thromboplastin time two to three times the control.[68] Regardless of which treatment regimen is used, intravenous therapy should be continued for 7 to 10 days.[62,68,69]

Several recent studies in nonpregnant women with thrombosis have demonstrated decreased morbidity when anticoagulant therapy has been continued for 3 months.[69] Several groups of investigators have recommended various protocols for administrating prolonged anticoagulant therapy to gravidas with deep vein thrombophlebitis for durations varying from 3 weeks to the entire gestational period and several weeks postpartum.[62,68-73] In light of the abovementioned findings in nonpregnant women and the physiologic changes of pregnancy, the recommendations of Kelton and Hirsch[62] appear most rational. These authors have recommended a moderate subcutaneous heparin dose (approximately 10,000 units twice daily, or 7000 units three times daily adjusted to maintain the serum heparin level between 0.2 and 0.3 units per ml, 6 hours after injection) for 3 months, followed by minidose subcutaneous heparin (5000 units twice daily) for the remainder of pregnancy, for women with antepartum deep venous thrombophlebitis. They have suggested intravenous heparin followed by warfarin for 3 months for women who develop thrombosis during labor, delivery, or the puerperium.[62] While the latter investigators have recommended discontinuing heparin during labor,[62] we favor continuing minidose heparin, with the omission of a single dose when delivery is imminent. There is general agreement that gravidas who experience pulmonary embolism during the antepartum period should receive anticoagulant therapy for the remainder of pregnancy.[62,68–73] Again, the regimen of Kelton and Hirsch appears appropriate. Oral warfarin may be utilized in the postpartum period.[62,68,69]

Bararacco and Vessey have demonstrated that women who have experienced a previous thromboembolic episode have a 12 percent risk of recurrence during the present pregnancy.[74] This observation has led some investigators to recommend that minidose prophylactic heparin be administrated to such gravidas from the 34th week of gestation until the patient is fully ambulatory postpartum.[72,73] A recent editorial has suggested that this practice be extended to include other high-risk groups such as women with advanced age, high parity, obesity or immobility, or concomitant diabetes, hypertension, cardiac disease, or severe varicose veins.[75]

Streptokinase, Urokinase

Streptokinase and urokinase are relatively recently developed medications which have been used to lyse clots in patients with thromboembolic disease. These agents exert their effect by activating plasmin, a proteolytic enzyme, from its precursor plasminogen. Plasmin, in turn, dissolves the clot.[68] Because of the significant risk of hemorrhage, these drugs are contraindicated during the puerperium.[68] They should also be avoided during the antepartum period, with the rare exception of patients at risk of death from pulmonary embolism who do not respond to heparin therapy.[68]

COLLAGEN VASCULAR DISORDERS

While any of the collagen vascular disorders may occur during pregnancy, rheumatoid arthritis and systemic lupus erythematosus are most common and perhaps most amenable to therapy. The prevalence of rheumatoid arthritis is 1 to 2 percent, and there is a two to three to one predilection for females over males.[76] The frequency of lupus is approximately one-tenth that of rheumatoid arthritis.[76] Approximately three-quarters of patients with rheumatoid arthritis experience symptomatic improvement during pregnancy.[76–79] Many of these women experience re-exacerbation in the postpartum period,[80,81] and occasionally de novo during pregnancy.[82] Rheumatoid arthritis does not cause any deleterious effect on pregnancy outcome.[76,79] The course of lupus during pregnancy is more variable. A proportion of patients remain stable or improve. Older studies suggested a tendency toward deterioration during the first half of pregnancy and the postpartum period.[76,79] In more recent studies, the incidence of flareups has been reduced dramatically.[83,84] Exacerbation of lupus nephritis is a particularly dangerous complication, and may be very difficult to differentiate from preeclampsia.[76,79] Patients with lupus experience higher frequencies of spontaneous abortion and stillbirths.[76,79] Some studies have noted increased frequencies of growth retardation and prematurity, although these have been observed inconsistently.[76,79]

Salicylates

Salicylates form the first line of pharmacologic therapy for rheumatoid arthritis, and may also be helpful for the control of minor symptoms in patients with systemic lupus.[76,79,85] These agents exert their anti-inflammatory effect by blocking prostaglandin synthesis through the inhibition of cyclooxygenase, an enzyme that metabolizes arachidonic acid to the unstable endoperoxides.[76,86] Enteric-coated acetylsalicylic acid is the preferable preparation.[76] The usual daily dose is 3.6 to 4 grains/day.[76] Potential maternal side effects include gastrointestinal irritation, platelet dysfunction (postpartum blood loss is occasionally increased, although severe hemorrhage is rare), and salicylism (tinnitus and deafness). Salicylism occurs at a level greater than 25 mg%,[76] and can be reversed with dose reduction.

Salicylates cross the human placenta.[86,87] While there have been occasional reports suggesting an increase in fetal malformations among salicylate users,[88–90] the overwhelming body of evidence has not demonstrated a teratogenic effect.[24,76,79,87,91,92] Extremely high-dose salicylate ingestion has been associated with decreased birthweight,[91] but this effect has not been noted at more moderate doses.[87,92] The length of gestation has been reported to be longer, the incidence of postdatism higher, and the duration of labor prolonged among mothers who have been treated with salicylates,[87,93,94] presumably due to the prostaglandin-inhibiting properties of these agents.[87,93] Premature closure of ductus arteriosus or neonatal pulmonary hypertension due to prostaglandin inhibition observed with other antiprostaglandin agents has not been reported to occur in humans due to salicylate ingestion. Maternal salicylate ingestion has been associated with neonatal platelet dysfunction.[95] Rumack and coinvestigators[96] have reported an increased frequency of intracranial hemorrhage among neonates of mothers who had ingested acetylsalicylic acid in comparison to controls.

Other nonsteroidal anti-inflamatory agents are frequently utilized in patients with rheumatoid arthritis who do not respond to salicylates, and in those with joint symptoms from lupus.[76,79] Their mechanism of action is identical to that of the salicylates.[76,87] These medications have been utilized for the prevention of premature labor in several investigational trials. Several authors have reported the occurrence of pulmonary hypertension, presumably due to the antiprostaglandin effects of these agents on the ductus arteriosus.[97–99] While other investigators have not noted the occurrence of this problem,[100.101] most authorities suggest that the use of these agents for treatment of collagen vascular disorders is contraindicated during pregnancy.[76,79]

Corticosteroids

Systemic corticosteroids are seldom indicated for the treatment of rheumatoid arthritis.[76] However, these drugs form the mainstay of therapy for the treatment of systemic lupus. These medications are utilized in the lowest possible dose to relieve symptoms and prevent recurrence.[76,79] A daily dose of 20 to 40 mg of prednisone may be utilized for flairs with nonmajor organ involvement. If major organ involvement (nephritis, central nervous system involvement, or vasculitis) is present, the daily dose should be increased to 40 to 80 mg.[76] The pharmacokinetics, mode of action, and potential maternal and fetal side effects of these agents have been discussed previously in this chapter. In the only controlled study of the use of corticosteroids in patients with lupus, those patients who received the medication had fewer exacerbations and less perinatal mortality than those who did not receive corticosteroids.[79,102]

Other Drugs

A number of other agents including gold, immunosuppressive medications, and penicillamine have been utilized to treat selected patients with collagen vascular disorders. Because of a lack of knowledge regarding potential fetal effects or substantial suggestion of fetal risk, however, most authorities recommend that these agents be avoided during pregnancy except in life-threatening situations when more traditional agents have failed.[76,79]

MIGRAINE HEADACHE

Migraine headaches are very common among women of childbearing age and are a frequent concern to these womens' physicians because of relationships to menstruation and oral contraceptive use. Approximately 60 percent of women afflicted with migraines note a relationship between their symptomatology and menstrual cycles, with headaches usually occurring just before or during menstruation.[103] These symptoms can sometimes be prevented or postponed by the administration of estradiol.[103] Migraine headaches are frequently exacerbated by oral contraceptive use, especially those preparations with high estrogen content.[104] This is of particular concern to the gynecologist because of evidence linking the occurrence of migraine headaches to a presumed increased risk of cerebral infarction among oral contraceptive users.

Most authors have noted a decrease in the frequency of migraine attacks during pregnancy.[104-106] This improvement generally occurs after the first trimester,[106] and appears to be more common among gravidas whose prior symptoms were related to menstruation.[107] Occasionally patients may note the onset or exacerbation of migraine headache, particularly during the first trimester.[107]

The administration of ergot alkaloids for their vasoconsticting properties, at the earliest indication of an attack, forms the cornerstone of pharmacologic therapy for migraine headache in nonpregnant individuals.[107] Most authors recommend that these agents be avoided during pregnancy due to their oxytocic effect.[107-109] To some extent, however, this recommendation may be more emotionally than scientifically based,[108] as several preparations are available containing ergotamine tartrate, which is devoid of oxytocic effect when administered orally.[108] The manufacturers' product information for all preparations containing ergotamine tartrate indicate that these drugs are contraindicated during pregnancy, and therefore it is obviously difficult for the practitioner to utilize these medications. Ergot alkoloids are also relatively contraindicated in the breastfeeding mother due to associated neonatal vomiting, diarrhea, and blood presure disturbances.[107]

Simple analgesics (Table 9–2), such as acetylsalicylic acid, acetaminophen, and codeine, are generally utilized for primary therapy during pregnancy.[107-109] By virtue of its analgesic and antiemetic effects, chlorpromazine in a dose of 25 to 50 mg every 6 to 8 hours may be helpful for treatment of chronic migraines or acute attacks.[108] For those patients with chronic migraine headaches who do not respond to the above medications, propranolol, 40 to 160 mg. in four divided daily doses, may be employed.[107,108] The pharmacology and potential side effects of propranolol are discussed in Chapters 6 and 10. Amitriptyline, 25 mg three times daily or 75 mg prior to sleep, may also be useful in patients with concomitant depression.[108]

MYASTHENIA GRAVIS

Myasthenia gravis is a chronic autoimmune disorder characterized by periods of remission and exacerbation. The disease is caused by a circulating antiacetycholine receptor immune globulin which binds to acetylcholine receptors at the myoneural junction and interferes with the action of acetylcholine.[110] This impairs the contractile capability of skeletal muscle and leads to clinical symptoms which include muscle weakness, particularly those innervated by the cranial nerves. Fatigue, opthalmoplegia, dysphagia, dysarthria, hypoventilation, and respiratory failure are characteristic symptoms.[107-109] Myasthenia

TABLE 9–2. DRUGS UTILIZED TO TREAT MIGRAINE IN PREGNANCY

Type	Drug	Dose	Route of Administration
Acute	Codeine	30 mg every 4 hrs	Oral or IM
	Acetysalicylic Acid with Codeine (Emprin Compound)	1 or 2 tablets every 6–8 hrs	Oral
	Acetaminophen with Codeine (Tylenol No. 3)	1 or 2 tablets every 4–6 hrs	Oral
	Chlorpromazine (Thorazine)	25–50 mg every 6–8 hrs	IM
		50–100 mg every 6–8 hrs	Rectal
Chronic	Propranolol (Inderal)	10–40 mg every 6 hrs	Oral
	Chlorpromazine	25 mg every 6 hrs	Oral

most commonly begins in the third decade of life, and among younger individuals, females being much more commonly affected than males.[107,108] Therefore, it is not rare for obstetricians to encounter gravidas with this disorder.

No study has compared the frequency of exacerbation among pregnant and nonpregnant women. Approximately 35 to 40 percent of myasthenic patients experience exacerbations during the antepartum period,[107,110] and an additional 30 percent of patients experience deterioration during the postpartum period.[110] Labor and delivery represent particularly dangerous periods, because many medications and anesthetic agents used at these times may adversely affect the myasthenic patient. Infection which is also potentially more common during pregnancy, labor, and delivery may promote deterioration. In the absence of maternal deterioration, myasthenia does not appear to exert adverse effects on pregnancy.[110] From 12 to 19 percent of infants born to mothers with myasthenia gravis develop neonatal myasthenia gravis,[110,111] presumably due to transplacental passage of maternal antibody.[112] This is a transient abnormality, although it may require therapy.[107–111]

Thymectomy is performed on selected patients with myasthenia gravis.[107–110,113] However, treatment with anticholinesterase agents forms the cornerstone of modern management of myasthenia gravis in both pregnant and nonpregnant individuals.[107–110] These preparations inhibit the enzyme cholinesterase, and allow for the accumulation of acetylcholine at the myoneural junction resulting in improved muscle contractile power.[107–110] However, a beneficial effect occurs only up to a certain dose. Thereafter, further dosage increments result in impaired neuromuscular transmission and cholinergic crisis.[107–111] The anticholinesterases to treat myasthenia gravis are the quarternary ammonium compounds, edrophonium, neostigmine, and pyridostigmine.[107,108,110] Edrophonium is employed for diagnostic testing and to assess the adequacy of treatment. In patients with myasthenia who have not yet received optimal anticholinesterase therapy, muscle power dramatically improves for approximately 5 minutes, beginning 30 seconds after a 10 mg intravenous injection.[107] Neostigmine and pyridostigmine are utilized for long-term therapy. Both are available in oral and parenteral forms with durations of action of 1 to 4 hours.[107–110] Neostigmine is perhaps the more widely used and time-tested of the two agents.[110] An initial dosage is 15 mg every 2 to 3 hours. Subsequent adjustment of the dose is necessary to optimize the patient's muscle strength.[110] Some clinicians prefer pyridostigmine because of the purported longer duration of action, reduced muscurinic side effects, and "smoother control."[107,110,114] An initial dose of 60 mg every 4 to 6 hours may be employed. The dosage is then adjusted by first reducing the interdose interval, and then increasing the quantity by 15 to 30 mg per dose until an optimum dose is reached.[110,115] A time-release capsule containing 180 mg of pyridostigmine is frequently utilized at bedtime to allow control during the sleeping hours.[107,110] However, pyridostigmine is inadequate for daily activities and should not be utilized during the waking hours.[107] The measurement of vital capacity and hand strength are useful techniques for assessing dosage adequacy.[107,110] Different muscle groups may exhibit different magnitudes of response to a given dose. In this situation, breathing and swallowing should be maximized.[107]

Injections must be utilized when oral administration is impossible, such as a morning dose in pregnancies complicated by hyperemesis. Injections should be utilized during labor, when oral absorption is unpredictable.[107,110] Equivalent oral and injectable doses are provided in Table 9–3.[107,110,114]

Common muscurinic side effects include bronchorrhea and gastrointestinal hypermotility. Atropine may be useful in controlling these symptoms.[107] The potentially most dangerous complication of anticholinesterase therapy, cholinergic crisis, occurs due to drug overdosage. Like a myasthenic crisis, it involves progressive muscle weakness and eventual respiratory failure. Therefore, the two forms of crisis are frequently difficult to differentiate.[110] Other muscurinic side effects such as tearing, ptyalism, abdominal cramping, diarrhea, nausea, and vomiting generally accompany cholinergic crisis.[110] Differentiation can be accomplished by the administration of edrophonium as outlined above.[107,110] If a cholinergic crisis is present, all anticholinergic agents must be discontinued, atropine should be administered to control muscurinic symptoms, and respiratory support instituted.[110]

TABLE 9–3. EQUIVALENT DOSES OF ANTICHOLINESTERASES

Drug	Route of Administration	Equivalent Dose
Neostigmine	Oral	15 mg
Neostigmine	Intravenous	0.5 mg
Neostigmine	Intramuscular	1.5 mg
Pyridostigmine	Oral	60 mg

Patients with myasthenia are adversely affected by a number of medications commonly used during pregnancy, labor, and delivery. They frequently develop respiratory depression when exposed to sedatives, narcotics, or tranquilizers,[107,110,115] and these medications should be avoided or used very sparingly. Curare-like drugs, ether, chloroform, trichlorethylene, and fluothane are contraindicated.[108,110] Regional anesthesia is the most appropriate form of pain control during labor and delivery.[107–110] Caution should be employed in utilizing procaine and its congeners, however, because cholinesterase is required for the metabolism of these agents, and the concomitant use with anticholinesterase agents may precipitate a generalized local anesthetic reaction.[110–116] Magnesium sulfate, aminoglycosides, quinidine, and quinine interfere with myoneural transmission and should be avoided.[107,110,116]

Placental transfer of the anticholinesterase agents is minimal.[117,118] The extent of secretion in breast milk is presently uncertain, but breastfeeding appears to be permissible.[107,110] Maternal rest should be encouraged to avoid the precipitation of a myasthenic crisis during and after pregnancy.

Corticosteroids and immunosuppressants have been utilized in patients with myasthenia gravis who do not respond adequately to the anticholinesterase agents.[107,110] However, to the author's knowledge the use of these agents in pregnant patients with myasthenia has not been reported to date.

REFERENCES

1. Weinstein A, Dubin B, Podleski W, et al.: Asthma and pregnancy. JAMA 241:1161, 1979
2. Hernandez E, Angell C, Johnson J: Asthma in pregnancy: Current concepts. Obstet Gynecol 55:739, 1980
3. deSwiet M: Maternal pulmonary disorders. In Creasy R, Resnik R (eds): Maternal—fetal Medicine Principles and Practice. Philadelphia, Saunders, 1984, pp 781–794
4. Greenberger P, Patterson R: Management of asthma during pregnancy. N Engl J Med 312:897, 1985
5. Gluck J, Gluck P: The effects of pregnancy on asthma. A prospective study. Ann Allergy 37:164, 1976
6. Gordon M, Niswander K, Berendes H, et al.: Fetal morbidity following potentially anoxigenic obstetric conditions, VII. Bronchial asthma. Am J Obstet Gynecol 106:421, 1970
7. Holbreich M: Care of the asthmatic during pregnancy. Contemp Ob-Gyn 21:155, 1983
8. Weinberger S, Weiss S, Cohen W, et al.: Pregnancy and the lung. Am Rev Respir Dis 121:559, 1980
9. Weinberger S, Weiss S: Pulmonary diseases. In Burrow G, Ferris T (eds): Medical Complications During Pregnancy, ed 2. Philadelphia, Saunders, 1982, pp 405–431
10. Hadjgeorgiov E, Kitsiov S, Psaroudakis A, et al.: Antepartum aminophylline treatment for prevention of the respiratory distress syndrome in premature infants. Am J Obstet Gynecol 135:257, 1979
11. Lipshitz J: Uterine and cardiovascular effects of aminophylline. Am J Obstet Gynecol 131:716, 1978
12. Arwood L, Dasta J, Freidman L: Placental transfer of theophylline: Two case reports. Pediatrics 63:844, 1979
13. Greenberger P, Patterson R: Safety of therapy of allergic symptoms during pregnancy. Ann Intern Med 89:234, 1978
14. Caritis S, Edelstone D, Mueller-Heubach E: Pharmacologic inhibition of preterm labor. Am J Obstet Gynecol 133:557, 1979
15. Gotten D, Strassner H, Lipson L, et al.: The effects of terbutaline on acid base, serum electrolytes, and glucose homeostasis during the management of preterm labor. Am J Obstet Gynecol 141:617, 1981
16. Smythe A, Sakakini A: Maternal metabolic alteration secondary to terbutaline therapy for premature labor. Obstet Gynecol 57:566, 1981
17. Katz M, Robertson P, Creasy R: Cardivascular complications associated with terbutaline treatment for preterm labor. Am J Obstet Gynecol 139:605, 1981
18. Caritis S, Toig G, Heddinger L, et al.: A double blind study comparing ritodrine and terbutaline treatment of premature labor. Am J Obstet Gynecol 150:7, 1984
19. McFadden E, Austen K: Asthma. In Petersdorf R, Adams R, Braunwald E, et al. (eds): Harrison's Principles of Internal Medicine, ed 10. New York, McGraw Hill, 1983, pp 1512–1518
20. Greenberger P, Patterson R: Beclomethasone dipropionate for severe asthma during pregnancy. Ann Intern Med 98:478, 1983
21. Fainstat T: Cortisone-induced congenital cleft palate in rabbits. Endrocrinology 55:502, 1954
22. Schatz M, Patterson R, Zeitz S, et al.: Corticosteroid therapy for the pregnant asthmatic patient. JAMA 233:804, 1975
23. Snyder R, Snyder D: Corticosteroids for asthma during pregnancy. Ann Allergy 41:340, 1978
24. Globus M: Teratology for the obstetrician: Current status. Obstet Gynecol 55:269, 1980
25. Warrell D, Taylor R: Outcome for the foetus of mothers receiving prednisolone during pregnancy. Lancet 1:117, 1968
26. Willoughby C, Truelove S: Ulcerative colitis and pregnancy. Gut 21:469, 1980.
27. Mogadam M, Dobbins W, Korelitz B, et al.: Pregnancy in inflammatory bowel disease: Effect of sulfasalazine and corticosteroids on fetal outcome. Gastroenterology 80:72, 1981
28. Vender R, Spiro H: Inflammatory bowel disease and pregnancy. J Clin Gastroenterol 4:231, 1982
29. Dubbins J, Spiro H: Gastrointestinal complications. In Burrow G, Ferris T (eds): Medical Complications during Pregnancy, ed 2. Philadelphia, Saunders, 1982, pp 259–277
30. Sorokin J, Levine S: Pregnancy and inflammatory bowel disease: A review of the literature. Obstet Gynecol 62:247, 1983
31. Murry-Lyon I, Powell-Tuck J: Gastrointestinal disorders. In Brudennell M, Wilds P, (eds): Medical and Surgical Problems in

Obstetrics. Bristol, John Wright, 1984, pp 160–74
32. Azad-Khan A, Truelove S: Placental and mammary transfer of sulphasalazine. Br Med J 2:1553, 1979
33. Leonard-Tucks J, Powell-Tuck J: Drug treatment of inflammatory bowel disease. Clin Gastroenterol 8:187, 1979
34. Cote C, Mevwissen H, Pickering R: Effects on the neonate of prednisone and azathioprine administered to the mother during pregnancy. J Pediatrics 85:324, 1974
35. Price H, Salaman J, Lawrence K, et al.: Immunosuppressive drugs and the foetus. Transplantation 21:294, 1976
36. Penn I, Makowski E, Harris P: Parenthood following renal transplantation. Kidney Int 18:221, 1980
37. Martin J, Morrison J, Files J: Autoimmune thrombocytopenia purpura: Current concepts and recommended practices. Am J Obstet Gynecol 150:86, 1984
38. Beer A: Discussion of an article by R Laros, R Kagan. Am J Obstet. Gynecol 148:905, 1984
39. Laros R, Kagan R: Route of delivery for patients with immune thrombocytopenic purpura. Am J Obstet Gynecol 148:901, 1984
40. O'Reilly R, Tabor B: Immunologic thrombocytopenic purpura and pregnancy. Obstet Gynecol 51:590, 1978
41. Schenker J, Polishuk W: Idiopathic thrombocytopenic purpura in pregnancy. Gynecologia 165:271, 1978
42. Laros R, Sweet R: Management of idiopathic thrombocytopenic purpura during pregnancy. Am J Obstet Gynecol 122:182, 1975
43. Jones W: Tissue-specific autoimmune diseases in pregnancy. Clin Obstet Gynecol 6:473, 1979
44. Horger E, Keane M: Platelet disorders in pregnancy. Clin Obstet Gynecol 22:843, 1979
45. Jones R, Asher M, Rutherford C, et al.: Autoimmune (idiopathic) thrombocytopenic purpura in pregnancy and the newborn. Br J Obstet Gynecol 84:679, 1977
46. Logaridis T, Doran T, Scott J, et al.: The effect of maternal steroid administration on fetal platelet count in immunologic thrombocytopenic purpura: Management of pregnancy and mode of delivery. Am J Obstet Gynecol 145:147, 1983
47. Scott J, Rote N, Cruishank D: Antiplatelet antibodies and platelet counts in pregnancies complicated by autoimmune thrombocytopenic purpura. Am J Obstet Gynecol 145:932, 1983
48. Cines D, Dusak B, Tomaski A, et al.: Immune thrombocytopenia purpura and pregnancy. N Engl J Med 306:826, 1982
49. Murray J, Harris R: The management of the pregnant patient with idiopathic thrombocytopenia purpura. Am J Obstet Gynecol 126:449, 1976
50. Levin J: Hematologic disorders of pregnancy, In Burrow G, Ferris T, (eds): Medical Complications During Pregnancy, ed 2. Philadelphia, Saunders, 1982, pp 62–87
51. Laros R, Swett R: Management of idiopathic thrombocytopenic purpura during pregnancy. Am J Obstet Gynecol 122:182, 1975
52. Karpatkin M, Porges R, Karpatkin S: Platelet counts in infants of women with autoimmune thrombocytopenia. Effect of steroid administration to the mother. N Engl J Med 305:936, 1981
53. Heys R: Childbearing and idiopathic thrombocytopenic purpura. J Obstet Gynecol Br Comm 73:205, 1966
54. Roboson H, Davidson L: Purpura in pregnancy with special referance to idiopathic thrombocytopenic purpura. Lancet 2:164, 1950
55. Thompson R, Moore R, Hess C: Idiopathic thrombocytopenic purpura: Long-term results of treatment and the prognostic significance of the response to corticosteroids. Arch Intern Med 13:730, 1972
56. Ahn Y, Harrington W: Treatment of idiopathic thrombocytopenic purpura (ITP). Ann Rev Med 28:299, 1977
57. Bierling P, Farcet J, Duedari N, et al.: Increased platelet IgG in patients on high dose gammaglobulin for autoimmune thrombocytopenia purpura. Lancet 2:388, 1982
58. Fehr J, Hoffman V, Kappeler V: Transient reversal of thrombocytopenia in idiopathic thrombocytopenic purpura by high-dose intravenous gammaglobulin. N Engl J Med 306:1254, 1982
59. Carroll R, Rosse W, Kitchens C: Intravenous immunoglobulin administration in the treatment of severe chronic immune thrombocytopenic purpura. Am J Med 76(2a):181, 1984
60. Warrier I, Lusher J: Intravenous gamma globulin treatment for chronic idiopathic thrombocytopenic purpura in children. Am J Med 76(2a):193, 1984

61. Tchernia G, Dreyfus M, Laurian Y, et al.: Management of immune thrombocytopenia in pregnancy: Response to infusions of immunoglobulins. Am J Obstet Gynecol 148:225, 1984
62. Kelton J, Hirsch J: Venous thromboembolic disorders. In Burrow G, Ferris T (eds): Medical Complications During Pregnancy, ed 2. Philadelphia, Saunders, 1982, pp 169–186
63. Gurll N, Helfand Z, Salzan E, et al.: Peripheral venous thrombophlebitis during pregnancy. Am J Surg 121:449, 1971
64. Friend J, Kakkar V: The diagnosis of deep vein thrombosis in the puerperium. J Obstet Gynecol Br Comm 77:820, 1970
65. Aaro L, Johnson T, Juergens J: Acute superficial venous thrombophlebitis associated with pregnancy. Am J Obstet Gynecol 97:514, 1967
66. Finnerty J, Mackay B: Antepartum thrombophlebitis and pulmonary embolism. Obstet Gynecol 19:405, 1962
67. Villasanta U: Thromboembolic disease in pregnancy. Am J Obstet Gynecol 93:142, 1965
68. Winnfield J: Anticoagulation for antenatal thrombolic disease. J Obstet Gynecol Br Comm 76:518, 1969
69. Knuppel R, Hoffman M, O'Brien W: Precautions on ob anticoagulant use. Contemp Ob/Gyn 25:53, 1985
70. Bolan J: Thromboembolic complications of pregnancy. Clin Obstet Gynecol 26:913, 1983
71. Laros R, Alger L: Thromboembolism and pregnancy. Clin Obstet Gynecol 22:871, 1979
72. deSwiet M: Management of thromboembolism in pregnancy. Drugs 18:478, 1979
73. Bonner J: Venous thromboembolism and pregnancy. Clin Obstet Gynecol 8:456, 1981
74. Bararacco M, Vessey M: Recurrence of venous thromboembolic disease and the use of oral contraceptives. Br Med J 1:215, 1974
75. Thromboembolism in pregnancy (editorial). Br Med J 1:1661, 1979
76. Urowitz M, Gladman D: Rheumatic diseases. In Burrow G, Ferris T (eds): Medical Complications During Pregnancy, ed 2. Philadelphia, Saunders, 1982, pp 475–497
77. Persellin R: The effect of pregnancy on rheumatoid arthritis. Bull Rheum Dis 27:922, 1977
78. Bulmash J: Rheumatoid arthritis and pregnancy. Obstet Gynecol Ann 8:276, 1978
79. Kitzmiller J: Autoimmune disorders: Maternal, fetal and neonatal risks. Clin Obstet Gynecol 21:385, 1978
80. Oka M, Vainio U: Effect of pregnancy on the prognosis and serology of rheumatoid arthritis. Rheum Scand 12:47, 1966
81. Neely N, Persellin R: Activity of rheumatoid arthritis during pregnancy. Tex Med 73:59, 1977
82. Oka M: Effects of pregnancy on onset and course of rheumatoid arthritis. Ann Rheum Dis 12:227, 1953
83. Tozman E, Urowitz M, Gladman D: Systemic lupus erythematosus and pregnancy. J Rheumatol 7:624, 1980
84. Zulman M, Talal N, Hoffman G, et al.: Problems associated with the management of pregnancy in patients with systemic lupus erythematosus. J Rheumatol 7:37, 1980
85. Scott J: Immunologic disorders. In Brudennell M, Wilds P (eds): Medical and Surgical Problems in Obstetrics. Bristol, John Wright, 1984, pp 1–11
86. Rudolph A: The effects of nonsteroidal antiinflammatory compounds on fetal circulation and pulmonary function. Obstet Gynecol 58:63S, 1981
87. Collins E: Maternal and fetal effects of acetaminophen and salicylates in pregnancy. Obstet Gynecol 58:57S, 1981
88. Richards I: Congenital malformations and environmental influences in pregnancy. Br J Prev Soc Med 23:218, 1969
89. Nelson M, Forfar J: Associations between drugs administered during pregnancy and congenital abnormalities of the fetus. Br Med J 1:253, 1971
90. Saxen I: Association between oral clefts and drugs taken during pregnancy. Int J Epidemiol 4:37, 1975
91. Turner G, Collins E: Fetal effects of regular salicylate ingestion in pregnancy. Lancet 2:338, 1975
92. Slone D, Siskind V, Heinonen O, et al.: Aspirin and congenital malformations. Lancet 1:1373, 1976
93. Lewis R, Schulman J: Influence of acetylsalicylic acid, an inhibitor of prostaglandin synthesis, on the duration of human gestation and labour. Lancet 2:1159, 1973
94. Collins E, Turner G: Maternal effects of regular salicylate ingestion in pregnancy. Lancet 2:335, 1975
95. Corby D, Schulman I: The effects of antenatal drug administration on aggregration of plate-

lets of newborn infants. J Pediatr 79:307, 1971
96. Rumack C, Guggenheim M, Rumack B, et al.: Neonatal intracranial hemorrhage and maternal use of aspirin. Obstet Gynecol 58:52S, 1981
97. Manchester D, Margolis H, Sheldon R: Possible association between maternal indomethacin therapy and primary pulmonary hypertension of the newborn. Am J Obstet Gynecol 126:467, 1967
98. Goudie B, Dossetor J: Effect on the fetus of indomethacin given to suppress labor. Lancet 2:1187, 1979
99. Csaba I, Sulyok E, Ertl T: Clinical note: Relationship of maternal treatment with indomethacin to the persistence of fetal circulation syndrome. J Pediatr 92:484, 1978
100. Wiqvist N, Kjellmer I, Thiringer K, et al.: Treatment of premature labor by prostaglandin synthetase inhibitors. Acta Biol Med Ger 37:923, 1978
101. Niebyl J, Blake D, White R, et al.: The inhibition of premature labor with indomethacin. Am J Obstet Gynecol 136:1014, 1980
102. Inanova A: Systemic lupus erythematosus and pregnancy. Akush Ginekol 5:55, 1974
103. Sommerville B: The role of estradiol withdrawal in the etiology of menstrual migraine. Neurology 22:355, 1972
104. Lance J, Anthony M: Some clinical aspects of migraine. Arch Neurol 15:356, 1966
105. Massey E: Migraine during pregnancy. Obstet Gynecol Surv 32:693, 1977
106. Somerville B: A study of migraine in pregnancy. Neurology 22:824, 1977
107. Donaldson J: Neurology of Pregnancy. Philadelphia, Saunders, 1978
108. Dalessio D: Neurologic diseases. In Burrow G, Ferris T (eds): Medical Complications During Pregnancy, ed 2. Philadelphia, Saunders, 1982, pp 435–473
109. Aminoff M: Maternal neurologic disorders. In Creasy R, Resnik R (eds): Maternal–Fetal Medicine Principles and Practice. Philadelphia, Saunders, 1984, pp 1012–1013
110. Plauche W: Myasthenia gravis in pregnancy: An update. Am J Obstet Gynecol 135:691, 1979
111. Namba T, Brown S, Grob D: Neonatal myasthenis gravis: Report of two cases and a review of the literature. Pediatrics 45:488, 1970
112. Keesey J, Lindstrom J, Cokely H, et al.: Anti-acetylcholine receptor antibody in neonatal myasthenia gravis. N Engl J Med 296:55, 1977
113. Eden R, Gall S: Myasthenia gravis and pregnancy: A reappraisal of thymectomy. Obstet Gynecol 62:328, 1983
114. Osserman K, Genkins G: Studies in myasthenia gravis: Review of a twenty-year experience in over 1200 patients. Mt Sinai J Med 38:497, 1961
115. McNall P, Jafarnia M: Management of myasthenia gravis in the obstetrical patient. Am J Obstet Gynecol 92:518, 1965
116. Donaldson J: Neurological disorders. In Brudennell M, Wilds P (eds): Medical and Surgical Problems in Obstetrics. Bristol, John Wright, 1984, pp 41–49
117. Edery H, Porath G, Zahavy J: Passage of 2-hydroximinomethyl-N-methyl-pyridium methanesulfonate to the fetus and cerebral spaces. Toxicol Appl Pharmacol 9:341, 1966
118. Roberts J, Thomas B, Wilson A: Placental transfer of pyridostigmine. Br J Pharmacol 38:202, 1970

10

Immunization During Pregnancy

Roger G. Faix and Thomas C. Shope

Immunization has proved to be an effective technique for preventing or ameliorating a variety of infectious diseases. Despite its efficacy, immunization is often underutilized among adults because of oversight or apprehension about possible side effects; as a result, potentially preventable infections may produce significant morbidity or mortality. Pregnant or possibly pregnant women frequently present special difficulties to the clinician since they are often exposed to preventable transmissible infections that may adversely affect their health or pregnancy outcome, yet the available immunizing agents are likewise not without some risk to the mother and fetus.

Decisions about immunization during pregnancy necessitate consideration of the severity of the disease in mother and fetus, significance of the exposure, incubation period for the disease, maternal immune status for the infection in question, allergic history, choice of available immunizing agents, and efficacy, toxicity, and side effects of the immunizing agents. Cost should not be an issue since most of these agents cost only a few dollars or can be obtained at minimal charge from public health agencies. If benefit clearly outweighs the risk, a careful discussion with the prospective mother should be initiated and immunization should be recommended. The purposes of this chapter are to discuss the relevant decision-making issues for immunization during pregnancy and to review how to most effectively immunize the gravid patient when that is warranted.

GENERAL CONSIDERATIONS FOR IMMUNIZATION

Active and Passive Immunization

Two types of immunization are available: active and passive. In active immunization, the immunizing antigen is administered to the patient to induce a long-lasting or permanent immune response. The antigen may be a whole organism (killed or live, following adequate attenuation to preclude pathogenicity), purified subcellular fraction of the organism, or an inactivated exotoxin (toxoid).

The desired protective immune response may take weeks or months to develop, which may be adequate if exposure has not yet occurred or if the incubation period exceeds the necessary interval for immunity to develop. Specific antibodies, cell-mediated immunity, and other immune effectors typically result from active immunization.

In passive immunization, the patient receives a preparation enriched with preformed antibody, harvested from carefully screened donors. Almost immediate protection is possible, but it is relatively short lived since the half-life of the IgG is only 20 to 30 days. Standard immune serum globulin (ISG) provides adequate specific antibody to protect against measles and hepatitis A but does not contain sufficient antibody for a variety of other infections.[1] Hyperimmune specific globulins are prepared from donors convalescing from acute infection (e.g., varicella-zoster immune globulin [VZIG]) or specifically immunized to develop high antibody titers (e.g., rabies immune globulin). Some preparations are derived from specially immunized horses (e.g., snake antivenin) and necessitate special precautions during administration to minimize the risk of serum sickness or anaphylaxis. Intravenous gamma globulin or plasma may be used in selected circumstances where use of the standard intramuscular preparations is undesirable. Currently available immunization preparations are listed in Tables 10–1 and 10–2.

TABLE 10–1. CURRENTLY AVAILABLE ACTIVE IMMUNIZING AGENTS

Bacteria	Viruses
Live	
*BCG[2]	Measles
Tularemia	Mumps Poliomyelitis, oral Rubella Yellow fever
Killed (or purified subcellular fraction)	
*Cholera[3]	Hepatitis B
Meningococcus, types A and C	Influenza
Pertussis	Poliomyelitis, inactivated
Yersinia pestis (plague)	Rabies
Pneumococcus	
*Typhoid[4,5]	
Hemophilus influenzae type b	
Toxoids	
Diphtheria	
Tetanus	
Anthrax	

* Controversial efficacy.

Side Effects and Toxicity

Both types of immunization may produce local swelling, redness, and discomfort. Active agents may also occasionally produce arthralgias or frank arthritis (e.g., rubella), high fever, irritability and encephalopathy (e.g., pertussis whole cell vaccine), transient mild depression of cutaneous markers of cell-mediated immunity (e.g., measles), and a variety of less common side effects. Immunodeficient or immunosuppressed individuals should not receive or be exposed to recipients of certain live vaccines, since they may develop life-threatening infection with the attenuated vaccine strain.[6] Passive agents usually require deep and often painful intramuscular injection of large volumes of fluid. Individuals with IgA deficiency and anti-IgA antibodies may develop anaphylaxis after exposure to immune globulin preparations which invariably contain small amounts of IgA.[7]

Both types of agents may contain preservatives, adjuvants, antibiotics, and residual proteins that may cause problems in hypersensitive individuals or patients who require multiple doses over prolonged periods. Thimerosal, a mercurial derivative, is a preservative found in immune globulin preparations that has been reported to produce mercury intoxication in hypogammaglobulinemic patients who required immune serum globulin

TABLE 10–2. CURRENTLY AVAILABLE PASSIVE IMMUNIZING AGENTS

General

- Immune serum globulin, for intramuscular use
- Gamma globulin in 10% maltose, for intravenous use
- Human plasma, fresh-frozen or single donor, for intravenous use

Specific

Antiviral

- Hepatitis B immune globulin (HBIG)
- Varicella-zoster immune globulin (VZIG)
- Varicella-zoster immune plasma (VZIP)
- Rabies immune globulin (RIG)
- Vaccinia immune globulin (VIG)

Antitoxin/Antivenin

- Tetanus immune globulin (TIG)
- Snake bite, coral and crotolid—horse serum
- Black widow spider—horse serum
- Diphtheria antitoxin—horse serum
- Tetanus antitoxin—horse serum
- Botulism antitoxin—horse serum

therapy for many years.[8] Residual antibiotics from culture media are present in only miniscule amounts in vaccines, but a history of hypersensitivity to neomycin should be sought prior to administration of measles, mumps, or rubella vaccine. A history of delayed-type hypersensitivity reactions is not a contraindication to receiving these vaccines. Penicillin is not a component of any currently marketed vaccines. Yellow fever, influenza, measles, and mumps vaccines are prepared from viruses grown in embryonated chicken eggs or chick embryo tissues. Individuals with anaphylactic hypersensitivity to eggs or inability to eat eggs without adverse effects should not receive these vaccines.[9]

Storage and Administration

Strict adherence to the manufacturer's recommendations for each vaccine are necessary for optimal results. Safety and efficacy testing have been based precisely on the conditions stated in the package insert. Reconstitution, storage conditions, dosing, and route of administration must be performed in accordance with these instructions. Multidose vials need to be dated and timed to prevent loss of potency associated with expiration. Such simple mistakes as storing vaccine in refrigerator doors—subject to many temperature fluctuations with each cycle of opening and closing—rather than in a better protected refrigerated area, may render a vaccine impotent.[10] Similarly, use of glass syringes for administration of live measles vaccine rather than the recommended plastic syringe has resulted in inactivation of the vaccine.[11] Exposure of measles, mumps, or rubella vaccines to light may destroy their immunogenicity.[12]

Administration of a vaccine or immune globulin should be considered to be an aseptic technique. Disposable sterile needles should be used for withdrawal from the vial and administration. Separate needles and syringes should be used for each patient. The site of administration should be selected to avoid active skin lesions and neurovascular structures. Preferred sites for intramuscular or subcutaneous administration include the anterolateral upper thigh and deltoid. Intradermal agents are usually administered on the volar surface of the forearm. The site should be carefully cleansed with either isopropyl alcohol or iodophor followed by isopropyl alcohol. Use of the Z technique for intramuscular administration will minimize the risk of vaccine or immune globulin seeping back into the subcutaneous, intradermal, or extracutaneous sites. Once the needle tip is judged to be in proper position, the syringe should be aspirated gently to be certain that a blood vessel has not been entered inadvertently. If vascular entry has occurred, the needle, syringe, and immunizing agent should be discarded, and new materials assembled.

Recent studies of hepatitis B vaccine have demonstrated that intramuscular administration in the deltoid is more effective than in the upper outer gluteal area.[13] This presumably reflects the large amount of fat in the gluteal area, which is often so deep that injections end up in fat rather than muscle even with a 1.5 inch or longer needle.[14] It seems advisable, therefore, to administer all intramuscular immunizing agents in the deltoid whenever possible, unless the volume to be administered is too great (e.g., small children, large doses of immune globulin). If an immune globulin and vaccine are to be administered at the same time, e.g., rabies, each should be administered with a separate syringe at a separate site. Administration of different live virus vaccines within 1 month of each other (but not on the same day) has been reported to decrease the immune response to the second vaccine and should therefore be avoided.[9]

When immunizing agents are administered, appropriate equipment and medication (airways, intravenous infusion equipment, 1:1000 epinephrine, oral and intravenous antihistamines, steroids) should be available to initiate promptly treatment for anaphylaxis or other acute immunization-related events. All recipients should be observed for 10 to 15 minutes to facilitate early detection and treatment if difficulties such as hives, bronchospasm, hypotension, or fainting arise.

SPECIAL CONSIDERATIONS DURING PREGNANCY

Immunization of the pregnant woman may impact upon the fetus as well as the mother. Antibodies induced in the mother may be transmitted across the placenta in increasing quantities as gestation progresses and may temporarily protect the infant. Such transient protection may also interfere with the development of the infant's own permanent antibody response, however, if sufficient maternal antibody remains when the child is immunized against the same pathogen.[15,16] Toxic effects of vaccine in the mother may include fever, cardiovascular compromise, or neurologic symptoms. These may affect the fetus by impairing blood flow and delivery of oxygen and nutrients to the uterus and placenta or by diminishing the capability of the mother to appropriately care for herself during pregnancy. Live vaccines harbor the theoretical risk of inducing maternal viremia, crossing the placenta, and infecting the fetus with resultant teratogenesis or destruction of fetal tissues. Whether vaccine use during pregnancy increases rates of spontaneous abortion or stillbirth is poorly studied for many vaccines, but is a theoretical possibility. Conscientious efforts to promote universal immunization during childhood would obviate the need for having to consider immunization during pregnancy, but unfortunately such compliance is not yet reality.

Prophylaxis Following Significant Exposure

For the above reasons, immunization is generally discouraged during pregnancy, but may be warranted if the mother has a significant exposure to a disease with a substantial risk of mortality or severe morbidity to herself or her fetus. Several preventable diseases are typically more severe among adults than children, e.g., measles and mumps, and some may inflict greater morbidity among pregnant than nonpregnant women, e.g., varicella-zoster and influenza, though confounding factors are difficult to exclude. If there is a significant chance of acquiring the disease and the risk associated with the disease is greater than that of an effective immunization agent, then immunization is warranted. Among the preventable diseases that fall into this category are rabies, hepatitis B, tetanus, yellow fever, measles, hepatitis A, tularemia, and possibly diphtheria and meningococcal disease.

Once the possibility of exposure is considered, the diagnosis in the sick person to whom the mother was exposed must be confirmed if at all possible, using clinical examination, culture, serology, or other specialized methods as necessary. If confirmed or indeterminate, the significance of the exposure must be assessed. Considerations for each disease vary according to routes of transmission, incubation period, and proximity and duration of exposure. If exposure was significant or indeterminate, and incubation time is greater than that required to induce an effective response, the mother's immune status for the pathogen should be checked. If already immune, immunization is unnecessary. Nonimmune mothers should be immunized.

The choice of active, passive, or a combination of both agents depends on the pathogen. Passive agents provide immediate protection and have less associated maternal and fetal side effects, but are not available or effective for all immunizable diseases. Among active agents, some killed vaccines are not as immunogenic as corresponding live vaccines but have less potential for transplacental infection. For prevention of poliomyelitis, many authorities recommend that nonimmune adults receive inactivated polio vaccine except in epidemic control circumstances because of a higher risk of vaccine-associated paralysis with oral polio vaccine among adults.[17] Toxoids cause virtually no risk to the mother. Active agents often take several weeks to induce an effective immune response. Although a number of polyvalent vaccines (i.e., directed against multiple pathogens) are available, the pregnant woman should receive the appropriate monovalent vaccine (if available) to avoid unnecessary risk associated with the superfluous agents.

For diseases where effective active and passive immunization agents are available, use of both agents may permit immediate protection while allowing time for a permanent endogenous response to be mounted. Combination regimens are not warranted in all immunizable diseases, since some live vaccines may pose unnecessary fetal risk and because exogenously administered antibody may interact with the vaccine antigen and prevent development of an active immune response. Combination active–passive immunization is recommended only in those conditions where the combination has been proved to be safe and effective. Administration of blood or blood products (plasma, serum, platelets, immunoglobulins) should be avoided for at least 14 days after active immunization since they may contain specific antibody against the vaccine antigen and thus interfere with the desired immune response.[9] If use of blood products is unavoidable, reimmunization may be required 3 months after the initial attempt. In all cases, the pregnant woman should be carefully advised of potential risks and benefits of the proposed immunization and should be an active participant in decision making. Considerations and recommendations following significant exposure of pregnant women to a variety of diseases for which immunizing agents are available are enumerated in Table 10–3.

If the potential risk of immunization is worth taking, all appropriate steps must be taken to insure that the immunization is performed properly. Assessing serologic response 4 to 6 weeks after active immunization is warranted to determine the need for additional steps or reimmunization if such tests are readily available. Specific cell-mediated immunity is also presumably induced by active immunization and may be the more critical factor for intracellular infections, but specific assays of cell-mediated immunity are rarely available.

Despite reports of increased infectious mortality and morbidity and generalized mild attenuation of immunologic responsiveness among pregnant women, most women who were immunocompetent before pregnancy are capable of developing an appropriate immune response during pregnancy.[38] Reported observations of declining antibody titers against a variety of viral and protozoal organisms during pregnancy have been interpreted by some to represent humoral immunosuppression, but more likely represent hemodilution caused by the physiologic increase in blood volume during pregnancy and transplacental IgG antibody transfer from mother to fetus.[39–42] The many well-documented series of successful gestational im-

TABLE 10–3. RECOMMENDATIONS FOR IMMUNIZATION OF SUSCEPTIBLE PREGNANT WOMEN FOLLOWING SIGNIFICANT EXPOSURE TO IMMUNIZABLE DISEASES

	Risk of Disease		
Disease	***Maternal***	***Fetal***	**Immunizing Agent of Choice**
Anthrax	Unchanged by pregnancy	Determined by severity of maternal illness	Vaccine, 0.5 ml SC, 3 doses at 2-wk intervals
Black widow spider bite	Unchanged by pregnancy	Determined by severity of maternal illness	Antivenin, equine 6000 U IM or slow IV, following sensitivity tests
Botulism	Unchanged by pregnancy	Determined by severity of maternal illness	Trivalent antitoxin, equine, following sensitivity tests
Cholera	Unchanged by pregnancy	Determined by severity of maternal illness	None
Diphtheria	Unchanged by pregnancy	Determined by severity of maternal illness	Exposure only: None For symptomatic patient: Antitoxin, equine, 10,000–100,000 U IV once, following sensitivity tests
Hemophilus influenzae type b	Unchanged by pregnancy	Determined by severity of maternal illness	None
Hepatitis A	Unchanged by pregnancy	Determined by severity of maternal illness; risk of neonatal hepatitis A if within 2 wk of delivery	Immune serum globulin, 0.02 ml/kg IM
Hepatitis B	Unchanged by pregnancy	Increased risk of chronic carrier state	Hepatitis B immune globulin, 5.0 ml IM; if recurrent exposure likely, monthly doses of HBIG *or* Vaccine, 1.0 ml IM with repeat doses 1 and 5 months later
Influenza	? Increased severity of pneumonia, risk of death	Rare transplacental transmission; ? increased nonspecific anomalies	Following exposure, none
Measles	? Increase in heart failure, pulmonary edema	Increased abortion, stillbirth, prematurity; rare congenital measles	Immune serum globulin, 0.25 ml/kg within 72 hours of exposure
Meningococcus	Unchanged by pregnancy	Determined by severity of maternal illness	If group A or C, monovalent or polyvalent vaccine, intradermal; If group B, none
Mumps	Unchanged by pregnancy	Abortion	None

Side Effects/Toxicity	Comments	References
Local Malaise	Contact with human case does not require immunization. Vaccination limited to those with occupational or daily exposure to high-risk animals or animal products. Vaccine available from Department of Immunobiologics, Centers for Disease Control (phone 404/329–3356)	18
Serum sickness Anaphylaxis Delayed neuritis	Administration should begin as soon as possible; supportive treatment with analgesics, calcium, anticholinesterases, and other agents also essential	
Serum sickness Anaphylaxis Delayed neuritis	Antitoxin available round-the-clock from Center for Disease Control: 404/329–3753 from 8:00 AM to 4:30 PM; 404/329–3644 at other times; concomitant administration of penicillin will kill organisms and reduce toxin production	
Local Fever, myalgia, malaise	Vaccine of dubious efficacy; immune response with postexposure vaccination takes too long to be protective	3, 19
Serum sickness Anaphylaxis Delayed neuritis	Immune response to postexposure immunization takes too long to be protective	
Local Unknown in pregnant women	Immune response to postexposure vaccine takes too long to be protective; risk to fetus of chemoprophylaxis with rifampin is unknown	
Local		20
Local Vaccine: fever, malaise, fatigue	HBIG most effective when given less than 24 hours after exposure	
Local Egg hypersensitivity Fever, malaise, myalgia	Immune response takes too long to be protective after exposure; high-risk individuals (see text) should receive appropriate vaccine for that year before influenza season, 0.5 ml IM single dose. Chemoprophylaxis with amantidine not recommended during pregnancy	21–23
Local	Live vaccine contraindicated because of theoretical risk of transplacental fetal injury	24
Local ? Theoretical induction of tolerance to other meningococcal strains	Serious consideration should be given to chemoprophylaxis with sulfonamides (? fetal effects of rifampin) for all groups of meningococci; immune response may take too long to be effective	25
—	Live vaccine contraindicated because of theoretical risk to fetus; vaccine not effective when given after exposure	26

(continued)

TABLE 10–3. (*Continued*)

Disease	Risk of Disease		Immunizing Agent of Choice
	Maternal	***Fetal***	
Pertussis	Unchanged by pregnancy	Determined by severity of maternal illness; ? increased risk of neonatal pertussis	None
Pneumococcus	Unchanged by pregnancy	Determined by severity of maternal illness; ? increased risk of neonatal sepsis	None
Poliomyelitis	Unchanged by pregnancy	Abortion Congenital polio (rare)	Inactivated polio vaccine, 1.0 ml SC, 3 doses at 4-wk intervals *or* Oral polio vaccine, 0.5 ml PO, 3 doses at 6-wk intervals
Rabies	Unchanged by pregnancy	Determined by severity of maternal illness	Rabies immune globulin, 20 IU/kg once—half infiltrated into wound site, half IM; if mucosal wound, all IM *and* Rabies vaccine, human diploid (Merieux), 1.0 ml IM once, then 3, 7, 14, and 28 days later at separate sites
Rubella	Unchanged by pregnancy	Teratogenesis Abortions Stillbirth	None (if abortion not an option some recommend immune serum globulin, 20 ml or 0.55 ml/kg IM)
Smallpox	Not applicable since natural disease no longer exists		None
Snake bite (coral and crotolid)	Unchanged by pregnancy	Determined by severity of maternal illness	Polyvalent antivenin, equine, 20–150 ml of reconstituted antivenin (depending on degree of envenomation) IV or IM, following sensitivity tests
Tetanus	Unchanged by pregnancy	Determined by severity of maternal illness	Tetanus toxoid, adsorbed, 0.5 ml IM, 3 doses at 3–8 wk intervals for primary immunization, one dose for booster if more than 5 yr since last dose *and*

Side Effects/Toxicity	Comments	References
—	Vaccine not recommended in adults because of mildness of adult disease and high incidence of unacceptable side effects	
—	Immune response takes too long for postexposure vaccine to be effective; should be administered pre-exposure to high-risk individuals (see text), 0.5 ml polyvalent vaccine SC or IM	
IPV: Local ? Increased risk of malignancy among infants born to mothers immunized in pregnancy OPV: Local Paralytic poliomyelitis	Controversial as to which agent should be used when immediate protection is needed: Advisory Committee on Immunization Practices recommends OPV, but IPV for all other circumstances among adults. Potential risk of transplacental infection, increased risk of paralysis among adults with OPV, and ? data to support more rapid immunity with OPV all justify IPV as an option	27–31
RIG: Local Fever, hives, angioedema (rare) Vaccine: Local Fever, nausea, emesis, myalgia, neuropathy	Recent reports of impaired immunogenicity with Wyeth vaccine suggest Merieux vaccine as agent of choice for now. Limited experience suggests vaccine well tolerated in pregnancy	32, 33
—	Vaccine should be avoided because of risk of fetal injury. ISG does not reliably prevent or modify disease, and may interfere with serologic testing if abortion is an option	34, 35
—	Vaccine should be avoided because of disease extinction and risk of fetal injury. If received or significantly exposed to vaccinee inadvertently, give vaccinia immune globulin (0.3 ml/kg IM). Globulin and consultation available from Centers for Disease Control: 404/329–3145 during day and 404/329-2888 evenings and weekends. If vaccinia infection develops, may require 0.6 ml/kg/24 hours globulin IM and adjunctive antiviral chemotherapy	50–55
Serum sickness Anaphylaxis Delayed neuritis	Administration within 4 hr of bite produces best results	
Toxoid: Local Fever, myalgia, malaise Polyradiculoneuropathy (rare) TIG: Local Fever, allergic reactions	Maternal immunization may be warranted to provide neonatal protection in parts of the world where neonatal tetanus is common. For treatment of active tetanus infection, use TIG 3000–6000 U IM	

(continued)

TABLE 10–3. *(Continued)*

Disease	Risk of Disease: *Maternal*	Risk of Disease: *Fetal*	Immunizing Agent of Choice
			If severe tetanus-prone wound, tetanus immune globulin 250–500 units IM once, repeat monthly if threat persists
Tuberculosis	Unchanged by pregnancy	If severe maternal dz: Miliary tuberculosis Stillbirth Abortion	None
Tularemia	Unchanged by pregnancy	Determined by severity of maternal illness	Live vaccine, 1 drop with multiple intradermal punctures
Typhoid	Unchanged by pregnancy	Determined by severity of maternal illness	None
Varicella-zoster	? Increased risk of pneumonia and death	Congenital varicella syndrome (rare)	Varicella-zoster immune globulin 625 U IM *or* Immune serum globulin, 0.6–1.2 ml/kg IM *or* None
Yellow fever	Unchanged by pregnancy	Determined by severity of maternal illness	17D live vaccine, 0.5 ml SC
Yersinia pestis (Plague)	Unchanged by pregnancy	Determined by severity of maternal illness	Killed vaccine, 1.0 ml IM, then 0.2 ml boosters 4 wk and 6 mo later with annual boosters thereafter

SC = subcutaneous; IM = intramuscular; IV = intravenous; ISG = immune serum globulin.

munizations, confirmed by seroconversion, attest to the immune responsiveness of the pregnant women.[43,44]

Occasionally immunization of a pregnant woman may be medically indicated before exposure to the pathogen. Conditions such as heart disease, chronic lung disease, chronic renal disease, diabetes, chronic severe anemia, or splenic insufficiency place a pregnant woman at increased risk of mortality and morbidity from influenza and pneumococcus. The reported increased susceptibility to mortality and morbidity from influenza in pregnant women without such conditions is controversial, but suggests that protection is even more imperative for pregnant women with predisposing conditions who have not previously been vaccinated.[21,45] Annual variations in influenza strains necessitate annual vaccine reformulations; consequently such women should be immunized before each influenza season (usually December through April) with the annually reformulated killed vaccine. Since influenza vaccine is usually designed for predicted influenza strains, it may not offer protection against the strain that actually enters the community. Even if the proper strain is included, the vaccine is often only 60 to 80 percent protective.[46] Consequently, recipients should still exercise common sense and caution to avoid unnecessary exposure to influenza.

Side Effects/Toxicity	Comments	References
—	Efficacy of BCG vaccine is controversial	2
Local Regional adenopathy	Vaccination of human case contacts unnecessary; vaccination only for high-risk exposure to infected animals and insects that bite them. Limited experience suggests no fetal risk associated with vaccine	36
—	Efficacy of vaccine is controversial; immune response after postexposure vaccine takes too long to be protective	4, 5
Local	VZIG use carefully regulated by American Red Cross because of limited supplies: unless patient immunosuppressed or immunodeficient, release of VZIG is unlikely and ISG may be only alternative. ISG may modify but not reliably prevent disease. Rarity of severe varicella complications and problems administering *large* volumes of ISG often makes no immunization the most attractive alternative	37
Local Headache, myalgia, fever Egg hypersensitivity	Exposure to infected person does not mandate vaccine; exposure to *Aedes aegyptii* mosquito vector in endemic area does	
Malaise, headache, adenopathy, fever	Vaccine efficacy indeterminate; ? immune response rapid enough for protection after single acute exposure	

Inadvertent Immunization During Pregnancy

Administration of immunizing agents to a woman whose pregnant state was not appreciated is another circumstance that requires consideration. In general, passive immunization agents pose no more threat than when administered to a nonpregnant woman. Toxoids similarly pose little additional risk, though it should be noted that primary vaccination with tetanus toxoid during pregnancy has been reported to increase the level of IgG antibody to blood groups A and B in women of blood group O and to induce a correspondingly higher rate of ABO hemolytic disease in the resultant infants.[47] In most circumstances, however, ABO disease is much less difficult to manage successfully than full-blown tetanus.

Inadvertent administration of live virus vaccines may carry some risk to the fetus. Polio, measles, mumps, and rubella may all theoretically infect the fetus, but among vaccine strains, only rubella has been demonstrated to do so. Though vaccine virus has been recovered from aborted products of conception and rarely from liveborn infants born to women who inadvertently received rubella vaccine shortly prior to conception or during the first trimester, no proven vaccine-caused cases of congenital rubella syndrome have been detected, even with the present, more potent RA27/3 vaccine.[48] Pregnant recipients of yellow fever vaccine have been reported to have no higher rate of teratogenesis, abortion, or stillbirth than nonimmunized pregnant women.[49] Vaccinia immunization for smallpox has been reported on several occasions to infect the fetus with devastating results.[49,50] Since the worldwide eradication of smallpox, there is no longer any valid indication for the use of this vaccine in any civilian population, except for rare selected laboratory workers with occupational exposure.[51] The United States armed forces routinely vaccinate all active duty, National Guard, and Reserve personnel upon entry and at 5-year intervals. In general, these vaccinations are performed at the start of basic training, summer camps, or other settings that minimize contact between recently vaccinated military personnel and the general public. Pregnant women are excused from active duty and would not ordinarily receive such vaccines. Inadvertent vaccination of female military personnel who do not yet know that they are pregnant or transmission of the vaccine virus to pregnant contacts of vaccinated personnel has not been reported, but is a possibility.[52–54]

The pregnant woman who has inadvertently received a live virus vaccine to which she is nonimmune should be counseled about potential risks and alternatives. With the possible exception of rubella vaccine, documented fetal risks following live virus vaccine seem miniscule enough that abortion for vaccine exposure alone is not warranted. In the case of rubella, present data strongly suggest that exposed fetuses will do well but enough doubt persists that abortion is still requested by a significant fraction of exposed mothers. Women who were immunized with rubella vaccine up to 3 months before conception should be included in the group at risk and also receive appropriate counseling. If a pregnant woman receives smallpox vaccine, vaccinia immune globulin (0.3 ml/kg IM) should be given as soon as possible to minimize the possibility of fetal infection.[55] The Centers for Disease Control provide this product as well as helpful advice in such circumstances (see Table 10–3). The problem of inadvertent live vaccine administration could be decreased if immunizing personnel routinely asked potential women vaccinees about the possibility of pregnancy before administration.

Women who are exposed to recipients of live virus vaccines, including rubella, have no greater risk of acquiring symptomatic infection or transmitting transplacental infection than pregnant women not so exposed.[56,57] One possible exception is smallpox vaccine.[52–54] Pregnant women should avoid contact with persons with active smallpox vaccination lesions. If significant contact with such a vaccinee occurs, consultation with public health authorities or the Centers for Disease Control should be sought and the administration of vaccinia immune globulin should be seriously considered. Individuals with immunodeficiency disorders may acquire life-threatening infection following exposure to recipients of vaccine viruses.[6] These individuals, their families, and their close contacts should receive only killed vaccines.

Travel Requirements

International travel occasionally raises the possibility of immunization during pregnancy, since many underdeveloped nations mandate a number of immunizations before entry is permitted. If the mother has not already received the necessary immunizations before pregnancy, travel to those nations should be postponed until the pregnancy is finished. If that is not possible, the required immunizations should be considered individually. If polio, yellow fever, or tetanus is endemic in the country and the woman has not been previously immunized, vaccine should be administered, since the actual risk of contracting the disease is much greater than the risk of the vaccine. Other vaccines, including cholera and typhoid, are of questionable efficacy and may have significant side effects. A certificate may be issued stating that these are contraindicated because of the pregnancy, but one should be aware that entry into some countries may be denied even with such a certificate. Consultation with the Centers for Disease Control or the World Health Organization about specific countries and situations may be helpful.

Postpartum Immunization

Once the pregnant woman has been delivered, serious consideration should be given to performing all indicated immunizations in the immediate 2 to 3 days after delivery. The mother is usually still hospitalized at this time and is available for vaccination and well-situated for observation of possible immediate side effects. A theoretical risk of transmission of live vaccine virus to her new infant by breast milk, nasopharyngeal secretions, or other body fluids does exist, but this actually happens very infrequently and even then rarely causes significant morbidity.[58] If multiple agents are required concurrently, use only those that have been shown to be effective when given in combination; others can be administered several months later.

Blood or blood products received within 2 weeks of these immunizations may interfere with their effectiveness. The one exception to this is Rhogam (Rh [D] immune globulin); though it could theoretically interfere with immunization, the usual administered volume is so small that interference has never been documented. If live vaccines are administered postpartum, the recipient mother should take steps to prevent conception for at least 3 months if possible. One should recall that even if immunization appears effective as documented by seroconversion, infection may still occur occasionally.[59,60]

NEW AND FUTURE VACCINES

Several new vaccines are at varying stages of development. It is unlikely that some, e.g., cytomegalovirus, varicella-zoster, will ever be considered safe for use during pregnancy except in the rarest of circumstances. Others may be useful in special situations, e.g., malaria vaccine prior to necessary travel in an area with endemic malaria. Some vaccines are being targeted for pregnant women, e.g., group B streptococcus type III vaccine, in an attempt to allow transplacental passage of maternally-induced antibody to protect the fetus or young infant from selected high-risk pathogens during the perinatal period.[61] Vaccines targeted against organisms causing major problems in children less than 1 year of age but not adequately immunogenic in such children, e.g., *Hemophilus influenzae* type b vaccine, might be modified to induce high antibody levels in expectant mothers and possibly facilitate transplacental delivery of sufficient antibody to later protect the child from infection until he reaches the age when he can mount his own vaccine response. Brazilian mothers vaccinated against meningococcus types A and C during an epidemic transmitted protective antibody to many of their offspring which persisted for up to 5 months; unfortunately, transmission was unreliable and impact on future immune response to vaccination against meningococcus in these infants is unknown.[62] New formulations of vaccines for influenza, hepatitis B, *Hemophilus influenzae* type b, and pertussis that are more immunogenic or have fewer side effects may be released soon. The availability of these new vaccines may alter immunization recommendations in the near future.

As long as humans interact with each other, the potential for transmission of infectious agents and resultant disease will exist. Use of effective vaccines and immune globulins may substantially decrease such transmission or ameliorate the severity of the disease. Further research will broaden the range of preventable diseases and decrease the probability of undesirable side effects to all recipients, pregnant or not.

REFERENCES

1. Fulginiti VA: Immune globulin. In Fulginiti VA (ed): Immunization in Clinical Practice. Philadelphia, Lippincott, 1982, pp 221–236
2. Tuberculosis Prevention Trial Madras: Trial of BCG vaccines in South India for tuberculosis prevention. Ind J Med Res 70:349, 1979

3. Finkelstein RA: Immunology of cholera. Curr Top Microbiol Immunol 69:138, 1975
4. Ray CG: Typhoid fever (*Salmonella septicemia*). In Fulginiti VA (ed): Immunization in Clinical Practice. Philadelphia, Lippincott, 1982, p 198
5. Anderson DC: Immunization: Active immunizing agents. In Feigin RD, Cherry JD (eds): Textbook of Pediatric Infectious Diseases. Philadelphia, Saunders, 1981, p 1751
6. Fulginiti VA: The scheduling of immunizations. In Fulginiti VA (ed): Immunization in Clinical Practice. Philadelphia, Lippincott, 1982, pp 66–67
7. Vyas GH, Perkins HA, Fudenberg HH: Anaphylactoid transfusion reactions associated with anti-IgA. Lancet 2:312, 1968
8. Matheson DS, Clarkson TW, Gelfand EW: Mercury toxicity (acrodynia) induced by long-term injection of gamma globulin. J Pediatr 97:153, 1980
9. Centers for Disease Control: General recommendations on immunization. Ann Intern Med 98:615, 1983
10. Lerman SJ, Gold E: Measles in previously vaccinated children. JAMA 216:1311, 1971
11. Fulginiti VA: Immunization practice: Some important guidelines. Postgrad Med 60:62, 1976
12. Krugman RD, Meyer BC, Enterline JC, et al.: Impotency of live-virus vaccines as a result of improper handling in clinical practice. J Pediatr 85:512, 1974
13. Centers for Disease Control: Suboptimal response to hepatitis B vaccine given by injection into the buttock. MMWR 34:105, 1985
14. Cockshott WP, Thompson GT, Howlett LJ, et al.: Intramuscular or intralipomatous injections? N Engl J Med 307:356, 1982
15. Yeager AS, Davis JH, Ross LA, et al.: Measles immunization: Successes and failures. JAMA 237:347, 1977
16. DiSant'Agnese PA: Combined immunization against diphtheria, tetanus, and pertussis in newborn infants, II. Duration of antibody levels. Antibody titers after booster dose. Effect of passive immunity to diphtheria on active immunization with diphtheria toxoid. Pediatrics 3:181, 1949
17. Centers for Disease Control: Poliomyelitis prevention. MMWR 28:510, 1979
18. Brachman SJ, Gold H, Plotkin SA, et al.: Field evaluation of human anthrax vaccine. Am J Public Health 52:632, 1962
19. Klein JD, Brunnel PA, Cherry JD, Fulginiti VA (eds): Report of the Committee on Infectious Diseases—1982, ed 19. Evanston, Ill, American Academy of Pediatrics, 1982, pp 62–64
20. Crumpacker CS: Hepatitis. In Remington JS, Klein JO (eds): Infectious Diseases of the Fetus and Newborn Infant. Philadelphia, Saunders, 1983, p 593
21. Braun G, O'Connor D, Schmidt R, et al.: Factors involved in immunization program for swine influenza. Am J Med 61:925, 1976
22. Yawn DH, Pyeatte J, Joseph M, et al.: Transplacental transfer of influenza virus. JAMA 216:1022, 1971
23. Yeager AS: Viruses uncommonly associated with infection of the fetus and newborn infant. In Remington JS, Klein JO (eds): Infectious Diseases of the Fetus and Newborn Infant, ed 2. Philadelphia, Saunders, 1983, pp 547–549
24. Christensen PE, Schmidt H, Barg HO, et al.: An epidemic of measles in southern Greenland, 1951. Measles in virgin soil, II. The epidemic proper. Acta Med Scand 144:430, 1953
25. Jones JF: Meningococcal infections. In Fulginiti VA (ed): Immunization in Clinical Practice. Philadelphia, Lippincott, 1982, p 213
26. Siegel M, Fuerst HT, Peress NS: Comparative fetal mortality in maternal virus diseases. N Engl J Med 274:768, 1966
27. Heinonen OP, Shapiro S, Monson RR, et al.: Immunization during pregnancy against poliomyelitis and influenza in relation to childhood malignancy. Int J Epidemiol 2:229, 1973
28. Roy CG: Poliomyelitis. In Fulginiti VA (ed): Immunization in Clinical Practice. Philadelphia, Lippincott, 1982, p 141
29. Amstey MS: Immunization in pregnancy. Clin Obstet Gynaecol 10:13, 1983
30. Bader ME: Polio vaccination during pregnancy (letter). JAMA 249:2018, 1983
31. Goodman RA, Orenstein WA, Hinman AR: Polio vaccination during pregnancy (letter). JAMA 249:2018, 1983
32. Centers for Disease Control: Rabies postexposure prophylaxis with human diploid cell rabies vaccine: Lower neutralizing antibody titers with Wyeth vaccine. MMWR 34:90, 1985
33. Varner MW, McGuiness GA, Galask RP: Rabies vaccination in pregnancy. Am J Obstet Gynecol 143:717, 1982
34. Fulginiti VA: Immune globulin. In Fulginiti VA (ed): Immunization in Clinical Practice. Philadelphia, Lippincott, 1982, pp 232–233

35. Klein JO, Brunell PA, Cherry JD, Fulginiti VA (eds): Report of the Committee on Infectious Diseases—1982, ed 19. Evanston, Ill, American Academy of Pediatrics, 1982, p 231
36. Albrecht RC, Cefalo RC, O'Brien WF: Tularemia immunization in early pregnancy. Am J Obstet Gynecol 138:1226, 1980
37. Klein JO, Brunnel PA, Cherry JD, Fulginiti VA (eds): Report of the Committee on Infectious Diseases—1982, ed 19. Evanston, Ill, American Academy of Pediatrics, 1982, pp 287–288
38. Scott JR, Beer A: Reproductive immunology. In Wynn RM (ed): Obstetrics and Gynecology Annual: 1974. New York, Appleton-Century-Crofts, 1974, p 109
39. Baboonian C, Griffiths P: Is pregnancy immunosuppressive? Humoral immunity against viruses. Br J Obstet Gynaecol 90:1168, 1983
40. Pasca AS, Pejtsik B: Impairment of immunity during pregnancy and antiviral effect of amniotic fluid. Lancet 1:330, 1977
41. Hutchins CJ: Plasma volume changes in pregnancy in Indian and European primigravidae. Br J Obstet Gynaecol 87:586, 1980
42. Studd J: The plasma proteins in pregnancy. Clin Obstet Gynaecol 2:285, 1975
43. Murray DL, Imagawa DT, Okada DM, et al.: Antibody response to monovalent A/New Jersey/8/76 influenza vaccine in pregnant women. J Clin Microbiol 10:184, 1979
44. Sumaya CV, Gibbs RS: Immunization of pregnant women with influenza A/New Jersey/76 virus vaccine: Reactogenicity and immunogenicity in mother and infant. J Infect Dis 140:141, 1979
45. Blanco JD, Gibbs RS: Immunizations in pregnancy. Clin Obstet Gynecol 25:611, 1982
46. Schiff GM: Active immunization for adults. Ann Rev Med 31:441, 1980
47. Gupta SC, Bahtia HM: Increased incidence of hemolytic disease of the newborn caused by ABO incompatibility when tetanus toxoid is given during pregnancy. Vox Sanguinis 38:22, 1980
48. Preblud S, William N: Fetal risks associated with rubella vaccine: Implications for vaccination of susceptible women. Obstet Gynecol 66:121, 1985
49. Levine MM, Edsall G, Bruce-Chwatt LJ: Live-virus vaccines in pregnancy: Risks and recommendations. Lancet 2:34, 1974
50. Hart RJC: Immunization. Clin Obstet Gynaecol 8:421, 1981
51. Centers for Disease Control: Smallpox vaccine. MMWR 34:341, 1985
52. Centers for Disease Control: Contact spread of vaccinia from a recently vaccinated Marine—Louisiana. MMWR 33:37, 1984
53. Centers for Disease Control: Contact spread of vaccinia from a National Guard vaccinee—Wisconsin. MMWR 34:182, 1985
54. Luisi M: Smallpox vaccination and pregnancy (letter). Am J Obstet Gynecol 128:700, 1977
55. Goldstein JA, Neff JM, Lane JM, et al.: Smallpox vaccinations, prophylaxis, and therapy of complications. Pediatrics 55:342, 1975
56. Fleet WF, Vaughn W, Lefkowitz IB, et al.: Gestational exposure to rubella vaccines. Am J Epidemiol 101:220, 1975
57. Centers for Disease Control: Rubella prevention. MMWR 30:37, 1981
58. Landes RD, Bass JW, Millunchick EW, et al.: Neonata rubella following postpartum maternal immunization. J Pediatr 97:465, 1980
59. Bott LM, Eizenberg DH: Congenital rubella after successful vaccination. Med J Aust 1:514, 1982
60. Enders G, Calm A, Schaub J: Rubella embryopathy after previous maternal rubella vaccination. Infection 12:56, 1984
61. Baker CJ, Edwards MS, Kasper DL: Immunogenicity of polysaccharides from type III group B streptococcus. J Clin Invest 61:1107, 1978
62. Carvalho AD, Giampaglia CM, Kimura H, et al.: Maternal and infant antibody response to meningococcal vaccination in pregnancy. Lancet 2:809, 1977

11

Glucocorticoids and Fetal Pulmonary Maturity

Frederick P. Zuspan and Leandro Cordero, Jr.

Respiratory distress is the major cause of death in the premature newborn. Fortunately, this respiratory distress lasts but 4 to 7 days in the newborn period. The use of antepartum glucocorticoids has been investigated by many and most results are consistent in demonstrating a lowered incidence and degree of severity of the res piratory distress syndrome (RDS) in the newborn. The established benefits of glucocorticoid therapy include: (1) a lowered incidence of RDS among infants less than 34 weeks' gestation; (2) a decrease in severity of RDS; (3) an increase in survival of premature infants; (4) a decreased incidence of intracranial hemorrhage; and (5) a significant savings in health care costs, coupled with decreased newborn morbidity.[1-6]

Until 34 weeks' gestation, the major survival problem for the very low birthweight baby is the development and maturation of the pulmonary tree, including the invasion of capillaries into the alveoli and the thinning of the alveoli to facilitate the transfer of oxygen. The development of type II pneumocytes in the terminal pulmonary tree is also important, since these specialized cells are responsible for pulmonary surfactant synthesis. The finding that glucocorticoids have an effect on fetal lung maturation through increased pulmonary surfactant production was discovered serendipitously. While studying the effects of corticosteroids to induce premature labor in sheep, Liggins observed in 1968 that dexamethasone injected directly into fetal lambs in utero resulted in a longer than expected survival after premature delivery.[7] Microscopic examination of the treated fetal lambs revealed partial aeration of the lung. Liggins postulated that dexamethasone might have enhanced the production of pulmonary surfactant prior to its normal biologic appearance. This finding was supported by De Lemos et al., who in 1970 reported that the in utero infusion of cortisol into one of twin lambs produced an advanced maturation of the pulmonary tree in the treated but not in the untreated twin.[8]

Having discovered the beneficial effects of prenatal steroid administration, other important observations which were made include: (1) the postnatal administration of steroids does not appear to influence the course of RDS,[9] (2) the prenatal administration of corticosteroids enhances the production of fetal pulmonary surfactant,[1] and (3) the biochemical effect of these steroids in animals does not necessarily correlate with the conditions observed in the human.[10-14]

MECHANISM OF ACTION OF GLUCOCORTICOIDS

The exact mechanism by which glucocorticoids induce pulmonary maturation is not fully understood, but is probably related to an increased enzyme activity for the biosynthesis of surface active phospholipids in the type II pneumocytes. Choline phosphotransferase and phosphatidic acid phosphatase (papase) are the primary enzymes responsible for the synthesis of the two principal surface-active phospholipids, phosphatidylcholine and phosphatidylglycerol (Fig. 11–1).[15,16] The choline pathway is thought to be the more important pathway for fetal lung development. Phosphatidic acid phosphatase catalyzes the hydrolysis of phosphatidic acid into diacylglycerol, which is a major substrate used in the biochemical pathway leading to the production of phosphatidylcholine. Phosphatidylcholine, phosphatidylglycerol, other lipids, and specific proteins are the primary constituents of lecithin, the major component of pulmonary surfactant.

Additionally, glucocorticoids in experimental animals increase the cellular population of β-receptors. The phenomenon is blocked by β-receptor blockers (propranolol). It is felt that the increased population of β-receptors on type II pneumocytes produces more surfactant.[17]

The type II pneumocyte in the alveolar space is considered to be the principal site of glucocorticoid action (Fig. 11–2). After crossing the cell membrane, the glucocorticoid binds to specific intracytoplasmic receptors for transfer to the nucleus.[14] It is within the nucleus that RNA is synthesized for the eventual enzyme production and surfactant synthesis.[11] Intracytoplasmic lamellar bodies store the surfactant until its release into the alveolar space. Although the lamellar bodies may be found as early as at 20 weeks' gestation, sufficient concentrations of surfactant to sustain lung stability are usually absent until about 33 weeks' gestation. Due to the pre-

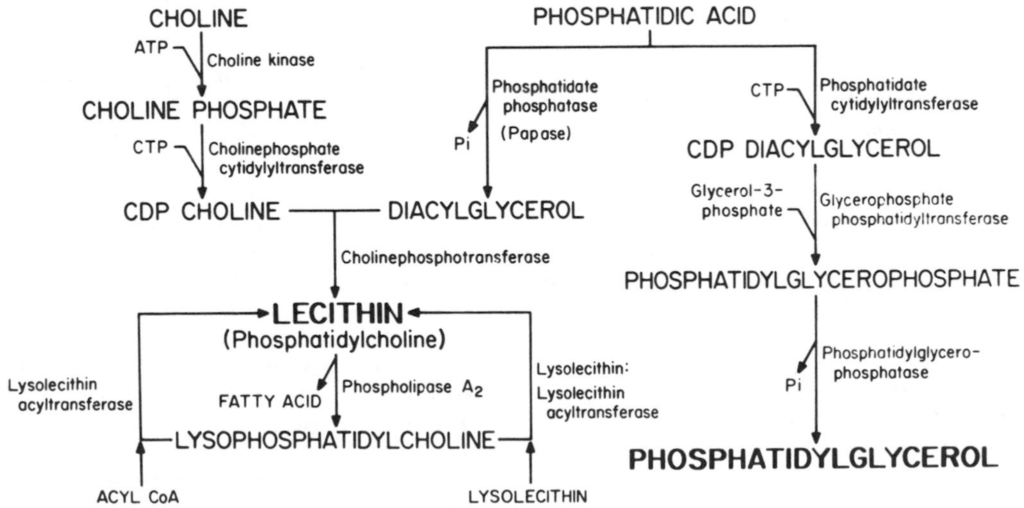

Figure 11–1. Pathways for lecithin and phosphatidylglycerol synthesis.

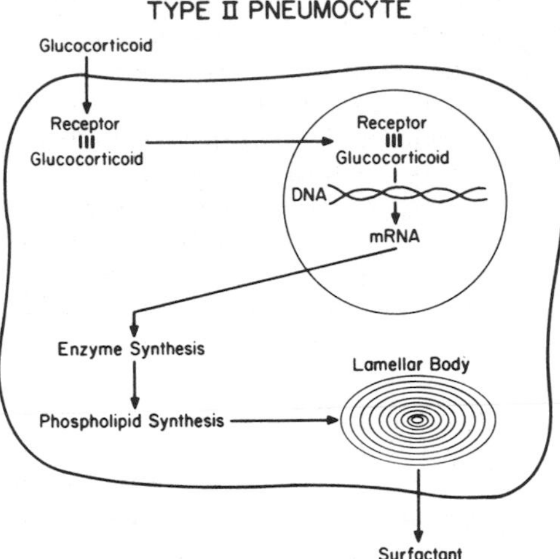

Figure 11–2. Model for glucocorticoid action in type II cells involving receptors and *de nova* synthesis of proteins.

requisite development of the pneumocytes, the ability of the fetal lung to respond to glucocorticoid administration is also dependent upon gestational age which is related to lung receptor population.

Exogenous glucocorticoids administered to the mother have been shown to cause diverse effects on the fetal lung within 24 to 48 hours. These changes include morphologic, biochemical, and physiologic alterations. Whatever the exact biochemical mechanism, the significant increases in the lecithin:spinogomyelin (L:S) ratio after therapy have been reported by several authors, including our own studies.[1,18] However, when administered to the mother, betamethasone apparently does not cause an increased L:S ratio, despite lowering the indicence and severity of respiratory distress.

PROBLEMS ENCOUNTERED IN STUDYING PULMONARY MATURATION

There are many variables involved in studies on pulmonary maturation in both animals and humans that makes it almost impossible to draw precise scientific conclusions. The problem is further clouded by the fact that the very low birthweight baby has a notoriously poor survival rate, and emotion often enters into therapy judgment. Some investigators state that the use of glucocorticoids to maturate fetal lungs may indeed be salutary, but its long-term safety has not been proven. It would be our contention, at this time, that there is no evidence of adverse newborn, infant, and long-term child effects. The proof would now seem to rest with those that use glucocorticoids and the contrary position must now be defended.[19,20]

The diagnosis of neonatal respiratory distress, even though standardized for the neonatologist, has some degree of uncertainty, and incidence figures depend upon the severity of the disease. Few studies in the literature are double-blind trials, and even in double-blind trials patient selection is not as precise as one would hope. Furthermore, the information is often not standardized or detailed enough to allow regular statistical comparison. Despite these limitations, the combined data from published double-blind trials reveal the incidence of respiratory distress to be three times lower for infants whose mothers were prenatally treated with glucocorticoids when compared to untreated, "control" groups. The data in Table 11–1 was assembled from the literature. The double-blind, collaborative, randomized clinical trial that began in 1976 on 696 women from 5 centers was published in 1981. The drug used, dexamethasone phosphate (5 mg every 12 hours) administered intramuscularly (IM), was compared to a placebo. The incidence of RDS in the control group was 18 percent compared to 12.6 percent in the treatment group ($p = 0.05$). The effect was attributed mainly to singleton female infants ($p = 0.001$).[21]

An example of trials which illustrate such problems would include the classic study of Liggins and Howie, published in 1972.[6] A group of 282 mothers were randomly selected to receive 12 mg of betamethasone IM. The rationale for the choice of cortisone acetate as a placebo which has one-fiftieth the relative corticosteroid potency of betametha-

TABLE 11–1. COMPARISON BETWEEN THE INCIDENCE OF RESPIRATORY DISTRESS AND NEONATAL MORTALITY FROM RESPIRATORY DISTRESS IN PREGNANCIES DELIVERING PREMATURELY WITH OR WITHOUT PRENATAL GLUCOCORTICOID TREATMENT

Condition	Total Incidence	Untreated	Treated
Respiratory distress*	142/703 (20.2%)	101/353 (28.8%)	41/350 (11.7%)
Neonatal mortality†	226/1431 (15.8%)	181/824 (21.9%)	45/607 (7.4%)

* Data based on five double-blind studies.

† Data based on 10 double-blind studies treated with betamethasone (8) or hydrocortisone (2).

sone is not discussed and would not make it a true control group. The study later included 884 patients through 1974, using a dosage of betamethasone that was doubled. There was no rationale for doubling this dosage; the results were essentially the same.

The criteria of patient selection is another important consideration, and a subset of patients with hypertension, edema, and proteinuria were included in the initial Liggins and Howie study. At least 24 hours intervened after the administration of the second dose of betamethasone before the delivery of a hypertensive or normotensive patient. The hypertensive group was found to have an increased incidence of antepartum and intrapartum fetal death, 12 of 47 in the hypertensive group as compared to 3 of 47 in the control group. Liggins and Howie concluded that patients with preeclampsia and other forms of hypertension should not be given betamethasone because of the increased fetal loss. When the report is analyzed more critically, it is apparent that the fetal loss is not directly related to the betamethasone administration as much as it is to the antepartum testing methods to determine the ideal time for delivery. Since that initial report, many studies have been reported showing no adverse effect on the hypertension when glucocorticoids are used. Hydrocortisone, dexamethasone, and betamethasone have all been used with similar results. We have now treated more than 125 hypertensive patients, both acute and chronic, and have not found a worsening of the hypertension.[22,23]

As scientists, we would all like to offer our patients the maximum protection learned from animal studies before trials in humans. Animal studies have used proportionally larger doses of glucocorticoids than in humans, and are therefore not comparable on that basis alone. Even if dosages were proportional, the extrapolation of data from the animal to the human is clearly not possible, since final proof always rests in the human. There are few dissenters that remain in not using glucocorticoids when the appropriate indication is present.

EFFECTS OF CORTICOSTEROIDS ON FETAL DEVELOPMENT

The classical assumption that toxic effects of medications are related to dosage and duration of therapy may lead to a false sense of security regarding corticosteroid therapy. Many animal studies involving corticosteroids involve therapies of relatively short duration with large doses. Glucocorticoids injected directly into the fetus for as short a time period as 3 days have resulted in somatic and lung growth retardation.

Particular concern has been expressed over data indicating that dendritic and synaptogenic growth has been altered in rats. Our research group studied brains of rat fetuses treated with hydrocortisone. Using a dosage scheme similar to human therapy, hydrocortisone was given intraperitoneally on days 12 and 15 of gestation in pregnant rats. The offspring were studied at days 20 to 21 of gestation and days 12 to 13 in the neonatal period. The amine systems of the hydrocortisone and saline groups showed equal cerebral maturation, and both groups demonstrated nerve cell bodies in areas A-1 to A-13 and axon terminals in all examined regions. The distribution in the fluorescent intensity in the brains did not show any differences in either group, and the cerebral concentrations of dopamine, epinephrine, and norepinephrine were also similar. These results indicate that hydrocortisone given during pregnancy does not influence the proliferation of amine cell bodies or the arrival of axon terminals in regions where formed in the fetus.[14]

Unlike that of the rat, the human cortex has developed more fully by the time glucocorticoid therapy would be given to promote pulmonary maturation. Neuronal multiplication in the human in the developing brain is followed by a migration to the outer cortical zones which occurs up to 24 weeks' gestation. It is unlikely that many neurons will enter the cerebral cortex beyond 24 weeks of gestation, but dendritic growth continues to 35 or 36 weeks and synaptogenesis probably continues through term. Glial development and myelinization are probably not completed until the second year of postnatal life. It is therefore possible that the different temporal patterns of brain development in the human may prevent some of the detrimental effects of glucocorticoid treatment observed in the rat. Prenatal glucocorticoid therapy treatment commits the physician team and the institution to careful and long-term follow-up, which is often unavailable outside tertiary-care-level facilities.

INDICATIONS FOR GLUCOCORTICOID THERAPY

The initiation of glucocorticoid therapy is based upon analysis of amniotic fluid. Unfortunately, not enough data are available to indicate the gestational age group that is most likely to respond favorably to corticosteroid therapy, but the fetus from 28 to 34 weeks probably has an optimum chance of response. Although infant survival rates are improving at 26 and 27 weeks' gestation, beneficial effects from glucocorticoid therapy before 28 weeks of gestation cannot be determined at the present time. The fetus beyond 34 weeks of gestation has a low incidence of respiratory distress.

A time lapse must exist between maternal treatment and fetal response of at least 24 hours after the last dose of steroid therapy.[24–27] If the underlying antepartum complication does not permit this period of nonintervention, glucocorticoid therapy should not be given, and delivery should take place. On the other hand, if the pregnancy continues for more than 10 days after therapy, an amniocentesis should be repeated, and the amniotic fluid should be reanalyzed prior to another course of therapy.

The cornerstone of therapy rests upon the prompt and accurate diagnosis of fetal pulmonary activity by amniotic fluid analysis. The four commonly used tests to analyze amniotic fluid for pulmonary surfactant production include the L:S ratio, phosphatidylglycerol determination, the "shake" test, and optical density OD_{650} determination. Although the L:S ratio and phosphatidylglycerol determination are performed at regional perinatal centers, the shake test and OD_{650} determination can be easily performed at any hospital and at awkward times such as at night, on weekends, and during holidays when specialized technicians are less accessible. Ideally, glucocorticoid therapy is to be administered after there is laboratory evidence of fetal pulmonary immaturity (L:S less than 2:1, OD_{650} less than 0.15, negative phosphatidylglycerol, or negative or suspicious shake test). If conditions remain favorable to delay delivery, an immature result using either the OD_{650} or shake test should be later confirmed with an L:S ratio determination. When using the OD_{650} to assess pulmonary maturity, we have not experienced a false-positive determination, that is, if the OD_{450} is greater than 0.15 at 650 mm, RDS has not been found, which confirms the observation by Sbarra who initially published the test.[29,30]

CONTRAINDICATIONS TO GLUCOCORTICOID THERAPY

The absolute and relative maternal and fetal contraindications for glucocorticoid therapy are straightforward (Table 11–2). Absolute contraindications are fortunately uncommon, but relative contrindications require individualization.

Premature Rupture of Membranes

Most authors conclude that there is no association between fetal–maternal infection and prenatal steroid treatment, since the dosage levels are quite small. Tauesch et al.,[31,32] however, reported maternal infections in 5 of 10 women treated as compared to 1 of 17 placebo patients. All patients studied had premature rupture of membranes greater than 48 hours, and none had signs of infection prior to corticosteroid or placebo therapy. No author has been able to document an increase in infant infections in corticosteroid-treated infants, but Schmidt et al.[25] have shown an increase in maternal infection in women treated with hydrocortisone to enhance pulmonary maturity. Although any decreased resistance to infection during corticosteroid therapy remains controversial, it is recommended that corticosteroid therapy be withheld in patients with amnionitis or other infections. Glucocorticoids are known to increase the white blood count, so cultures and clinical criteria remain the best methods to monitor for any infection.[33] A Gram stain and search for white cells in amniotic fluid may also be helpful.

A review of the data at Ohio State University has not confirmed the fact that premature rupture of membranes promotes an acceleration of pulmonary surfactant, but controversy continues.[34–36] It is our practice that if the patient has premature rupture of membranes, amniotic fluid is obtained from either the vaginal pool or from ultrasound-guided amniocentesis for pulmonary maturity testing. A culture of the material and microscopic examination with Gram stain are also done. Any advantage to the use of glucocorticoids in the conservative management of this complication remains unclear. Randomized double-blind studies at Ohio State University[37] and University of Virginia[38] confirmed the original study of Garite et al.[39] that glucocorticoids do not alter the incidence of respiratory distress syndrome in patients with premature rupture of membranes. Why this is different when membranes are intact remains obscure.

Hypertensive Disorders

There has been speculation but no data that glucocorticoids may compromise placental function in hypertensive patients. This speculation is based on urinary and serum estriol values diminishing precipitously after glucocorticoid therapy. This decreased value is instead a reflection of maternal adrenal

TABLE 11–2. CONTRAINDICATIONS TO PRENATAL GLUCOCORTICOID THERAPY

	Absolute	Relative
Maternal	Tuberculosis Viral keratitis Active herpes, type II Febrile illness or infection	Hypertensive disorder Diabetes mellitus Hyperthyroidism Uterine bleeding Peptic ulcer
Fetal	Amnionitis Imminent delivery Mature amniotic fluid test result Inability to monitor the fetus	Premature rupture of membranes (PROM) Placental insufficiency

suppression from the corticosteroids. The analysis of Liggins' original data indicates that the increased perinatal death rate in preeclamptic patients is closely related to the degree of proteinuria and the severity of the disease. As an example, patients excreting more than 3 g of protein had a perinatal mortality rate of 43 percent, while those with less proteinuria had a perinatal mortality rate of only 14 percent.[40] It probably was not the glucocorticoid, but the severity of the disease that resulted in these stillbirths.

At least four different investigators have treated hypertensive patients with glucocorticoids, with all reporting similar results of hypertension not exacerbated and fetal mortality not increased.

The group at Ohio State University recently evaluated 32 hypertensive gravidas who were treated in the third trimester of pregnancy with intravenous hydrocortisone to enhance fetal lung maturity. Blood pressure was determined throughout the 24 hours of steroid therapy, and no significant increase in maternal blood pressure was found.[22] The two antepartum fetal deaths in our study group were similar to those in the Liggins and Howie control group. In addition, 15 different studies utilizing various drugs such as betamethasone, hydrocortisone, and dexamethasone have treated 1214 patients with only 22 stillbirths following prenatal glucocorticoid therapy, or a 2 percent fetal mortality for these high-risk patients. The fear of steroid-induced exacerbation of maternal hypertension has therefore not been supported as a valid reason to withhold steroid therapy in hypertensive patients if indications are present for its use and the maternal condition is stable. We have shown that glucocorticoids do not worsen the hypertension.

Diabetes Mellitus

Glucocorticoids increase insulin requirements by inhibiting glucose utilization, by mobilizing amino acids for their conversion to glucose and glycogen, and by the induction of liver enzymes involved in gluconeogenesis. This increase in insulin requirement occurs within minutes after initiation of therapy. β-adrenergic tocolytic agents (terbutaline, isoxsuprine, ritodrine) are often used concurrently with glucocorticoids and may also increase circulating glucose levels. Thus, the concurrent administration of β-sympathomimetics and corticosteroids may compound the management problem of the diabetic mother and requires diligent monitoring of maternal blood glucose levels. Glucocorticoid therapy is not recommended if the woman's diabetes is poorly controlled.

Bleeding

Glucocorticoid therapy may decrease the platelet number and function. A negative history of excessive bleeding and a normal platelet count are desirable before therapy. Severe vaginal bleeding necessitates prompt delivery, but a pregnancy complicated by placenta previa may be a candidate for glucocorticoid therapy if conservative treatment is successful. Once therapy has begun it is repeated on a weekly basis usually until 34 weeks of gestation.

DRUG CHOICE AND DOSAGE SCHEDULE

The specific drug of choice and the dosage of drug are presently unknown. No agent has been shown to offer any advantages in promoting pulmonary maturity, but there are certain differences in their pharmacology which deserve consideration.

The durations of anti-inflammatory effects based on approximately equivalent onetime doses may be used as a guideline and are shown in Table 11–3. Since anti-inflammatory effects may reflect immunosuppressant capability, hydrocortisone may offer some advantage to decrease the risk of infections for both mother and child. A potential disadvantage of hydrocortisone is the significant mineralocorticoid activity with associated fluid retention which is not present

TABLE 11–3. COMPARISONS BETWEEN ANTI-INFLAMMATORY EFFECTS WITH HYDROCORTISONE, DEXAMETHASONE, AND BETAMETHASONE

Drug	Dose (mg)	Duration of Anti-Inflammatory Effect (Days)
Hydrocortisone	250	1.25–1.5
Dexamethasone	5	2.75
Betamethasone	6	3.25

with dexamethasone and betamethasone therapy.

The most expedient route of administration is intravenous, and the slower intramuscular absorption of betamethasone and dexamethasone would appear to be less desirable unless time is not a factor.

The transport of glucocorticoids across the placenta and to the fetal pulmonary target tissue is worthy of consideration. All agents rapidly cross the placenta, and any difference in metabolic conversion by the 11-dehydrogenase enzyme system is thought not to be significant. In addition, any 11-keto compound metabolite formed during placental transfer may also be effective in promoting type II pneumocyte stimulation. Steroid binding to carrier proteins in the fetus is less with dexamethasone and betamethasone (to albumin only) as compared to hydrocortisone (to albumin and cortisol-binding globulin). If urinary estriol excretion is identified as an index of suppression of the fetal adrenal activity, hydrocortisone shows the most rapid effect, that is, maximum depression of urinary estrogen is seen in less than 12 hours, whereas with betamethasone 24 hours is required.

A therapy regimen utilizing the minimal effective dose for the shortest duration is not established for any of the glucocorticoids. Table 11–4 identifies dosage regimens that have been used at many institutions. An advantage of hydrocortisone is that the L:S ratio has been shown to increase in 80 percent of treated cases, while no change has been reported with betamethasone.

A time lapse of at least 24 hours after the last dose until delivery is necessary for the corticoid to activate the type II pneumocyte to produce surfactant. If more than 7 days have elapsed after completion of therapy, amniotic fluid testing may be repeated before administering another course of therapy. The effectiveness of the second weekly dose has not been proved to be effective.

In conclusion, the short-term benefits from the use of prenatal glucocorticoid therapy to promote fetal lung maturity has been established from animal and human investigations. The appropriate agent and dosage regimen, and the proper selection of prospective candidates remain unclear. Absolute safety to the mother and fetus requires that there be further short- and long-term inves-

TABLE 11–4. GLUCOCORTICOID DOSAGE REGIMENS USED TO PROMOTE FETAL LUNG MATURATION

Drug	Dosage Schedule	Total Dose (mg)
Betamethasone (6 mg acetate/6 mg phospate—Celestone)	12 mg IM every 12 hr for two doses	24
Dexamethasone (Decadron, Deronil)	4 mg IM every 8 hr for six doses	24
Hydrocortisone (Cortisol, Cortef, Cortril, etc.)	500 mg IV every 8 hr for four doses	2000

tigation. Glucocorticoid therapy should be initiated only after informed patient consent has been obtained and after amniotic fluid testing suggests fetal pulmonary immaturity or if the fetus is known to be less than 30 weeks' gestation.

REFERENCES

1. Zuspan FP, Cordero L, Semchyshyn S: Effects of hydrocortisone on lecithin-sphinogomyelin ratio. Am J Obstet Gynecol 128:571, 1977
2. Farrell PM, Zachman RD: Induction of choline phosphotransferase and lecithin synthesis in the fetal lung by corticosteroids. Science 179:297, 1973
3. Grub L: Administration of cortical steroids to induce maturation of fetal lung. Am J Dis Child 130:976, 1976
4. Ballard RA, Ballard PL: Use of prenatal glucocorticoid therapy to prevent respiratory distress syndrome. Am J Dis Child 130:982, 1976
5. Ballard PL, Ballard RA: Corticosteroid and respiratory distress syndrome: Status 1979. Pediatrics 63:163, 1979
6. Liggins GC, Howie RN: A controlled trial of antepartum glucocorticoid treatment for prevention of the respiratory distress syndrome in premature infants. Pediatrics 50:515, 1972
7. Liggins GC: Premature delivery of fetal lambs infused with glucocorticoids. J Endocrinol 45:515, 1969
8. De Lemos R, Shermeta D, Knelson J, et al.: Acceleration of appearance of pulmonary surfactant in the fetal lamb by administration of corticosteroids. Am Rev Resp Dis 102:459, 1970
9. Buckingham S, McNary WF, Sommers SC, et al.: Is lung an analog of Moog's intestine? Phosphatase and pulmonary alveolar differentiation in fetal rabbits (abstr). Fed Proc 27:328, 1968
10. Hallman M, Grub L: Development of the fetal lung. J Perinat Med 5:3, 1977
11. Taeusch HW, Heitner M, Avery ME: Acceleration of lung maturation and increased survival in premature rabbits treated with hydrocortisone. Am Rev Resp Dis 105:971, 1972
12. Schapiro S, Salas M, Vukovich K: Hormonal effects on the ontogeny of swimming ability in the rat: Assessment of CNS development. Science 168:147, 1970
13. De Lemos RA: Glucocorticoid effect: Organ development in monkeys. In Proceedings of the 70th Ross Conference on Pediatric Research. Columbus, Ohio, Ross Laboratories, 1975, pp 77–80
14. Van Geijn H, Copeland K, Vorys A, et al.: The Effects of Hydrocortisone on the Development of the Amine Systems in the Fetal Brain (abstr). Society for Gynecologic Investigation, 1979
15. Ballard P, Benson B, Brehier A: Glucocorticoid effects in the fetal lung. Am Rev Resp Dis 115 (suppl):29, 1977
16. Weischel M: Glucocorticoid effect upon thymidine kinase in the developing cerebellum. Pediatr Res 8:361, 1974
17. Ayromlooi J, Bandyopadhyay S, Neogi A, et al.: Effect of aminophylline on fetal lung maturation. Proceed SGI 1983, (abstr) 378
18. Morrison JC, Whybrew WE, Bucovaz ET, et al.: Injection of corticosteroids into mother to prevent neonatal respiratory distress syndrome. Am J Obstet Gynecol 131:358, 1978
19. Collaborative Group: Effects of antenatal dexamethasone administration in the infant: Long-term follow-up. J Pediatr 104:259, 1984
20. Avery ME: The argument for prenatal administrative of dexamethasone to prevent respiratory distress. J Pediatr 104:240, 1984
21. Collaborative Group on Antenatal Steroid Therapy: Effect of antenatal dexamethasone administration on prevention of respiratory distress syndrome. Am J Obstet Gynecol 141:276, 1981
22. Iams JD, Semchyshyn S, O'Shaughnessey R, et al.: Blood pressure response in hypertensive pregnancies treated with cortisol. Clin Exp Hypertension 2:923, 1980
23. Lamont RF, Dunlop PDM, Levene MI, Elder MG: Use glucocorticoids in pregnancies complicated by severe hypertension and proteinuria. Br J Obstet Gynecol 90:199, 1983
24. Kennedy JL: Antepartum betamethasone in the prevention of RDS (abstr). Pediatr Res 8:447, 1974
25. Schmidt PL, Sims ME, Strassner HT, et al.: Effect of antenatal glucocorticord administration upon neonatal respiratory distress syndrom and perinatal infection. Am J Obstet Gynecol 148:178, 1984
26. Caspi E, Schreyer P, Weinraub Z, et al.: Prevention of the respiratory distress syndrome in premature infants by antepartum glucocorticoid therapy. Br J Obstet Gynecol 83:187, 1976

27. Ballard RA, Ballard PL, Granberg JP, et al.: Prenatal administration of betamethasone for prevention of respiratory distress syndrome. J Pediatr 94:97, 1979
28. Thornfeldt RE, Franklin RW, Pickering NA, et al.: The effect of glucocorticoids on the maturation of premature lung membranes. Am J Obstet Gynecol 131:143, 1978
29. Copeland W Jr, Stempel L, Lott J, et al.: Assessment of a rapid test on amniotic fluid for estimating fetal lung maturity. Am J Obstet Gynecol 130:225, 1978
30. Michlewitz H, Selvaraj RJ, et al.: Correlation between amniotic fluid density and L:S ratio. Obstet Gynecol 48:613, 1976
31. Taeusch HW, Frigoletto F, Kitzmiller J, et al.: Risk of respiratory distress syndrome after prenatal dexamethasone treatment. Pediatrics 63:64, 1979
32. Taeusch HW, Wang NS, Baden M, et al.: A controlled trial of hydrocortisone therapy in infants with RDS: II. Pathology. Pediatrics 52:850, 1973
33. Ferguson II JE, Hensleigh PA, Gill P: Effects of betamethasone on white blood cells in patients with premature rupture of the membranes and preterm labor. Am J Obstet Gynecol 150:439, 1984
34. Berkowitz RL, Bontz BW, Warshaw JE: The relationship between premature rupture of the membranes and the respiratory distress syndrome. Am J Obstet Gynecol 124:712, 1976
35. Thibeault DW, Emmanouilides GC: Prolonged rupture of fetal membranes and decreased frequency of respiratory distress syndrome and patent ductus arteriosus in preterm infants. Am J Obstet Gynecol 129:43, 1977
36. Christensen KK, Christensen P, Ingermarsson I, et al.: A study of complications in preterm deliveries after prolonged premature rupture of the membranes. Obstet Gynecol 48:670, 1976
37. Iams JD, Barrows H: Management of preterm prematurely ruptured membranes: A retrospective comparison versus use of steroids and timed delivery. Am J Obstet Gynecol 150:977, 1984
38. Simpson G, Marbert G: Use of β-methasone in management of preterm gestation with premature rupture of membranes. Obstet Gynecol 66:168, 1985
39. Garite TJ, Freeman RK, Linzey EM, et al.: Prospective randomized study of corticosteroids in the management of premature rupture of the membranes and the premature gestation. Am J Obstet Gynecol 141:508, 1981
40. Liggins GC: Prenatal glucocorticoid treatment: Prevention of respiratory distress syndrome. In Proceedings of the 70th Ross Conference on Pediatric Research. Colombus, Ohio, Ross Laboratories, 1975 pp 97–105

12

Drugs to Inhibit Premature Labor

William F. Rayburn, Donald M. DeDonato, and William K. Rand, III

Despite the remarkable success achieved in neonatal intensive care units, most perinatal morbidity and mortality occurs in premature infants. Although less than 10 percent of all infants are delivered before term, 75 percent of perinatal deaths are directly related to premature birth.[1] Significant neonatal morbidity, such as permanent intellectual and physical handicaps, also occurs more commonly in premature infants. The prevention of premature delivery is therefore a primary objective of prenatal care. When premature labor occurs, the use of pharmacologic agents to suppress labor is an alternative to delivery. A delay for even 1 or 2 weeks may offer psychologic, financial, and physical advantages, and may avoid death or significant central nervous system handicaps for some infants.

Premature labor is usually defined as the onset of labor before the 38th week of amenorrhea. The incidence of premature delivery varies with the population studied. In American women the incidence of premature birth is estimated to be 8 to 10 percent.[2] Only 3.3 percent of infants in East Germany are born prematurely, in contrast to nearly one-fourth being premature in impoverished areas of India.[3]

Events leading to the onset of labor are poorly understood. The etiology is most likely multifactorial: conditions associated with an increased incidence of premature labor are listed in Table 12–1. The difference between true and false labor is often subtle and may be so unclear that it is too late for therapy to be successful. The most widely accepted criteria for the clinical diagnosis of premature labor requires palpable contractions occurring every 10 minutes for at least 30 minutes and lasting 30 seconds or more.[4] When using these criteria, 40 to 70 percent of patients who are managed with sedation and bedrest alone will not deliver prematurely. Unless contraindicated, a drug to inhibit uterine contractions (tocolytic drug) should be administered early, even though some patients may be treated for false labor.

The earliest gestational age at which premature labor is to be arrested is controversial. Attempts at precise determination of gestational age must be obtained from pertinent clinical information and ultrasonographic

TABLE 12–1. CONDITIONS ASSOCIATED WITH PREMATURE LABOR

MATERNAL
Acute severe systemic illness
Chronic severe systemic illness
Pyelonephritis
Chronic hypertension
Hyperthyroidism
Hyperparathyroidism
Hyperadrenocorticism
Previous history of premature labor
Fever
Inadequate nutrition
Age (under 16, over 40 years)
Excess smoking

UTERINE
Polyhydramnios
Multiple gestation
Foreign body (IUD)
Trauma
Cervical incompetence or trauma
Uterine anomalies
Amniocentesis
Surgery
Chorioamnionitis, overt, or "silent"

FETOPLACENTAL
Fetal death
Placenta previa
Abruptio placenta
Fetal anomalies
Multifetal gestation
Preterm ruptured amniotic membranes

findings. The frequency of anomalies occurring in pregnancies with spontaneous labor before 20 weeks may preclude tocolysis. Arresting labor after the 36th week is not beneficial, since perinatal morbidity and mortality have not been shown to decrease. Amniocentesis to assess fetal pulmonary maturity is helpful, especially when fetal age is uncertain, so that the risks of neonatal respiratory distress can be predicted better before tocolytic therapy is begun.

The arrest of premature labor may not benefit all fetuses. Certain underlying fetal or maternal conditions may predispose to premature labor or may be deleterious if intrauterine existence is continued. Commonly accepted criteria for selecting patients for tocolytic therapy are listed in Table 12–2. Most women in premature labor have no other discernible antepartum complication and therefore qualify for inhibition of uterine contractions. Vaginal cultures for gonorrhea and group B β-streptococci are performed routinely when determining whether the amniotic membranes are ruptured. A sufficient period of time (usually 30 minutes or more) is necessary in monitoring uterine activity and the fetal heart rate and in allowing maternal hydration and rest on her left side. Bedrest is necessary with the mother lying on her side in a Trendelenburg position.

Tocolytic drugs may be identified by their presumed mechanisms of action. Premature labor may be arrested by using agents that prevent the synthesis or release of a uterine stimulant (ethanol, antiprostaglandin) or by suppressing the contractile response at the target organ, the myometrial cells (magne-

TABLE 12–2. STANDARD CRITERIA FOR SELECTING PATIENTS FOR TOCOLYTIC THERAPY

Clinical Diagnosis
- Gestational age between 20 and 36 weeks
- Estimated fetal weight less than 2500 g
- Uterine contractions every 10 min, lasting 30 sec or more, for 30 min or more
- Cervical dilation of 4 cm or less

No Remarkable Antepartum Complication
- Maternal
  - Cardiac disease, symptomatic
  - Hypertension, moderate or severe
  - Symptomatic hypotension
  - Diabetes mellitus, uncontrolled
  - Thyrotoxicosis
  - Fever or disseminated infection
- Fetoplacental
  - Intrauterine infection
  - Placenta previa or placental abruption
  - Suspected severe fetal growth retardation
  - Fetal anomaly
  - Polyhydramnios
  - Fetal demise

No Evidence of Fetal Pulmonary Maturity

sium sulfate, β-adrenergic agents). More specific mechanisms of actions of each drug group remain uncertain but are shown in Figure 12–1. Dose regimens, side effects, and contraindications for use are described in Tables 12–3 and 12–4. More detailed comments and the relative effectiveness of each drug group are described further.

TOCOLYTIC AGENTS

Ethanol

Ethanol has been the most widely used tocolytic agent in the past for inhibiting premature labor. Despite its former widespread use, the effectiveness of ethanol in improving perinatal outcome is debatable and maternal side effects make it undesirable. The intravenous administration of ethanol became popular after a clinical trial by Fuchs and associates was published in 1967.[5] Ethanol was thought to act on the central nervous system by blocking the release of oxytocin, and on the myometrium by a direct suppressant action. Intravenous ethanol was reported to prolong pregnancy in 67 percent of the cases for greater than 72 hours, when the membranes were intact and the cervix was dilated less than 4 cm. A randomized study in 1972 by Zlatnick and Fuchs reported a delay in delivery for at least 72 hours in 81 percent of women treated with ethanol as compared to 31 percent of those treated with placebo.[6] Subsequent nonrandomized studies with control populations and with comparisons to other tocolytic agents have reported widely different success rates, ranging from no better than placebo to 81 percent success.[7,8] Some of these differences in success are explained by differing criteria for diagnosis and success and differing ethanol dosages and durations of therapy. Two recent, randomized, controlled studies have shown ethanol to be less effective than magnesium sulfate or ritodrine in delaying premature delivery.[9,10] Furthermore, seldom has ethanol been shown to stop labor for more than 48 hours in patients with ruptured membranes, and it is likely to be no more effective than conservative management with bedrest.

Intravenous ethanol may cause side effects in the mother. Inebriation should be expected when ethanol is infused at dosages described in Table 12–4 since the usual serum level of alcohol is above the legal definition of intoxication (100 mg%). Serum ethanol concentrations at the standard infusion rates range from 100 to 210 mg%.[11] Serum concentrations of 250 mg% may be anesthetic, and concentrations above 300 mg% may cause coma or death.[12] Because of a depressed consciousness and an impaired gag reflex, the risk of aspiration pneumonitis (Mendelson's syndrome) is increased. The monitoring of the woman's mental status and the administration of antiemetics and antacids may minimize this hazard. Metabolic al-

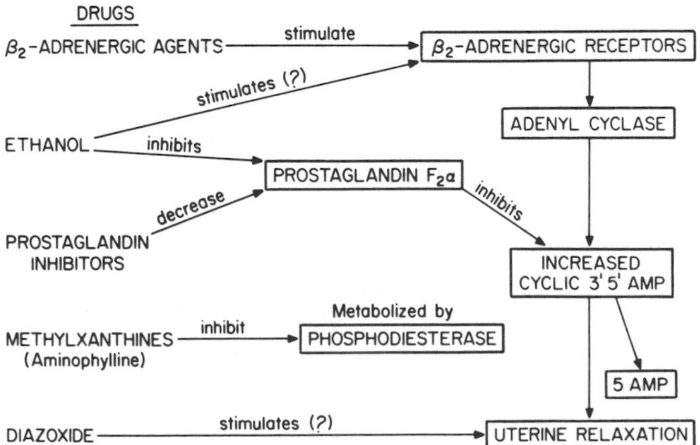

Figure 12–1. Proposed sites for pharmacologic action of drugs to inhibit preterm uterine contractions.

TABLE 12-3. DOSAGE REGIMENS FOR TOCOLYTIC DRUGS

Drug	Preparation	Loading Dose	Maintenance Dose	
			Short-term	*Long-term*
Ritodrine (Yutopar)	0.03% solution in 5% dextrose and 0.45 normal saline (150 mg/500 ml)	None	0.1–0.35 mg/min IV for 12 hr (20–70 ml/hr)	10 mg po every 2 hr *or* 10–20 mg po every 4–6 hr
Terbutaline (Brethine, Bricanyl)	0.001% solution in 5% dextrose and 0.45 normal saline (10 mg/liter)	0.25 mg IV over 1–2 min	0.01–0.025 mg/min IV for 12 hr (60–150 ml/hr)	0.25 mg SC every 4 hr; 2.5–5.0 mg po every 4–6 hr
Isoxsuprine (Vasodilan)	0.02% solution in 5% dextrose and 0.45 normal saline (200 mg/liter)	0.2–1.0 mg IV over 10 min	0.1–0.3 mg/min IV for 12 hr (30–90 ml/hr)	10–20 mg po every 4–6 hr
Magnesium sulfate	40 g in 1000 ml in 5% dextrose in water and 0.45 normal saline (40 g/liter)	4 g in 100 cc over 20 min	1–4 g IV/hr for 8–12 hr (25–100 cc/hr)	No oral administration (use oral β-adrenergic drug)
Ethanol	10% solution in dextrose 5% solution in dextrose	7.5 ml/kg/hr IV for 2 hr	1.5 ml/kg/hr IV for 6–12 hr	Oral administration not advised

terations resulting from ethanol exposure include hypoglycemia and lactic acidemia with an inhibition of gluconeogenesis.

Despite its rapid transfer across the placenta, the adverse effects of ethanol on the premature fetus have been more theoretical than real. Some newborns exhibit transient signs of lethargy, hypotonia, and intoxication at birth, but significant depression and respiratory difficulties are surprisingly rare. The fetal alcohol syndrome (Chap. 2) is not associated with acute alcohol exposure in late pregnancy.

Magnesium Sulfate

Along with its anticonvulsant properties in managing toxemia, parenteral magnesium sulfate has also been found to inhibit uterine contractions.[13] Ionic magnesium is thought to antagonize calcium flow and to exert its effects on myometrial cells in three possible ways: (1) decrease the frequency of muscle-cell action potentials, (2) uncouple the excitation and contraction of smooth muscles, and (3) relax the contractile elements. Clinical studies in patients with premature labor are scarce. Observations have been primarily by Spisso et al.[14] and Steir and Petrie.[9] The data from Steir and Petrie[9] suggest that magnesium sulfate is superior to ethanol for the management of premature labor. The inhibition of uterine contractions is dose related and a serum concentration of 4 to 8 mg/dl of magnesium should effectively reduce uterine contractions.

Much of the current literature about magnesium use in halting premature labor deals with its adjunctive use with ritodrine or when a β-adrenergic drug is contraindicated.[15,19] For effective tocolysis, magnesium sulfate is to infused at maintenance doses of

TABLE 12–4. SIDE EFFECTS AND CONTRAINDICATIONS FOR TOCOLYTIC AGENTS

Drug	Side Effects: Maternal	Side Effects: Fetal	Contraindications
β-adrenergics	Tachycardia	Tachycardia	Heart disease (A)*
	Hypotension	Transient hypoglycemia	Hyperthyroidism (R)†
	Hyperglycemia	Hypotension	Hypertension
	Restlessness		Diabetes mellitus
	Headache		Poorly controlled (A)
	Nausea and vomiting		Well controlled (R)
	Palpitations		
	Tremor, anxiety		
	Hypokalemia		
	Angina (occult cardiac disease)		
	Pulmonary edema		
Magnesium sulfate	Cutaneous flushing	Depression (rare)	Heart block (A)
	Nausea and vomiting		Myocardial damage (A)
	Respiratory depression		Impaired renal function (R)
	Depressed reflexes		
	Intracardiac conduction delays (cardiac arrest)		
Antiprostaglandins (Indomethacin, Naproxen)	GI bleeding and ulceration	Premature closure of the ductus arteriosus‡	Active or recurrent GI lesion (A)
	Nausea and vomiting	Pulmonary hypertension	Epilepsy (R)
	Allergic rashes	Coagulopathy	Psychiatric disturbances (R)
	Bone marrow depression	Hyperbilirubinemia	
Ethanol	Intoxication	Intoxication	Liver disease (A)
	Nausea and vomiting	Depression	Alcoholism (A)
	Aspiration		Diabetes mellitus (R)
	Restless		
	Hypoglycemia		
	Lactic acidemia		
	Diuresis with dehydration		
	Headache		
	Tachycardia		

* A = Absolute contraindication.
† R = Relative contraindication.
‡ Limited data.

2 g (1.5–3 g/hr) or more per hour after a 4 g loading dose. This use is not FDA approved, however, and lower doses (1 g/hr) for seizure prophylaxis are likely to be ineffective in inhibiting uterine contractions. The monitoring of maternal serum magnesium levels is recommended when these higher doses are prescribed.

Clinical signs of hypermagnesemia in the mother are not infrequent. Her knee reflexes, urine output, and respiratory rate must be closely monitored.[4] The knee-jerk reflex disappears at serum concentrations of 10 to 12 mg/dl. Respiration is depressed when the serum magnesium level reaches 12 to 15 mg/dl. Abnormalities in electrocardiograph tracings (increased P-R interval, prolonged QRS interval, increased T wave) have been related to serum concentrations as low as 6 mg/dl. Cardiac arrest does not occur until the serum magnesium concentration is 30 mg/dl or greater.[20] Cardiovascular actions of magnesium are similar to but less pronounced than β-adrenergic drugs.

The maternal administration of magnesium sulfate usually does not compromise the neonate.[21] Magnesium does cross the placenta promptly by active diffusion and can produce fetal serum concentrations which are comparable to the mother's.[22,23] However, only isolated reports of neonatal depression have appeared, and these cases are associated with perinatal asphyxia or decreased urinary output in the neonate. Apgar scores do not relate to serum concentrations of magnesium in the cord blood. Respiratory depression from hypermagnesemia can be reversed in the mother (calcium gluconate 10 ml of 10 percent solution IV) but not in the neonate.

Prostaglandin Synthetase Inhibitors

Prostaglandins have been implicated in the onset of uterine contractions. Their synthesis in the uterus is dependent on prostaglandin synthetase, an enzyme complex necessary for the conversion of arachidonic acid to prostaglandins (Chaps. 13 and 25). Antiprostaglandin agents are thought to inhibit spontaneous uterine contractions in pregnant rats and subhuman primates by reducing the amount of prostaglandins synthesized and released by the myometrial cells.[24-26] Human investigations by Lewis and Schulman[27] and by Zuckerman and co-workers[28] have involved pregnancies undergoing therapeutic abortion. Large doses of aspirin or indomethacin were found to either inhibit or prolong labor. Evidence from animal studies has revealed that aspirin, indomethacin, and naproxen are effective in prolonging gestation and labor.[29] Their use in clinical obstetrics has largely been as prophylaxis to avoid the onset of recurrent premature labor. Niebyl et al. found indomethacin to be effective in inhibiting premature labor in a prospective, randomized, double-blind study involving 30 patients.[30] The lowest effective dose for each drug has not yet been determined.

Prostaglandin synthetase inhibitors are not approved by the Food and Drug Administration for inhibiting uterine contractions. Potential side effects in the mother and fetus may result from acute or chronic exposure. Adverse effects in the mother include peptic ulceration, bleeding, bone marrow depression, and gastrointestinal perforation and are usually related to the dose and duration of the specific drug. Theoretic effects on the human fetus include closure of the ductus arteriosus, decreased platelet aggregation, and diminished uteroplacental circulation.[31-33] Dudley et al. have reported no serious effects on the fetus or neonate when a short course of indomethacin was used in 167 cases of premature labor before 35 weeks.[34] Adaptive adjustments from fetal to neonatal life may be impaired.[35] Double-blind, controlled, prospective studies are necessary to establish the effectiveness of prostaglandin synthetase inhibitors in inhibiting the onset or duration of premature uterine contractions.

Progesterone

Progesterone, which is synthesized in the placenta, has been proposed by Csapo to block uterine activity.[36] The onset of labor in several animal species may result from decreasing the placental production of progesterone. In contrast, increasing levels of estrogen during pregnancy may promote uterine contractions, perhaps by increasing the release of or sensitivity to oxytocin. The direct injection of progesterone into the uterine wall or the intravenous infusion of the progesterone precursor, pregnenolone, or of dexamethasone may inhibit drug-induced uterine contractions.[37] In contrast, several studies by Fuchs and Stakemann[38] and by Brenner and Hendricks[39] have failed to demonstrate any labor-inhibiting effect of progesterone in women with premature labor. The prescribed dosages of progesterone may have been inadequate to supplement the placental production for inhibiting the onset of labor. Progesterone is probably ineffective after the onset of labor in avoiding preterm delivery. Kauppila et al. reported an improved delay in delivery and greater birthweights of infants in mothers treated with apparent premature labor using IV cortisol for 3 days followed by weekly intramuscular injections of 17-α-hydroxyprogesterone caproate. This finding requires further investigation elsewhere.[40]

The most promising work has been by Johnson et al. reported in 1975.[41] The prospective, double-blind study involved the prophylactic weekly injections of 250 mg of 17-α-hydroxyprogesterone caproate (Delalutin) begun *after* the 14th week of gestation.[41] Premature delivery did not occur in the 18 patients receiving the progestational agent, whereas 9 of the 22 patients receiving placebo had premature delivery. Yemini et al. in Israel also reported promising results using 17-α-hydroxyprogesterone in the same prophylactic manner.[42] The rate of premature delivery was lower in the treated group (16 percent) than the placebo group (38 percent). The mean birthweight was also significantly higher in the treatment group. The safety and effectiveness of these prophylactic injections require further investigation at other institutions before FDA approval can be obtained for this indication.

β-Adrenergic Drugs

β-Adrenergic drugs have gained the attention of many investigators during recent years because of their efficacy in inhibiting spontaneous or induced uterine contractions. These agents are structurally similar to epinephrine and act by binding to adrenergic receptors on uterine smooth muscle cells. Rucker, in 1925, was the first investigator to report the inhibiting effect of infused epinephrine on the gravid uterus;[43] however, the transient nature and unwanted cardiovascular side effects limited its clinical use. Being structurally similar to catecholamines and capable of stimulating adrenergic receptors, isoxsuprine was later found to diminish uterine contractile activity with fewer cardiovascular side effects. Other adrenergic drugs such as terbutaline and ritodrine were soon studied, and adrenergic receptor function became better understood.

Pharmacology

Adrenergic receptors in many tissues were initially categorized by Ahlquist in 1944 according to their vasoactive properties.[44] α-receptor stimulation caused vasoconstriction, while β-receptor stimulation provoked vasodilation and tachycardia. In 1967 Lands et al. further subdivided β-receptor function into β_1 and β_2 groups.[45] Specific effects from stimulation of these three types of adrenergic receptors (α, β_1, β_2) are listed in Table 12–5. A betamimetic drug with primarily β_2 adrenergic activity is most desirable in inhibiting premature labor. A subset of β_2 receptor stimulants acting on uterine smooth muscle receptors rather than on blood vessel or bronchial receptors would be ideal.

β_2-adrenergic drugs bind to specific receptors on the outer smooth-muscle cell membrane to activate the enzyme, adenylcyclase.[46] Adenosine 5′-triphosphate (ATP) is then rapidly converted to cyclic adenosine 5′-monophosphate (cAMP) which causes protein kinases to phosphorylate cell membrane proteins. The phosphorylated proteins sequester intracellular calcium to prevent the activation of muscle cell contractile elements for uterine smooth muscle contraction.

All β-adrenergic drugs are metabolized in the liver and eliminated primarily through the kidneys in either unchanged or inactive, conjugated forms. They are also eliminated by transplacental transfer but in limited amounts. The intervillous and umbilical circulations are maintained during short-term administration in normotensive mothers.[47]

Preparations and Dosages

All preparations that have been used clinically are structurally similar to epinephrine (Fig. 12–2). Observed effects relate to differ-

TABLE 12–5. EFFECTS FROM ADRENERGIC RECEPTOR STIMULATION

Adrenergic Receptor	Tissue	Observed Effect
α	Uterus	Uterine contractions
	Blood vessels	Hypertension
β_1	Heart	Tachycardia
	Adipose	Lipolysis
	Small intestine	Gastrointestinal relaxation
β_2	Uterus	Uterine relaxation
	Bronchioles	Bronchial relaxation
	Blood vessels	Hypotension
	Muscles	Glycogenolysis
	Liver	

ences in substitutions on the aromatic ring, the α- and β-carbons, and the terminal amine group. Isoxsuprine (Vasodilan), terbutaline (Brethine, Bricanyl), and ritodrine (Yutopar) have been used in the United States. Fenoteral, hexoprenaline, and salbutamol are other β-adrenergic drugs which have been used for tocolysis. Reports of their use have been limited to mostly centers in the United States.[48,49] Only ritodrine has been approved by the FDA for inhibiting preterm labor, and it has been studied for more than 15 years at various medical centers in the United States and Europe. The wholesale cost of ritodrine is considerably higher than the cost of an equivalent dose of terbutaline.

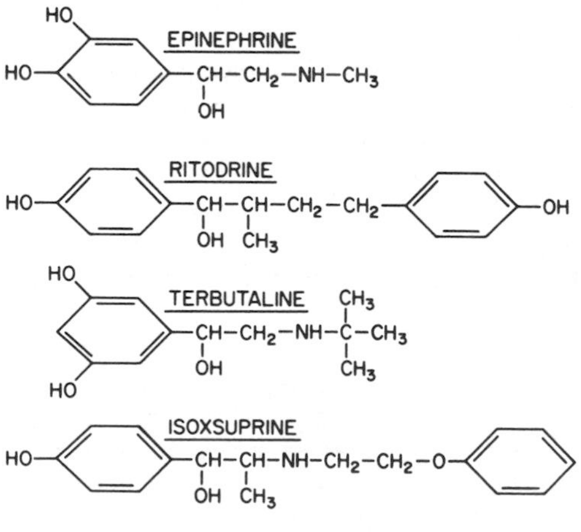

Figure 12–2. Structures of the β-adrenergic agents.

The preparations and dose regimens for initial and maintenance therapy are listed in Table 12–3. Unlike many other tocolytic agents, the β-adrenergic drugs may be administered by intravenous, subcutaneous, or oral routes. The parenteral dose is titrated according to contraction frequency and side effects. Intravenous treatment should be continued for approximately 6 to 12 hours after contractions cease. Oral therapy may then be started during SC injections or IV therapy. Therapy can be reinstituted if labor returns after successful tocolysis, but the persistence of labor despite the maximal recommended IV dose warrants discontinuation of the drug. Because side effects outweigh the benefits, β-adrenergic therapy is discontinued by the 37th gestational week, or if fetal pulmonary maturity has been established.

ISOXSUPRINE. Reports from controlled studies by Das[50] and by Csapo and Herczeg[51] have supported the use of isoxsuprine in arresting premature labor. This gained further acceptance from studies by Bishop and Woutersz[52] and by Hendricks.[53] Success rates judged by a delay in delivery of 3 days or more were 80 percent. Frequent severe side effects including maternal tachycardia and hypotension from α- and β-receptor stimulation have limited the routine use of isoxsuprine. The average maternal blood pressure decreased by 8 mm Hg and average maternal heart rate increased by 10.9 beats/min in the isoxsuprine-treated group. There was a slight average increase in fetal heart rate (FHR) of 6 beats/min,[54] in addition to some patients developing transient dizziness, weakness, nausea, sweating, and headaches.

Glycogenolysis from β_2-receptor stimulation in the liver and muscles can cause hyperglycemia, lactic acidemia, and elevated levels of free fatty acids. Transient increases in insulin secretion and a moderate decrease in serum potassium levels may occur. As a result of fetal hyperinsulinemia in response to the hyperglycemia, transient hypoglycemia may be seen in the neonate. No increase in neonatal morbidity has been reported in a 2-year follow-up after ritodrine use.

TERBUTALINE. Terbutaline is a selective β_2-agonist which has wide clinical use in the treatment of bronchial asthma. Most of the initial studies on terbutaline's effectiveness in the therapy of premature labor were done by Anderson and Ingemarsson in Sweden.[55,56] In 1975 Anderson demonstrated that intravenous terbutaline in concentrations of 0.2 to 1.0 mcg/ml inhibited spontaneous contractile activity of isolated strips of myometrium in vitro from seven patients undergoing cesarean section at term. The effects of terbutaline were inhibited by propranolol (β_1 and β_2-blocker); however, a selective β_1-blocker had no effect on the actions of terbutaline in vitro. A small number of patients in labor received a terbutaline infusion of 10 to 15 mcg/min for 20 to 40 minutes, which inhibited both spontaneous and oxytocin-induced labor. The intensity and frequency of the contractions were diminished in all patients.

The safety of terbutaline has been supported by animal studies by Caritis et al.[57] Terbutaline suppressed spontaneous and oxytocin-augmented uterine activity in the pregnant baboon when administered intravenously. Mean maternal arterial pressures were not significantly changed, although a mild maternal tachycardia occurred which was dose related. Significant alterations in maternal or fetal acid-base status did not occur despite the presence of hyperglycemia. Using infusion rates in excess of labor-inhibiting doses in pregnant ewes, terbutaline did not cause adverse changes in uterine blood flow.[58] Akerlund and Andersson determined that intravenous terbutaline caused an inhibition of myometrial activity and an increase in local endometrial blood flow in the human uterus at all phases of the menstrual cycle.[55]

In 1974, Andersson et al. administered intravenous terbutaline at a rate of 10 to 20 mcg/min to 14 patients in normal term labor.[59] In all pregnancies studied, uterine contractions were inhibited with a decrease in amplitude and frequency of contractions. Inhibition was not affected by the use of oxytocin, and no rebound was noted after discontinuation of the drug. Most patients had an increase in systolic pressure but a decrease in diastolic pressure, thereby increasing the pulse pressure.[60] The most significant change was an increase in maternal heart rate while on terbutaline. The fetal heart rate also increased up to a maximum rate of 160 beats/min.

This study was followed by the first double-blind, placebo-controlled study with terbutaline by Ingemarsson.[61] Thirty patients in premature labor with intact membranes were randomized and matched. Cervical dilation in all women was less than 4 cm. In the terbutaline-treated group, 12 of 15 (80 percent) of the patients delivered at week 37 or beyond, while only 3 patients (20 percent) in the placebo group reached term. No serious side effects occurred with terbutaline. Maternal tachycardia occurred in all patients treated with terbutaline with an average increase of 30 percent, and fetal tachycardia was also observed.

Wallace et al.[62] performed an uncontrolled study of 50 women in premature labor. An initial IV bolus of 250 mcg of terbutaline was followed by a maintenance infusion of 10 to 80 mcg/min. Success, as defined by a prolongation of gestation for 72 hours or more, involved 78 percent of the study group. There was an average prolongation of gestation of 3.7 weeks, with 48 percent of patients reaching 36 weeks or more.

Caritis et al. compared 100 women in preterm labor who were randomly treated with either ritodrine or terbutaline in a double-blind fashion.[63] Both drugs were comparably effective during IV therapy. Side effects were most likely to occur with either drug during periods when the infusion rate was increased than when the rate was constant. The terbutaline-treated women were more likely to have a serum glucose level in excess of 140 mg percent. A maternal heart rate of greater than 130 bpm was more common during IV therapy for those women receiving ritodrine than terbutaline (20 of 31 versus 8 of 27, $p < 0.05$).

Most side effects encountered with IV terbutaline are mild, and careful attention must be placed on monitoring the maternal blood pressure and pulse rate. The patient must be well hydrated before administration of the drug. There have been some isolated reports of pulmonary edema occurring in women treated simultaneously with terbutaline and steroids to enhance lung maturity.[64,65] Orally administered terbutaline produces no significant maternal biochemical or biophysical changes or any side effects on the fetus.[65]

RITODRINE. Ritrodrine hydrochloride is the most studied β-adrenergic agonist for inhibiting premature labor. The preferential affinity for β_2-receptors for inhibiting uterine contractions is present. It is a weak β_1-agonist and has no α-sympatholytic effects; therefore, direct cardiovascular effects should be minimal. It is presently the only drug approved by the FDA for use in premature labor. Its safety and patient acceptance of the drug have been proven in extensive worldwide clinical trials. Evidence for its efficacy in improving neonatal outcome is attested to by some but not all individual studies of the agent.

Trials of ritodrine in the United States were judged as providing sufficient evidence of efficacy and safety for the FDA approval in 1980. The study was a collaborative attempt to assemble data from 11 investigators in a prospective, randomized or double-blind manner by comparing ritodrine to either ethanol or placebo.[66] Unfortunately, only a partially standardized protocol was used. Over a 5-year period (1975–1979), 313 pregnancies with premature labor were evaluated. Neonatal deaths and respiratory distress were significantly less in the treated versus the control groups. The average number of days gained prior to delivery was 32.6 in the ritodrine group and 21.3 days in the control group. Significantly, more infants in the treated group obtained birthweights of greater than 2500 g or gestation ages of 36 weeks or more. In all categories the most benefit was gained by the neonates whose estimated gestational age at the onset of treatment was less than 33 weeks.

The pharmacokinetics of ritodrine have been studied extensively in animals and humans.[67] Animal studies show that between 50 and 80 percent of the drug is excreted in the urine. Ninety percent of the drug is excreted in 24 hours, the majority in the form of inactive metabolites. Almost twice as much of the drug is excreted unchanged when given intravenously. In sheep, the drug crosses the placenta and reaches 20 percent of the maternal concentration. In the two most sensitive animal species, the lethal dose (LD_{50}) has been found to be 80 times the effective therapeutic level in humans.

No ill effects have been noted in animals during short or protracted courses of therapy, and the only fetal effect in most species has been an increase in fetal weight. Uterine blood flow studies have not shown consistent results but indicate either no or only slight decreases in intervillous and umbilical vein blood flow which are not associated with acid-based changes in the fetus.[68]

Human studies revealed that 32 percent of the drug is bound to albumin. Most of the drug (71 to 93 percent) is eliminated in the urine with maximum rate of excretion being 1 hour after oral administration. As in animal studies, approximately 20 percent of the drug crosses the placenta. The monitoring of maternal ritodrine levels does not seem to be useful clinically. However, there is a direct correlation between neonatal drug concentration and major neonatal complications. Gross et al. have reported that the concentration of ritodrine in both maternal and umbilical vein was found to vary inversely with the length of time the drug was discontinued before delivery.[69] The maternal ritodrine dose within 24 hours before delivery and the drug discontinuance to delivery interval were both related to umbilical vein ritodrine concentrations. The frequency of respiratory distress is thought to be increased in the neonate whose umbilical vein ritodrine concentrations are greater than 10 mg/ml compared with those whose umbilical vein levels range from 3 to 10 mg/ml.

Several maternal cardiovascular effects with IV ritodrine include a dose-related increase in maternal heart rate of 19 to 40 bpm, a widening of the pulse pressure by 3 to 18 mm Hg, and a slight increase in cardiac output. The mean fetal heart rate increases slightly but consistently. M-mode echocardiography performed before and during IV β-adrenergic therapy has shown a significant increase in maternal heart rate, fraction shortening, and cardiac output.[70] Side effects such as maternal hypertension, vomiting, chest discomfort, and shortness of breath are most commonly observed when the infusion rate and concentration of ritodrine are increasing.[71] Temporary electrocardiographic evidence has suggested myocardial ischemia may be found in persons in whom chest pain has been reported. This has involved T-wave inversion and ST-T segment depression.[72,73]

These cardiovascular effects may be blocked with β-blocking agents or by decreasing the dose or discontinuing the infusion. Side effects are rare, but two maternal deaths have been reported.[67] One woman had suspected idiopathic pulmonary hypertension, while the other was taking multiple medications which included corticosteroids. Pulmonary edema has been reported in women who were also receiving corticosteroids, usually when excessive fluids were administered intravenously. Fluid retention, left-sided heart failure, and elevated hydrostatic pressures have been postulated, using the baboon model, as the etiology of induced pulmonary edema.[74] Discontinuation of the β-adrenergic therapy, oxygenation, and administration of diuretics with or without digoxin should be successful in reversing the process. Anemia, multiple gestation, and excess intravenous fluids have also been associated risk factors.[75]

Metabolic changes in the mother during ritodrine therapy have included transient increases in glucose, free fatty acids, lactic acid, and insulin with a moderate decrease in potassium and calcium.[76–78] These have been reported when ritodrine has been administered IV but not intramuscularly or orally.[79] If untreated, these metabolic changes are self-limited and not associated with adverse effects although not absolutely innocuous.[80] The routine administration of potassium is not thought to be necessary. Diabetic women in premature labor may still be prescribed IV ritodrine as long as their glucose control is strict.[81]

Unpleasant but probably physiologically insignificant side effects include tremor (10 to 15 percent), palpitations (33 percent), and nervousness or restlessness (20 percent). There have been no reports of an increase in postterm pregnancies, abnormal labor, or uterine atony.

No increase in neonatal morbidity has been noted in a 2-year follow-up of infants delivered during these trials.[82] Although transient hypoglycemia and respiratory distress may be more common in infants delivered by mothers receiving ritodrine, no significant differences have been found in umbilical cord pH, Apgar scores, head circumference, and neurologic conditions compared with matched controls.[83] Differences in childhood growth, neurologic findings, and psychometric testing are not thought to be significant between fetuses exposed to ritodrine in utero and those who were not.[84]

The dosage of ritodrine in treating premature labor is begun at 100 mcg/min IV and usually increased in increments of 50 mcg/min up to 350 mcg/min as needed to inhibit contractions (see Table 12–3). Accurate fluid balance is necessary, and isotonic saline solutions should be avoided. The manufacturer recommends continuing IV treatment for 12 hours after contractions cease. Subcutaneous therapy is seldom used. Instead, oral maintenance therapy is started 30 minutes before discontinuing the IV regimen. The initial oral therapy consists usually of 10 mg every 2 hours or 20 mg every 4 hours. The maximum maintenance oral dose should not exceed 120 mg/day.

Guidelines for IV ritodrine therapy for women with twin gestations are the same as for singleton pregnancies.[85-86] Compared with a matched group of singleton pregnancies, increases in maternal and fetal heart rates, and decreases in maternal blood pressures are not significantly different from twin gestations (Figs. 12–3 and 12–4).[85] Undesired cardiovascular effects are also not more common with close monitoring and usually occur during the initial infusion period. The duration of therapy, averaged maximum doses, and delays in deliveries are also expected to be similar between the twin and singleton groups (Fig. 12–5). In contrast, the prophylactic use of oral ritodrine is not thought to be more beneficial than a placebo in prolonging pregnancy for women with twin gestations. Maternal tachycardia should be considered as an index of patient responsiveness to the betamimetic treatment.

If labor recurs and there are no contraindications to tocolysis, the infusion may be restarted. Continuous long-term IV β-adrener-

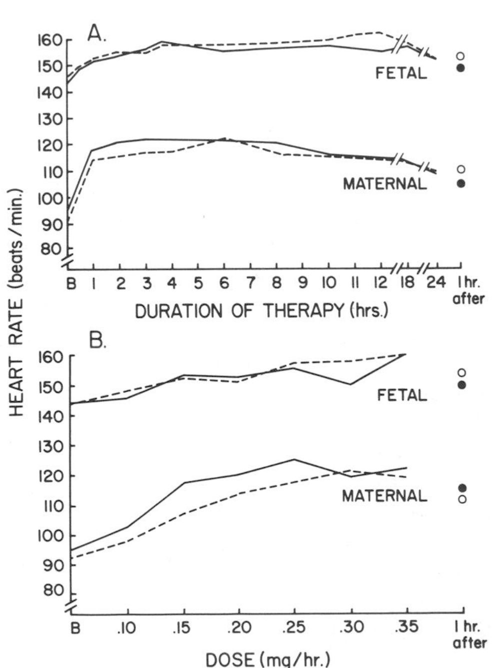

Figure 12–3. Maternal and fetal heart rate responses to intravenous ritodrine therapy for twin (—) and singleton (---) pregnancies. *(From Rayburn W et al, with permission.[85])*

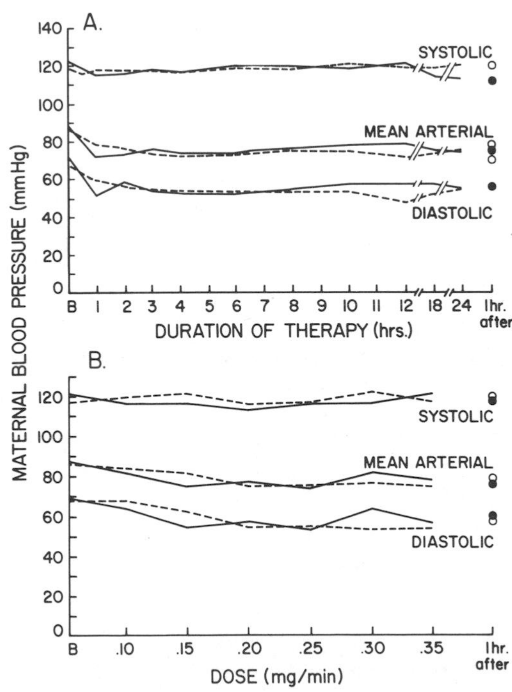

Figure 12–4. Maternal blood pressure responses to intravenous ritodrine therapy for twin (—) and singleton (---) pregnancies. *(From Rayburn W et al, with permission.[85])*

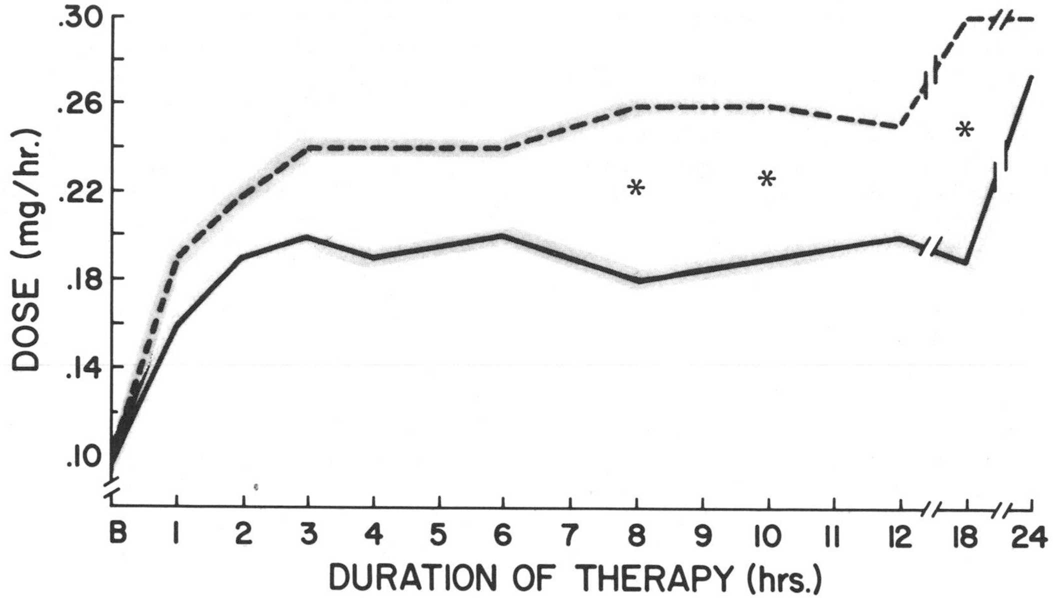

Figure 12–5. Doses of intravenous ritodrine used to inhibit premature labor in twin (—) and singleton (---) pregnancies. * represents a significant difference between the two groups. *(From Rayburn W et al, with permission.[85])*

gic tocolysis is seldom necessary for several days. The maternal cardiovascular and metabolic effects during IV therapy are thought to return to pretreatment values after the first 4 days. Prolonged infusion of ritodrine may lead to decreased responsiveness in β-adrenergic mechanisms regulating maternal plasma metabolities and hormone levels.[86] A similar unresponsiveness in the fetus, although less well-understood, may increase hazards during delivery and newborn adaptation. The drug may be discontinued without the need for tapering once fetal lung maturity is evident or the gestational age reaches 37 weeks.

OTHER DRUGS WITH UTERINE INHIBITORY ACTIVITY

Calcium Channel Blockers

Calcium channel blockers such as nicardipine and nifedipine are calcium antagonists which constitute a new approach to tocolysis. These drugs inhibit the entry of calcium into muscle cells and diminish uterine contractility in various animal studies.[88–92] The control of uterine activity may affect not only the pregnant myometrium but also the nonpregnant myometrium in cases of severe dysmenorrhea. The wide use of such drugs during pregnancy is questionable, however, and several aspects of the actions of calcium antagonists including any negative effects in the fetus must be clarified.[93,94] The limited use of these drugs in pregnant humans may be considered only after no explanation for the premature labor is apparent and a failure from use of ritodrine and magnesium sulfate therapy has taken place.

Diazoxide (Hyperstat)

Diazoxide is a potent vasodilating agent which is a nondiuretic thiazide. It may markedly inhibit uterine activity when used to treat a hypertensive crisis during pregnancy.[95] The mechanism for tocolysis is uncertain but may be a direct effect on uterine smooth muscle or through the release of catecholamines.[96] Cardiovascular (tachycardia, hypotension) and metabolic (hypoglycemia) effects from diazoxide are similar to those of the β_2-adrenergic agents, but they are not reversed by β-blocking agents (propranolol) and are more pronounced. Uterine blood flow was not reduced in sheep during a slow infusion.[97] Studies in humans with doses that inhibited contractions resulted in only mild tachycardia and a small reduction in blood pressure. Controlled, convincing studies of the effectiveness of diazoxide are lacking and are unlikely to be undertaken, since β_2-adrenergic agonists have been shown to be effective and probably less hazardous.

Aminophylline

Aminophylline is a xanthine derivative used to treat asthma during pregnancy. It has been postulated that aminophylline may indirectly inhibit uterine motility by its phosphodiesterase inhibitory action.[98] The inhibition of phosphodiesterase may cause an accumulation of cAMP, which is an important regulator in myosin light-chain phosphorylation for smooth muscle contractility. A study by Coutinho and Lopes supported this theory by infusing aminophylline to 60 women at various phases of their menstrual cycles.[99] Uterine activity was decreased in all patients. Aminophylline is not approved by the FDA for premature labor therapy, and a paucity of data supports its effectiveness.

Recent evidence in rabbit, rat, and human investigations has suggested that phosphodiesterase inhibitors may offer another benefit by promoting an increase in alveolar surfactant concentration and synthesis.[100,101] The principal result is thought to be an increase in phosphatidylcholine levels.

GUIDELINES FOR SELECTING TOCOLYTIC AGENTS

Once early premature labor is diagnosed, the use of tocolytic drugs to temporarily delay delivery until at least 33 gestational weeks is thought to be cost effective.[102]

The proper choice of an appropriate tocolytic agent is not often easy. Many agents described in this chapter (ethanol, magnesium sulfate, isoxsuprine, diazoxide, aminophylline) were found to have tocolytic potential only as a result of incidental use. The mechanism of uterine contraction has become better understood in recent years, and β_2-adrenergic drugs are the most useful because of their more specific interaction with myometrial receptors. They are effective and may be used repetitively and chronically as oral agents. Ritodrine is the only such drug that is currently FDA approved for tocolysis and is the drug of choice in the majority of pregnancies treated for premature labor.

No group of drugs described in this chapter has been proven to be ideal for inhibiting uterine contractions. Adverse effects to the mother and fetus must be considered as cases are selected for tocolysis. Close monitoring is a prerequisite, and package inserts describing each drug must be provided for patient understanding.

The choice of tocolytic agent must be tailored to the individual clinical situation. Anticipated side effects from each drug may require a change in drugs or a discontinuation of therapy. This is especially true if heart disease, hypertension, thyroid disease, liver disease, impaired renal function, diabetes mellitus, or vaginal bleeding is present. Magnesium sulfate may be preferred. It does not apparently alter uterine perfusion pressure and may have a beneficial effect on uterine hemodynamics. Ritodrine, terbutaline, and magnesium sulfate were compared recently for their relative safety and efficacy.[63,102] No differences in efficacy could be demonstrated, but a markedly higher risk of maternal side effects was found with the β-adrenergic drugs, especially terbutaline. A well-supervised delivery near an intensive care nursery may be preferred to inhibiting uterine contractions, especially when fetal lung maturity is evident.

Very little information is available about the combined use of tocolytic agents. Uterine contractions may be more effectively inhibited, while unwanted side effects may not be increased or may be reduced, if smaller dosages can be administered. The concomitant administration of a β-adrenergic drug and magnesium sulfate may be done if the initial attempt at tocolysis with a β-adrenergic drug alone is unsuccessful or associated with cardiac complications. Maximum doses of both drugs may be used with caution, and signs for pulmonary edema should be sought. Decreasing the ritodrine infusion may be necessary to eliminate maternal or fetal tachycardia.[103,104]

Further clinical investigation is necessary to better understand the etiology of premature labor, endocrinology of parturition, and effectiveness of the various tocolytic drug regimens. Double-blind, prospective studies involving control groups must be continued at regional perinatal centers. Along with determining what percentage of pregnancies remain undelivered within a few days or several weeks after initiating therapy, long-term effects on the fetus and infant must be assessed. The practicality of tocolytic therapy also requires further investigation for conditions in which preterm rupture of amniotic membranes are present or in which prophylactic therapy may decrease the risk of subsequent premature labor.

Lastly, tocolytic drugs have also been used for other conditions besides inhibiting premature labor. Both magnesium sulfate and β-adrenergic drugs have been used during external cephalic version.[105,106] Uterine relaxation to correct uterine inversion after delivery has been reported with terbutaline sulfate.[107] Evidence for acute fetal distress intrapartum, especially severe fetal bradycardia associated with uterine hypertonus, has been alleviated with the administration of a bolus of ritodrine or magnesium sulfate.[108-111]

REFERENCES

1. Fuchs F: Prevention of prematurity. Am J Obstet Gynecol 126:809, 1976
2. Creasy R: Preterm labor and delivery. In Creasy R, Resnik R (eds): Maternal–Fetal Medicine. Philadelphia, Saunders, 1984, pp 415–443
3. Wynn M, Wynn A: The Prevention of Preterm Birth. London, Foundation for Education and Research in Child-Bearing, 1977
4. Caritis SN, Edelstone DI, Mueller-Heubach E: Pharmacologic inhibition of preterm labor. Am J Obstet Gynecol 133:557, 1979
5. Fuchs F, Fuchs AR, Poblete VF Jr, Risk A: Effect of alcohol on threatened premature labor. Am J Obstet Gynecol 99:627, 1967
6. Zlatnick FJ, Fuchs F: A controlled study of ethanol in threatened premature labor. Am J Obstet Gynecol 112:610, 1972
7. Watring WG, Benson WL, Wiebe RA, Vaughn DL: Intravenous alcohol—a single blind study in the prevention of premature delivery: A preliminary report. J Reprod Med 16:35, 1976
8. Castren O, Gummerus M, Saarikoski S: Treatment of imminent premature labour. Acta Obstet Gynecol Scand 54:95, 1975
9. Steir CM, Petrie RH: A comparison of magnesium sulfate and alcohol for the prevention of premature labor. Am J Obstet Gynecol 129:1, 1977
10. Lauersen NH, Merkatz IR, Tejani N, et al.: Inhibition of premature labor: A multicenter comparison of ritodrine and ethanol. Am J Obstet Gynecol 127:837, 1977
11. Fuchs F: Prevention of prematurity. Am J Obstet Gynecol 126:809, 1976
12. Ritchie JM: The aliphatic alcohols. In Goodman LS, Gilman A (eds): The Pharmacologic Basis of Therapeutics, ed. 5. New York, Macmillan, 1975, pp 137–151
13. Kumar D, Zourlas PA, Barnes AC: In vitro and in vivo effects of magnesium sulfate on human uterine contractiligy. Am J Obstet Gynecol 86:1036, 1963
14. Spisso K, Harbert G, Thiagarajah S: The use of magnesium sulfate as the primary tocolytic agent to prevent premature delivery. Am J Obstet Gynecol 142:840, 1982
15. Ogburn P, Hansen C, Williams P, et al.: Magnesium sulfate and β-mimetic dual-agent tocolysis in preterm labor after single-agent failure. J Reprod Med 30:583, 1985
16. Ferguson J, Hensleigh P, Kredenster D: Adjunctive use of magnesium sulfate with ritodrine for preterm labor tocolysis. Am J Obstet Gynecol 148:166, 1984
17. Hatjis CG, Nelson LH, Meis PJ, et al.: Addition of magnesium sulfate improves effec-

tiveness of ritodrine in preventing premature delivery. Am J Obstet Gynecol 150:142, 1984
18. Valenzuela G, Cline S: Use of magnesium sulfate in premature labor that fails to respond to β-mimetic drugs. Am J Obstet Gynecol 144:718, 1982
19. Elliott JP: Magnesium sulfate as a tocolytic agent. Am J Obstet Gynecol 147:277, 1983
20. Wacker WEC, Parisi AF: Magnesium metabolism. N Engl J Med 278:658, 1968
21. Stone SR, Pritchard JA: Effect of maternally administered magnesium sulfate on the neonate. Obstet Gynecol 35:574, 1970
22. Lipsitz PJ: The clinical and biochemical effects of excess magnesium in the newborn. Pediatrics 47:501, 1971
23. Pritchard JA: The use of magnesium sulfate in pre-eclampsia–eclampsia. J Reprod Med 23:107, 1979
24. Aiken JW: Aspirin and indomethacin prolong parturition in rats: Evidence that prostaglandins contribute to expulsion of foetus. Nature 240:21, 1972
25. Csapo AI, Csapo EF, Fay E, et al.: The delay of spontaneous labor by naproxen in the rat model. Prostaglandins 3:827, 1973
26. Novy MJ, Cook MJ, Manaugh L: Indomethacin block of normal onset of parturition in primates. Am J Obstet Gynecol 118:412, 1974
27. Lewis RB, Schulman JD: Influence of acetylsalicyclic acid, an inhibitor of prostaglandin synthesis, on the duration of human gestation and labour. Lancet 2:1159, 1973
28. Zuckerman H, Reiss U, Rubinstein I: Inhibition of human premature labor by indomethacin. Obstet Gynecol 44:787, 1974
29. Johnson WL, Harbert GM, Martin CG: Pharmacologic control of uterine contractility. Am J Obstet Gynecol 123:364, 1975
30. Niebyl JR, Blake DA, White RD, et al.: The inhibition of premature labor with indomethacin. Am J Obstet Gynecol 136:1014, 1980
31. Starling MB, Elliott RB: The effects of prostaglandins, prostaglandin inhibitors, and oxygen on the closure of the ductus arteriosus, pulmonary arteries and umbilical vessels in vitro. Prostaglandins 8:187, 1974
32. Haslam RR, Ekert H, Gilliam GR: Hemorrhage in a neonate possibly due to maternal ingestion of salicylate. J Pediatr 84:556, 1974
33. Naden R, Iliya C, Arant B, et al.: Hemodynamic effects of indomethacin in chronically instrumented pregnant sheep. Am J Obstet Gynecol 151:484, 1985
34. Dudley D, Hardie M: Fetal and neonatal effects of indomethacin used as a tocolytic agent. Am J Obstet Gynecol 151:181, 1985
35. Bleyer WA, Breckenridge RT: Studies on the detection of adverse drug reactions in the newborn: II. The effects of prenatal aspirin on newborn hemostasis. JAMA 213:2049, 1970
36. Csapo AI: The regulatory interplay of progesterone and prostaglandin F_2 in the control of the pregnant uterus. In Josimovich JB (ed): Uterine Contraction, New York, Wiley 1973, pp 223–255
37. Tomasi A, Tseng H, Scommegna A, Burd L: The effect of medroxyprogesterone acetate on premature labor in the sheep. Am J Obstet Gynecol 151:694, 1985
38. Fuchs F, Stakemann G: Treatment of threatened premature labor with large doses of progesterone. Am J Obstet Gynecol 79:172, 1960
39. Brenner WE, Hendricks CH: Effect of medroxyprogesterone acetate upon the duration and characteristics of human gestation and labor. Am J Obstet Gynecol 83:1094, 1962
40. Kauppila A, Hartikainen-Sorri A, Janne O, et al.: Suppression of threatened premature labor by administration of cortisol and 17 α-hydroxyprogesterone caproate: A comparison with ritodrine. Am J Obstet Gynecol 138:404, 1980
41. Johnson JWC, Austin KL, Jones GS, et al.: Efficacy of 17-hydroxyprogesterone caproate in the prevention of premature labor. N Engl J Med 293:675, 1975
42. Yemini M, Borenstein R, Dreasen Z, et al.: Prevention of premature labor by 17 α-hydroxyprogesterone caproate. Am J Obstet Gynecol 151:574, 1985
43. Rucker MP: The action of adrenalin on the pregnant human uterus. South Med J 18:412, 1925
44. Ahlquist RP: A study of the adrenotropic receptors Am J Physiol 153:586, 1948
45. Lands AM, Luduena FP, Buzzo HJ: Differentiation of receptors responsive to isoproterenol. Life Sci 6:2241, 1967
46. Steer ML, Atlas D, Levitzki A: Inter-relations between α-adrenergic receptors, adenylate cyclase and calcium N Engl J Med 292:409, 1975
47. Sodha RJ, Schneider H: Transplacental transfer of β-adrenergic drugs studied by an in vitro perfusion method of an isolated human

placental lobule. Am J Obstet Gynecol 147:303, 1983

48. Marivate M, de Villiers K, Fairbrother P: Effect of prophylactic outpatient administration of fenoterol on the time of onset of spontaneous labor and fetal growth rate in twin pregnancy. Am J Obstet Gynecol 128:707, 1977
49. Fredericksen MC, Grayson K, Depp R, et al.: A comparison of the metabolic effects of hexaprenaline and ritodrine. Soc Gynecol Invest, San Francisco, March 21 – 24, 1984, Abs. #37
50. Das RK: Isoxsuprine in premature labour. J Obstet Gynaecol India 19:1076, 1965
51. Csapo AI, Herczeg J: Arrest of premature labor by isoxsuprine. Am J Obstet Gynecol 129:482, 1977
52. Bishop EH, Woutersz TB: Arrest of premature labor. JAMA 178:116, 1961
53. Hendricks CH: The use of isoxsuprine for the arrest of premature labor. Clin Obstet Gynecol 7:687, 1964
54. Stander RW, Barden TP, Thompson JF, et al.: Fetal cardiac effects of maternal isoxsuprine infusion. Am J Obstet Gynecol 89:792, 1964
55. Akerlund M, Andersson K-E: Effects of terbutaline on human myometrial activity and endometrial blood flow. Obstet Gynecol 47:529, 1976
56. Andersson K-E, Bengisson L Ph, Gustafson I, Ingemarsson I: The relaxing effect of terbutaline on the human uterus during term labor. Am J Obstet Gynecol 121:602, 1975
57. Caritis SN, Morishima HO, Stark RI, et al.: Effects of terbutaline on the pregnant baboon and fetus. Obstet Gynecol 50:56, 1977
58. Caritis SN, Mueller-Heubach E, Morishima HO, Edelstone DI: Effect of terbutaline on cardiovascular state and uterine blood flow in pregnant ewes. Obstet Gynecol 50:603, 1977
59. Andersson K-E, Ingemarsson I, Persson CGA: Effects of terbutaline on human uterine motility at term. Acta Obstet Gynecol Scand 54:165, 1975
60. Schwartz R, Retzke U: Cardiovascular effects of terbutaline in pregnant women. Acta Obstet Gynecol Scand 62:419, 1983
61. Ingemarsson I: Effect of terbutaline on premature labor. Am J Obstet Gynecol 125:520, 1976
62. Wallace RL, Caldwell DL, Ansbacher R, Otterson WN: Inhibition of premature labor by terbutaline. Obstet Gynecol 51:387, 1978
63. Caritis S, Toig G, Heddinger L, et al.: A double-blind study comparing ritodrine and terbutaline in the treatment of preterm labor. Am J Obstet Gynecol 150:7, 1984
64. Jacobs MM, Knight AB, Areas F: Maternal pulmonary edema resulting from betamimetic and glycocorticoid therapy. Obstet Gynecol 56:56, 1980
65. Jovanic R: Serial serum potassium and glucose levels during treatment of premature labor with oral terbutaline. Int J Gynaecol Obstet 28:399, 1985
66. Merkatz IR, Peter JB, Barden TP: Ritodrine hydrochloride: A betamimetic agent for use in preterm labor. Obstet Gynecol 56:7, 1980
67. Barden TP, Peter JB, Merkatz IR: Ritodrine hydrochloride: A betamimetic agent for use in preterm labor. Obstet Gynecol 56:1, 1980
68. Jouppila P, Kirkinen P, Koivula A, et al.: Ritodrine infusion during late pregnancy: Effects on fetal and placental blood flow, prostacyclin, and thromboxane. Am J Obstet Gynecol 151:1028, 1985
69. Gross T, Kuhnert B, Kuhnert P, et al.: Maternal and fetal plasma concentrations of ritodrine. Obstet Gynecol 149:798, 1984
70. Finley J, Katz M, Rojas-Perez M, et al.: Cardiovascular consequences of β-agonist tocolysis: An echocardiographic study. Obstet Gynecol 64:787, 1984
71. Caritis S, Lin L, Toig G, et al.: Pharmacodynamics of ritodrine in pregnant women during preterm labor. Am J Obstet Gynecol 147:752, 1983
72. Michalak D, Klein V, Marquette G: Myocardial ischemia: A complication of ritodrine tocolysis. Am J Obstet Gynecol 146:861, 1983
73. Ying YK, Tejani NA: Angina pectoris as a complication of ritodrine hydrochloride therapy in premature labor. Obstet Gynecol 60:385, 1982
74. Hauth JC, Hankins GD, Kuehl TJ, et al.: Ritodrine hydrochloride infusion in pregnant baboons. Am J Obstet Gynecol 146:916, 1983
75. Nimrod C, Rambihar V, Fallen E, et al.: Pulmonary edema associated with isoxsuprine therapy. Am J Obstet Gynecol 148:625, 1984
76. Richards S, Chang F, Stempel L: Hyperlactacidemia associated with acute ritodrine infusion. Am J Obstet Gynecol 146:1, 1983
77. Cano A, Tovar I, Parrilla J, et al.: Metabolic disturbances during intravenous use of ritodrine: Increased insulin levels and hypokalemia. Obstet Gynecol 65:356, 1985
78. Spellacy WN, Cruz AC, Buhi WC, et al.: The

acute effects of ritodrine infusion on maternal metabolism: Measurement of levels of glucose, insulin, glucagon, triglycerides, cholesterol, placental lactogen and chorionic gonadotropin. Am J Obstet Gynecol 131:673, 1978
79. Schreyer P, Caspi E, Snir E, et al.: Metabolic effects of intramuscular and oral administration of ritodrine in pregnancy. Obstet Gynecol 57:730, 1981
80. Young D, Toofanian A, Leveno K: Potassium and glucose concentrations without treatment during ritodrine tocolysis. Am J Obstet Gynecol 145:105, 1983
81. Miodovnik M, Peros N, Holroyde J, Siddiqi T: Treatment of premature labor in insulin-dependent diabetic women. Obstet Gynecol 65:621, 1985
82. Freysz H, Willard D, Lehr A, et al.: A long-term evaluation of infants who received a betamimetic drug while in utero. J Perinat Med 5:94, 1977
83. Huisjes H, Touwen B: Neonatal outcome after treatment with ritodrine: A controlled study. Am J Obstet Gynecol 147:250, 1983
84. Polowczyk D, Tejani N, Lauersen N, et al.: Evaluation of seven- to nine-year-old children exposed to ritodrine in utero. Obstet Gynecol 64:485, 1984
85. Rayburn W, Piehl E, Schork M, et al.: Intravenous ritodrine therapy: A comparison between twin and singleton gestations. Obstet Gynecol 66: 243, 1985
86. Bassett J, Burks A, Levine D, et al.: Maternal and fetal metabolic effects of prolonged ritodrine infusion. Obstet Gynecol 66:755, 1985
87. Cetrulo CL, Freeman RK: Ritodrine HCL for the prevention of premature labor in twin pregnancies. Acta Genet Med Gemellol 25:321, 1976
88. Forman A, Gandrup P, Andersson KE, Ulmsten U: Effects of nifedipine on spontaneous and methylergometrine-induced activity post partum. Am J Obstet Gynecol 144:442, 1982
89. Lirette M, Holbrook H, Katz M: Effect of nicardipine HCI on prematurely induced uterine activity in the pregnant rabbit. Obstet Gynecol 65:31, 1984
90. Forman A, Gandrup P, Andersson K, Ulmsten U: Effects of nifedipine on oxytocin- and prostaglandin F_2 α-induced activity in the postpartum uterus. Am J Obstet Gynecol 144:665, 1982
91. Golichowski A, Hathaway D, Jose M, et al.: Tocolytic and cardiovascular effects of nifedipine in the ewe. Soc Gynecol Invest, 1983, abstr 447
92. Holbrook RH, Lirette M, Katz M: Nicardipine tocolysis of preterm labor in the pregnant rabbit. Soc Perinatal Obstet, San Antonio, TX, 1984, abstr 100
93. Forman A, Andersson K, Ulmsten U: Inhibition of myometrial activity by calcium antagonists. Semin Perinatal 5(3):288, 1981
94. Huszar G, Janis R, Sakamoto H, et al.: Calcium entry blockers and the control of labor. Soc Gynecol Invest, 1983, abstr 448
95. Pennington JC, Picker RH: Diazoxide and the treatment of the acute hypertensive emergency in obstetrics. Med J Aust 2:1051, 1972
96. Wohl AJ, Hausler LM, Roth FE: Studies on the mechanism of antihypertensive action of diazoxide: In vitro vascular pharmacodynamics. J Pharmacol Exp Ther 158:531, 1967
97. Caritis SN, Morishima HO, Stark RI, James LS: The effect of diazoxide on uterine blood flow in pregnant sheep. Obstet Gynecol 48:464, 1976
98. Polson JB, Krzanowski JJ, Fitzpatrick DF, et al.: Studies on the inhibition of phosphodiesterase-catalyzed cycle AMP and cycle GMP breakdown and relaxation of canine tracheal smooth muscle. Biochem Pharmacol 27:254, 1978
99. Coutinho EM, Vieira Lopes AC: Inhibition of uterine motility by aminophylline. Am J Obstet Gynecol 110:726, 1971
100. Brinkman CR, Nuwayhid B, Assali NS: Renal hypertension and pregnancy in sheep. I. Behavior of uteroplacental vasomotor tone during mild hypertension. Am J Obstet Gynecol 121:931, 1975
101. Karotkin EH, Kido M, Cashore WJ, et al.: Acceleration of fetal lung maturation by aminophylline in pregnant rabbits. Pediatr Res 10:722, 1976
102. Korenbrot C, Aalto L, Laros R: The cost effectiveness of stopping preterm labor with β-adrenergic treatment. N Engl J Med 310:691, 1984
103. Beall M, Edgar B, Paul R. et al.: A comparison of ritodrine, terbutaline, and magnesium sulfate for the suppression of preterm labor. Am J Obstet Gynecol 153:854, 1985
104. Frederiksen M, Toig R, Depp R: Atrial fibrillation during hexoprenaline therapy for

premature labor. Am J Obstet Gynecol 145:108, 1983
105. Cantrell C, Clark S, Golde S, et al.: Is magnesium sulfate an effective uterine relaxant for external cephalic version? Soc Perinatal Obstet, Las Vegas, Nev, Feb 1985, abstr 237
106. Van Dorsten J, Schifrin B, Wallace R: Randomized control trial of external cephalic version with tocolysis in late pregnancy. Am J Obstet Gynecol 141:417, 1981
107. Kovacs B, DeVore G: Management of acute and subacute puerperal uterine inversion with terbutaline sulfate. Am J Obstet Gynecol 150:784, 1984
108. Sheybany S, Murphy J, Evans D, et al.: Ritodrine in the management of fetal distress. Br J Obstet Gynaecol 89:723, 1982
109. Hutchon DJR: Management of severe fetal bradycardia with ritodrine. Br J Obstet Gynaecol 89:671, 1982
110. Lipshitz J, Shaver D: Use of hexoprenaline in the management of fetal distress in labor. Soc Perinatal Obstet, San Antonio, TX, 1984, abstr 108
111. Barrett JM: Fetal resuscitation with terbutaline during eclampsia-induced uterine hypertonus. Am J Obstet Gynecol 150:895, 1984

13

Uterine Stimulants

William F. Rayburn and John S. Russ

Many theories concerning uterine stimulation during pregnancy exist, and explanations have paralleled knowledge about uterine physiology. Despite our inability to completely explain the mechanisms involved in uterine contractility, nature continually illustrates the process. At some critical time, which almost always seems appropriate and purposeful, the uterus is stimulated for the evacuation of its contents. Almost unerringly the process begins and ceases, being timed perfectly for mother and child.

The initiation and maintenance of uterine activity involves a complex interaction between maternal, uterine, and fetal factors. Progress in understanding the mechanisms for initiation of parturition have led to advances in uterine stimulation by pharmacologic agents. With continued clinical application these uterine stimulators have been modified and improved for use during the intrapartum and postpartum periods.

The three major groups of drugs to induce uterine stimulation include oxytocin, ergot alkaloids, and prostaglandins. An appreciation of their properties, indications, and effects on the target tissues should increase the clinician's competence in managing the induction of labor and in diminishing uterine blood loss in the postpartum period.

OXYTOCIN

In 1906 Dale was the first person to describe the chemical properties and elucidate the pharmacology of oxytocin from pituitary extracts.[1] It was not until the early 1950s, however, that duVigneaud and co-workers did the pioneering and Nobel prize-winning work on the structure of oxytocin.[2] Once commercially prepared quantities became available, knowledge about oxytocin paralleled advances in the comprehension of mechanisms of labor and the effects of labor on the uterus and on the fetus. Oxytocin is now the most widely used uterine stimulant and the most potentially harmful agent, if used improperly.

Pharmacology

Oxytocin is an octapeptide which is synthesized in the supraoptic and paraventricular nuclei of the hypothalamus. It is transported by carrier proteins from the hypothalamus to the posterior pituitary, where it is eventually released. Oxytocin has a half-life of 3 to 4 minutes and a duration of action of approximately 20 minutes. It is rapidly metabolized and degraded by oxytocinase.[3] The component amino acids are either redistributed or eliminated via the kidneys.

The mechanism wherein oxytocin facilitates smooth muscle contraction is not fully understood. Oxytocin is thought to bind to receptors on myometrial cell membranes, where cyclic adenosine 5′-monophosphate (cAMP) is eventually formed for a dose-dependent increase in amplitude and frequency of uterine contractions.[4] Bound intracellular calcium near the cell membrane is eventually mobilized from the sarcoplasmic reticulum to activate the contractile proteins. Oxytocin is also thought to act with prostaglandins. The uterine response to oxytocin stimulation depends on the uterine threshold of excitation, with the sensitivity of the uterus to oxytocin increasing gradually during gestation and sharply increasing before parturition.[5] Oxytocin is secreted in increasing amounts as labor progresses.

Clinical Use

Oxytocin is used to induce or augment uterine contractions in term and preterm pregnancies requiring uterine evacuation (Fig. 13–1). Pregnancy complications requiring uterine evacuation with oxytocin and uterine curettage would include incomplete or inevitable abortion, missed abortion, trophoblastic disease, and elective abortion. The uterine sensitivity to oxytocin infusion increases with gestational age and stage of labor.

Oxytocin may also be used during the intrapartum period to augment uterine contractions which are mild or infrequent (hypotonic contractions).[6] Postpartum hemorrhage is reduced when oxytocin is given with uterine massage. In our experience, an emptied uterus which does not contract well at cesarean section may respond to a direct 10-unit intramyometrial injection. Except for small hematomas, no immediate adverse effects have been observed.

Oxytocin may be administered as a nasal spray to stimulate impaired milk ejection. One spray in each nostril 3 to 4 minutes before breast pumping is helpful in relieving breast engorgement.

Oxytocin is either contraindicated or should be used with extreme caution when certain obstetric complications exist (Table 13–1). The drug may be used during a trial of labor in women with a previous cesarean section. The risk of instrumental vaginal delivery, uterine scar dehiscence, transfusion, birth trauma, or poor neonatal outcome is not increased if oxytocin is used to augment or induce labor as long as uterine activity is monitored closely. The risks and benefits must be carefully considered on an individual basis. Careful uterine and fetal monitoring is essential with close labor and delivery personnel supervision. Oxytocin should not be used to force cervical dilation.

Preparations and Doses

When taken orally, oxytocin is rapidly degraded in the gastrointestinal tract. Ampules of 10 units/ml of oxytocin (Pitocin, Syntocinon) are currently available for parenteral use. Tablets for application to the buccal cavity are no longer available, since the variable absorption caused unpredictable uterine understimulation and overstimulation.

The administration of oxytocin by intramuscular (IM) injection, intravenous (IV) bolus, or nasal drip is to be discouraged during labor. Compared to these routes of administration, the slow, continuous IV infusion has more predictable absorption, distribution, and response patterns.

One liter solutions for IV use usually contain 10 units of oxytocin (10 mU/ml). More concentrated solutions are possible when appropriate monitoring of the dose can be ar-

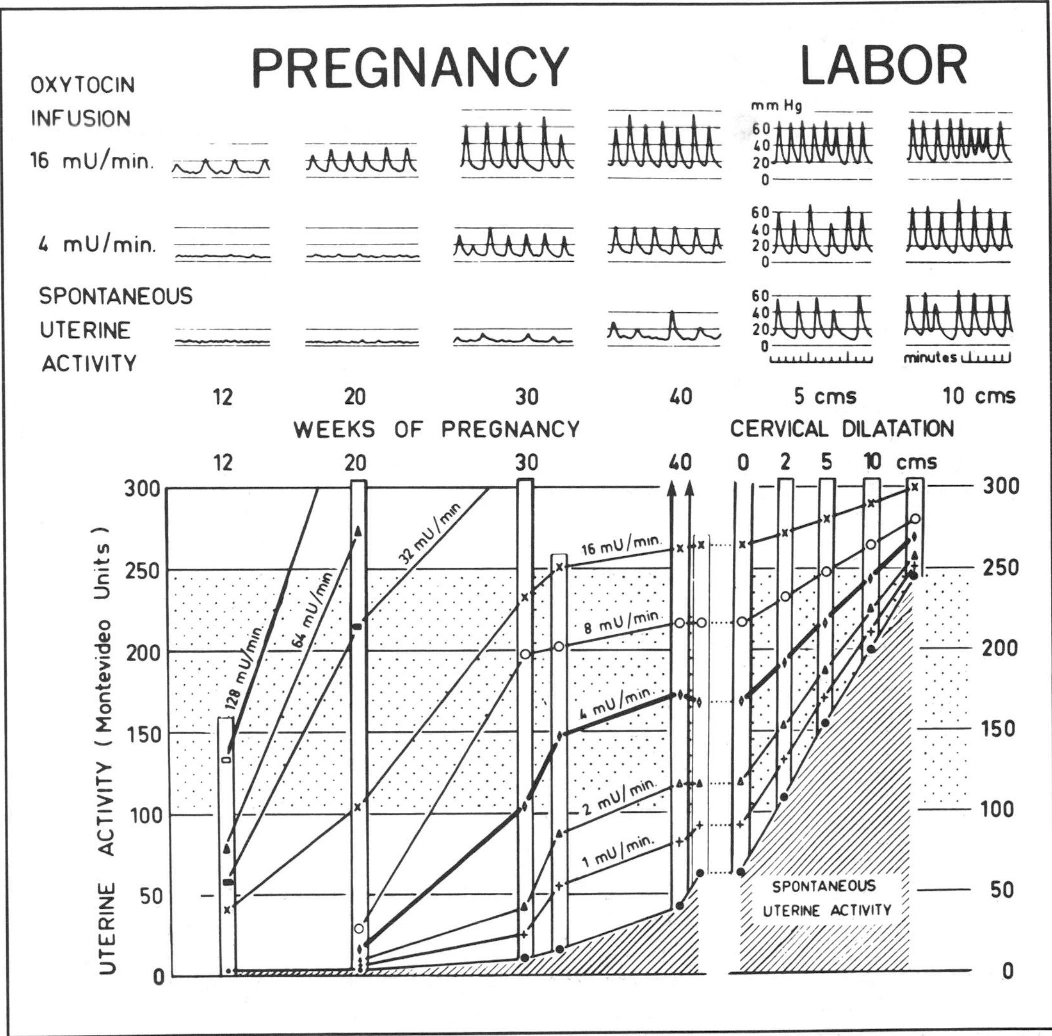

Figure 13–1. Sensitivity of the human uterus to oxytocin during pregnancy. Uterine activity tracings in the upper section illustrate the increasing sensitivity of the human uterus to oxytocin. The mean values of the uterine response to increasing doses are plotted against the duration of pregnancy and cervical dilation. (*From Caldeyro-Barcia R, Heller (eds): Oxytocin. Oxford, Pergamon, 1961, with permission.*)

ranged. Infusion pumps are recommended for the accurate control of the rate of infusion. Automatic infusion of oxytocin in a closed loop system for the induction of labor is not thought to have any advantage over the traditional manual administration of oxytocin by peristaltic infusion.[7] The dosage of the latter is derived from an intrauterine catheter or by clinical assessment of uterine activity.

The goal of induction is the presence of

TABLE 13–1. CONDITIONS IN WHICH OXYTOCIN IS EITHER USED WITH CAUTION OR IS CONTRAINDICATED

Used with caution
- Cephalopelvic disproportion
- Multiple fetuses
- Polyhydramnios
- Cardiac disease (with fixed cardiac output)
- Suspected fetal distress
- Grand multiparity
- Delivery of second twin
- Severe hypertension
- Breech
- Repeat cesarean section
- Other uterine-stimulating drugs

Contraindicated
- Unfavorable fetal position (transverse lie)
- Placenta previa
- Fetal distress where delivery not imminent
- Hypertonic uterine contractions

uterine contractions occurring every 2 to 3 minutes and lasting approximately 45 to 60 seconds.[8] When an intrauterine pressure catheter is used, a 50 mm H_2O recording is considered to be reasonable evidence of an adequate contraction. The infusion is begun at 2 mU/min and increased at 2-mU/min increments every 15 to 20 minutes until adequate contractions are palpated and observed.

The maximal rate of infusion for delivery purposes should generally not exceed 20 mU/min and the uterine response generally will not improve if a rate of 30 mU/min or more is administered.[8] An abdominal pregnancy should be considered if a very large dose (more than 50 mU/min) does not cause uterine contractions. With labor augmentation, the rate of infusion and maximal rate necessary are also less than for induction.[9,10] Once sufficient uterine activity has led to adequate progress of labor, the dosage of oxytocin should be decreased or stopped to allow labor to continue spontaneously. Table 13–2 lists the IV infusion schedules of oxytocin using a 10 units/liter solution mixture.

Following delivery, 10 U of oxytocin may be given IM or 5 U slowly IV. Postpartum hemorrhage associated with uterine atony requires a strong infusion of oxytocin (50 U in 500 ml of 5 percent dextrose in lactated Ringer's solution) at 25 mU/min and increased up to 50 mU/min.

Side Effects

Side effects from oxytocin use are usually easily predicted. Adequate supervision with monitoring of the uterine contractions, the fetus, and the infusion is necessary. Hyperstimulation with strong (hypertonic) or prolonged (tetanic) contractions, or a resting tone above 15 to 20 mm H_2O between contractions can lead to uterine rupture, uteroplacental hypoperfusion, and fetal distress from hypoxia. Under these circumstances the infusion should be stopped immediately. Uterine rupture is rare, being found most often in multiparous women with high doses of oxytocin.

Cardiovascular side effects including premature ventricular contractions may occur when an IV bolus of one or more units is given.[11] Hypotension from direct peripheral vasodilation may also occur, especially when oxytocin is given rapidly in a concentrated solution used in combination with a general anesthetic such as cyclopropane. The vasopressor effect of oxytocin administered during the treatment for postpartum hemorrhage is mild, and any hypertension is usually mild and transient.

Natural and synthetic oxytocin is structurally similar to antidiuretic hormone (ADH), and fluid reabsorption from the glomerular filtrate may cause fluid retention (Fig. 13–2). To avoid this, large quantities of IV solutions are not to be infused with high concentrations of oxytocin. The infusion of 20 mU/min may lead to a decrease in urine output, while 40 mU/min or more of oxytocin with excessive nonelectrolyte fluid infusion has led to fluid overload and convulsions or coma.[12] The antidiuretic effect may be observed after the use of 40 units of oxytocin.[13]

TABLE 13–2. INTRAVENOUS INFUSION SCHEDULE OF OXYTOCIN (USING A 10 mcg/LITER SOLUTION MIXTURE)*

Infused Oxytocin (mU/min)[†]	Eyeball (drops/min)	IVAC (drops/min)	IMED (ml/hr)
2	2	2	12
4	4	4	24
6	6	6	36
8	8	8	48
10	10	10	60
12	12	12	72
14	14	14	84
16	16	16	96
18	18	18	108
20	20	20	120

* In the prescribed mixture, 1 drop contains 1 mU of pitocin and 1 ml of solution contains 10 drops or 10 mU of pitocin.
† Oxytocin infusion is routinely begun at 2 mU/min and increased at 2 mU/min increments every 15 to 20 min as necessary. Hyperstimulation and water intoxication are to be avoided, and infusion at 16 mU/min or more is discouraged.

Avoiding a prolonged induction and infusing no more than 1 liter of fluid (10 U oxytocin) should not cause water intoxication. Oral fluids do not contribute to the problem because this is regulated by the patient. Hypoglycemia and decreased circulating triglyceride levels have also been associated with prolonged oxytocin use, although the mechanism is unclear.[14]

Oxytocin does not cross the placenta, so no direct effects on the fetus have been observed. However, uterine hypertonicity from overzealous oxytocin use may lead to variable decelerations of the fetal heart rate and fetal hypoxia. Trauma to the fetal head leading to intracranial hemorrhage is not thought to be associated with cephalopelvic disproportion or oxytocin, rather from forceps. A greater incidence of hyperbilirubinemia has been reported in infants delivered after oxytocin was used during labor.[15] This was found when large amounts of oxytocin had been given and

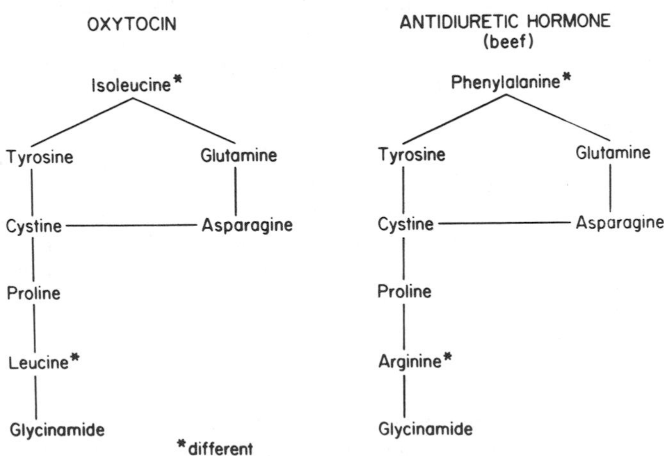

Figure 13–2. Chemical structures of oxytocin and antidiuretic hormone.

may have resulted from fetal hemorrhage during the birthing process rather than directly from the drug. This risk of hyperbilirubinemia has also been refuted recently.

Breastfeeding may begin despite oxytocin administration, since little of the drug crosses into breast milk.

ERGOT ALKALOIDS

The earliest report of ergot alkaloid use for uterine stimulation was in the 1582 *Kreuterbuch* by Adam Lonicer. In the 1700s, the grain source of this stimulant was identified, and by the early 1800s, John Stearns introduced ergot into obstetric practice. It was not until the beginning of the 1950s that the contractile properties of the ergots became well understood. Work on the purification of these compounds and advancements in receptor pharmacology have resulted in the practical use of the ergots for uterine stimulation.

Pharmacology

The natural ergot alkaloids are derived from a fungus (*Claviceps purpurea*) which is grown commercially. The semisynthetic derivatives contain a chemical modification which causes more specific actions with fewer side effects. The ergots affect many organ systems, particularly the cardiac, nervous, and uterine organs. The mechanism of action is by direct smooth-muscle cell receptor stimulation. The uterus is very sensitive to ergot stimulation, and powerful contractions may persist for hours. Vasoconstriction from direct smooth muscle stimulation is usually observed. The ergot alkaloids are detoxified in the liver and eliminated in the urine.

Most currently used drugs are semisynthetic derivatives of the ergot alkaloids. Each consists of a lysergic acid amide moiety combined with a condensed polypeptide. The amine alkaloids are of particular interest because of their direct stimulation of the uterine smooth muscle.

The uterine response to ergot alkaloid stimulation increases steadily during pregnancy. The characteristic uterine activity pattern in the preterm period consists of frequent, weak contractions with hypertonus, while hypercontractility is more evident at term.[16] During labor, this uncoordinated pattern of uterine activity during ergot administration is more similar to that observed with sparteine sulfate rather than with oxytocin use.[17]

Clinical Uses

Because of the potential for sustained uterine contractions and fetal compromise, which are not pharmacologically reversible, ergot products should not be used during labor.[16] Fetal and maternal injuries and deaths have been reported from such violent uterine contractions.[18] Therefore, ergot preparations are used in obstetrics only to promote uterine involution in the postabortion or postpartum periods. Although not used routinely, ergometrine given intramuscularly provides sustained uterine contractility in combination with the more rapid action of oxytocin.

Preparations and Doses

The two amine alkaloids used for uterine stimulation include ergonovine maleate (Ergotrate) and methylergonovine maleate (Methergine). Both drugs are prepared in tablet or solution forms and, unlike most ergot derivatives, they have the advantage of being well absorbed in the gastrointestinal tract. The 0.2-mg tablets are used three or four times each day for 2 days up to 1 week to diminish bleeding after uterine evacuation. Immediate effects are seen with a 0.2 mg IV infusion given over at least 1 minute or a 0.2-mg IM injection. The onset of action is usually 40 seconds with IV infusion and 7 minutes with IM injection.[3]

Side Effects

Ergonovine and methylergonovine have relatively poor vasoconstrictive properties. Hypertension and signs of cardiac ischemia occur rarely in the postpartum period, but transient elevations in blood pressure may be severe and are most prominent after IV infusion.

Central nervous system effects are variable, but the dramatic results in preventing or treating migraine headaches with certain ergot alkaloids are not seen with ergonovine and methylergonovine. Nausea and vomiting may occur.

Along with serious injuries to the fetus and mother, ergot alkaloids are not to be used for labor induction, since eclampsia and cardiovascular collapse have been reported.[19,20] Pregnancies complicated by hypertension should therefore not receive ergot preparations. In addition, the placenta may become trapped if the ergot is given too early after delivery.

PROSTAGLANDINS

Prostaglandins are the most recent addition to the uterine stimulants. More than 3000 original publications and 10 years of clinical experience have led obstetricians to realize the enormous potential of these compounds on human parturition.

Prostaglandins were first discovered in 1935, when von Euler found substances in seminal fluid which promoted smooth muscle stimulation and relaxation, especially on the uterus.[21] With the recent development of synthetic processes to make prostaglandins, our understanding of their pharmacology and uses has increased greatly. Within the last decade, the Food and Drug Administration has approved the use of prostaglandins for abortion and experimental use during labor.

Pharmacology

Prostaglandins are 20-carbon compounds formed by the action of the enzyme prostaglandin synthetase on the precursor, arachidonic acid (Chap. 26). Enzymes for prostaglandin synthesis are present in most cells, and prostaglandins are formed rapidly in response to physiologic changes. All prostaglandins are structurally similar, and individual variations in chemical structure would explain differing binding characteristics to cell receptors and different effects.

Prostaglandins released from decidual and myometrial cells are thought to act on specific cell receptors to alter or inhibit the action of adenylcyclase, subsequently inhibiting formation of cAMP, the mediator of most hormone action.[22] It is also postulated that calcium release is influenced by these compounds.[4] The observed effects result primarily from changes in smooth muscle tone and modulation of hormonal activity. While their action is influenced by estrogen and progesterone, prostaglandins can effect uterine contractions at any stage of pregnancy.[3] The effect on uterine smooth muscle is not completely specific, and systemic use of these compounds can also overstimulate the gastrointestinal, circulatory, and respiratory tracts. The subsequent degradation of prostaglandins is usually rapid, since many tissues are capable of utilizing and converting these compounds. The metabolites are considered to be biologically inactive.

Preparations

Although many prostaglandins exist, the major types important in reproduction are prostaglandin E_2 (PGE_2) and F_2 (PGF_2). They differ from the parent compound, prostanoic acid, by the substitution at C-9 and C-11 of the cyclopentane ring and the addition of a double bond (Fig 13–3).

PGF_2 (Prostin) is commercially available in 5 mg/ml concentrations in 20- and 40-mg ampules. It is administered by intra-amniotic instillation, rather than by IV or IM routes, since systemic effects are less pronounced. The IM injection of PGF_2 does not offer any advantages over the direct intra-amniotic route.

PGE_2 is prepared in a 20-mg vaginal suppository. Advantages to the suppository preparation are the ability to efface the cervix and the rapid reversal of undesired effects by removal of the suppository.

The relative cost difference between

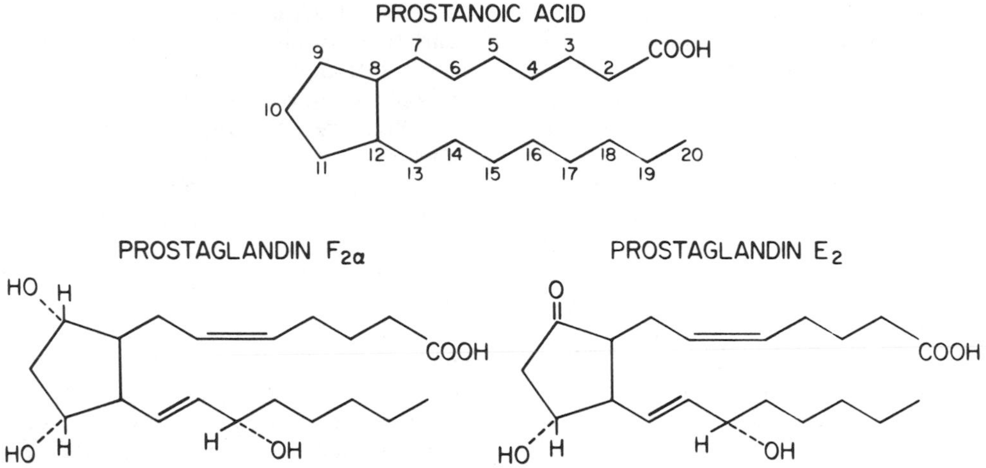

Figure 13–3. Chemical structure of the parent prostaglandin compound (prostanoic acid), prostaglandin $F_{2\alpha}$, and prostaglandin E_2.

PGF_2 and PGE_2 for the desired effect is negligible.

Clinical Uses

Pregnancy Termination

Both PGE_2 and PGF_2 are used only for the stimulation of uterine contractions for pregnancy termination. Their effectiveness during the first trimester and the high incidence of gastrointestinal effects preclude first trimester use. PGF_2 is FDA approved for intra-amniotic instillation in terminating pregnancies from 13 to 20 weeks' gestation. PGE_2 is also marketed for the termination of pregnancies complicated by intrauterine fetal demise, missed abortion (up to 28 weeks), nonmetastatic gestational trophoblastic disease, and therapeutic abortion between the 12th and 27th weeks.[23] The use of prostaglandins for the induction of labor in uncomplicated pregnancies is not recommended until investigations on uterine and fetal effects are better understood and the drugs are proven safe.

Preinduction Cervical Ripening

The unfavorable or unripe cervix is an impediment to the successful induction of labor. Oxytocin administration under such circumstances is largely ineffective, resulting in many induction failures and a high incidence of cesarean section. Certain pregnancy complications such as postdates, hypertension, suspected fetal compromise, and diabetes would indicate the need for a trial of labor.

Various methods have been used to promote cervical ripening before labor or mechanical dilation before surgical termination during the first and second trimesters. Estradiol and laminaria tents have been used with variable success.[24-28] Prostaglandin compounds given vaginally, orally, intravenously, or extra-amniotically have been given on a prospective, randomized basis.[28-40] This drug is not presently licensed for this purpose in the United States and is used on a hospital-approved investigational protocol basis.

The intracervical or vaginal application of a prostaglandin-containing viscous gel has gained the widest interest.[29-40] Cervices so ripened have led to shorter labors, lower cesarean section rates, and more favorable perinatal outcomes. The prostaglandin PGE_2 gel has been prepared by mixing 40 ml of cellulose gel with a thawed out 20-mg PGE suppository (Prostin). The final concentration (2 mg/4 ml) of prostaglandin gel may be stored in a plastic syringe in a refrigerator at −20C.

It has been our practice to examine the patient the afternoon or evening before the scheduled induction. A Bishop's score of 4 or less would qualify that person for the vaginal instillation of the gel. The cervix is wiped clean before gel insertion. She should be placed in a lithotomy position and instructed to remain supine for approximately 15 minutes following infusion of 4 ml of gel into the posterior vaginal fornix or external cervical os. It is our custom for a fetal heart rate monitor to be attached with continuous recordings being carried out for the next 2 hours. Any subsequent uterine contractions should also be monitored.

Our preliminary experience has been the same as others that the PGE_2 vaginal preparation is favorable in changing the Bishop's score, rate of cervical dilation, and percentage of successful inductions compared to no treatment.[41-43] No correlation has been found between drug effectiveness and gravidity, gestational age, and duration of action.[40] The need for oxytocin for induction or augmentation of labor is less.[34,43] Furthermore, the maximum concentration of oxytocin and duration at this concentration is significantly less with preinduction PGE_2 therapy.[34,42] Once the cervix becomes riper, amniotomy is recommended and oxytocin infusion may be started or continued. Uterine pressure monitoring is necessary, although uterine rupture is rare.[44]

PGE_2 has also been applied within the intracervical region. Less drug is required (0.25 mg intracervically versus 2 to 4 mg intravaginally).[29-43] Gastrointestinal side effects and myometrial activity are thought to be less common with intracervical gel application. These findings require further documentation at other hospitals where there are institutional protocols for investigation.

Postpartum Hemorrhage

The use of prostaglandins in the management of postpartum hemorrhage from uterine atony is a logical extension of clinical experiences with prostaglandins in pregnancy termination and term labor induction trials. Approximately 5 percent of all pregnant women are anticipated to undergo severe postpartum hemorrhage which is defined as hemorrhage associated with either an episode of hypotension or blood loss of 1000 ml or more. Those persons who may benefit from prostaglandin therapy have failed to respond to conventional treatment with oxytocin, methylergonovine, uterine massage, and uterine curettage. The possibility of genital tract lacerations and retained placental fragments must also be ruled out.

Although IV infusion or instillation of vaginal PGE_2 suppositories has been described, most reported cases involving successful management of uterine atony has been with IM administration of 15-methyl $PGF_{2\alpha}$.[44-51] Recurrent inversion of the puerperal uterus has also been managed with $PGF_{2\alpha}$ and uterine packing.[52] A 1 ml ampule (1.25 mg) may be injected IM in an open fashion. Up to five repeated injections at intervals of 1.5 hours or longer may be permissible. The $PGF_{2\alpha}$ has also been administered transabdominally directly into the myometrium. Successful control of such hemorrhage has been reported to occur in 86 percent of trials, thereby avoiding surgical therapy. Mild transient side effects such as nausea, vomiting and diarrhea, mild temperature elevation, and headaches have been described infrequently.

Dose and Effectiveness

Before the instillation of intra-amniotic PGF_2, laminaria tents may be used to dilate the cervix. After starting a precautionary IV line, a 5-mg (1-ml) intra-amniotic test dose should be instilled using a 20-gauge spinal needle under local anesthesia to search for any systemic reactions such as dyspnea, tachycardia, nausea, or vomiting. These undesired effects would indicate intravascular injection and are reversed only by discontinuation of the medication and expectant management. In the absence of these effects after 5 minutes, the remaining 35-mg (7-ml) dose is slowly instilled (Table 13–3). If amniocentesis is unsuccessful, the PGF_2 may be administered by an extraovulatory, transcervical route, using an infant feeding tube

TABLE 13-3. AGENTS USED FOR SECOND TRIMESTER PREGNANCY TERMINATION (13-24 weeks)

Agent	Preparation	Dose Regimen	Initiation-to-Abortion Time
Prostaglandin $F_{2\alpha}$	20- and 40-mg ampules (5 mg/ml)	40 mg (8 ml) intra-amniotically every 24 hr	12-19 hr (mean: 17 hr)
Prostaglandin E_2	20-mg vaginal suppository	One suppository every 3-5 hr	10-22 hr (mean: 14 hr)
Hypertonic saline	20% saline solution	200 ml intra-amniotically every 24 hr	16-43 hr (mean: 29 hr)
Urea	40-80-g solution	40 g intra-amniotically every 24 hr	>48 hr

Note: Laminaria tents are useful in dilating the cervix to avoid extensive laceration, and oxytocin may be used to augment uterine contractions and decrease the dose required for each agent.

or pediatric Foley catheter. Strong uterine contractions may become readily apparent. A second dose may be necessary if abortion has not occurred and the membranes remain intact after 24 hours. Oxytocin may also be infused at approximately 40 mU/min for 2 hours after each injection.

If PGE_2 suppositories are to be used, laminaria tents may also be inserted in the cervical canal; premedication using an antinauseant (prochlorperazine 10 mg IM) and an antidiarrheal agent (Lomotil 5 mg orally) is recommended 1 hour before the suppository insertion. A narcotic (Meperidine 50 mg IM) and an antipyretic (acetaminophen 325 mg rectal suppository) are often necessary to relieve pain from the uterine contractions and to control elevated temperatures (38C or more). Hypertonic saline or urea has also been instilled to decrease the likelihood of delivering a viable fetus. In addition, urea (40 mg) instilled with PGF_2 should decrease the necessary effective dose of PGF_2.

The initiation-to-abortion time using PGF_2 or PGE_2 is approximately the same and ranges between 12 and 23 hours (mean: 16 hours) (Table 13-3). The use of laminaria and an increased gestational age are associated with a shorter initiation-to-abortion time.[53-54] Failures are uncommon with either preparation but have been reported to occur in 2 to 8 percent of all cases.[53-54] The risk of failed abortion is greatest among nulliparous patients before 16 weeks' gestation. A dilation and evacuation procedure or a hysterotomy may then be necessary.

Side Effects

Side effects from PGF_2 are similar to those with PGE_2 but may be more prominent. The major complications associated with prostaglandin use involve gastrointestinal complaints which occur in less than half of the patients. Elevated temperatures requiring medication may occur in 29 percent of those patients being treated with PGE_2 suppositories. Perhaps the greatest concern with prostaglandin use is the delivery of a viable fetus, which has been reported to occur in 3 to 4 percent of the PGE_2 group and less than 1 percent of the PGF_2 group.[55]

Absolute contraindications to prostaglandin use include hypersensitivity to the compound acute pelvic inflammatory disease, and asthma. (Table 13-4). Although not absolutely contraindicated, prostaglandins should be used with caution in patients with a history of hypertension, cardiovascular disease, renal disease, peptic ulcer disease, anemia, jaundice, or diabetes. It is necessary that these medical conditions be sufficiently treated before attempting to evacuate the uterus. Prostaglandin E_2 is neither a cerebral

TABLE 13–4. CONDITIONS WHERE PROSTAGLANDINS SHOULD BE USED WITH CAUTION OR ARE CONTRAINDICATED

- Used with caution
  - Asthma
  - Hypertension
  - Cardiovascular disease
  - Renal disease
  - Peptic ulcer disease
  - Anemia
  - Jaundice
  - Diabetes mellitus
  - Seizure disorder
  - Prior uterine surgery
- Contraindications
  - Hypersensitivity
  - Pelvic inflammatory disease
  - Unfavorable fetal position (transverse lie)
  - Placenta previa

irritant nor bronchoconstrictor. If these diseases become manifest, the anticonvulsant or bronchodilator medication is inadequate.

Prostaglandin therapy is not absolutely contraindicated in the presence of a uterine scar. Signs of uterine rupture or extensive cervical tears should be sought when prostaglandins are used on patients who have had uterine surgery or overdistention. Although rare, uterine rupture with PGE_2 has been reported in women with a prior unscarred uterus. Uterine monitoring during labor and exploration of the uterine cavity after delivery are recommended. The patient should also be advised before treatment that uterine emptying is sometimes incomplete and may require curetting.

Systemic effects vary according to the type of prostaglandin and the route of administration. Although nausea, vomiting, diarrhea, and headaches are particularly common, organic causes must be considered.

The use of each prostaglandin has its own special precautions. When using intra-amniotic prostaglandins, care should be taken to avoid intramyometrial (myonecrosis) or IV (systemic reactions) injection. The risk of subsequent endometritis and parametritis is greater with the intra-amniotic instillation of any abortifacient.[55] Uterine exploration after evacuation is routine. The patient should be given a prescription for a 3- to 7-day course of a broad-spectrum antibiotic (doxycycline, tetracycline, ampicillin) following a pharmacologically induced abortion.

The use of PGE_2 suppositories requires careful monitoring of uterine contractions. Placement of an intrauterine pressure catheter may be necessary if intense and sustained contractions are suspected by external monitoring methods. They are active on the myometrium at any stage of pregnancy. Low-dose oxytocin may be used in conjunction. To minimize any risk of a uterine rupture, removal of the suppository and infusion of a β-adrenergic tocolytic drug (Chap. 9) may be necessary.

OTHER UTERINE STIMULANTS

Other uterine stimulants such as urea and hypertonic saline have been used for pregnancy termination. Despite their extensive use in the past, these agents will probably have limited application in the future with the advent of more specific stimulators (prostaglandins).

Hypertonic Saline

This hypertonic solution is assumed to act as an irritant to promote uterine contractions by drawing fluid from the extravascular space. These injections are thought to increase the prostaglandin $F_{2\alpha}$ stimulating action of oxytocin which may be responsible for the enhanced contractile response to the hormone.[56] The procedure is performed for therapeutic abortion, usually between 16 and 22 weeks, or as soon as the uterus is large enough for safe injection. After removing approximately 100 ml of amniotic fluid using a 20-gauge spinal needle under local anesthesia, 200 ml of a 20 percent solution of sodium chloride is instilled over a 10-minute period. If abortion has not occurred and the membranes remain intact at 24 hours, reinstillation is necessary using the same dose.

Advantages of hypertonic saline over other agents would include the greater likelihood of stillbirth, the higher percentage of complete uterine evacuation, and less uterine bleeding.[57,58] The time of the abortion process is not shortened with saline injection, and potential cardiovascular effects may result from the sodium load. A coagulopathy from thromboplastin release into the maternal circulation may occur in less than 1 percent of the cases. When compared to the prostaglandins with or without oxytocin laminaria tents, or urea, intra-amniotic saline was not found to be more effective.[59]

Urea

Urea was originally used as a single agent for intra-amniotic instillation to terminate second trimester pregnancies. Because of its long instillation-to-abortion time (2 to 5 days), urea is instead instilled with PGF_2 (2.5–10 mg), so that less PGF_2 is necessary and the abortion and fetal death processes are accelerated.[60] The usual dose of urea is 40 to 80 g in 35 ml of 5 percent dextrose in water. Like hypertonic saline, a disadvantage of urea instillation is myonecrosis if injection is in the uterine muscle. Other side effects include nausea and vomiting and a transient increase in blood urea nitrogen (BUN) levels.

Dextrose

Large volumes of high-dextrose concentrations (50 percent dextrose in water) have been used as an intra-amniotic agent for pregnancy termination. A long instillation-to-abortion time combined with an increased risk of infection or metabolic problems have curtailed its use.[61]

REFERENCES

1. Dale HH: Some physiologic actions of ergots. J Physiol 34:163, 1906
2. duVigneaud V, Ressler C, Tripett S: The sequence of amino acids in oxytocin, with a proposal for the structure of oxytocin. J Biol Chem 205:949, 1953
3. Rall T, Schleifer L: Oxytocin, prostaglandins, ergot alkaloids, and other agents. In Gilman AF, Goodman LS, Gilman A (eds): The Pharmacological Basis of Therapeutics, ed 6. New York, Macmillan, 1980, pp 935–950
4. Huszar G: Cellular Aspects of Labor. In Premature Labor. Mead Johnson Symposium on Perinatal and Developmental Medicine, no 15. 1980, pp 16–25
5. Tepperman HM, Beydoun SN, Abdul-Karim FW: Drugs affecting myometrial contractility in pregnancy. Clin Obstet Gynecol 20:423, 1977
6. Hendricks CH, Eskes TK, Saameli K: Uterine contractility at delivery and in the puerperium. Am J Obstet Gynecol 83:890, 1962
7. Gibb D, Arulkumaran S, Rathnam S: A comparative study of methods of oxytocin administration for induction of labor. Br J Obstet Gynecol 92:688, 1985
8. Friedman EA: Labor: Clinical Evaluation and Management, ed 2. New York, Appleton-Century-Crofts, 1978, p 336
9. Seitchik J, Castillo M: Oxytocin augmentation of dysfunctional labor: 1. Clinical data. Am J Obstet Gynecol 144:899, 1982
10. Seitchik J, Amico J, Robinson A, et al.: Oxytocin augmentation of dysfunctional labor. Am J Obstet Gynecol 150:225, 1984
11. Hendricks CH, Brenner WE: Cardiovascular effects of oxytocic drugs used postpartum. Am J Obstet Gynecol 108:5, 1970
12. Abdul-Karim R, Assali NS: Renal function in human pregnancy: V. Effects of oxytocin on renal hemodynamics and water and electrolyte excretion. J Lab Clin Med 57:522, 1961
13. Petrie RH: The pharmacology and use of oxytocin. Clin Perinatol 8:35, 1981
14. Burt RL, Leake NH, Dannenburg WN: Effect of synthetic oxytocin on plasma nonesterified fatty acids, triglycerides, and blood glucose. Obstet Gynecol 21:708, 1963
15. D'Souza SW, Black P, MacFarlane T, Richards B: The effect of oxytocin in induced labour on neonatal jaundice. Br J Obstet Gynecol 86:133, 1979
16. Cibils LA, Hendricks CH: Effect of ergot derivatives and sparteine sulfate upon the human uterus. J Reprod Med 3:147, 1969
17. Hendrick CH, Reed DW, Praagh IV, et al.: Effect of sparine sulfate upon uterine activity

in human pregnancy. Am J Obstet Gynecol 91:1, 1965
18. Browning DJ: Serious side effects of ergometrine and its use in routing obstetric practice. Med J Aust 19:741, 1957
19. Berde B: Pharmacology of ergot alkaloids in clinical use. Med J Aust (special Suppl) 11/78:3, 1978
20. Valentine BH, Martin MA, Phillips NV: Collapse during operation following I.V. ergometrine. Br J Anaesth 49:81, 1977
21. Csaky TZ: Cutting's Handbook of Pharmacology: The Actions and Uses of Drugs, ed 6. New York, Appleton-Century-Crofts, 1979, p 338
22. Challis JR: Endocrinology of parturition. In Huszar G: Cellular Aspects of Labor. Mead Johnson symposium on Perinatal and Developmental Medicine, no 15, 1980, pp 8–15
23. Prostin E_2 Vaginal Suppository. The Upjohn Company, October 1977
24. Lackritz R, Gibson M, Frigoletto F: Preinduction use of laminaria for the unripe cervix. Am J Obstet Gynecol 134:349, 1979
25. Brenner W, Zuspan K: Synthetic laminaria for cervical dilation prior to vacuum aspiration in midtrimester pregnancy. Am J Obstet Gynecol 143:475, 1982
26. Kazzi GM, Bottoms SF, Rosen MG: Efficacy and safety of laminaria digitata for preinduction ripening of the cervix. Obstet Gynecol 60:440, 1982
27. Gower RH, Toraya J, Miller JM: Laminaria for preinduction cervical ripening. Obstet Gynecol 60:617, 1982
28. Killick S, Williams C, Elstein M: A comparison of prostaglandin E_2 pessaries and laminaria tents for ripening the cervix before termination of pregnancy. Br J Obstet Gynaecol 93:518, 1983
29. Lauersen NH, Den T, Iliescu C, et al.: Cervical priming prior to dilation and evacuation: A comparison of methods. Am J Obstet Gynecol 144:890, 1982
30. Arias F: Efficacy and safety of low-dose 15-methyl prostaglandin $F_{2\alpha}$ for cervical ripening in the first trimester of pregnancy. Am J Obstet Gynecol 149:100, 1984
31. Troffater K, Bowers D, Galls S, et al.: Preinduction cervical ripening with prostaglandin E_2 (Prepidil) gel. Am J Obstet Gynecol 153:268, 1985
32. Prins RP, Bolton RN, Mark C, et al.: Cervical ripening with intravaginal prostaglandin E_2 gel. Obstet Gynecol 61:459, 1983
33. Edman G, Forman A, Marsal K, et al.: Intravaginal versus intracervical application of prostaglandin E_2 in viscous gel for cervical priming and induction of labor at term in patients with an unfavorable cervical state. Am J Obstet Gynecol 147:657, 1983
34. Jagani N, Schulman H, Fleischer A, et al.: Role of prostaglandin-induced cervical changes in labor induction. Obstet Gynecol 63:225, 1984
35. Neilson DR, Prins RP, Bolton RN, et al.: A comparison of prostaglandin E_2 gel and prostaglandin $F_{2\alpha}$ gel for preinduction cervical ripening. Am J Obstet Gynecol 146:526, 1983
36. Nimrod C, Currie J, Yee J, et al.: Cervical ripening and labor induction with intracervical triacetin base prostaglandin E_2 gel: A placebo-controlled study. Obstet Gynecol 64:476, 1984
37. Hunter I, Cato E Ritchie J: Induction of labor using high-dose or low-dose prostaglandin vaginal pessaries. Obstet Gynecol 63:418, 1984
38. Ulmsten U, Wingerup L, Andersson K: Comparison of prostaglandin E_2 and intravenous oxytocin for induction of labor. Obstet Gynecol 54:581, 1979
39. Lorenz RP, Botti JJ, Chez RA, et al.: Variations of biologic activity of low-dose prostaglandin E_2 on cervical ripening. Obstet Gynecol 64:123, 1984
40. Borten M, DiLeo LA, Friedman EA: Low-dose prostaglandin E_2 analogue for cervical dilation prior to pregnancy termination. Am J Obstet Gynecol 150:561, 1984
41. Buchanan D, Macer J, Yonekura M: Cervical ripening with prostaglandin E_2 vaginal suppositories. Obstet Gynecol 63:659, 1984
42. Lange I, Collister C, Johnson J, et al.: The effect of vaginal prostaglandin E_2 pessaries on induction of labor. Am J Obstet Gynecol 148:621, 1984
43. Macer J, Buchanan D, Yonekura M: Induction of labor with prostaglandin E_2 vaginal suppositories. Obstet Gynecol 63:664, 1984
44. Claman P, Carpenter RJ, Reiter A: Uterine rupture with the use of vaginal prostaglandin E_2 for induction of labor. Am J Obstet Gynecol 150:889, 1984
45. Hertz RH, Sokol RJ, Dierker LJ: Treatment of postpartum uterine atony with prostaglandin E_2 vaginal suppositories. Obstet Gynecol 56:129, 1980
46. Jacobs M, Arias F: Intramyometrial prostaglandin $F_{2\alpha}$ in the treatment of severe postpartum hemorrhage. Obstet Gynecol 55:665, 1980

47. Hayashi RH, Castillo MS, Noah ML: Management of severe postpartum hemorrhage due to uterine atony using an analogue of prostaglandin $F_{2\alpha}$. Obstet Gynecol 58:426, 1981
48. Toppozada M, El-Bossaty M, El-Rahman HA, et al.: Control of intractable atonic postpartum hemorrhage by 15-methyl prostaglandin $F_{2\alpha}$. Obstet Gynecol 58:327, 1981
49. Andrinopoulos GC, Mendenhall HW: Prostaglandin $F_{2\alpha}$ in the management of delayed postpartum hemorrhage. Am J Obstet Gynecol 147:217, 1983
50. Henson G, Gough J, Gillmer M: Control of persistent primary postpartum haemorrhage due to uterine atony with intravenous prostaglandin E_2: Case report. Br J Obstet Gynecol 90:280, 1983
51. Hayashi RH, Castillo MS, Noah ML: Management of severe postpartum hemorrhage with a prostaglandin $F_{2\alpha}$ analogue. Obstet Gynecol 63:806, 1984
52. Heyl PS, Stubblefield PG, Phillippe M: Recurrent inversion of the puerperal uterus managed with 15(s)-15-methyl prostaglandin $F_{2\alpha}$ and uterine packing. Obstet Gynecol 63:263, 1984
53. Grimes DA, CatesW: The comparative efficacy and safety of intraamniotic prostaglandin $F_{2\alpha}$ and hypertonic saline for second-trimester abortion. J Reprod Med 22:248, 1979
54. Methods of Midtrimester Abortion: ACOG Technical Bulletin no 56, Dec 1979
55. Robins J, Surrogo E: Alternatives in midtrimester abortion induction. Obstet Gynecol 56:716, 1980
56. Fuchs A, Rasmussen A, Rehstrom J, et al.: Prostaglandin $F_{2\alpha}$, oxytocin, and uterine activation in hypertonic saline-induced abortions. Am J Obstet Gynecol 150:27, 1984
57. Grimes DA, Cates W Jr: The brief for hypertonic saline. Contemp Obstet Gynecol 15:29, 1980
58. Kerenyi TD, Mandelman N, Sherman DH: Five thousand consecutive saline inductions. Am J Obstet Gynecol 116:593, 1973
59. Binkin N, Schultz K, Grimes D, et al.: Urea-prostaglandin versus hypertonic saline for instillation abortion. Am J Obstet Gynecol 146:947, 1983
60. Burnett L, King T, Atienza M, et al.: Intraamniotic urea as a midtrimester abortifacient: Clinical results and serum and urinary changes. Am J Obstet Gynecol 121:7, 1975
61. Pritchard J, Whalley P: Abortion complicated by *Clostridium perfringens* infection. Am J Obstet Gynecol 111:484, 1971

14

Management of Pain During Labor

Joseph J. Kryc

Relief of pain during labor and delivery has been a topic of interest since the banishment of Adam and Eve from the Garden of Eden. Pain during childbirth was Eve's punishment for her role in the fall of mankind and was to be suffered by all her descendents. In the Middle Ages, any attempts to relieve the pain and suffering associated with childbirth was considered blasphemous by the Church. Despite these prevailing religious attitudes, many psychologic and physical techniques were devised to comfort the patient in labor.

The discovery of nitrous oxide by Joseph Priestley in 1772 marked the introduction of modern analgesia and anesthesia. However, the utilization of these techniques in obstetrics did not occur for approximately 70 years. Ether was first administered in 1847 to a patient in labor by James Y. Simpson, a professor of midwifery at the University of Edinburgh. Because of strong religious teachings, acceptance was delayed until 1853, when Queen Victoria received chloroform analgesia for the birth of her eighth child. Obstetric analgesia and anesthesia have since evolved into a complex science utilizing many pharmacologic agents and anesthetic techniques. Presently the relief of pain during labor may be accomplished by one or more of the following methods: Psychologic preparation, systemic medication, regional analgesia, and inhalation agents (Table 14–1).

Since fear and anxiety can contribute to the pain experienced during labor, recent emphasis has been placed on educating and preparing women for childbirth. Psychologic techniques such as hypnosis, Lamaze, LeBoyer, and acupuncture may result in excellent analgesia in selected patients. These techniques rely on a positive conditioning response to produce analgesia. Although psychoprophylaxis reduces the amount of pharmacologic agents required, between one-third and two-thirds of patients still require supplemental analgesia.[1] Obvious advantages of this technique include an awake patient capable of maintaining laryngeal reflexes and the avoidance of drug depression to the mother and fetus.

TABLE 14–1. ANALGESIC/ANESTHETIC TECHNIQUES USED FOR PAIN RELIEF DURING LABOR

- Psychologic
  - Hypnosis
  - Lamaze—psychoprophylaxis
  - Acupuncture
- Systemic analgesics and sedatives
  - Narcotics
  - Barbiturates
  - Benzodiazepines
  - Phenothiazines
  - Amnesic agents
- Regional anesthesia
  - Minor conduction
    - Local infiltration
    - Paracervical block
    - Pudendal block
  - Major conduction
    - Spinal (subarachnoid) block
    - Lumbar/caudal epidural block
- Inhalation anesthesia
  - Nitrous oxide
  - Halogenated agents

SYSTEMIC ANALGESICS AND SEDATIVES

Systemically administered medications are used frequently to relieve pain and anxiety during labor. Narcotics, sedatives, and tranquilizers are the pharmacologic agents most commonly used. Dissociative and amnesic agents are used less often. There is no ideal drug, and maternal and fetal depression are related to the route of administration, the dose, and the timing of administration during labor of the specific agent as well as any underlying obstetric complication.

Sedatives, hypnotics, and tranquilizers are used during labor to decrease fear and anxiety and to induce sleep. Their differentiation is based on the degree of action, which is generally dose dependent. Tranquilizers produce a decrease in anxiety without a sedative effect. Sedatives relieve tension and anxiety by producing a calmness that allows the patient to fall asleep. Hypnotics are central nervous system (CNS) depressants that enable patients to fall asleep. These agents are all capable of depressing the vasomotor and respiratory centers; however, they have no analgesic activity.

Narcotics

Narcotics are the most widely used systemic medications used to reduce pain during the first and second stages of labor. Many narcotic agents are currently available (Table 14–2), but their pharmacologic properties and observed effects are similar. The exact mechanism by which narcotics exert their effects remains unknown. Highly specific opiate receptors have been identified within the CNS of vertebrates. The receptors are located in the thalamus, hypothalamus, and substantia gelatinosa of the spinal cord. Currently, four specific opiate receptors have been identified: μ (mu), δ (delta), κ (kappa), and σ (sigma). These specific opiate receptor sites are known to have different affinities for various agonists and antagonists. They, therefore, produce different physiologic effects depending upon the agent(s) used.[2] The most studied receptors are the μ (mu) morphine-

TABLE 14–2. CLASSIFICATION OF NARCOTIC DRUGS

- Natural alkaloids
  - Morphine
  - Codeine
- Semisynthetic compounds
  - Diacetyl morphine (Heroin)
  - Dihydromorphinone (Dilaudid)
  - Oxymorphone (Numorphan)
- Synthetic compounds
  - Meperidine derivatives
    - Meperidine (Demerol)
    - Alphaprodine (Nisentil)
  - Methadone and derivatives
  - Fentanyl
  - Pentazocine (Talwin)
- Agonist/antagonist
  - Nalbuphine
  - Pentazozine

preferring and δ (delta) enkephalin-preferring receptors.

The μ receptor produces supraspinal analgesia, euphoria, depression of ventilation, and physical dependence. It is activated by β-endorphin and morphine and antagonized by naloxone and pentazocine (Talwin). The δ receptor apparently modulates μ activity and produces some supraspinal analgesia. Its agonists include β-endorphine and leu-enkephalin. It is antagonized by naloxone and met-enkephalin. The κ receptor produces spinal analgesia, sedation, meiosis, and limited ventilatory depression. It is activated by morphine, nalbuphine, and pentazocine and antagonized by naloxone. The σ receptor produces hallucinations and dysphoria. Its agonists include ketamine and pentazocine and is antagonized by naloxone. Endogenous polypeptides, called endorphins, have been identified as having potent analgesic action.[3] These compounds are capable of modifying pain impulses traveling to the central nervous system and are considered to bind to the opiate receptors.

Maternal Effects

Effects from narcotic use are seen in a variety of organ systems. In small to moderate doses, narcotics produce drowsiness, changes in mood, mental clouding, and analgesia without loss of consciousness. They also raise the pain threshold and dampen pain perception. Large doses cause a greater depression of the central nervous and respiratory systems and may lead to apnea. CNS effects may be potentiated by other depressants and can result in a decrease in all respiratory parameters (respiratory rate, minute volume, tidal volume).

Cardiovascular parameters such as blood pressure, central venous pressure, and cardiac output remain essentially unchanged with usual doses. Slight bradycardia may occur from vagal stimulation with larger doses. Peripheral vasodilation following large-dose administration results from histamine release and can result in orthostatic hypotension.

Narcotics decrease gastric motility and emptying, and may induce nausea and vomiting by stimulating the chemoreceptor trigger zone of the medulla.

The effects of narcotics on uterine contractility during labor are variable and depend on the severity of pain and apprehension, the dose, the route of administration, and the stage or labor. In studies where narcotics have been reported to shorten labor, the major mechanism is related to a decrease in anxiety and pain, rather than to a direct uterine effect.[4,5] Narcotics may actually prolong labor and impair the mother's ability to voluntarily assist in the delivery.

Fetal and Neonatal Effects

All narcotics are capable of easily crossing the placenta. CNS depression of the fetus is a major concern, since respiratory efforts and neurobehavioral adjustments may be delayed.[6,7] These effects have been studied most extensively using meperidine. Decreased beat-to-beat variability of the fetal heart rate, decreased respiratory motion, and altered electroencephalograms in the fetus have been reported. It is postulated that intravenous (IV) injection during a uterine contraction will slow narcotic transfer to the fetus. Theoretically, blood flow through the placental bed is slowed, thereby allowing the bolus of medication to bypass this area.

Neonatal respiratory depression is uncommon and usually mild and transient. Its presence and severity are related to the dose, the time from administration to delivery, and the use of other depressant agents (e.g., barbiturates).[6] The risk of neonatal depression after intramuscular (IM) meperidine is not great if delivery occurs within 1 hour of administration. If delivery occurs 2 to 3 hours after administration, the incidence of neonatal depression is increased. The reason for this delay is uncertain, but may be due to an active metabolite unique to meperidine.[8] The metabolites show a slow rise in serum levels with gradual elimination that may be as long as 3 to 6 days. Meperidine metabolites include normeperidine, meperidinic acid, and normeperidinic acid. Normeperidine is an active metabolite and has been implicated as the agent causing neurobehavioral or respiratory depression in the neonate for up to 48 to 72 hours after delivery. Naloxone (Narcan) may be given to the infant to reverse any depression from narcotic use (Chap. 15).

Selecting the Proper Narcotic

The selection of an appropriate narcotic is dependent upon the effects desired. The various narcotics differ with respect to the dosage range, onset of action, duration of action, and side effects (Table 14–3). Meperidine (Demerol) is the most widely accepted narcotic for pain relief during labor and delivery. Other narcotics seem to offer no distinct advantage, and neonatal depression may be greater.[9]

Morphine is the most important alkaloid extracted from opium and represents the parent compound of the narcotic analgesics. Like meperidine, it is absorbed rapidly after IV or IM administration. Biotransformation in the liver is by oxidation and conjugation with glucuronic acid. The conjugated compound is then excreted into the urine. Morphine provides no better analgesic effect than equipotent doses of meperidine and may have more of a respiratory depressent effect on the fetus.[10]

Pentazocine (Talwin) is a weak synthetic analgesic agent that has not been used extensively in labor. It does not seem to have any advantages when compared to meperidine, except for a slight decrease in the incidence of nausea and vomiting. When given in large doses (60 mg or more), pentazocine has been associated with hallucinations and nightmares.[11] Narcotic antagonist properties make this agent dangerous in the narcotic-

TABLE 14–3. COMPARATIVE EFFECTIVENESS OF NARCOTIC ANALGESICS

	70–90% Relief of Pain with Sedation and Euphoria				
Efficacy	***Morphine***	***Meperidine (Demerol)***	***Alphaprodine (Nisentil)***	***Pentazocine (Talwin)***	***Fentanyl (Sublimaze)***
Obstetric					
Dosage IM (mg)	5–10	50–100	30–40	20–30	50–100 mcg
IV (mg)	2–5	25–50	10–20	10–20	25–50 mcg
Onset of action					
IM (min)	10–20	10–20	10–20	5–20	7–8
IV (min)	3–5	3–5	3–5	2–3	Immediate
Duration of action					
IM (hr)	2–4	2–3	1½–2	3–4	1–2
IV (hr)	1–2	1½–2	1½–2	2–3	½–1
Side effects Maternal	—Large doses–Orthostatic, hypotension, respiratory depression, nausea and vomiting, delayed gastric emptying, histamine release with morphine			—Minimal cardiovascular effects —Minimal nausea and vomiting —Psychotropic effects with pentazocine	
Fetal	Mild to marked depression dependent upon dosage. Neurobehavioral effects of up to 72 hr				
Placental transfer	Rapid for all narcotic agents				
Active metabolites	No	Yes (normeperidine)	No	No	No

dependent mother. Alphaprodine (Nisentil) is a synthetic narcotic with a rapid onset and short duration of action, which makes this a popular drug. It may also be given subcutaneously. In equianalgesic doses, there seems to be no advantage of alphaprodine over meperidine. Respiratory arrest and fetal sinusoidal heart rate patterns have been associated with alphaprodine use.[12]

Fentanyl (Sublimaze) is a relatively new synthetic narcotic agent that is extremely potent, with a rapid onset and a short duration of action. Respiratory depression has been reported to outlast its analgesic properties, so its use during labor has been very limited.[13]

Agonist/antagonists are agents that are capable of producing agonist activity similar to other classic narcotics, yet, at the same time, are capable of demonstrating antagonist activity. Nalbuphine is one such agent, demonstrating activity at both the μ- and κ-receptors. On a weight basis, nalbuphine is equal to or slightly more potent than morphine in analgesic activity. It is also capable of reversing mild to moderate amounts of morphine-induced respiratory depression without reversing the analgesic properties.[14,15] It does, however, produce a more marked sedation effect. Nalbuphine and other agonist/antagonist agents have not been adequately evaluated in the pregnant patient to date. Recommendations concerning their use is therefore limited.

Barbiturates

Barbiturates are sedative-hypnotics; these are no longer popularly used during labor. Their primary indication is for sedation during the early stages of labor. The four major groups of barbiturates have the same pyrimidine derivation, and an intimate relation exists between their structures and activities.

Pharmacology

In sedative and hypnotic doses, barbiturates are thought to act by interfering with the transmission of impulses to the cortex at the thalamus and ascending reticular formation. Barbiturates are well absorbed orally and most compounds are biotransformed within the liver and eliminated in the kidneys. With repeated usage, they are capable of inducing liver enzymes.

With standard oral doses, there are minimal cardiovascular effects including a slight decrease in blood pressure and heart rate. The medullary vasomotor center is depressed, but reflexes remain intact. When used as an induction agent for anesthesia, thiopental causes direct myocardial depression in proportion to the concentration and dose used. It is also associated with histamine release and vasodilation, a decrease in cardiac output and cerebral blood flow, and either an increase or no change in heart rate.

Barbiturates may affect the respiratory system by influencing neurogenic, chemical, and hypoxic mechanisms for maintaining breathing.[16] The neurogenic center for breathing is located in the reticular activating system and is important in the normal awake state. Its function is extremely sensitive to the hypnotic effects of barbiturates. The respiratory control center is influenced by cerebral spinal fluid, pH, and $Pa{CO_2}$, and is located in the medulla. The chemical drive for respiration is depressed at about three to four times the usual barbiturate dose. The hypoxic driving mechanism is the least sensitive to barbiturate exposure. Although extreme respiratory depression can occur, barbiturates do not obtund protective reflexes such as laryngeal reflexes.

Preparations

Barbiturates are characterized by their duration of action including ultrashort, short, intermediate, and long acting. The various preparations are described in Table 14–4.

Thiopental sodium (Pentothal) is an ultrashort-acting barbiturate used IV for the induction of anesthesia. The rapid recovery from the original dose is explained by its lipid solubility and redistribution properties. Following a bolus injection of a thiobarbiturate, blood concentrations in richly perfused organs, including the brain, are high. After a

TABLE 14-4. ONSET AND DURATION OF ACTION OF BARBITURATES AFTER IM INJECTION

	Ultrashort	Short	Intermediate	Long
Onset of action	Seconds	Minutes	1 hr	1+ hr
Duration	Minutes	4–8 hr	6–8 hr	10–12 hr
Preparations	Thiopental (Pentathal)	Secobarbital (Seconal) Pentobarbital (Nembutal)	Amobarbital (Amytal)	Phenobarbital (Luminal)

few circulations, it is then redistributed to other areas of the body, such as muscle and adipose tissue, resulting in lower levels in vital organs and a subsequent loss of activity. Although very little drug has been metabolized or excreted during this brief time interval, its clinical action has been terminated because of the lowered plasma concentration.

Secobarbital (Seconal) and pentobarbital (Nembutal) are short-acting agents which provide brief hypnosis and mild sedation. Amobarbital (Amytal) and phenobarbital have longer onsets of action and durations and are therefore not used after the onset of uterine contractions.

Maternal Effects

In the usual prescribed oral doses, barbiturates should have no adverse effects on the mother. They exhibit no known inhibitory effects on uterine tone or contractility. The central nervous system, however, is exquisitely sensitive to these drugs, and depression varies from mild sedation to coma.[16] Effects are dependent on the type of barbiturate, the dose, and the route of administration.[17] Orally administered barbiturates cause drowsiness for a few hours, followed by subtle alterations in mood, impairment of judgment, and diminished fine motor skills for up to 24 hours. Unlike gaseous and volatile anesthetic agents, barbiturates do not obtund pain sensation. With small doses, they increase the reaction to painful stimuli, possibly by depressing some inhibitory pathways in the brain. In larger anesthetic doses, all barbiturates exhibit anticonvulsant activity. Phenobarbital is especially popular in this regard because of its selective anticonvulsant activity without producing anesthesia (Chap. 5). Although overdose during labor is rare, severe respiratory depression may require ventilatory assistance.

Fetal and Neonatal Effects

Barbiturates rapidly cross the placenta. Fetal serum levels of the highly lipid-soluble, short-acting barbiturates approach maternal levels in only a few minutes.[18,19] With excessive use or in high doses, prolonged CNS depression can occur and lead to respiratory depression and neurobehavioral abnormalities during the first 48 hours of life. The neonate's attention span may be shortened and feeding problems may be evident, even with small doses. All these undesired effects may be further accentuated with combined narcotic use during labor.[6] Induction of fetal hepatic microsomal enzymes with these agents has already been discussed in Chapter 1.

Benzodiazepines

The benzodiazepines are tranquilizers which include diazepam (Valium), chlordiazepoxide (Librium), and flurazepam (Dalmane). Their use for relief of maternal anxiety during labor has become less popular and is not considered to be any more effective than barbiturates. Any direct muscle relaxant action is not appreciable during labor. Diazepam has been most widely used and is most effective during the antepartum and intrapartum periods to control seizures from grand mal epilepsy or eclampsia (Chap. 5).

The mechanism of action of benzodiazepines is unknown. Serotonin and catecholamines are not released, and monoamine oxidase inhibitors (MAO) are unaffected. Accumulation may occur, since excretion is usually delayed. Toxic reactions are uncommon but include ataxia, vertigo, syncope, and drowsiness. Hypotension and respiratory depression may occur with rapid IV infusion.

Although the margin of safety is great in the mother, IV diazepam easily crosses the placenta and fetal serum levels may be equal to or greater than the mother's (Chap. 1). Desmethyldiazepam, an active metabolite of diazepam with a biologic half-life of greater than 90 hours, may accumulate and cause CNS toxicity.[20] Acid-base derangements are uncommon with diazepam, however, a loss of variability of the fetal heart rate may be seen in IV doses as small as 5 to 10 mg. In larger doses (30 mg or more), lethargy, poor feeding, and poor temperature control may persist for several days.[21] Diazepam has also been associated with hyperbilirubinemia of the newborn. Sodium benzoate, a buffer of the injectable form, has been implicated as a bilirubin albumin uncoupler, which may cause increased levels of free bilirubin.[22] All of these undesired effects may be compounded further with the administration of a systemic analgesic.

Phenothiazines and Hydroxyzine

The phenothiazines represent a large group of tranquilizers used primarily in treating psychiatric disorders. Their common use during labor has been to control nausea and vomiting, to sedate, and to prolong the effects from narcotics. Phenothiazines are three ringed amino compounds with a basic configuration, shown in Figure 14–1. Substitutions at positions R_1 and R_2 independently alter the pharmacologic activity of these agents. Substitutions at the R_2 position tend to depress motor activity and increase antipsychotic and antiemetic properties. Substitutions at position R_1 result in three major groups: (1) The dimethylamino group, which includes promethazine (Phenergan) and propiomazine (Largon); (2) the piperidine group, which includes thioridazine (Mellaril); and (3) the piperazine group, which includes perphenazine (Trilafon).

The primary mechanism of action of phenothiazines is to inhibit uptake of norepinephrine and 5-OH-tryptophan on the CNS. As a group, they are very similar pharmacologically and therapeutically. Promethazine (Phenergan) 25 mg or propiomazine (Largon) 10 mg are commonly given parenterally with meperidine. They are absorbed well and distributed widely. Biotransformation is within the liver, and excretion in the kidneys or feces is partly as sulfoxide.

Toxic effects using recommended dosages in the mother are quite uncommon. Therapeutic doses usually result in sedation and indifference to surroundings with a concomitant loss of anxiety. For this reason, reduced narcotic doses are usually necessary to relieve pain. Phenothiazines also lower the seizure threshold and should be used with extreme caution in patients with a history of a seizure disorder. Extrapyramidal effects such as parkinsonian movements are prominent and thought to result from a blockage of dopamine receptors in the brain. The phenothiazines in general and chloropromazine (Thorazine) in particular are potent antiemetics and directly inhibit the chemoreceptor trigger zone. The cardiovascular effects of these agents are complex. Direct depression of myocardial contractility and hypotension from α-adrenergic blockade of the blood vessels are possible.

Placental transfer varies between the different groups of phenothiazines but is usually rapid. In recommended doses, promethazine and propiomazine are not responsible for any detrimental effects on the fetus or neonate, even though a loss of fetal heart rate beat-to-beat variability may occur.[23]

The antihistamine hydroxyzine (Atarax, Vistaril) is another rapidly acting, mild sedative. Unlike the barbiturates, its effects are not dose dependent. Along with its antihistamine properties, the use of hydroxyzine during labor is similar to the phenothiazines.

DIMETHYLAMINO GROUP

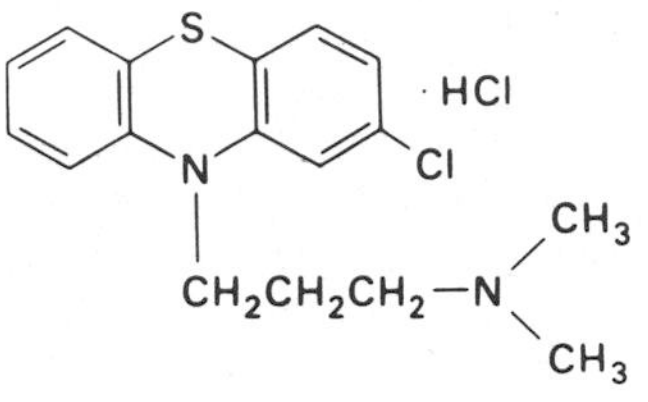

CHLORPROMAZINE (Thorazine)

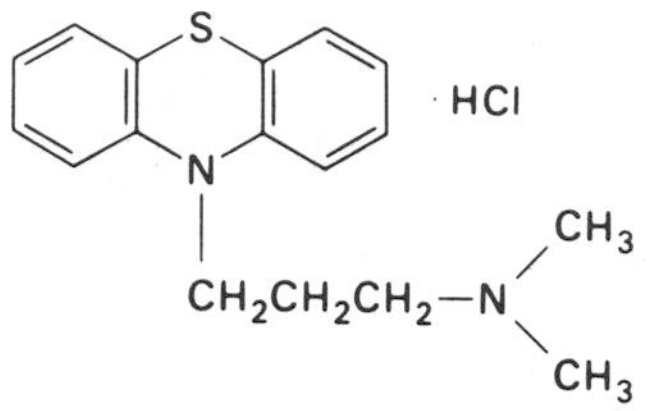

PROMAZINE (Sparine)

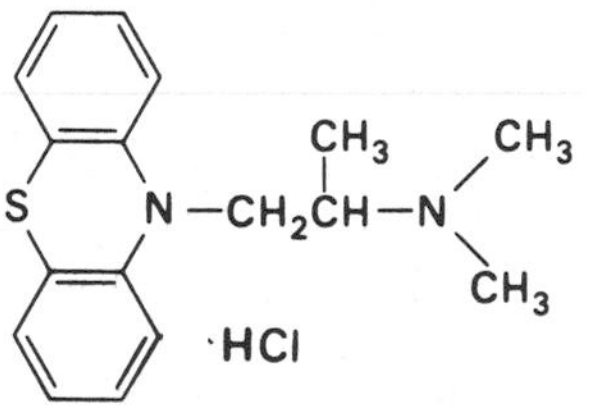

PROMETHAZINE (Phenergan)

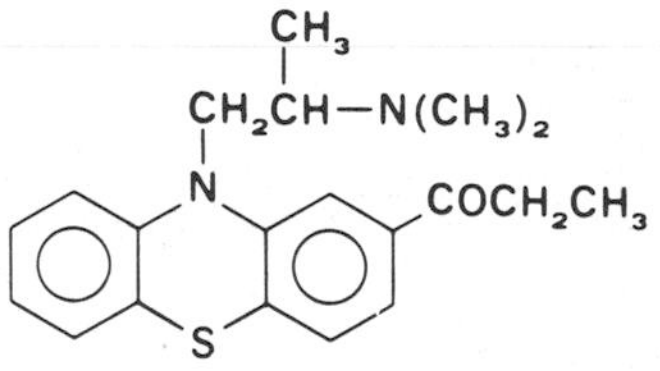

PROPIOMAZINE

PIPERIDINE GROUP

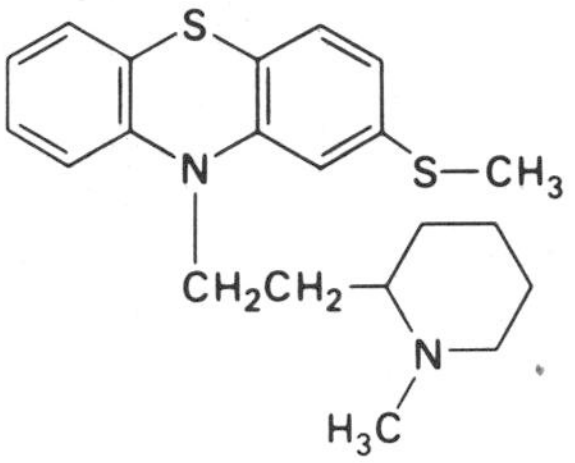

THIORIDAZINE (Mellaril)

PIPERAZINE GROUP

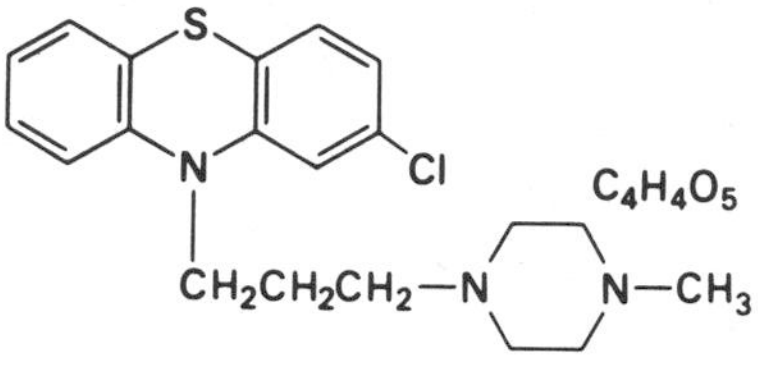

PROCHLORPERAZINE (Compazine)

Figure 14–1. Chemical structure of the phenothiazine drugs. *(From Csáky TZ Barnes BA: Cutting's Handbook of Pharmacology: The Actions and Uses of Drugs, ed. 7. New York, Appleton-Century-Crofts, 1984, pp 374, 677–680, with permission.)*

Hydroxyzine may relieve anxiety and reduce the dose of narcotics needed without increasing the risk of neonatal depression.[24] This drug is very irritating to tissues and should be given by deep IM injection in the buttocks. Intravenous, subcutaneous, or prolonged intravenous injections are not recommended.

Amnesia Drugs

Amnesic or dissociative drugs include ketamine and scopolamine and are no longer popular or recommended for sedation during labor. In low IV doses, these drugs can cause a dream-like state, which is no longer desired by most patients. The analgesic effect of ketamine is not observed with scopolamine, and narcotic supplementation is required. Transient hallucinations and delirium may occur with high or excessive dosages of either agent.

Ketamine (Ketalar, Ketaject)

Ketamine is an IV administered anesthetic which is a cyclohexanone compound similar in structure to phencyclidine (PCP). Intravenous doses of 1 to 2 mg/kg produces anesthetic and sedative effects similar to the ultrashort-acting barbiturates (thiobarbiturates). The mechanism of action is unknown. The onset of action and clearance are usually rapid. Systemic vasopressor effects of ketamine do not apparently reduce uterine blood flow. In the low doses (0.25 to 0.5 mg/kg), uterine contractions are unaffected; however, with doses greater than 0.5 mg/kg, there is an increase in the frequency of contractions.[24] Low-dose ketamine may be administered every 2 to 5 minutes to achieve the desired effect. A total dose of 100 mg over 30 minutes is to be avoided. Placental transfer is rapid, but neonatal depression is seen only after high doses (> 1 mg/kg body weight or > 100 mg total dose). The frequency of low Apgar scores is not significantly greater with low-dose ketamine than with regional, local, or general anesthesia.[25]

Scopolamine (Hyoscine)

Like atropine, scopolamine is a belladonna alkaloid. It acts centrally by inhibiting the uptake of acetylcholine at binding sites on postganglionic receptors. The distribution is wide and may be prolonged, but dangerous toxicity to the mother is very uncommon. After the intravenous administration of 0.3 to 0.6 mg, maternal amnesia occurs and may be intense. Pain suppression and further sedation require the addition of a narcotic to produce "twilight sleep." Physostigmine has been used to reverse sedative and delirium effects from scopolamine. Scopolamine has no apparent effect on uterine contractility and can cross the placenta rapidly. Fetal tachycardia and a loss of beat-to-beat variability may be readily apparent and may last for 60 to 90 minutes.[26] Respiratory depression in the newborn is not common after scopolamine use alone.

LOCAL ANESTHETICS

Regional anesthesia provides a temporary interruption of painful impulses from any portion of the body without a loss of consciousness. Local infiltration and major regional blocks using local anesthetics are used frequently for pain relief during labor and delivery. Local anesthetics are capable of reversibly inhibiting the transmission of impulses in neural tissue. These agents exhibit marked selectivity, since they can inhibit neural transmissions from one part of the body without significantly affecting other areas. This selectivity and the reversibility of action make their use in obstetrics ideal.

Cocaine, the first naturally occurring local anesthetic identified, was isolated from the coca shrub in 1860 by Albert Niemann. It was not utilized as an anesthetic agent for 25 years. Because of extreme toxicity, its clinical usefulness was limited. A search for a less toxic material led to the discovery of procaine in 1904 by Einhorn. This drug remained the cornerstone of local anesthetics for almost 50 years, until Löfgren, a Swedish chemist, discovered the amide local anesthetic, lidocaine, in 1948. This discovery led to the development of other amide agents that are more potent, longer acting, and less toxic.

Physiology of Neural Transmission

Neural tissue has the unique capability of transferring messages in the form of electrical potentials from one area of the body to another. These electrical potentials are initiated by mechanical, electrical, or thermal stimuli. Each nerve cell or neuron consists of a cell body, axon, and multiple dendrite extensions. The axon or nerve fiber is a cylinder of axoplasm which is encased in a semipermeable membrane. (A diagram of the nerve fiber membrane is shown later in Figure 14–2.) The membrane consists of a double-thickness layer of phospholipid molecules. This structure is thinly covered by inner and outer layers of protein. A larger portion of the protein molecule is distributed in the bimolecular phospholipid layer, giving rise to a mosaic-type pattern on the surface. The nerve membrane also contains small channels which connect the extracellular and intracellular spaces. These channels vary in size and are

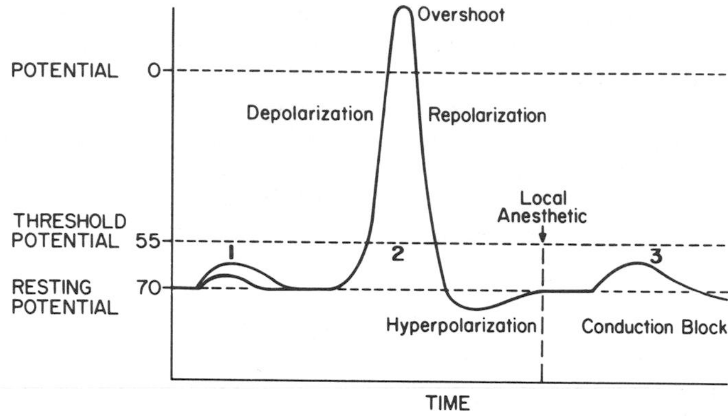

Figure 14–2. Electrochemical events in nerve cell stimulation: (1) subthreshold stimulus—no action potential generated, (2) threshold stimulus—action potential generated, (3) effect of local anesthetic—no action potential generated.

selective for either sodium or potassium. Located on the internal portion of the channel are voltage-dependent "gates" which open and close to either block or allow ionic migration (Fig. 14–3I). The ionic separation created by the semipermeability of the membrane gives rise to an electrochemical gradient known as the resting membrane potential. At rest, the sodium channel is relatively impermeable to the passage of sodium ions. The potassium channel is considerably more permeable, allowing the easy passage of potassium between the extracellular and intracellular spaces. During the resting state, a small amount of ionic leakage occurs which allows sodium to enter and potassium to exit from the cell. Since potassium is more permeable, it flows out of the cell leaving larger, negatively charged ions behind. These negative ions impart a net negative charge to the interior of the cell and eventually halt the outward flow of potassium. In an effort to maintain this electrochemical gradient, sodium is also transported out of the cell by an energy-dependent system known as the sodium-potassium pump.

When a stimulus is applied to the nerve, the generated electrical field causes the gates in the sodium and potassium channels to open. This results in an inward surge of sodium ions with a change in electrical potential (Fig. 14–3II). If the stimulus is weak, only a few gates will open, and the sodium will be quickly pumped out of the cell. With a larger stimulus, many gates are opened, and a threshold is eventually reached where sodium influx matches sodium efflux (firing threshold). When this is reached, depolarization and sodium influx occur at an extremely rapid rate (see Fig. 14–2). For a short period, the interior of the cell is more positive than the exterior of the cell, until potassium efflux begins. This process of depolarization gives rise to an impulse or action potential and is rapidly followed by repolarization of the nerve membrane. During repolarization, the sodium channels close, and sodium is actively pumped out of the cell to reestablish the original resting membrane potential. If the process of depolarization is interrupted along the axon, an impulse cannot be transmitted and the nerve becomes blocked.

Many nerve fibers are surrounded by a fatty material known as myelin. The myelin sheath is interrupted at regular intervals by gaps, known as nodes of Ranvier, at which a small portion of the nerve membrane is exposed to the surrounding medium. The myelin sheath acts as an electrical insulator which enables the nerve to conduct an impulse at a faster rate than an unmyelinated nerve of comparable width.

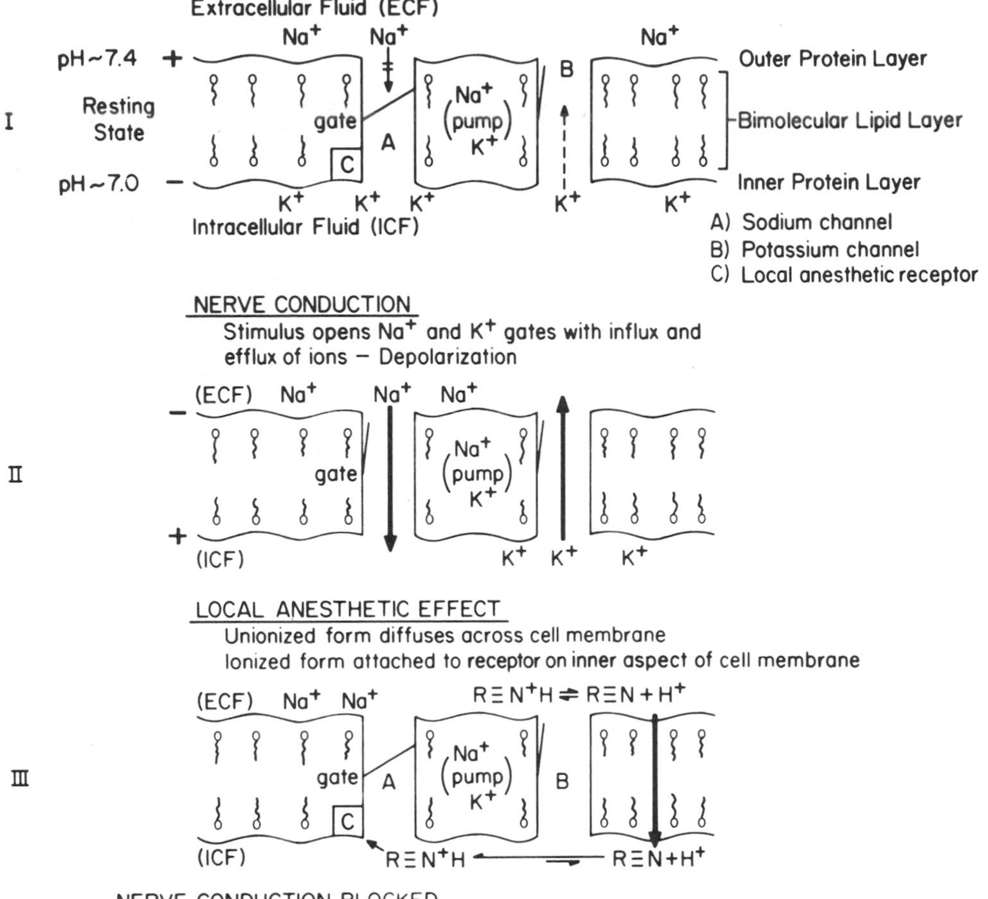

Figure 14–3. Local anesthetic effect on nerve fiber membrane function.

Mechanism of Action

Local anesthetics are thought to obstruct the inward surge of sodium ions associated with depolarization.[27] When a local anesthetic is applied to a nerve, impulse conduction occurs gradually to progressively lower the height of the action potential, reduce its rate of rise, elevate the threshold level, and eventually block conduction.

There is no change in the resting potential. Local anesthetics therefore prevent depolarization. The site of action of local anesthetic agents is the internal surface of the cell membrane at a receptor site located on the opening of the sodium channel (see Fig. 14–3III). Some binding also occurs at the potassium channel, but the receptor-binding affinity is much less.

Although it is generally agreed that local anesthetics bind to receptor sites, the mechanism for impulse blockade remains controversial.[28] One potential mechanism of action involves a change in the surface charge of the sodium channel which prevents the sodium ion from entering the channel. A second mechanism may involve membrane expansion to decrease the size of the sodium channel.

Sensitivity to local anesthetics is also influenced by fiber width and myelin thickness. The wider and more myelinated the nerve, the more excitable and rapidly it conducts an impulse. Small, thin, unmyelinated nerves which transmit pain, temperature, and autonomic effects are slowly conducting and not easily excitable.

The minimum anesthetic concentration (C_M) is the lowest concentration of an anesthetic agent necessary to cause an impulse blockade within a specified time.[28] A nerve will not be solidly blocked until this concentration is reached. Each local anesthetic agent has its own C_M. Nerve fibers also have different C_M's, based on their size and amount of myelin present. Thin, unmyelinated nerves which transmit pain are adequately blocked, while thicker, myelinated fibers transmitting motor or touch remain unblocked. This selectivity or differential nerve block is clinically important, since motor function, touch, and pressure sensation may remain intact during regional anesthesia even though pain has been completely abolished.

Preparations

Local anesthetics have pharmacologic properties that are influenced by their structure, pKa, lipid solubility, and protein-binding. Although many agents are commercially available, as a group they are quite similar.

Local anesthetics contain three structural portions: (1) a hydrophilic amino portion, which is almost always a tertiary amine; (2) an intermediate chain, which is either an ester or an amide; and (3) a lipophilic aromatic residue (Fig. 14–4). Based on the type of linkage between the aromatic residue and the intermediate chain, the local anesthetics can be classified as either esters or amides. Changes in any portion of the molecule result in a change in anesthetic properties.

Amides and esters are biotransformed differently.[28] The ester agents are metabolized by plasma pseudocholinesterase, while the amide agents are metabolized in the liver. The amide agents therefore have a longer half-life than the esters.

Although local anesthetics can be classified as either esters or amides, each possesses a substituted amine group and therefore is considered to be a weak base. In the free-base form these local anesthetics are unstable and only slightly soluble in water. Therefore, to confer stability to the parent compounds and to generate water-soluble drugs suitable for injection, the local anesthetics such as amine hydrochloride salts are generally used. When salts are formed, an uncharged tertiary amine is converted to a quaternary ammonium salt:

$$\text{(1) Local anesthetic}-\underset{\text{(weak base)}}{N\langle} + \underset{\text{(acid)}}{HCl} \longrightarrow \text{local anesthetic}-NH^+Cl^{\ominus}$$

When placed in an aqueous solution, the salt dissociates into a cation and anion:

$$\text{(2) Local anesthetic}-\underset{\text{(salt)}}{NH^+Cl^-} \rightleftharpoons \text{local anesthetic}-\underset{\text{(cation)}}{NH^+} + \underset{\text{(anion)}}{Cl^{\ominus}}$$

and establishes an equilibrium with the unionized base:

$$\text{(3) Local anesthetic}-\underset{\text{(cation)}}{NH^+} \overset{pKa}{\rightleftharpoons} \text{local anesthetic}-\underset{\text{(base)}}{N\langle} + H^+$$

The amount of dissociation is dependent upon the dissociation constant (pK_a) of the cation and on the pH of the solution. When the pK_a of the anesthetic is equal to the pH, there is an equal concentration of ionized and nonionized molecules. As the pH is increased

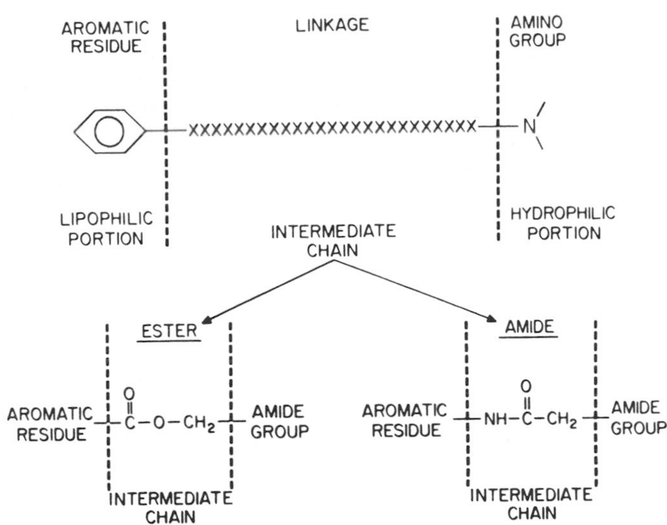

Figure 14–4. Chemical structure of the ester and amide local anesthetics.

(less H^+ available), equation (3) is forced to the right, and a higher concentration of the nonionized drug is apparent. Conversely, as the pH is lowered (more H^+ available), equation (3) is forced to the left, producing a higher concentration of the ionized form.

The site of action of local anesthetics is on the interior of the nerve cell membrane.[27] At this location, the positively charged molecule (cation) is the active form. This ionized molecule is not lipid soluble and as such cannot traverse the cell membrane. It has been demonstrated that a local anesthetic at a nerve exists in both a charged and uncharged form, as described by equation (3). The uncharged form is extremely lipid soluble and diffuses easily through the cell membrane. Since the interior of the cell is slightly more acidic than the exterior, more hydrogen ions are available to interact with this uncharged molecule. This causes the molecule to become charged and "trapped" to bind with a receptor at the opening of the sodium channel.

Following injection of a local anesthetic, its subsequent uptake and distribution is dependent on the site of injection, dosage, agent, and addition of any vasoconstrictor. Table 14–5 lists the local anesthetics in common use in obstetrics. Agents that are highly lipid soluble and not strongly protein bound will be absorbed by the target tissues and removed slowly into the bloodstream. This results in lower blood levels. Vasoconstrictors are also very useful in slowing vascular absorption and prolonging the duration of action. The use of epinephrine may, however, interfere with uterine activity when used with epidural analgesia.[28] Because of the marked amount of vasoconstriction produced by this agent, its use with paracervical block is contraindicated.

The distribution of local anesthetics occurs in two phases. The first or α-phase is very rapid (less than 1 hour) and relates to the rapid redistribution of the anesthetic agent throughout the body. The second or β-phase is much slower (several hours) and relates to metabolism and excretion of the drug.

Bupivacaine is the preferred local anesthetic of choice for obstetric anesthesia. Its onset of action is reasonably rapid, and the duration of action is long (3 to 5 hours). Because of its high pK_a (8.1) and its high protein-binding property (95 percent protein bound), bupivacaine is less likely to cross the placental barrier and affect the fetus (Table 14–5). Both xylocaine and carbocaine have rapid onsets of action, but each is only 50 to 70 percent protein bound and has a lower pK_a. There-

TABLE 14–5. THERAPEUTIC PROPERTIES OF LOCAL ANESTHETICS

Agent	Concentrations (%)	Class	pK[a]	Relative Potency	Maximum Dose (mg)	Duration (min)
I. Low potency, Short duration						
Procaine (Novacaine)	1.0–2.0	Ester	8.9	1	1000	45–90
Chloroprocaine (Nesacaine)	2.0–3.0	Ester	8.9	1	1000	45–69
II. Intermediate Potency, Intermediate Duration						
Mepivacaine (Carbocaine)	1.0–2.0	Amide	7.6	2	500	120–140
Lidocaine (Xylocaine)	1.0–2.0	Amide	7.9	2	500	90–200
III. High potency, Long duration						
Tetracaine (Pontocaine)	0.15–0.25	Ester	8.5	8	200	180–600
Bupivacaine (Marcaine)	0.25–0.75	Amide	8.1	8	300	180–600
Etidocaine (Duranest)	0.5–1.5	Amide	7.7	6	300	180–600

fore, fetal effects are more apparent than with bupivacaine and may last up to 24 to 48 hours after delivery.[29]

Chloroprocaine (Nesacaine) has until recently been widely popular in obstetric units. It represents the "ideal" agent for use in obstetric conditions because of its rapid onset and short duration. Since it is an ester compound which is metabolized by plasma pseudocholinesterase, the effective half-life in the fetus is 45 seconds. Recently, choloroprocaine has been associated with prolonged neural blockade and adhesive arachnoiditis with inadvertent subarachnoid injections of large volumes. Neural toxicity is believed to be related to sodium bisulfite which is employed as an antioxidant in the chloroprocaine solution. If an inadvertant subarachnoid injection of chloroprocaine occurs, current recommendations are to aspirate at least 10 ml of cerebral spinal fluid and, if possible, irrigate the subarachnoid space with preservative-free lactated Ringer's or normal saline.[30,31]

Etidocaine is a new amide agent very similar to bupivacaine. It is much more lipid soluble and approximately equal in protein binding to bupivacaine. However, etidocaine use for regional anesthesia is associated with more pronounced and prolonged muscle relaxation than analgesia.[32] This can interfere with the patient's ability to bear down and the dynamics of the second stage of labor, making it a less than ideal agent for use in obstetrics.

Maternal Effects

Since local anesthetics block conduction of nerve impulses, they may interfere with any organ where impulse transmission occurs. Effects on the central nervous and cardiovascular systems are particularly noteworthy. When local anesthetics are absorbed systemically, they can easily cross the blood–brain barrier. Toxic levels produce central nervous stimulation followed by marked depression or coma. Circulatory support and assisted ventilation may be necessary. Other signs of local anesthetic toxicity include tinnitus, drowsiness, slurred speech, tremors, and convulsions. Respiratory arrest can also occur with large doses. The apparent stimulation and subsequent CNS depression observed is related to the extreme sensitivity of inhibitory cortical neurons to local anesthetics. With inhibitory pathways blocked, excitatory neuronal pathways are unopposed, and excitation and convulsions may occur. As the local anesthetic concentration increases, the excitatory pathways also become blocked.

CNS toxicity usually follows inadvertent intravascular injection and is dependent on the potency of the agent being used (see Table 14–5). The susceptibility of the brain can be altered by the prophylactic administration of benzodiazepines or barbiturates. Neither sedative is routinely used in obstetric practice, so meticulous technique should be used to prevent an intravascular injection of a local anesthetic.

Local anesthetics may affect the cardiovascular system by acting directly on the heart and peripheral vasculature and indirectly on sympathetic blockade. When applied directly to the myocardium, local anesthetics decrease the electrical excitability, the rate of conduction, and the force of contractility.

In 1973, isolated reports of cardiac arrest requiring prolonged resuscitative efforts appeared in the literature. These reports involved obstetric patients who had received 0.75 percent bupivacaine for epidural anesthesia and had experienced an intravascular injection. It was speculated by a few that the longer acting local anesthetics, such as bupivacaine and etidocaine, were relatively more cardiotoxic than the shorter acting local anesthetics, such as lidocaine. Recent studies in sheep and rabbits indicate that this is indeed true. The most likely mechanism for bupivacaine cardiotoxicity relates to its actions on the cardiac sodium channels. Although lidocaine and bupivacaine both produce a fast block of the cardiac sodium channels, it has been found that recovery is approximately five times longer with bupivacaine. Cardiac toxicity, therefore, is approximately 16 times greater for bupivacaine as compared to lidocaine.

Correct administration requires meticulous care to avoid IV injections. Small fractionated doses should be given rather than rapid bolus injections if used in epidurals.[30,31] Vasodilation is seen when an anesthetic is injected into peripheral vessels, including the pudendal artery. However, when injected into the uterine artery, intense vasospasm which is dose dependent occurs.[33]

Allergic reactions to local anesthetics are uncommon. Localized edema, urticaria, and pruritis are related to breakdown products of metabolized esters and should be treated with antihistamines. Anaphylactic reactions are rare and require epinephrine injection and supportive care. Allergic reactions rarely occur with amide use. Most allergic phenomena are associated with para-amino benzoic acid (PABA), the metabolic byproduct of the ester-type local anesthetics.

Fetal Effects

Direct fetal effects may occur following the injection of a local anesthetic in a highly vascular space (epidural, pudendal, paracervical) and may result in significant maternal serum concentrations. Despite metabolism in the liver and elimination in the kidneys, local anesthetics may reach the intervillous space. Their ability to cross the lipid placental membrane is related to the drug's chemical properties (Chap. 1). Since fetal blood is more acidic than maternal blood, local anesthetics become ionized and therefore "trapped" in the fetal circulation. This "trapping" phenomenon is more pronounced in the presence of fetal acidosis. The binding of these drugs to fetal protein is not well understood, but fetal tissue affinity for local anesthetics is high. The fetus is capable of detoxifying local anesthetics by hepatic microsomes, but not to the extent of the maternal counterpart.

Indirect fetal effects of these agents are produced by alterations of maternal homeostasis that secondarily involve the fetus. This includes alterations in uterine blood flow, caused by their direct action on the uterine arteries and myometrium, and maternal hypotension secondary to autonomic blockade.[34]

Despite the possibility of adversely affecting the maternal–fetal unit, the local anesthetics have been used extensively and safely in obstetrics. The route of administration and the specific agent used is extremely important. Paracervical blocks pose a greater threat to the fetus than do either epidural or subarachnoid blocks. The incidence of significant fetal bradycardia with paracervical blocks varies from 25 to 75 percent. Lidocaine and mepivacaine tend to produce fetal bradycardia more frequently than bupivacaine, but bupivacaine can produce fetal bradycardias of extremely long duration (90 minutes to 2 hours).[35] These effects are not dependent on the concentration of the anesthetic used.

No fetal deaths have been reported when epidural anesthesia has been used. However, certain agents may cause neonatal depression, which principally involves transient motor retardation that is not reversed with any drug.[36] Lidocaine and mepivacaine are more likely to cause these transient effects because of their described chemical properties. Bupivacaine produces fewer, if any, of these transient effects.

INHALATION AGENTS

Inhalation agents are occasionally used for pain relief during labor, even though their popularity has declined in recent years. With close supervision, analgesia may be obtained in subanesthetic doses, so that the patient will remain conscious and cooperative. In higher concentrations, delirium and a progressive loss of vital function may become apparent. Inhalation agents may also be used when uterine relaxation is necessary. Conditions requiring uterine relaxation would include delivery of a second twin (intrauterine manipulation), manual removal of an adherent placenta, or replacement of an inverted uterus.

All inhalation agents are inspired and absorbed as gases, metabolized to some degree and eliminated in the lungs and kidneys. Their mechanisms of action remain unclear.

The risks of inhalation agents used during labor and delivery are several. In anesthetic doses, respiratory depression to the mother may cause inadequate oxygenation, loss of laryngeal reflexes, and aspiration of gastric contents. Halogenated agents produce uterine relaxation, which is dose dependent, and may increase uterine bleeding. All inhalational agents rapidly cross the placental barrier, and cause a transient depression of the fetal central nervous, cardiovascular, and respiratory systems. This depression is directly proportional to the duration and depth of maternal anesthesia, since fetal concentrations rapidly approach the mother's as the anesthetic is continued. The properties of each agent are discussed in the sections which follow. A comparison of their effects is given in Table 14–6. Techniques used for administration of these agents must be performed by qualified personnel and are described in several standard anesthesiology texts.[37]

Nitrous Oxide

Nitrous oxide is the most commonly used inhalation agent for analgesia because of its relative safety, rapid onset, and short duration of activity. It is an inert, colorless gas which is nonflammable and stored in a tank as a liquid. It is relatively nonirritating, nontoxic, and rapidly reversible. Concentrations may vary up to 70 percent, but inhalation of 50 percent nitrous oxide with 50 percent oxygen is standard. At this concentration, maternal or fetal depression is unlikely.[38] Analgesic effects are obtained with intermittent use prior to the onset of each contraction or with continuous use during labor. Continuous analgesia is often more reliable, since the onset

TABLE 14-6. COMPARATIVE EFFECTS OF INHALATION AGENTS

Agent	Analgesia (Subanesthetic Dose)	Uterine Relaxation	Neonatal Depression	Toxicity
Nitrous oxide	+++	—	±	Cardiac (if heart disorder), nausea, leukocyte suppression
Methoxyflurane	+++	±	±	Cardiodepression, hypotension, hepatotoxicity, nephrotoxicity
Halothane	—	+++	++	Cardiodepression, hypotension, hepatotoxicity
Enflurane	—	+++	++	Cardiodepression, hypotension, hepatotoxicity
Isoflurane	—	+++	++	Cardiodepression, hypotension, hepatotoxicity

+++ = pronounced effect; ± = negligible effect; ++ = moderate effect.

of uterine contractions may be unpredictable. The self-administration of 50 percent nitrous oxide with 50 percent oxygen (Nitronox) has been used successfully during the late first stage and the second stage of labor.

Methoxyflurane (Penthrane)

Methoxyflurane is a potent inhalation agent which is an effective analgesic in subanesthetic doses. It is a halogenated (F and Cl) methylethyl ether and is nonexplosive. A concentration of 0.35 percent administered intermittently is ideal. The analgesic effect is comparable to nitrous oxide, and the two agents have been used in combinations of lesser concentrations to produce a greater analgesic effect.[39]

Renal effects from methoxyflurane may be a concern. Its metabolic products, inorganic fluoride and oxalic acid, may be associated with subclinical renal toxicity with an increase in blood urea nitrogen (BUN), creatinine, and uric acid values during 48 hours after delivery.[40] Serum inorganic fluoride levels have also been increased in the neonate. What effect this may have on the renal and central nervous systems is presently unknown. Methoxyflurane should be avoided if pre-existing renal disease or nephrotoxic drugs are being used.

Halothane (Fluothane)

Halothane is a potent, halogenated anesthetic agent with depressant effects on the respiratory and cardiovascular system. Induction of anesthesia is rapid when inhaled concentrations of 3 to 4 percent are used. Relaxation of the uterus at these concentrations is extremely rapid, but analgesia is obtained only in anesthetic doses.[41] Because of its associated hepatic toxicity, halothane is not recommended in patients with hepatic dysfunction.

Other Agents

Enflurane and Isoflurane are other halogenated inhalational agents. Their use for pain relief during labor is very limited, since their properties are similar to halothane (myometrial depression, hypotension, myocardial depression, analgesia in anesthetic doses).

INTRATHECAL AND EPIDURAL OPIOIDS

New approaches to pain relief in the obstetric patient were heralded by Wang and associates in 1979, with their report of the use of intrathecal opioids in man.[42] The major obstetric advantages of selectively blocking the transmission of pain impulses by spinal opioids included the possibility of good analgesia with minimal amounts of drug, an absence of sympathetic blockade with associated hypotension, and the avoidance of cardiovascular and neurologic complications inherent with the use of local anesthetics.[43] This selective blockade, accompanied by a long duration of analgesia following spinal administration of opioids, has, however, been tempered by incomplete analgesia during the second stage of labor and a host of side effects of which late respiratory depression is the most serious.

The physiochemical properties and actions of spinal opioids are similar to those of the local anesthetics. The opioids have similar molecular weights and pK_a's and considerable overlap of partition coefficients when compared to local anesthetics. Onset of action and duration of action are dependent upon lipid solubility and the degree of ionization at physiologic pH, which is also similar to the local anesthetic agents.[43]

Meperidine, fentanyl, and lofentanil (phenylpiperidine derivatives) are structurally similar to local anesthetics. Therefore, the rate of absorption and onset of action is comparable to that of lidocaine. Meperidine in high concentrations is also capable of producing a profound peripheral nerve block.[44] In contrast, morphine is much less lipid soluble and chemically has a higher degree of water solubility than the other opioids. This results in a slow efflux from the spinal cord and allows for greater migration of the molecule in the spinal fluid to the brain. This may explain its greater propensity for respiratory depression when compared to the other opioids.

In contrast to the local anesthetics which act by axonal blockade, the spinal opioids function at both the presynaptic and postsynaptic receptors in the substantia gelatinosa of the dorsal horn of the spinal cord.

Effective analgesia during the first stage of labor can be achieved by either the intrathecal injection of small amounts of morphine (0.25 to 0.5 mg)[45] or the epidural injection of larger amounts of morphine (5 to 10 mg)[46] with more consistent results being achieved with the larger dose. Effective analgesia during the second stage of labor, however, is not satisfactorily achieved with spinal opioids alone.

Although there appears to be no effect on labor and neonatal outcome is good, there are extensive maternal side effects that tend to limit the clinical usefulness of these agents. Recently, Bromage et al.[47] studied the nonrespiratory side effects of epidurally injected morphine and observed the appearance and resolution of these side effects. All subjects tested experienced some degree of one or more of the following complications: generalized pruritis, nausea and vomiting, urinary retention, meiosis, and slight cardiovascular depression.

In an effort to alleviate these annoying side effects, various authors have suggested treatment with benadryl and/or naloxone. This, however, introduces more, not fewer, agents for the obstetric patient and, therefore, defeats the purpose of spinal opioids. Additional efforts are presently focused on the combined use of local anesthetics and opioids administered epidurally to try to achieve prolonged duration and minimal side effects.[48] Neither the ideal agent(s) nor the ideal method of administration has not been adequately identified at this time.

In contrast to their use in the laboring patient, spinal opioids have achieved a great degree of success in the postoperative period. Most of the narcotic agents have been studied and all demonstrate a good level of analgesia in the postoperative patient.

REFERENCES

1. Shnider SM, Levinson G: Psychological anesthesia for obstetrics. In Shnider SM, Levinson G (eds): Anesthesia for Obstetrics. Baltimore, Williams & Wilkins, 1979, p 67
2. Martin WR: History and development of mixed opioid agonists, partial agonists and antagonists. Br J Clin Pharmacol 7:273S, 1979
3. Stoelting RK: Opiate receptors and endor-

phins: Their role in anesthesiology. Anesth Analg 59:874, 1980
4. DeVoe SJ, DeVoe K Jr, Rigsby WC, et al.: Effect of meperidine on uterine contractility. Am J Obstet Gynecol 105:1004, 1969
5. Filler WW Jr, Hall WC, Filler NW: Analgesia in obstetrics. Am J Obstet Gynecol 96:832, 1967
6. Shnider SM, Moya F: Effects of meperidine on the newborn infant. Am J Obstet Gynecol 89:1009, 1964
7. Brackbill Y, Kane J, Manniello RL: Obstetric meperidine usage and assessment of neonatal status. Anesthesiology 40:116, 1974
8. Morrison JC, Whybrew WD, Rosser SI, et al.: Metabolites of meperidine in the fetal and maternal serum. Am J Obstet Gynecol 126:997, 1976
9. Flowers CE: Obstetrical Analgesia and Anesthesia. New York, Harper & Row, 1967, p 76
10. Way WL, Costley EC, Way EL: Respiratory sensitivity of the newborn infant to meperidine and morphine. Clin Pharmacol Ther 6:454, 1965
11. Paddock R, Beer EG, Bellville JW, et al.: Analgesic and side effects of pentazocine and morphine in a large population of postoperative patients. Clin Pharmacol Ther 10:355, 1969
12. Gray JH, Cudmore DW, Luther ER, et al.: Sinusoidal fetal heart rate patterns associated with alphaprodine administration. Obstet Gynecol 52:678, 1978
13. Kaulman RD, Aqleh KQ, Bellville TW: Relative potencies and durations of action with respect to respiratory depression of intravenous meperidine, fentanyl, and alphaprodine in man. J Pharmacol Exp Ther 208:73, 1979
14. DiFazio CA, Moscicki JC, Magruder MR: Anesthetic potency of nalbuphine and interaction with morphine in rats. Anesth Analg 60:629, 1981
15. Magruder, MR, Delaney RD, DeFazio CA: Reversal of narcotic-induced respiratory depression with nalbuphine hydrochloride. Anesthesiol Rev 9:34, 1982
16. Frost E: Update on therapeutic barbiturate coma. Curr Rev Clin Anesthesiol 1:1, 1980
17. Myers R, Meyers S: Use of sedative, analgesic and anesthetic drugs during labor and delivery: Bane or boon. Am J Obstet Gynecol 133:83, 1979
18. Root B, Eichner E, Sunshine I: Blood secobarbital levels and their clinical co-relation in mothers and newborn infants. Am J Obstet Gynecol 81:948, 1961
19. Kosaka Y, Takahashi T, Mark LC: Intravenous thiobarbiturate anesthesia for cesarean section. Anesthesiology 31:849, 1969
20. Cree IE, Meyer J, Hailey DM: Diazepam in labour: Its metabolism and effect on the clinical condition and thermogenesis of the newborn. Br Med J 4:251, 1973
21. Yeh SY, Paul RH, Cordero L, et al.: A study of diazepam during labor. Obstet Gynecol 43:363, 1974
22. Schiff D, Chan G, Stern L: Fixed drug combinations and the displacement of bilirubin from albumin. Pediatrics 48:139, 1971
23. Powe CE, Kiem IM, Fromhagen C, et al.: Propiomazine hydrochloride in obstetrical analgesia. JAMA 181:290, 1962
24. Zsigmond EK, Patterson RL: Double blind evaluation of hydroxyzine hydrochloride in obstetric anesthesia. Anesth Analg 46:275, 1967
25. Downing JW, Mahomedy MC, Jeal DE, et al.: Anaesthesia for caearean section with ketamine. Anaesthesia 31:883, 1976
26. Boehm FH, Smith BE, Egilmez A: Physostigmine's effect on diminished fetal heart rate variability caused by scopolamine. In Abstracts of Scientific Papers. Annual Meeting, Society for Obstetric Anesthesia and Perinatalogy, Philadelphia, 1975, p 18
27. Dejong R: The Neural Target in Local Anesthetics, ed. 2. Springfield, Ill, Thomas, 1977, p 10
28. Covino BG: Pharmacology of local anesthetic agents. Surg Rounds, pp 32–51, July, 1978
29. Brown WU, Bell GC, Jurie AO, et al.: Newborn blood levels of lidocaine and mepivacaine in the first postnatal day following maternal epidural anesthesia. Anesthesiology 42:698, 1975
30. Levenson G: Selecting the agent for regional analgesia and anesthesia in obstetics. Lecture 132. ASA Annual Refresher Course Lectures, 1984
31. Covino B: Toxicity of local anesthetic agents. Lecture 109. ASA Annual Refresher Course Lectures, 1984
32. Phillips G: A double-blind trial of bupivacaine (Marcaine) and etidocaine (Duranest) in extradural block for surgical induction of labour. Br J Anaesth 47:1305, 1975
33. Ralston DH, Shnider SM: The fetal and neonatal effects of regional anesthesia in obstetrics. Anesthesiology 48:34, 1978
34. Usubiaga JE: Neurologic complications follow-

ing epidural analgesia. Int Anesthesiol Clin 13:1, 1975
35. Salts L, Orr M, Walson PD: Local anesthetic agents—pharmacologic basis for use in obstetrics: A review. Anesth Analg 55:829, 1976
36. Tronick E, Wise S, Als H, et al.: Regional obstetrical anesthesia and newborn behavior: Effect over the first ten days of life. Pediatrics 58:94, 1976
37. Shnider SM, Levinson G: Anesthesia for Obstetrics. Baltimore, Williams & Wilkins, 1979
38. Marx GF, Joshi CW, Orkin LR: Placental transmission of nitrous oxide. Anesthesiology 32:429, 1970
39. Jones PL, Rosen M, Mushin WW, et al.: Methoxyflurane and nitrous oxide as obstetric analgesics: II. A comparison by self-administered intermittent inhalation. Br Med J 3:259, 1969
40. Creasser CW, Stoelting RK, Krishna G, et al.: Methoxyflurane metabolism and renal function after methoxyflurane analgesia during labor and delivery. Anesthesiology 41:62, 1974
41. Munson ES, Embro WJ: Enflurane, isoflurane, and halothane and isolated human uterine muscle. Anesthesiology 46:11, 1977
42. Wang JK, Nauss LA, Thomas JE: Pain relief by intrathecally applied morphine in man. Anesthesiology 50:149, 1979
43. Cousins MJ, Mather LE: Intrathecal and epidural administration of opioids. Anesthesiology 61:276, 1984
44. Way, EL: Studies on the local properties of isonipecaine. J Am Pharm Assoc 35:44, 1946
45. Nordberg G, Hedner T, Mellstrand T, et al.: Pharmacokinetic aspects of intrathecal morphine analgesia. Anesthesiology 60:448, 1984
46. Booker PD, Wilkes RG, Bryson THL, et al.: Obstetric pain relief using epidural morphine. Anaesthesia 35:377, 1980
47. Bromage PR, Camporesi EM, et al.: Non-respiratory side effects of epidural morphine. Anesth Analg 61:490, 1982
48. Justins DM, Francis D, Houlton PG, Reynolds F: A controlled trial of extradural fentanyl in labour. Br J Anaesth 54:409, 1982

15

Drug Therapy for Immediate Care of the Newborn

Craig W. Anderson

From the time of conception, the fetus is frequently exposed to drugs and drug metabolites which cross the placenta from the mother. Nearly 95 percent of all babies make the transition from intrauterine to extrauterine life without difficulty. A small percentage may require resuscitation and need certain pharmacologic agents within the first few minutes of life. Regardless of the newborn's condition, routine eye and bleeding prophylaxis should be performed. Thus, from conception to after delivery, the developing fetus and newborn are repeatedly exposed to various pharmacologic agents in the perinatal period. The discussion in this chapter includes those drugs used for both routine care of the newborn as well as pharmacologic agents utilized in emergency situations during immediate postnatal life.

EYE PROPHYLAXIS

Prophylaxis against gonococcal ophthalmia neonatorum in the first hour of life remains mandatory. This action is supported by the known increase in asymptomatic genital gonococcal infection and the estimated 28 percent occurrence of gonococcal ophthalmia in untreated infants born to infected mothers.[1] Silver nitrate ophthalmic drops, tetracycline and erythromycin ointments, and penicillin G intramuscularly have all been given for gonococcal eye prophylaxis.

Silver Nitrate

Silver nitrate is a water-soluble, colorless crystal and is known to be directly germicidal against *Neisseria* gonorrhea.[2] The 1 percent opthalmic solution in single-dose ampules is instilled into the conjunctiva immediately after birth. Irrigation of the eyes with water is unnecessary and does not apparently reduce the incidence of chemical conjunctivitis commonly seen in the first week of life.[3] Since the silver ions precipitate with the chloride ions, flushing with saline will produce a temporary black staining of surrounding tissues. Although silver nitrate may theoretically postpone eye-to-eye maternal–infant bonding, its value in preventing eye damage from gonococcal infection is well substantiated and would appear to outweigh the temporary inconvenience.[2] Silver nitrate has been the major therapeutic drug for gonococcal prevention until recently when antibiotic ointments became more easily available.

Tetracycline and Erythromycin Ointments

Erythromycin ointment (0.5 percent) and tetracycline ointment (1 percent) are topical antibiotics which have been recently approved and recommended for eye prophylaxis by the Centers for Disease Control and the American Academy of Pediatrics.[3] They are supplied in single-use tubes and are effective against *Neisseria* gonorrhea. In addition, both antibiotics have been shown to be effective in vitro against *Chlamydia trachomatis*, an important organism contributing to neonatal conjunctivitis and subsequent respiratory illnesses. Clinical trials have revealed an appreciable decrease in chlamydial conjunctivitis with erythromycin ointment but not with tetracycline ointment.[4] Erythromycin ointment has become the treatment of choice for newborn eye prophylaxis in most perinatal centers.[5]

Penicillin G

The intramuscular use of 50,000 units of aqueous penicillin G given intramuscularly within the first 30 minutes of life for prophylaxis against gonococcal conjunctivitis is another aternative. This mode of therapy cannot be recommended, however, until the incidence of disease from evolving penicillin-resistant organisms, including *Neisseria* gonorrhea, is more clearly delineated.[4] Furthermore, penicillin sensitization within the first year has been reported, and a greater incidence of penicilloyl-sensitive IgM antibodies has been shown in those treated with single-dose penicillin at birth as compared to those receiving local eye prophylaxis. These differences in penicillin sensitivity were no longer present by 5 years of age.[6]

BLEEDING PROPHYLAXIS (VITAMIN K)

The newborn, especially the premature infant, has only 20 to 40 percent of the normal adult level of the vitamin K-dependent clotting factors II (prothrombin), VII (proconvertin), IX (Christmas or Plasma thromboplastin component), and X (Stuart-Prower). The administration of exogenous vitamin K is therefore necessary to arrest the further physiologic decline of these vitamin K-dependent factors which occurs during the first few days of life.[7] Following the establishment of the normal enteric flora, bacterial synthesis and oral intake provide an adequate supply of vitamin K.[8]

A failure to administer this vitamin soon after birth may result in hemorrhagic disease of the newborn, which occurs within the first 48 hours of life. This condition presents as bleeding from the gastrointestinal tract, umbilical cord, circumcision site, nose or intracranial structures.[8] Newborns who are breastfed are also susceptible to this deficiency if untreated, since human milk contains 15 mcg/liter of vitamin K in comparison to 60 mcg/liter found in cow's milk. The calculated daily requirement of vitamin K is 15 mcg/day for the first 3 years of life.[9]

Vitamin K consists of a group of lipid-soluble structures that are cofactors for the activation of clotting factor precursors. Biochemically, the glutamic acid peptide residue is converted to γ-carboxyglutamic acid in the microsomal enzyme system. This alteration then allows calcium ion binding and phospholipid surface binding which are important steps for the activation of the clotting factor cascade.[2]

The three forms of vitamin K are shown in Figure 15–1. Vitamin K_1 or phytonadione. (2-methyl-3-phytyl-1,4-naphthoquinone) is present in plants and is the only natural vi-

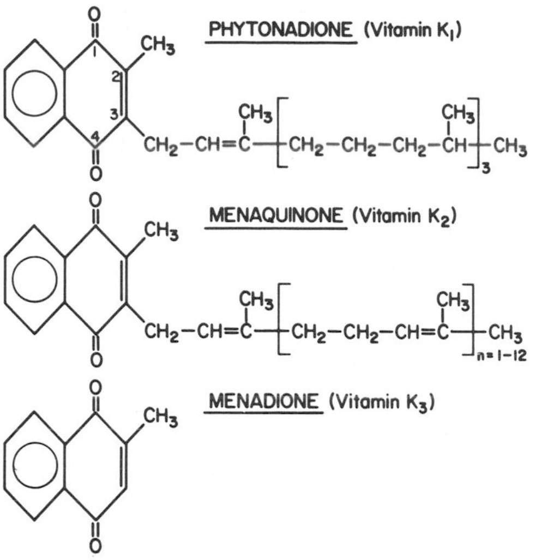

PHYTONADIONE (Vitamin K_1)

MENAQUINONE (Vitamin K_2)

MENADIONE (Vitamin K_3)

Figure 15–1. Chemical structure of three vitamin K compounds.

tamin used therapeutically. Vitamin K_2 or menaquinone is synthesized by bacteria and represents a group of compounds where a side chain of prenyl units is substituted for the phytyl side chain. Vitamin K_3 or menadione (2-methyl-1,4 naphthoquinone) is the most biologically active of the synthetic derivatives.[1]

Hemorrhagic disease of the newborn from vitamin K deficiency is easily prevented by the intramuscular administration of 1 mg of phytonadione (vitamin K_1) preparation. Aquamephyton (neonatal) is a yellow, viscous liquid containing phytonadione (1 mg/0.5 ml) dispersed in polyoxyethylated fatty acid derivatives, dextrose, sterile water, and benzyl peroxide (0.9 percent). Konakion uses polysorbate and propylene glycol to disperse phytonadione.[2]

Certain synthetic analogues of menadione or vitamin K_3 (Hykione and Synkonite) should not be administered during the neonatal period because of potentially serious sequelae. Hemolytic anemia, hyperbilirubinemia, kernicterus, and an increase in mortality may occur with excessive doses, which may be partly related to competition between vitamin K_3 and bilirubin for the albumin binding sites.[8]

PHARMACOLOGY OF RESUSCITATION

Several informative and helpful articles on resuscitation of the newborn are available.[10,11] The prevention of birth asphyxia and the knowledge of proper resuscitative techniques can often preclude the use of a pharmacologic agent in the first minutes of life. The appropriate use of drugs in the newborn will depend on the experience of medical personnel and the condition of the neonate at 1 and 5 minutes after birth, as evaluated by the Apgar scoring system[12] (Tables 15–1 and 15–2). If the newborn's status reflects significant hypoxia (Apgar score 0 to 4), thermal neutrality must be maintained (drying and placing the infant under a radiant warmer), the head and neck must be correctly extended, the airway should be gently cleared of secretions and ventilated by mouth-to-mouth resuscitation, and bag breathing and/or endotracheal intubation must be performed. Pharmacologic intervention after these crucial basic steps may then be instituted. Comparison of Apgar score does not necessarily reflect degree of hypoxia as measured by cord pH unless Apgar is less than 3.

Oxygen

Since oxygen's discovery in the late 1700s by Priestley, oxygen therapy has become a major pharmacologic agent. This colorless, odorless, therapeutic gas is required in all delivery rooms where potential resuscitation of a newborn may be necessary. Although most newborns do well without the use of oxygen (including those with peripheral cyanosis or acrocyanosis), asphyxiated infants with hypoxia and acidosis greatly benefit from its administration. In those emergency situa-

TABLE 15–1. EVALUATION OF THE NEWBORN USING THE 1- AND 5-MINUTE APGAR SCORING SYSTEM: POINTS ASSIGNED

Sign	Score 0	Score 1	Score 2
Heart rate	Absent	≤100	>100
Respiratory effort	Absent	Weak, irregular	Good, crying
Muscle tone	Flaccid	Some flexion of extremities	Well flexed
Reflex irritability (catheter in nose)	No response	Grimace	Cough and sneeze
Color	Blue, pale	Body pink, extremities blue	Pink

tions where oxygen is needed, a 5- to 7-liter flow of warmed, humidified oxygen is placed in front of the infant's face. The prerequisite of warmed oxygen eliminates the potential for cold stimulation of the trigeminal nerve which may cause reflex apnea and bradycardia. Excessive flow of the gas may cause marked turbulence and jeopardize optimal oxygenation of the patient. Oxygen is supplied through both pressurized wall outlets or from pressurized cylinders, which must be well supported for safety precautions. Regulators, flow meters, humidifers, and heating units should be understood by responsible persons.

The importance of minimizing and reversing hypoxia by oxygen administration in the acute situation at birth clearly outweighs any potential toxicity seen in the newborn intensive care unit. (Retrolental fibroplasia and bronchopulmonary dysplasia are usually associated with chronic exposure to oxygen.) The normal physiologic adjustments involving fetal transitional structures are facilitated by oxygenation at birth. The ductus arteriosus, although influenced by various vasoactive substances, responds principally to an increasing arterial blood oxygen tension (> 80 mm Hg). Additional effects of oxygen on the central nervous system, pulmonary system, and peripheral receptors in the neonate continue to be an area of intense investigation.[13]

Intravenous Fluids

Parenteral fluid administration is paramount in certain neonatal conditions such as prematurity, diabetic progeny, small-for-gestational age, septic shock, and severe birth asphyxia. Both water and glucose supplementation support important critical functions.

TABLE 15–2. DEGREE OF HYPOXIA AND CLINICAL APPEARANCE OF THE NEWBORN USING THE APGAR SCORING SYSTEM

Degree of Hypoxia	1-Minute Apgar Score	pH	Clinical Presentation
None	7–10	≥7.25	Heart rate >100, good respirations, well flexed, reflex irritability present, acrocyanosis/pink color
Moderate	4–6	7.10–7.25	Heart rate >100, gasping respirations, some flexion, some reflex irritability, pale blue color
Severe	0–3	≤7.10	Heart rate <100, apneic, flaccid, poor to no reflex irritability, pale color

From 32 weeks gestational age until term, water constitutes roughly 80 percent of the total body weight in the newborn. In the sick infant, for whom oral feedings are unwise and potentially dangerous, intravenous (IV) solutions are needed to replace fluid losses (insensible, urine, and stool) and to support intravascular volume.

Glucose is known to be the major substrate utilized for metabolic processes in the neonate. It is necessary for continued function and preservation of the cardiovascular and central nervous systems and to prevent hypoglycemia and its serious sequelae. A reduction in tissue catabolism[14] and an improvement in survival rate in prematures[15] have been documented following early IV administration of water and glucose. Ten percent dextrose (10 g of dextrose/100 ml water) without electrolytes is used for all term newborns and low birthweight infants (1000 to 2500 g) who require IV fluids within the first 24 hours of life.

In very low birthweight (VLBW) infants (< 1000 g), 7.5 percent dextrose in water (7.5 g dextrose/100 ml water) or 5 percent dextrose in water (5 g dextrose/100 ml water) should be used to avoid hyperglycemia and the subsequent rise in serum osmolarity. An appropriate fluid load is to 80 to 100 ml/kg/day, although VLBW infants may require more to counteract their increased insensible water loss. Fluid therapy is regulated by frequent evaluations of body weight, urine output, urine specific gravities, and degree of insensible water losses, quite variable depending on gestational age. All affected infants should have serum sodium, potassium, and chloride levels measured within 24 hours after birth and prior to adding electrolytes to the IV fluids.

Sodium Bicarbonate

Cardiovascular support in asphyxiated, high-risk infants requires a patent airway, supplemental oxygen, and IV fluids (water and glucose). Occasionally, a buffering agent is necessary to combat lactic acidosis. Sodium bicarbonate ($NaHCO_3$) is a sterile, hypertonic solution used intravenously as a systemic alkalizer. The 4.2 percent solution (infant dosage) contains 0.5 mEq/ml of sodium, 0.5 mEq/ml of bicarbonate, with an osmolality of 1000 mOsm and a pH of 8.0.

This agent is used in the newborn to increase the buffering capacity of the blood which is diminished following such situations as anemia, hypoxemia, and ischemia. An appropriate dosage of $NaHCO_3$ is 2 mEq/kg, diluted in equal volumes with sterile water to reduce the osmolality. Infusion should occur over a minimum of 10 to 15 minutes through a peripheral IV or central umbilical catheter line. An upper limit of 6 to 8 mEq/kg over a 24-hour period is recommended.[3] The bicarbonate buffering system is based on the following equation:

$$H^+ + HC_3^- \rightleftharpoons H_2CO_3 \rightleftharpoons H_2O + CO_2$$

Elimination of carbon dioxide (CO_2) is required in order for bicarbonate to work effectively and is symbolized on the right side of the above equation. Obviously, proper ventilation of the newborn is a prerequisite to bicarbonate administration.

The complications associated with the use of this drug in the newborn include hypernatremia, increased osmolality, fluid overload, hypocalcemia, respiratory acidosis, and intra-cranial hemorrhage in the premature infant. Administration concomitantly with calcium mixtures should be avoided because of the precipitation of calcium-bicarbonate ad-mixtures.[16]

Naloxone Hydrochloride (Narcan)

Narcotic-induced depression of the newborn is uncommon, but to ensure sufficient oxygenation and to prevent hypercarbia and acidosis, early recognition and prompt resuscitation are required. Proper technique in resuscitation and adequate supportive care diminish significantly the need for a narcotic-antagonist.

Naloxone (Narcan) is an almost pure antagonist of opioid-like compounds with virtually no agonistic effects. It is this characteristic which makes naloxone the drug of choice for narcotic-induced depression when compared to other antagonists that have combined actions (nalorphine hydrochloride and levallorphan tartrate). The neonatal preparation of naloxone (0.02 mg/ml) is recommended at a dose of 0.01 mg/kg IV. Less predictable absorption occurs with subcutaneous, intramuscular, and intralingual administration. Due to its short-lasting action, naloxone may be readministered within 5 minutes if the initial positive response of rhythmic respirations is not sustained.[17]

Naloxone and other narcotic-antagonists act centrally by direct competition for the opiate receptor sites. These receptors seem to be intimately involved with the enkephalin neurotransmitters distributed with the spinal cord, brain stem, pituitary, thalamus, and amygdala.[18] Further studies of these peptide structures and receptor sites may lead to the development of synthetic nonaddicting analgesics.

Naloxone should be used very discriminately in the newborn. Although short-term side effects seem to be negligible, the long-term safety of naloxone is still being investigated. Acknowledgment of the role of endogenous polypeptides (endorphins and enkephalins) in the central nervous system has raised serious questions about the routine use of a narcotic-antagonist. Alterations in release of prolactin, growth hormone, luteinizing hormone and follicle-stimulating hormone have been documented in animals following naloxone administration.[17] It should not be given to infants of narcotic-dependent mothers wherein withdrawal may be abrupt.

The use of naloxone to reverse hypotension caused by endorphine release in septic shock has been reported.[19] However, naloxone is unreliable in stabilizing arterial pressures and may cause severe adverse reactions emphasizing the need for further controlled studies.

Additional Drugs

Critically ill newborns who continue to have difficulty adjusting to extrauterine life despite oxygenation, ventilation, IV glucose, volume expansion, and bicarbonate may need additional pharmacologic agents to support their heart rate, blood pressure, and cardiac output. These drugs are summarized in Table 15–3 and described below.

Epinephrine

Effects from epinephrine, a mediator of the adrenergic nervous system, are directly related to the stimulation of α- and β-adrenergic receptor sites.[20] During resuscitation, this drug raises blood pressure through vasoconstriction of the precapillary vascular beds and increases cardiac output by its direct stimulation of the myocardium. An increase in the strength of ventricular contraction (positive inotropic effect) and an increase in heart rate (positive chronotropic effect) further contributes to the improvement in arterial blood pressure. Epinephrine (1 ml) in a 1:10,000 dilution (0.1 mg/ml) should be administered intravenously or via the endotracheal tube to the asphyxiated newborn when bradycardia (heart rate $<$ 80 beats/min) continues despite proper resuscitation. If this is unsuccessful in improving the heart rate, intracardiac administration using a subxiphoid approach should be attempted.

Catecholamines appear to work less effectively in an acid medium; therefore buffering with sodium bicarbonate may increase their effectiveness. Epinephrine and bicarbonate should not be given simultaneously in the identical IV line however, since their interaction may cause precipitation, and thus inactivate the catecholamines.[21]

Atropine

By inhibition of vagal effects on the sinoatrial node, atropine may increase heart rate during newborn resuscitation. Known as an antimuscarinic agent, atropine competes directly with the neurotransmitter acetyl-

TABLE 15–3. DRUGS FOR RESUSCITATION OF THE NEONATE

Drug	Dose	Route	Indication	Complications
Sodium bicarbonate (4.2% solution)	2 mEq/kg* (dilute 1:1 with sterile water)	IV slowly	Severe asphyxia, metabolic acidosis	Hypernatremia, hyperosmolarity, volume overload, intraventricular hemorrhage, respiratory acidosis
Epinephrine	1ml 1:10,000 dilution	IV, IC, ET*†	Bradycardia (HR < 80) despite ventilation	Ventricular fibrillation
Volume expander (saline, blood, plasma)	10 ml/kg	IV slowly	Hypotension, volume depletion	Volume overload, intraventricular hemorrhage
Narcan (neonatal)	0.01 mg/kg	IV or IM	Depression, with maternal narcotic history	Minimal; antagonism with enkephalins
Atropine	0.01 mg/kg	IM, SC, ET*†	Continued bradycardia	Marked tachycardia
Isoprel	1 amp (0.2 mg) per 50 ml D_5W Dose: 0.1–0.4 mcg/min	IV	Low cardiac output, bradycardia	Arrhythmias, reduced cardiac output if heart rate > 200
Dopamine	5-10 mcg/kg/min	IV	Low cardiac output	Arrhythmias; gangrene, increased pulmonary artery pressure

* IV = intravenous, IC = intracardiac, IM = intramuscular, SC = subcutaneous, ET = endotracheal. Calculated dose mEq $NAHCO_3$ = 0.3 × weight (kg) × base deficit.

† Endotracheal with epinephrine and atropine.

choline at the postganglionic receptor sites. Subcutaneous administration of 0.01 mg/kg will inhibit parasympathetic effects and allow sympathomimetic pharmacologic agents to elevate the contraction frequency of the heart. Atropine may also be given down the endotracheal tube.

Dopamine

Dopamine, an endogenous catecholamine, stimulates β_1-adrenergic receptors and, at higher doses, α-adrenergic receptors. Its unique characteristics have made it the drug of choice in critically ill infants needing continued cardiovascular support. Dopamine selectively dilates renal, coronary, splanchnic, and cerebral vessels by causing a decrease in their vascular resistance.[22] Its positive inotropic and chronotropic effects increase cardiac output, support arterial blood pressure, and allow perfusion of vital organs.[23] Potential complications include increased pulmonary arterial pressure and peripheral ischemia.

Isoproterenol

Isoproterenol, a β_1- and β_2-adrenergic agonist, causes significant inotropic and chronotropic cardiac stimulation. However, its powerful chronotropic effect often prevents improvement in cardiac output. Additionally, its strong β-stimulation of the periphery leads to vasodilation and subsequent hypotension. Unlike dopamine, isoproterenol fails to selectively increase flow to vital organ systems.[23] Further investigation into the pharmacologic actions of dopamine, isoproterenol, and dobutamine is necessary.

REFERENCES

1. Davidson HH, Hill J, Eastman JJ: Penicillin in the prophylaxis of opthalmic neonatorum. JAMA 145:1052, 1951
2. Harvey S: Antiseptics and disinfectants; fungicides; ectoparasiticides. In Gilman AG, Goodman LS, Gilman A (eds): The Pharmacological Basis of Therapeutics, ed. 6 New York, Macmillan, 1980, pp 976–977
3. Segal S, Brann A, Mortimer E, et al.: Prophylaxis and treatment of neonatal gonococcal infections. Pediatrics 65:1047, 1980
4. Siegel JD, McCracken GH, Threlkeld N, et al.: Single-dose penicillin prophylaxis against neonatal group B streptococcal infections. N Engl J Med 303:769, 1980
5. Hammerschlag, M, Chandler, J, Alexander, E, et al.: Erythromycin ointment for ocular prophylaxis of neonatal chlamydial infection. JAMA 244:2291, 1980
6. Fellner MJ, Klaus MV, Baer RL, et al.: Antibody production in normal children receiving penicillin at birth. J Immunol 107:1440, 1971
7. Owen GM, Nelson EC, Baker GL, et al.: Use of vitamin K_1 in pregnancy. Am J Obstet Gynecol 99:368, 1967
8. Oski FA: Hematologic problems. In Avery GB (ed): Neonatology: Pathophysiology and Management of the Newborn, ed 2. Philadelphia, Lippincott, 1981, pp 569–571
9. Anderson TA, Foman SJ: Vitamins. In Foman SJ (ed): Infant Nutrition, ed 2. Philadelphia, Saunders, 1974, pp 222–223
10. Anderson CW, Iams J: Resuscitation of the newborn infant. In Zuspan FP, Quilligan EJ (eds): Practical Manual of Obstetrical Care, ed 1. St Louis, Mosby, 1981,
11. Fisher DE, Paton JB: Resuscitation of the newborn infant. In Klaus MH, Fanaroff AA (eds): Care of the High-Risk Neonate, ed 2. Philadelphia, Saunders, 1979, pp 23–44
12. Apgar V: A proposal for a new method of evaluation of the newborn infant. Anesth Analg (Paris) 32:260, 1953
13. Nelson NM: Respiration and circulation after birth. In Smith CA, Nelson NM (eds): The Physiology of the Newborn Infant, ed 4. Springfield, Ill, Thomas, 1976, pp 143-152
14. Auld PA, Bhangananden P, Mehta S: The influence of an early caloric intake with IV glucose on catabolism of premature infants. Pediatrics 37:592, 1966
15. Cornblath M, Forbes AE, Pildes RS, et al.: A controlled study of early fluid administration on survival of low birth weight infants. Pediatrics 38:547, 1966
16. Bowen FW, Lewis WJ: The use and abuse of bicarbonate in neonatal acid-base derangements. Resp Care 23:5, 1978
17. Segal S, Anyan WR, Hill RM, et al.: Naloxone use in newborns. Pediatrics 65:667, 1980
18. Snyder S: Opiate receptors in the brain. N Engl J Med 296:5:266, 1977
19. Rock P, Silverman H, Plump D, et al.: Efficacy and safety of naloxine in septic shock. Crit Care Med 13:28, 1985
20. Weiner N: Norepinephrine, epinephrine and the sympathomimetic amines. In Gilman AG, Goodman LS, Gilman A (eds): The Phamacological Basis of Therapeutics, ed 6. New York, Macmillan, 1985, pp 66–99
21. Holbrook PR, Mickell J, Pollack MM, et al.: Cardiovascular resuscitation drugs for children. Crit Care Med 8:588, 1980
22. Goldberg L: Dopamine—Clinical uses of an endogenous catecholamine. N Engl J Med 291:707, 1974
23. Driscoll DJ, Gillette PC, Lewis RM, et al.: Comparative hemodynamic effects of isoproterenol, dopamine and dobutamine in the newborn dog. Pediatr Res 13:1006, 1979

16

Rho(D) Immune Globulin

Melanie S. Kennedy

Isoimmune hemolytic disease of the newborn is the destruction of the red blood cells of the fetus and neonate by antibodies produced by the mother. The mother can be stimulated to form the antibodies in any of a number of ways (Table 16–1). Previously, about 95 percent of the cases of hemolytic disease of the newborn were due to antibodies in the mother directed against the red blood cell antigens called Rh (previously Rho).[1] In the United States, the incidence of the disease due to Rh decreased from 40.5 cases per 10,000 total births in 1970 to 14.3 per 10,000 in 1979.[2] Currently, less than 50 percent of cases are due to Rh incompatibility. This decreased incidence can be attributed to the development and release in 1968 of the hyperimmune globulin called Rho(D) immune globulin [Gamulin Rh (Armour), HypRho-D (Cutter), MICRhoGAM (Ortho), Mini-Gamulin Rh (Armour), Rho(D) Immune Globulin (Human) (Cooper/Connaught), RhoGAM (Ortho)].

MECHANISM OF ACTION

The prevention of active immunization by the simultaneous administration of red cell antigen and antibody was first observed in 1909.[3] However, it was not until the late 1950s that the application of this principle was investigated for the prevention of Rh immunization by the use of anti-D. During pregnancy and at delivery, the mixing of fetal and maternal blood occurs. If the mother is Rh negative and the infant is Rh positive, the mother has a 5 to 13 percent chance of being stimulated to form anti-D.[3] As little as 1 ml of fetal red blood cells can elicit a response.[4] Antepartum, the risk of sensitization is 1.5 to 2.0 percent of susceptible women,[5] indicating that a significant amount of fetal red blood cells can enter the maternal circulation during pregnancy. However, the greatest risk is at delivery. It has been theorized but not proven that an Rh-negative fetus could be immunized to the mother's Rh-posi-

TABLE 16–1. CAUSES OF MATERNAL IMMUNIZATION TO Rh

1. Previous pregnancy of Rh-positive fetus
   a. No Rho(D) immune globulin
   b. Insufficient Rho(D) immune globulin
   c. Immunization during gestation
2. Previous transfusion of Rh-positive blood
3. Current pregnancy of Rh-positive fetus
   a. Spontaneous fetomaternal hemorrhage
   b. Amniocentesis
   c. Spontaneous or induced abortion
   d. Ectopic pregnancy
   e. Trauma
4. Rh-positive mother (grandmother theory)

tive red cells during gestation (grandmother theory).[5]

The passively administered Rho(D) immune globulin attaches to the fetal Rho(D)-positive red blood cells in the maternal circulation. The antibody coated red cells are trapped in the maternal spleen where they take up more antibody from the circulating plasma. This stimulates immune suppression by suppressor cells and/or the production of anti-idiotypic antibody.[6] The amount of antibody necessary for the suppressor effect has been determined empirically and is known to be less that that required to saturate all D antigen sites.[6]

DRUG PREPARATION

The only source of Rho(D) immune globulin is plasma from Rh-negative women immunized by pregnancy and Rh-negative men deliberately immunized by repeated Rh-positive red blood cell injections.[7] In the United States, the immune globulin is prepared by the Cohn cold ethanol fractionation method from pooled raw plasma from at least 20 different human donors. All immune globulins prepared by this method cannot be injected intravenously unless further modified or prepared by other methods. Rho(D) immune globulin has not been produced for intravenous use in the United States, but has been available elsewhere.[5,8] Although immune globulins, regardless of the method of preparation, cannot be pasteurized, they do not transmit hepatitis B or other viral diseases for unknown reasons. (See Chap. 10.)

Each regular single-dose vial contains sufficient anti-D to protect against 15 ml of Rh-positive, packed red blood cells. This is about 300 mcg when compared to the WHO Rho(D) immune globulin reference material. The microdose vial contains sufficient anti-D to protect against 2.5 ml of red cells. A multiple dose vial is also available (RhoGAM, Ortho). The products also contain 0.3 M glycine as a stabilizer and 0.01 percent thimerosal as a preservative. Rho(D) immune globulin should be stored between 2 and 8C and must not be frozen.

INDICATIONS

At Delivery

Because the highest risk for Rh immunization occurs at the time of delivery, the unsensitized mother should receive Rho(D) immune globulin soon after delivery of an Rh-positive infant. The original studies of the efficacy of the product in prisoners were carried out using 72 hours between the injection of the Rh-positive red blood cells and the injection of the Rho(D) immune globulin. The 72-hour time interval was selected because of weekends and the usual postpartum stay.[5] Complete protection from immunization was shown for the 72-hour time period, although administration beyond 72 hours probably is protective as well, and is certainly not contraindicated.[5]

The mother should be D negative as well as D^u negative (Fig. 16–1). The great majority of D^u positive individuals are genetically D positive but have weakened antigenic expression of D by gene interaction.[5] The rare individuals who actually are missing part of the D antigen may react strongly or weakly

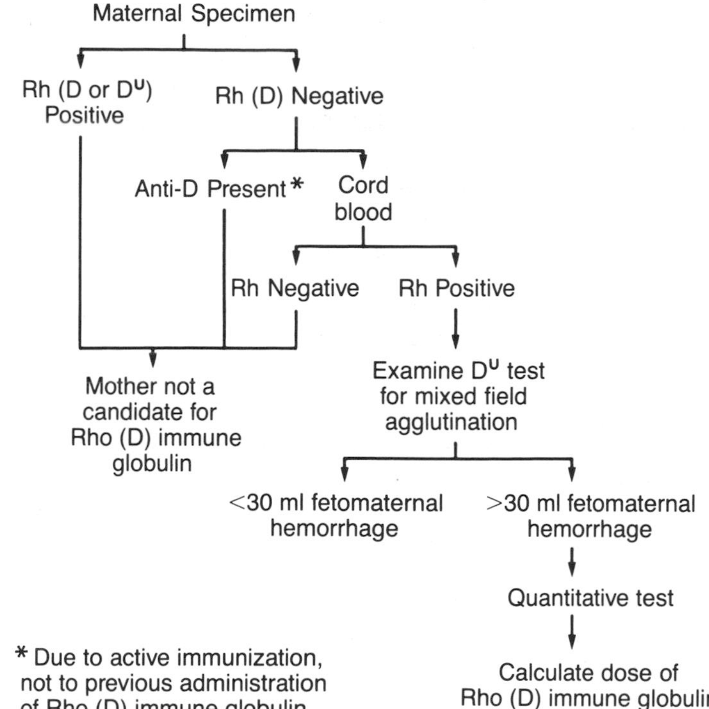

Figure 16–1. Decision tree for the indications and dose of Rho(D) immune globulin as determined by laboratory test results. The maternal blood specimen, collected after delivery, is essential. If the cord or neonatal blood specimen is unavailable, assume that the fetus is D- or D^u-positive.

with routine Rh typing sera.[9] About half of these individuals type as "D" (immediate reaction with reagent sera) and cannot be detected unless anti-D is produced.[9,10] The infant should be Rh (D or D^u) positive. Rho(D) immune globulin should also be administered if the Rh type of the infant is unknown (e.g., stillborn or abortus.)[5] Whether or not an unsensitized mother undergoing postpartum sterilization should receive Rho(D) immune globulin is controversial because tubal reanastomosis procedures are becoming more popular.

Routine Antepartum Prophylaxis

Because there is some risk of immunization during pregnancy, the use of antepartum Rho(D) immune globulin has been recommended to reduce this risk.[5,11] Most obstetricians have accepted this practice. In Winnipeg, Canada, the investigation of the prenatal injection of Rho(D) immune globulin, which was begun in 1968,[5] has shown that single injections at 28 weeks' gestation and again at delivery are effective in preventing nearly all cases (>98 percent) of Rh immunization.

According to a recent technical bulletin by the American College of Obstetricians and Gynecologists (ACOG Technical Bulletin #79, August 1984), an Rh-negative unsensitized woman should receive 300 mcg of Rho(D) immune globulin at approximately 28 weeks of gestation and again postpartum (if the infant is Rh positive). Clinical data are lacking to support the administration of a second dose if the pregnancy exceeds 40 weeks; however, there is a theoretical risk (see below).[3] Anti-D antibody titers are not recommended because the amount of circulating Rho(D) immune globulin does not correlate with effectiveness of immune suppression.

It would seem that the administration of

Rho(D) immune globulin would pose a risk to an Rh-positive fetus, because maternal IgG is actively transported across the placenta during pregnancy.[12] However, a full dose of Rho(D) immune globulin causes an albumin titer of 1:1 or 1:2 in the mother,[3] which is below the level to cause hemolytic disease of the newborn, although a positive direct antiglobulin test (Coombs') may be observed in the newborn.

The half-life of IgG is about 25 days, so that 300 mcg administered at 28 weeks' gestation would be expected to be about 30 mcg at 40 weeks. This may not be sufficient to protect against the possible fetomaternal hemorrhage at delivery. An additional regular dose must be administered after delivery if the infant is Rh positive. The blood bank or transfusion service must be informed of any woman receiving Rho(D) immune globulin during gestation, because the remaining anti-D in the maternal circulation after delivery may be detected by the routine blood bank type and screen. This could be interpreted erroneously as active rather than passive immunization and further administration of Rho(D) immune globulin considered contraindicated. The omission of an additional dose may lead to active Rh sensitization.

Routine antepartum use has been debated,[5,7,13,14] considering the low incidence of immunization (5 to 13 percent per pregnancy) and the fact that a single dose after delivery will prevent more than 60 to 80 percent of these cases. Nusbacher and Bove[7] pointed out that approximately 40 percent of Rh-negative women will be carrying Rh-negative fetuses, so that the amount of antenatal Rho(D) immune globulin would be almost twice that required at delivery.

Whether an additional dose during pregnancy is cost beneficial is controversial.[11,15] In addition, because humans are the only source of the product, the risks to the donors—hepatitis, immunization to leukocyte and platelet antigens, immunization to non-Rho(D) antigens, inadvertent pregnancy in "boosted"women,[16] and death due to mixup in the red cells returned—must be considered.[7]

Amniocentesis

Several authors[5,17] have recommended the administration of Rho(D) immune globulin after amniocentesis in the nonimmunized Rho(D)-negative woman, because the risk of fetomaternal hemorrhage is increased. Administration at 28 weeks and postpartum should be considered if a dose is given after amniocentesis.

Abortion and Ectopic Pregnancy

About 2 to 5 percent of Rh-negative women who abort spontaneously or therapeutically will become sensitized, with a higher risk from therapeutic abortion.[5] The risk of immunization is about twice that of antenatal sensitization during a normal pregnancy, so administration is clearly indicated. Fetal red blood cells are formed at about the sixth week of gestation.[18] Abortions and ectopic pregnancy before 12 weeks' gestation can receive the microdose, which is sufficient to protect against 2.5 ml of packed red blood cells. The regular dose, should be given for terminations after 12 weeks' gestation.

Accidental or Inadvertent Transfusion

Rh-positive red blood cells accidentally transfused to a Rh-negative woman of childbearing age can cause immunization in those 70 to 80 percent who are "good responders."[4,5] Platelet concentrates and leukocyte concentrates contain variable amounts of red blood cells. The use of Rh-positive donors may be necessary because of such considerations as supply and HLA matching.

Modifying Alloimmunization

It has been proposed that the administration of Rho(D) immune globulin to sensitized Rh-negative women could suppress the production of anti-D. However, prospective studies giving Rho(D) immune globulin at 6-week intervals to pregnant Rh immunized women did not suppress further antibody production.[19]

DOSE AND ADMINISTRATION

The regular vial in the United States contains sufficient anti-D to protect against 15 ml of packed red blood cells, or 30 ml of whole blood (Table 16–2). Although the standardization in the United States is not based on micrograms, the regular dose vial is equivalent to 300 mcg of WHO reference material. The regular vial in the United Kingdom contains about 100 mcg, whereas in most other countries each vial contains between 200 and 300 mcg.[4] The 100 mcg dose appears to be adequate for postpartum prophylaxis.[20] Less than 1 percent of women delivering after 20 weeks' gestation will have fetomaternal hemorrhages of more than 30 ml of whole blood.[5] These massive hemorrhages can lead to sensitization if adequate Rho(D) immune globulin is not administered. The existence of a possible massive fetomaternal hemorrhage may be detected by the routine use of the indirect antihuman globulin (Coombs' reagent) test, reading the result microscopically. This test is the same as the D^u test (Fig. 16–1), and can detect 10 ml of Rh-positive fetal red blood cells in the maternal circulation. Other tests are available for screening purposes. Quantitation of the actual amount of hemorrhage must be done by a quantitative test, such as the Kleihauer-Betke test. In this test, a thin smear of the maternal blood is subjected to acid and then stained. The fetal cells contain hemoglobin that is resistant to acid and will remain dark. The maternal hemoglobin is eluted by the acid, and therefore maternal cells will appear as ghosts. After several hundred cells are counted, the percentage of fetal cells is determined, and the volume of fetal hemorrhage is calculated using the formula:

$$\frac{\text{No. of fetal cells} \times \text{Maternal blood volume}}{\text{Number of maternal cells}} = \text{Volume of fetomaternal hemorrhage}$$

The calculated volume of fetomaternal hemorrhage is then divided by 30 to determine the number of required vials of Rho(D) immune globulin.

The microdose is sufficient for abortions up to 12 weeks' gestation because the total fetal blood volume is estimated at less than 5 ml at 12 weeks. The use of the microdose vial will save the patient from 45 to 55 percent of the cost of the regular vial.

The number of vials for transfusion accidents is calculated by dividing the volume of Rh-positive packed red blood cells transfused by 15 ml, the amount of red blood cells covered by one vial. The amount of Rho(D) immune globulin required can be large, so that the entire dose is often divided and administered in several injections at separate sites. Another approach is to perform an exchange transfusion and then calculate the dose based on the number of Rh-positive red cells remaining in the circulation.[5] For platelet concentrates, one vial is sufficient for 30 or more units (bags), because each unit con-

TABLE 16–2. INDICATIONS AND DOSE

Indications	Dose
Gestational age <12 weeks	Microdose
Abortion, spontaneous or induced	
Ectopic rupture	
Amniocentesis	
Gestational age >12 weeks	Regular
Abortion, spontaneous or induced	
Ectopic rupture	
Amniocentesis	
Delivery spontaneous, induced, section, or stillbirth	
Sterilization postpartum	
Massive fetomaternal hemorrhage >30 ml whole blood	Calculate by quantitative test

tains less than 0.5 ml red blood cells. The dose for leukocyte concentrates can be calculated by obtaining the hematocrit and volume of the product from the supplier.

Rho(D) immune globulin, prepared by the Cohn fractionation technique, as available in the United States, must be injected intramuscularly only. Intravenous injections can cause severe anaphylactic reactions due to the anticomplementary activity of the product. The entire calculated dose should be administered within 72 hours of delivery or accidental transfusion, since nearly all clinical studies use this time span. It is unknown how much delay would still allow complete protection, but if the administration of the Rho(D) immune globulin is inadvertently delayed beyond 72 hours, the dose should still be given. One group gives the Rho(D) immune globulin up to 28 days later.[5]

With antepartum use, a second dose must be given about 12 weeks later, and/or postpartum. The low level at delivery after a previous dose may actually enhance the immune response to form antibody.[6]

PRECAUTIONS

Contraindications

Rho(D) immune globulin is of no benefit once a person has been actively immunized and has formed anti-D. If anti-D is identified in the potential recipient, administration of Rho(D) immune globulin is not indicated, unless it can be shown that the presence of anti-D is due to the previous administration of Rho(D) immune globulin.

According to recommendations by the FDA (manufacturers' circulars of information) and the American Association of Blood Banks,[21,22] Rho(D) immune globulin is not indicated for mothers who are D- or D^u-positive, because the product is incompatible with their red blood cells and would cause their rapid destruction. This conflicts with the 1981 recommendation of the American College of Obstetrics and Gynecology that D^u-positive women also receive Rho(D) immune globulin.[23] This was later modified by a statement that "a woman who is *genetically* D^u-positive is Rh-positive and administration of Rh immune globulin is unnecessary.[22] The apparent intent of the original recommendation was to avoid misinterpretation of the typing of women with massive fetomaternal hemorrhage. It is important that fetal red blood cells in the maternal circulation not be interpreted as maternal, because the mother would then be assumed to be D^u-positive. The difference can be distinguished by examining the D^u test microscopically, because the presence of Rh-positive fetal cells in the Rh-negative maternal blood would have the typical "mixed field" appearance. Confirmation should then be made with a quantitative test.

Rho(D) immune globulin is not indicated for the mother if the infant is found to be D- and D^u negative. This is usually not possible to determine for abortions, stillbirths, and ectopic pregnancies; therefore, Rho(D) immune globulin should be administered in these circumstances.

Rho(D) immune globulin is not to be given to the newborn infant.

Adverse Effects

There is no risk of transmission of viral diseases including hepatitis B and AIDS.[24] Local reactions to the injections are frequent, and fever occurs occasionally. Rarely, severe anaphylactic reactions may occur. Individuals receiving Rho(D) immune globulin may be stimulated to form antiglobulin antibodies, which may be due to aggregated IgG formed in the Cohn fractionation process.[13] The clinical significance of these antibodies is unknown.

A case of serum sickness has been reported that occurred after the second injection of Rho(D) immune globulin and worsened after the third injection. Eight months later the patient was well, with evidence of mild inactive mesangial glomerulonephritis on renal biopsy.[25]

Rho(D) immune globulin has also been reported to contain antibody to both hepatitis A and B and thus may cause false-positive hepatitis serology.[26]

Transmission of non-A and non-B hepatitis by intravenous immune globulin has recently been reported by several investigators.[27] However, other viral diseases (including AIDS) have not been transmitted.

Failures

The level of antibody at the time of delivery may be too small to detect except by very sensitive techniques. Thus the mother would be considered unsensitized, given Rho(D) immune globulin, and then termed a "failure" at the next pregnancy. Although the Rh type can be misinterpreted due to massive fetomaternal hemorrhage, another source of failure is an error in reporting the Rh type of the mother. Schmidt et al.[27] found an error rate of about 3 percent in mothers who were reportedly Rh negative. A similar error rate has been observed in a national survey. Thus we can assume a similar rate for reportedly Rh-positive women.[28]

The cause of the largest group of "failures" is the failure to give the Rho(D) immune globulin when indicated. About half of the women sensitized in the series by Tovey[13] were due to failures of administration. Table 16–3 lists these and additional causes of apparent failure.

TABLE 16–3. CAUSES OF APPARENT FAILURES OF Rho(D) IMMUNE GLOBULIN

1. Antepartum immunization
2. Inadequate dose
3. Misinterpretation of maternal Rh type
4. Error in Rh typing
5. Previous Rh-positive transfusion
6. Failure of administration when indicated
7. Immunization to cross-reacting antigen (G or C + D)
8. Delay in administration

FUTURE DIRECTIONS

The development and marketing of Rho(D) immune globulin prepared for intravenous injection would allow a lower dose. Use during gestation requires care to administer a second dose at delivery only if the newborn is Rh positive. Educational efforts and increased surveillance should decrease any failures of administration, and thus further reduce the incidence of Rh hemolytic disease of the newborn.[2]

REFERENCES

1. Rh hemolytic disease, United States, 1968–1977. Morbid Mortal Wkly Rep 27:487, 1978
2. Adams MM, Gustafson J: Epidemiology of Rh hemolytic disease of the newborn, United States, 1960–1979. Prog Clin Biol Res 70:213, 1981.
3. Pollack W: Rh hemolytic disease of the newborn: Its cause and prevention. Prog Clin Biol Res 70:185, 1981
4. Mollison PL: Blood Transfusion in Clinical Medicine, ed 6. Oxford, Blackwell, 1979, pp 292–352
5. Bowman JM: Controversies in Rh prophylaxis: Who needs Rh immune globulin and when should it be given? Am J Obstet Gynecol 151:289, 1985
6. Pollack W: Recent understanding for the mechanism by which passively administered Rh antibody suppresses the immune response to Rh antigen in unimmunized Rh-negative women. Clin Obstet Gynecol 25:255, 1982
7. Nusbacher J, Bove JR: Rh immunoprophylaxis: Is antepartum therapy desirable? N Engl J Med 303:935, 1980
8. Walsh TJ, O'Riordan JP: A review of the production and clinical use of intravenous anti-D immunoglobulin. Irish Med J 75:243, 1982
9. Lacey PA, Caskey CR, Werner DJ, Moulds JJ: Fatal hemolytic disease of a newborn due to anti-D in an Rh-positive D^u variant mother. Transfusion 23:91, 1983

10. White CA, Stedman CM, Frank S: Anti-D antibodies in D- and D^u-positive women: A cause of hemolytic disease of the newborn. Am J Obstet Gynecol 145:1069, 1983
11. Tovey LAD, Townley A, Stevenson BJ, Taverner J: The Yorkshire antenatal anti-D immunoglobulin trial in primigravidae. Lancet ii:244, 1983
12. Mollison PL: Haemolytic syndromes due to alloantibodies. In Gell PGH, Coombs RRA, Lachman PJ (eds): Clinical Aspects of Immunology, ed 3. Oxford, Blackwell, 1975, pp 1043–1060
13. Tovey GH: Should anti-D immunoglobulin be given antenatally? Lancet ii:466, 1980
14. Nusbacher J, Nichols EE: Routine antepartum Rh immune globulin administration. JAMA 252:2763, 1984
15. Adams MM, Marks JS, Koplan JP: Cost implications of routine antenatal administration of Rh immune globulin. Am J Obstet Gynecol 149:633, 1984
16. Fisher MM: Pregnancy in anti-D donors. Lancet ii:618, 1982
17. Murray JC, Karp LE, Williamson RA, et al.: Rh isoimmunization related to amniocentesis. Am J Med Genetics 16:527, 1983
18. Oski FA, Schwartz E: Hematology of the newborn. In Williams WJ, Beutler E, Erslev AJ, Rundles RW (eds): Hematology. New York, McGraw-Hill, 1972, p 52
19. Bowman JM, Pollock JM: Reversal of Rh alloimmunization: Fact or fancy? Vox Sang 47:209, 1984
20. Tabor A, Bock JE, Jerne D, Jacobsen JC: Dose of rhesus immunoprophylaxis. Lancet i:121, 1983
21. Standards for blood banks and transfusion services, ed 11. Arlington, Va, American Association of Blood Banks, 1984
22. Konugres AA, Polesky HF, Walker RH: Rh immune globulin and the Rh-positive, D^u variant mother. Transfusion 22:76, 1982
23. The selective use of Rho(D) immune globulin (RhIG). ACOG Technical Bull 61, March, 1981
24. Recommendations for protection against viral hepatitis. Morbid Mortal Wkly Rep 34:313, 1985
25. Jones BF, Trevillian PR, Nanra RS: Serum sickness due to Rh(anti-D) immunoglobulin. Aust NZ J Obstet Gynaecol 24:49, 1984
26. Tabor E, Smallwood LA, Gerety RJ: Antibodies to hepatitis A and B virus antigens in Rho(D) immune globulin. Lancet i:46, 1985
27. Webster ADH, Lever AML, Trepo C, et al.: Non-A, non-B hepatitis after intravenous gamma globulin (letters). Lancet i:322, 1986
28. Schmidt PJ, Pautler K, Samia CT: Prenatal Rh typing errors. Am J Obstet Gynecol 145:884, 1983

17

Lactation Suppressants

William E. Copeland, Jr.

Despite the resurgence of interest in breastfeeding, there is a significant number of women who choose not to nurse or are unable to do so due to various maternal or neonatal factors. Pharmacologic methods for lactation suppression offer an option to traditional, symptomatic measures of breastbinding, ice packs, fluid restriction, and analgesics. The concepts involved in the complex mechanism of lactation have only recently been understood. This information has significantly influenced the development of specific therapeutic modalities for lactation suppression.

PHYSIOLOGY OF LACTATION

Anatomically, the mature mammary gland is comprised of 15 to 25 lobes, arranged in a radial fashion and separated by fat. Each lobe is made up of several lobules, which are composed of large numbers of alveoli. Each alveolus is lined by a layer of milk-secreting epithelial cells and covered by a layer of contractile myoepithelial fibers. The alveolus secretes milk into the lumen, which subsequently drains into connecting intralobular ducts and finally, into the major lactiferous ducts for each lobule. The growth of this ductal system is estrogen dependent, while alveolar growth and development are stimulated by progesterone. Although ovarian hormones are primarily involved in breast development, complete differentiation requires an integrated effect from insulin, cortisol, thyroxine, prolactin, and growth hormone, along with human placental lactogen in pregnancy.

During pregnancy, there are progressive increases in the levels of circulating prolactin, estrogen, and progesterone. Prior to parturition and during the early puerperium, only nonmilk colostrum is produced. Colostrum contains desquamated epithelial cells and a transudate, which contains higher levels of fat, protein, and immunoglobulins and less lactose than normal breast milk. Despite the high levels of prolactin, milk production is absent. This is thought to be the result of an inhibitory effect of placental estrogen and progesterone, which exert local effects on the breast.[1-4] Following parturition, circulating levels of estrogen and progesterone fall precipitously. Prolactin levels initially remain elevated and fall more slowly to normal levels. This process is prolonged in the nursing mother. Breast engorgement and milk secretion usually begin on the third or fourth postpartum day. These events probably reflect the loss of inhibitory effects from estrogen and progesterone on the breast. Engorgement is a self-limited phenomenon in the puerperium, lasting 48 to 72 hours, and manifested by swollen, firm, tender breasts.

Lactation is a complex process involving multiple neuroendocrine functions (Fig. 17–1). Suckling or breast stimulation signals tactile sensors in the areola, to activate hypothalamic centers via a neural arc. These centers may also be activated by the mother thinking of the newborn, seeing the baby, or hearing a cry. The hypothalamic centers synthesize and transport oxytocin to the posterior pituitary gland. Oxytocin is then released to stimulate the alveolar myoepithelial fibers to contract; this results in the emptying of the alveoli and lactiferous ducts and the ejection of milk from the nipple and is known as milk "let-down."

Suckling also activates a similar feedback mechanism resulting in the inhibition of prolactin inhibitory factor (PIF) secretion from the hypothalamus, which leads to an increased production of prolactin from the anterior pituitary gland. Prolactin stimulates the breast to produce milk composed of proteins, casein, fatty acids, and lactose. Prolactin secretion also controls the volume of milk produced through a supply-and-demand system triggered by suckling. The absence of suckling results in cessation of let-down and restoration of normal levels of PIF production in nonnursing mothers. Breast engorgement diminishes, and milk secretion ceases within a few days. Suckling stimulates let-down and milk production long after serum prolactin levels have returned to normal in nursing women (Fig.17–2). This may result from transient elevations in prolactin associated with suckling in the early puerperium. Later, milk secretion will continue despite normal serum levels of prolactin when suckling is

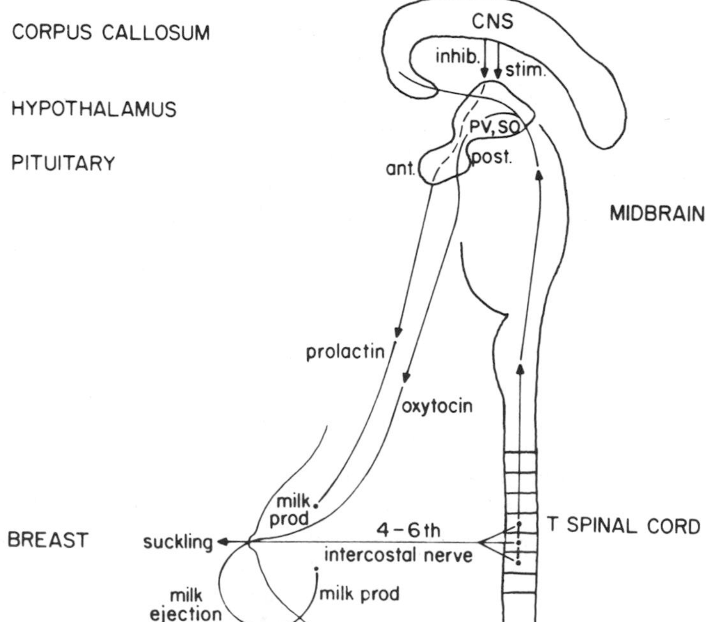

Figure 17–1. Neuroendocrine reflexes involved in lactation. (*From Tulchinsky D: The postpartum period. In Tulchinsky D, Ryan K, (eds): Maternal–Fetal Endocrinology. Philadelphia, Saunders, 1980, with permission.*)

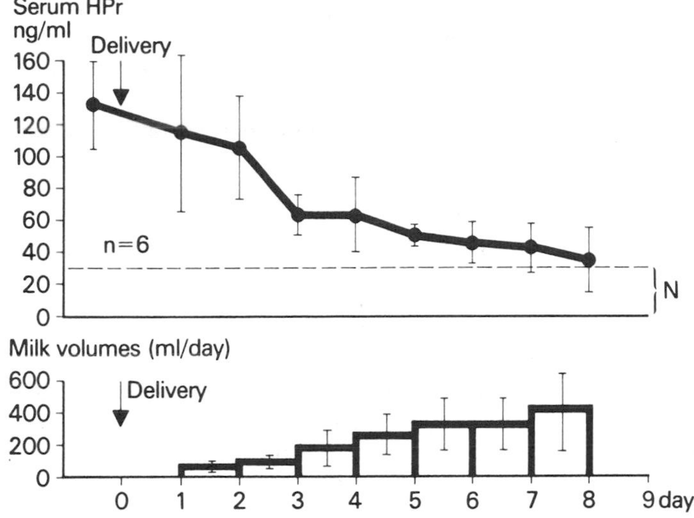

Figure 17-2. Suckling stimulates let-down and milk production long after serum prolactin levels have returned to normal in nursing women. *(From Brun del Re R et al., with permission.[3])*

continued. It is hypothesized that this event involves increased sensitivity of the breast to lower levels of prolactin.

TREATMENT FOR LACTATION SUPPRESSION

A significant percentage of patients will experience symptomatic breast engorgement, lactation, and breast pain during the first few days postpartum. Studies on the incidence of symptoms vary widely but reveal a range of subjective and objective symptomatology of 25 to 80 percent in placebo-controlled populations.[5-9] Marked symptoms in these individuals ranged from 15 to 49 percent for engorgement, 15 to 33 percent for breast pain, and 15 to 20 percent for excessive lactation.[5-8] While these numbers are significant, many patients are asymptomatic, or require modest symptomatic treatment, and have an uncomplicated resolution of symptoms. Pharmacologic agents demonstrated to be effective for lactation suppression during the puerperium include chlorotrianisene, the combination of estradiol valerate and testosterone enanthate, and bromocriptine mesylate.

Chlorotrianisene (TACE)

Chlorotrianisene is a synthetic, orally effective, nonsteroidal substance. This compound (tri-*p*-anisylcholoroethylene) is classified as a proestrogen, as it is presumably altered in the body prior to exerting its effect. The prolonged estrogenic effect results from storage in adipose tissue and gradual release into the systemic circulation. The recommended dosage is one tablet (72 mg) orally twice daily for 2 days, beginning within 8 hours of delivery. Alternative dosages include 12 mg orally four times daily for 7 days or 24 mg orally four times daily for a total of six doses. The mechanism of lactation suppression by estrogenic substances is felt to result from local effects on breast tissue. Animal studies have shown that estrogen implants in rat breast tissue decreased milk secretion, while similar implants in the pituitary gland and median eminence stimulated a release of prolactin.[1] Subsequent human clinical trials failed to show reductions in serum prolactin levels during therapy with exogenous estrogens despite demonstrable lactation suppression.[2,3] These data suggest a localized inhibitory effect at the breast.

Chlorotrianisene has been demonstrated

to be significantly better than a placebo in the prevention of breast engorgement, pain, and lactation.[5-7] These findings were present in 10 to 35 percent of women receiving chlorotrianisene, but symptoms were severe in less than 10 percent of treated individuals. A rebound phenomenon of engorgement and lactation following completion of therapy was found in early studies,[6] but these findings were not substantiated by other investigators.[7] Lochial flow, uterine involution, and return of menstrual function were not significantly altered when compared to a placebo group.[5,7]

Testosterone Enanthate and Estradiol Valerate (Deladumone OB, Ditate-DS)

This compound contains the long-acting steroid esters testosterone enanthate (360 mg) and estradiol valerate (16 mg). The recommended dose is a single 2-ml IM injection administered at the beginning of the second state of labor or within the first hour following parturition. The mechanism of action is considered to be due to local inhibitory effects of estrogen on breast tissue rather than a central effect. Previous experience suggested a reduction in estrogenic side effects when these substances were combined with androgenic compounds.[8] Androgens alone suppress lactogenesis, but are unsatisfactory therapy due to their side effects. Other double-blind studies have demonstrated more effective lactation suppression with combined androgen-estrogen preparations when compared to estrogen alone.[6,7]

In previous controlled studies, testosterone enanthate and estradiol valerate were found to be significantly more effective than a placebo in the prevention of breast engorgement, pain, and lactation.[6-10] These symptoms were present in 1 to 20 percent of patients in pooled series, but most studies demonstrated an incidence of severe symptoms which was less than 5 percent. Initial concerns regarding maternal effects from the androgenic component were unfounded, since virilization has not occurred when the androgen is administered with estrogen. No statistical difference was found in the occurrence of rebound lactation, amount of lochial flow, progress of uterine involution, or return of menstrual function when this compound was compared to a placebo.[7-9] Local discomfort and the risks associated with IM injection must be taken into account prior to administration.

Bromocriptine Mesylate (Parlodel)

Bromocriptine is a nonestrogenic, nonhormonal agent, whose action is systemic rather than local. Bromocriptine is a dopamine receptor agonist with a direct effect on the anterior pituitary gland resulting in an inhibition of prolactin secretion.[11] Some experimental evidence also suggests a hypothalamic effect that increases PIF.[12]

The recommended dosage is one tablet (2.5 mg) orally twice daily for 14 days, with an additional 7 days of treatment should rebound effects occur. Bromocriptine has been found to be significantly better than a placebo in the prevention of breast engorgement, pain, and lactation in clinical trials.[12,13] The specific effect of bromocriptine is demonstrated by a prompt decrease in prolactin suppression during treatment (Fig. 17–3).[3] The transient rise in prolactin levels in response to suckling is also abolished by bromocriptine therapy (Fig. 17–4).[3] Bromocriptine has even been demonstrated to suppress previously initiated lactation in a high percentage of patients.[11,13] This condition is unresponsive to hormonal therapy.

The absence of symptoms with bromocriptine use for postpartum women has been reported in 98 to 99 percent for engorgement, 77 to 85 percent for lactation, and 94 to 95 percent for rebound mammary congestion with pain when compared to placebo controls.[3,11-13] Side effects from the medication are infrequent but include headache, nausea, and dizziness. A potentially significant side effect was the occurrence of hy-

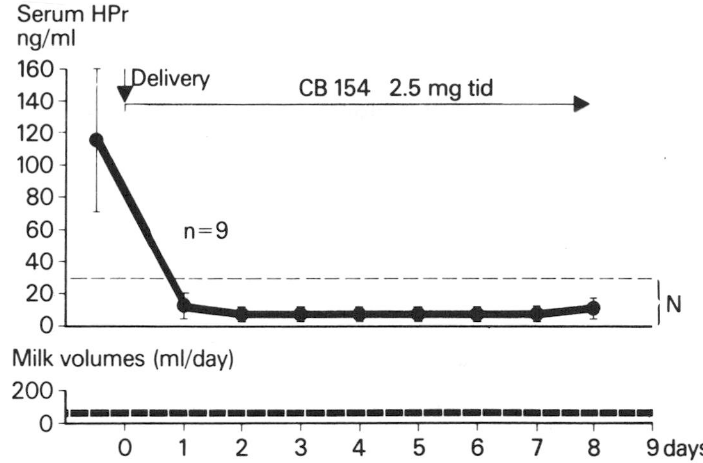

Figure 17–3. Prompt suppression of prolactin secretion with bromocriptine. (*From Brun del Re R et al., with permission.*[3])

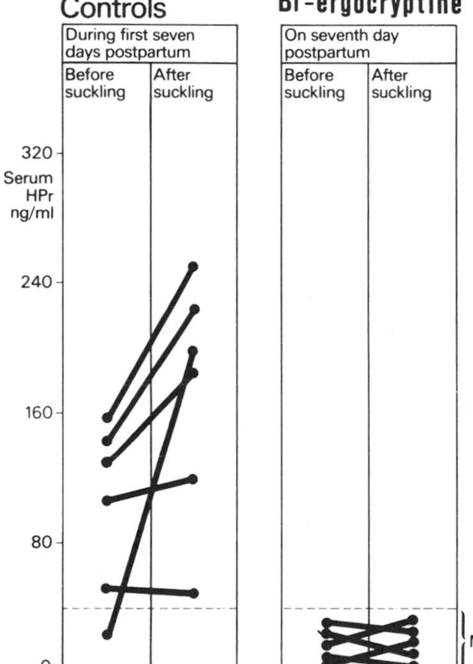

Figure 17–4. The transient rise in prolactin levels in response to suckling is also abolished by bromocriptine therapy. (*From Brun del Re R et al., with permission.*[3])

potension in over 25 percent of cases in earlier studies, though syncopal episodes were noted in less than 1 percent of cases (product insert). A recommendation has subsequently been adopted to delay administration of the drug until vital signs are stable and a minimum of 4 hours has elapsed since delivery.

A recent revision in the product labeling has occurred due to reports of postpartum hypertension, seizures, and cerebrovascular accidents associated with bromocriptine.[14] A cause-and-effect relationship has not been established, yet these postpartum vascular events have been described with other ergot alkaloid derivatives. The Food and Drug Administration has requested further reports of postpartum incidents to further elucidate the possible relationship. Mild to moderate rebound breast symptoms have been reported in 18 to 40 percent of cases, but these effects are controlled by continuation of treatment for an additional 7 days.

Gynecologic uses for bromocriptine include the treatment of various amenorrhea-galactorrhea syndromes, induction of ovulation, and symptomatic relief of the premenstrual syndrome (Chap. 21).[15,16]

TABLE 17–1. DOSAGES, ROUTES OF ADMINISTRATION, AND COST CONSIDERATIONS AMONG LACTATION SUPPRESSANTS

Drug	Route of Administration	Dose	Cost
Chlorotrianisene (TACE)	Oral	72 mg twice daily for 2 days	Equal
Testosterone enanthate/ estradiol valerate (Deladumone OB, Ditate-DS)	IM	2 ml IM	Equal
Bromocriptine mesylate (Parlodel)	Oral	2.5 mg twice daily for 14 days	3–4X other substances

Special Considerations

Thromboembolism with Lactation Suppressants

Significant concern has arisen over the use of estrogens in the puerperium and the possible potentiation of thromboembolic events. An epidemiologic review indicates that the risk of thromboembolism during pregnancy and postpartum is greater than five times that for nonpregnant control subjects.[17] The pathophysiology of puerperal thromboembolism is a complex entity involving numerous contributing factors, particularly advanced maternal age and an operative vaginal or abdominal delivery.

The additive effect of estrogens utilized for lactation suppression seemed to contribute toward an increased risk of thromboembolic disease in British studies.[17–19] The incidence of deep vein thrombophlebitis (DVT) was not statistically different in women under the age of 25 having pharmacologic lactation suppression following normal spontaneous vaginal deliveries when compared to a similar, untreated group. Women over the age of 25 and those patients undergoing operative delivery were found to have a higher incidence of thromboembolic disease. The incidence of DVT and embolism ranged from two- to tenfold higher in the group treated with estrogen when compared to an untreated control group. The studies indicate an increase from a baseline of 1 to 2 cases of thromboembolism per 1000 deliveries of lactating mothers to 6 to 10 thromboembolic events per 1000 deliveries treated with estrogens for lactation suppression. Women over the age of 35 undergoing cesarean section were at highest risk. It should be emphasized that the estrogens studied were ethinyl estradiol and diethylstilbestrol, but that similar concerns must be applied to all estrogens used for lactation suppression. The decision for use of estrogenic compounds in the puerperium must have the potential benefit of lactation suppression weighed against the possible risk of thromboembolic disease.

Bromocriptine is nonestrogenic and is not associated with an increased risk for thromboembolic disease or in any demonstrable alteration in coagulation factors studied to date.[11,13]

Cost Comparison

Presently, chlorotrianisene and the testosterone-estradiol compounds are comparably priced. Bromocriptine is three to four times this cost, depending on length of treatment (Table 17–1).

REFERENCES

1. Bruce JO, Ramirez VD: Site of action of the inhibitory effect of estrogen upon lactation. Neuroendocrinology 6:19, 1970
2. L'Hermite M, Stavric V, Robyn C: Human pituitary prolactin during pregnancy and post-

partum as measured in serum by a radioimmunoassay. Acta Endocrinol (KBH) 159 (Suppl):37, 1972

3. Brun del Re R, del Pozo E, de Grandi P, et al.: Prolactin inhibition and suppression of puerperal lactation by a Br-ergocryptive (CB-154). Obstet Gynecol 41:884, 1973
4. Turkington RW, Hill RL: Lactose synthetase: Progesterone inhibition of the induction of α-lactalbumin. Science 153:1458, 1969
5. Tyson JEA: A high-dosage estrogen for lactation suppression. Obstet Gynecol 27:729, 1966
6. Schwartz DJ, Evans PC, Garcia C-R, et al.: A clinical study of lactation suppression. Obstet Gynecol 42:599, 1973
7. Morris JA, Creasy RK, Hohe PT: Inhibition of puerperal lactation. Obstet Gynecol 36:107, 1970
8. Womack WS, Smith SW, Allen GM, et al.: A comparison of hormone therapies for suppression of lactation. South Med J 55:816, 1962
9. Iliya FA, Safon L, O'Leary JA: Testosterone emanthate (180 mg) and estradiol valerate (8 mg) for suppression of lactation: A double-blind evaluation. Obstet Gynecol 27:643, 1966
10. Markin KE, Wolst MD: A comparative controlled study of hormones used in the prevention of postpartum breast engorgement and lactation. Am J Obstet Gynecol 80:128, 1960
11. Cooke I, Foley M, Lenton E, et al.: The treatment of puerperal lactation with bromocriptine. Postgrad Med J 52:75, 1976
12. Rolland R, Schellekens, L: A new approach to the inhibition of puerperal lactation. J Obstet Gynaecol Br Commonw 80:945, 1973
13. Nilsen PA, Meling A-B, Abildgaard U: Study of the suppression of lactation and the influence on blood clotting with bromocriptine (CB-154) (Parlodel): A double-blind comparison with diethylstilboestrol. Acta Obstet Gynecol Scand 55:39, 1976
14. ADR Highlight No. 83-12, FDA (HFN-730), 5600 Fishers La., Rockville, MD 20857
15. Parkes D: Drug therapy—bromocriptine. N Engl J Med 301:873, 1979
16. Elsner CW, Buster JE, Schindler RA, et al.: Bromocriptine in the treatment of premenstrual tension syndrome. Obstet Gynecol 56:723, 1980
17. Jeffcoate TNA, Miller J, Roos RF, Tindall VR: Puerperal thromboembolism in relation to the inhibition of lactation of oestrogen therapy. Br Med J 4:19, 1968
18. Turnbull AC: Puerperal thromboembolism and suppression of lactation. J Obstet Gynaecol Br Commonw 75:1321, 1968
19. Tindall VR: Factors influencing puerperal thromboembolism. J Obstet Gynaecol Br Commonw 75:1324, 1968

18

Drugs in Breast Milk

Debra K. Gardner and William F. Rayburn

The prevalence of breastfeeding has increased dramatically during the past decade. The Ross National Mothers Survey of 10,000 women indicated that the number of mothers that breastfeed at the time of hospital discharge had increased from 33 percent in 1975 to 43 percent in 1977.[1] The 1984 *Report of the Surgeon General on Breastfeeding and Human Lactation* stated that 61 percent of American women now breastfeed their newborns. The emergence of this trend coincides with an increased awareness of the advantages of breastfeeding by a more health conscious society. Psychologists have demonstrated the importance of the maternal–infant bond during the early days of life, and the advantages of breastfeeding are well documented.[2] Members of all health care professions are involved in educating parents on breastfeeding, and organizations have been formed to encourage nursing mothers.

As a result of the increased interest in breastfeeding, knowledge about drug therapy and exposure to environmental pollutants during lactation are becoming more important. The long-term consequences to infants being fed breast milk containing drugs and other chemicals remain unknown. To alter the practice of routine weaning as a precaution during drug therapy, accurate information must be available to evaluate the risks and benefits of therapy to both the mother and the infant.

Only within the last 5 to 10 years have sound pharmacokinetic principles been applied in research on drug excretion in human breast milk. Older studies were of variable quality and often contradictory with most human data including only a small number of patients or a single case report. Single determinations of a drug in breast milk are of limited value. Animal studies may be misleading due to species variations in pH, milk composition, and metabolic differences. Certain drug assay procedures in the past lacked sensitivity and specificity, and extraction from either the aqueous or lipid phase was often not quantitative.

Many important drugs still have not been adequately studied and information regarding drug effects on infants is generally lacking. Manufacturer's unpublished data and the use of phrases such as "may" or "might" when referring to the possible effect of the drug on the nursing infant are often understood to mean the drug is contraindicated in nursing mothers. An understanding of the pharmacokinetic properties of the drug and serial measurements of drug levels in maternal plasma, breast milk, and infant plasma are necessary. Drug therapy that is beneficial for the mother and not detrimental to the infant is the ultimate goal.

SYNTHESIS AND COMPOSITION OF MILK

Mammary glands are morphogenetically similar to sweat glands. They are composed of alveolar cells, which produce and secrete milk into a lumen, and myoepithelial cells, which have contractile properties that permit expulsion of milk from the alveoli into the duct system. Milk in the lumen is separated from the extracellular space by a semipermeable lipoid membrane similar to other biologic membranes in the body.

Breast milk resembles an oil-in-water emulsion consisting of fat droplets suspended in an isotonic aqueous medium in which lactose, inorganic salts, and protein are dissolved. Casein, the primary milk protein, is assembled in the ribosomes of the rough endoplasmic reticulum. Other proteins in milk include serum albumin, α-lactalbumin, β-lactoglobulins, immunoglobulins, and other glycoproteins. Total milk protein concentration is approximately 0.9 g/dl.[3] The predominant carbohydrate nutrient in milk is lactose, which is synthesized from maternal glucose and galactose in the Golgi apparatus by the enzyme, lactose synthetase. Lactose creates an osmotic gradient drawing water into the alveoli, forming the aqueous phase of milk and therefore regulating milk volume. Protein is combined with its carbohydrate complement within the Golgi apparatus prior to its secretion into the alveolar lumen.

Lipid droplets in milk are primarily composed of cholesterol and its esters, phospholipids, triglycerides, and free fatty acids. These droplets are engulfed in the apical membrane and are eventually discharged into the lumen. Ions are either free in solution or bound to milk proteins, and are usually transported into alveolar cells by passive diffusion. A low sodium concentration is maintained in milk by active extrusion of sodium ions by the basal portion of the secretory cell back into plasma.[4] Calcium, magnesium, and amino acids appear to be actively transported into the alveolus.[5]

Variations in milk composition and yield become important when dealing with drug excretion, as the distribution will depend on their degree of solubility in either the aqueous or lipid fraction of milk and their degree of binding to milk proteins. As colostrum progresses to mature milk, the profile of protein and lipid content changes. Total lipid content increases and protein decreases. Milk from mothers who deliver prematurely contains significantly higher concentrations of protein, sodium, chloride, and lactose than milk of mothers delivering at term.[6] The milk the infant receives initially during a feeding (fore-milk) differs in composition from that received during the latter part of a feeding (hind-milk). The rate of fat production and fat concentration, along with protein concentration, increases during the last half of feeding. Fat excretion has diurnal variations, with its minimum content being the first morning feeding and its highest concentration being the midmorning feeding with a progressive decline throughout the day.[7]

There is a direct relationship between blood flow to the breast and milk yield. The amount of milk produced is also dependent upon the age and needs of the infant. Average daily milk yield is in the range of 600 to 840 ml.[8]

PRINCIPLES OF DRUG TRANSFER INTO MILK

Principles of drug transfer into milk and the effect on the infant encompass absorption, distribution, metabolism, and elimination of a drug in both the mother and the infant. This concept is illustrated in Figure 18–1, and is described in detail in the sections that follow.

Drugs and pollutants present in maternal blood must cross the capillary endothelium, extracellular spaces, and the hydrophobic barrier created by the alveolar cell membrane before entering the milk. Most drug transfer occurs by passive diffusion, in which the concentration gradient governs solute movement. As maternal plasma levels decrease, the drug concentration in the milk decreases by back diffusion.[7] Some ionized particles and small hydrophilic drugs with molecular weights less than 200 penetrate the membrane through aqueous channels or pores.[9] Facilitated diffusion, an uncommon method of drug transfer, explains the passage of water-soluble substances too large to pass through membrane pores.[10] Active transport mechanisms requiring energy provide a process whereby substances are carried from a lower concentration to a higher concentration. Substances that are actively transported include glucose, amino acids, calcium, and magnesium, but very few drugs have been found to use this mechanism of transfer.[4] Pinocytosis and reverse pinocytosis are involved in the transport of very large molecules and proteins.

Drug transfer and concentration in breast milk is influenced by the drug's physical and chemical properties (molecular weight, degree of ionization, solubility characteristics, and protein-binding). Compounds with very high molecular weights such as heparin cannot pass through cell membranes into milk. Most clinically useful drugs have molecular weights between 250 and 500, and their passage into breast milk depends on their lipid solubility and degree of ionization, since usually the unionized lipid-soluble form passes through the cell membrane.

The degree of ionization of weak acids and bases is related to the pH of the medium and to the drug dissociation constant (pKa) and is described by the Henderson–Hasselbach equation.[11]

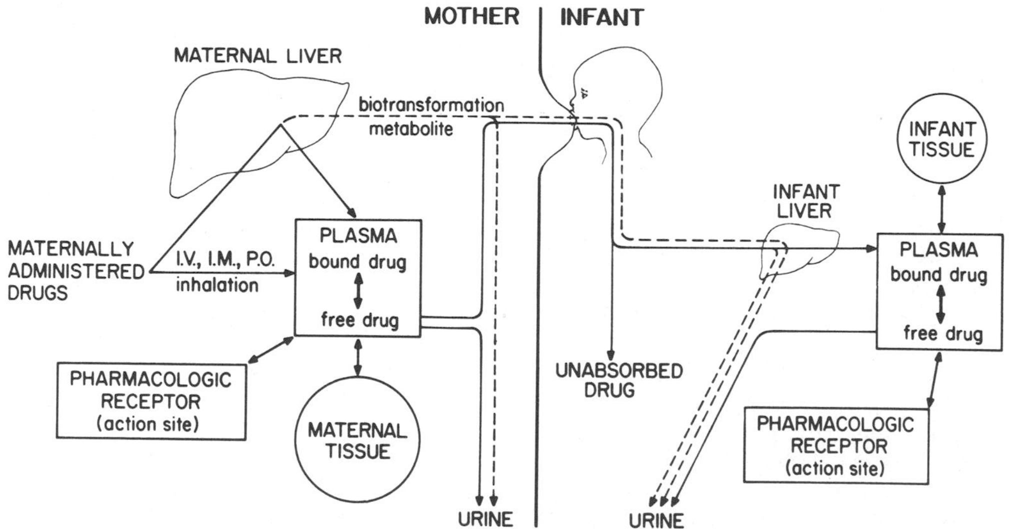

Figure 18–1. Drug disposition in the maternal infant unit. *(From Giacoia GP, Catz CS, 1979, with permission.[10])*

$$\text{pH} = \text{pKa} + \log \frac{\text{(proton acceptor)}}{\text{(proton donor)}}$$

The breast milk pH ranges from 6.6 to 7.3 which is lower than plasma and interstitial fluid.[12] The unionized drug concentration in plasma establishes equilibrium across the alveolar cell membrane and is equivalent to the unionized drug concentration in milk. Weak bases are more unionized in the higher pH of the plasma and pass readily into the more acidic milk where they become ionized and "trapped," creating a higher concentration in milk than in plasma. Weak acids such as barbiturates, organic acids, sulfonamides, diuretics, and benzyl penicillin have an equal or lower concentration in milk than in plasma. Drug dissociation constants for commonly prescribed medications can be found in Appendix I.

Since milk contains a lipid phase, highly lipophilic drugs may partition into milk fat and achieve higher concentrations in milk than in plasma. However, this is a relatively minor determinant of total drug concentration in milk. Lipid-soluble drugs diffuse more rapidly across the hydrophobic alveolar cell membrane, attaining higher peak milk concentrations. Therefore, the important consequence of lipid solubility is the rate at which the drug appears in milk rather than the extent of its passage into milk.[13] The blood flow to the breast is another factor that determines the rate of a drug's presentation to the milk.

Protein binding characteristics of a compound also govern the amount of drug in breast milk, since the unbound fraction is readily excreted into milk. Most drugs are much less highly bound to milk proteins than plasma proteins.[8] Equilibrium is established between the free (unbound) drug concentration in plasma and the milk ultrafiltrate (aqueous portion excluding milk proteins and fat). Therefore, drugs that are highly protein bound in plasma will generally achieve low milk concentrations. The extent of plasma protein binding of certain drugs appears in Appendix I.

The following example illustrates how these pharmacokinetic principles can be applied to calculate the approximate milk concentration that a drug might achieve.

Phenytoin (Dilantin), a weak acid with a pKa of 8.3, is approximately 90 percent bound to plasma proteins and for the purpose of this example, its binding to milk proteins is assumed to be negligible. The total (bound + unbound) steady-state serum concentration (Cp_{total}) of phenytoin in a lactating woman is 12 mcg/ml.

Free phenytoin plasma concentration (Cp_{free})

$$\begin{aligned} Cp_{free} &= Cp_{total} \times \text{fup} \\ &\quad \text{(fraction unbound in plasma)} \\ &= 12 \text{ mcg/ml} \\ &= 1.2 \text{ mcg/ml} \end{aligned}$$

Unionized phenytoin milk concentration [(unionized) m] at equilibrium

$$\text{pH} = \text{pKa} + \log \frac{\text{(ionized) p}}{\text{(unionized) p}}$$

$$7.4 = 8.3 + \log \frac{\text{(ionized) p}}{\text{unionized) p}}$$

$$\text{(unionized) p} = 1.07 \text{ mcg/ml}$$

Unionized phenytoin milk concentration [(unionized) m] at equilibrium

$$\text{(unionized) m} = \text{(unionized) p} = 1.07 \text{ mcg/ml}$$

Total phenytoin milk concentration (Cm_{total}) assuming breast milk pH is 6.8

$$6.8 = 8.3 + \log \frac{\text{(ionized) m}}{\text{(unionized) m}}$$

$$31.6 = \frac{\text{(unionized) m}}{\text{(ionized) m}}$$

$$\begin{aligned} \text{(ionized) m} &= 0.034 \text{ mcg/ml} \\ Cm_{total} &= \text{(unionized) m} + \text{(ionized) m} \\ &= 1.104 \text{ mcg/ml} \end{aligned}$$

The phenytoin milk concentration may be somewhat higher due to binding to milk proteins and partitioning into the lipid phase of milk.

The milk/plasma (M:P) ratio represents the relative drug concentrations in milk and plasma when both fluids are measured simultaneously after equilibrium has been established. Milk/plasma ratios that are calculated based on the physicochemical properties of the drug rather than measured are considered to be theoretical. When comparing M:P ratios of drugs, it is important to note whether the value is theoretical or measured.

When drug therapy is essential in a lactating woman, selection of an agent within a therapeutic class should be based on physicochemical properties that will minimize drug concentration in milk. Compounds that are weak acids and extensively bound to plasma proteins do not favor partitioning into milk. A short half-life and a high maternal clearance are pharmacokinetic parameters that are advantageous, since rapid elimination from the mother's body prevents accumulation in breast milk. Drugs with extremely long half-lifes may accumulate in both maternal plasma and breast milk with chronic dosing. Combination products that may contain unnecessary drugs should generally be avoided while priority should be given to hydrophilic compounds and agents with low M:P ratios. The smallest potential for adverse effects on the infant is, of course, one of the most important factors in drug selection.

The amount of drug present in the milk and consumed by the infant depends on the dose, frequency and duration of exposure, route of administration, and the time of drug administration relative to infant feedings. The lowest effective dose should be prescribed and alternative dosage regimens can be employed when they are known to be equally effective, such as administering the total daily dose of phenytoin at bedtime. Patients on chronic drug therapy should be counseled to schedule doses in such a way that the infant is not fed at times of peak milk levels of the drug (generally 1 to 1.5 hours after dose). Administering medications after infant feedings or just prior to the infant's longest sleep period will generally achieve this goal.

ABSORPTION AND ELIMINATION OF DRUGS BY THE NURSING INFANT

The nursing infant is constantly maturing and the manner in which it absorbs, tolerates, and metabolizes drugs can vary within a short period of time. The bioavailability of compounds ingested by the infant depends on the functional readiness of the gastrointestinal tract.

Drugs that are normally too large to be absorbed or that are usually destroyed in the gastrointesinal tract, such as hormones and parenterally administered antibiotics, may reach the neonate's systemic circulation to a greater degree than in an older infant. This may be due to higher gastric pH and increased permeability of the gastrointestinal mucosa in the newborn. Gastric emptying time is generally prolonged and a slower transit time in the upper small intestine may also enhance absorption of certain drugs. Some drugs (e.g., tetracycline) form complexes with components in the milk, which limits their absorption.

Drug distribution in the neonate differs from that of an adult in that the neonate has a larger extracellular fluid volume and a smaller deposition of fat.[10] Drugs that are confined to extracellular fluid (aminoglycosides, ampicillin, ticarcillin) have larger distribution volumes in newborns.[14] Total serum protein concentrations are lower in newborns than in adults, which limits available protein binding sites. Only free (unbound) drug diffuses across cell membranes and exerts pharmacologic activity. Therefore, a neonate may exhibit a more profound response secondary to an elevated free fraction of drug (phenyltoin, theophylline, diazepam) despite low total drug concentrations.[8] Jaundice may occur when drugs (sulfonamides) displace bilirubin from plasma protein binding sites.

During the first few months of life, drug-metabolizing pathways and kidney function are not fully developed. The half-lifes of certain drugs are prolonged and make the infant susceptible to toxicity from drug accumulation (Chap. 1). Hepatic glucuronyl transferase is deficient in the neonate which accounts for the slower elimination of chloramphenical[14] and cases of hyperbilirubinemia when certain drugs (estrogens, progestins) are ingested by the nursing infant.[15] The rate of drug metabolism and excretion develops rapidly during the first 6 months of life.[8]

Another concern is idiosyncratic reactions precipitated by compounds in milk that are not dose related or allergic in nature. Red blood cell hemolysis occurs in glucose-6-phosphate dehydrogenase (G6PD)-deficient infants and occasionally in preterm infants after ingestion of agents such as nitrofurantoin, sulfonamides, probenecid, and chloramphenicol.[16] Drug sensitization can also occur via breast milk and the possibility of allergic reactions exists, particularly to penicillins.

Estimates of the dose received by the infant through breast milk can be made if the M:P ratio, maternal plasma level (Cp_{avg}), and the total amount of milk consumed are known.

$$\text{Infant dose(mg/kg/day)} = Cp_{avg} \times \text{M:P} \times \text{milk volume (ml/kg/day)}.$$

There is considerable variation in infant milk consumption, and daily intake can range from 130 to 180 ml/kg depending on age, weight, and sex.[13] The estimated dose ingested by the infant can be compared to recommended pediatric dosages when available to assess the possibility of pharmacologic activity. Monitoring infant plasma levels is indicated if adverse effects are exhibited or if the drug has a very narrow therapeutic range. When a course of a potentially hazardous drug must be prescribed, breastfeeding may have to be discontinued temporarily. During this time the mother can manually or mechanically express and discard milk to maintain her milk supply. After drug discontinuation, breastfeeding may be reinstituted when five half-lifes of the drug have elapsed.

ASSAY TECHNIQUES

Studies of drug excretion in breast milk conducted before the 1970s often reported the amount in milk to be "undetectable" or "trace" because of insensitive assay techniques. Research on many of these drugs has not been repeated with the more sensitive assays now available and inaccurate data still remain in the literature. Milk concentrations of many compounds are only a fraction of that in plasma and assay methods that are commonly employed to measure therapeutic plasma concentrations are not adequate to quantify the amount in milk. The greater sensitivity of high performance liquid chromatography (HPLC) is better suited to the low concentration of drugs that do not readily pass into breast milk.

Breast milk differs from other commonly analyzed body fluids because high concentrations of fatty acids and lipids reduce extraction efficiency and interfere with certain analyses. Analysis of compounds with a high lipid solubility therefore requires multiple solvent extractions. The removal of lipids by washing with a low polarity solvent (e.g., hexane) may lower recovery of the drug.[4] A control of breast milk containing no drugs must be used rather than plasma in making reference standards for calibrating breast milk drug assays. Special buffering techniques may be necessary to accommodate the lower pH of milk.

Assay techniques commonly employed for breast milk include gas liquid chromatography, gas chromatography-mass spectometry, and radioimmunossay as well as HPLC. Drug manufacturers are usually willing to assay milk for their drug products and will provide information for proper storage and transport of the sample.

DRUGS THAT AFFECT THE PRODUCTION OF MILK

Mammary blood flow determines the rate of drug presentation to the breast. Factors regulating mammary blood flow include the metabolic activity in the mammary gland, the release of lactogenic hormones in response to suckling, a decrease in intramammary pressure due to the removal of accumulated secretions in the alveoli as sucking occurs, and the use of certain drugs. Mammary blood vessels are extremely sensitive to vasoconstrictors. Drugs with sympathomimetic activity (stimulants, decongestants) can decrease blood flow and milk yield. Large amounts of nicotine in mothers who smoke heavily (one to two packs/day) can decrease milk supply.[9] Vasodilating drugs can increase the rate of excretion of substances that are rapidly excreted by the alveolar epithelium, since their transport is flow dependent.

Prolactin secretion is susceptible to drug modification. Levodopa, ergocriptine, bromocriptine, pyridoxine, and monoamine oxidase inhibitors cause stimulation of dopamine receptors either directly or indirectly in the hypothalamus, which increases the release of prolactin inhibitory factor (Chap. 14). Conversely, drugs acting on the hypothalamus to suppress prolactin inhibitory factor secretion include phenothiazines, cimetidine, metoclopramide, methysergide, and certain antihypertensive agents (reserpine, clonidine, and methyldopa).[17] Metoclopramide, a potent stimulator of prolactin release, increases milk yield and enhances the rate of transition from colostrum to mature milk[18] and has been used to restore milk flow in women whose volume has decreased.[19]

COMMONLY ENCOUNTERED DRUGS DURING LACTATION

Physicians often encounter the following classes of drugs when treating nursing mothers or answering their questions. Specific information concerning individual drugs is found in the Appendix at the end of this chapter and discussed in further detail as follows.

Alcohol, Caffeine, and Nicotine

Most babies are periodically or chronically exposed to alcohol through breastfeeding. Ethanol in plasma rapidly equilibrates in breast milk, and the M:P ratio is 0.9.[4] Almost every source of information dealing with the presence of alcohol in breast milk recounts a case report published in 1936 involving a mother who ingested 750 ml of port wine during a 24-hour period. The affected infant displayed unarousable sleep with snoring, deep respiration, and no reaction to pain.[20] If a moderate social drinker (two to three cocktails, two to three glasses of wine, or two to three 340-ml bottles of beer) had a blood alcohol concentration of 50 mg/dl, the nursing infant would receive about 82 mg of alcohol, which would produce insignificant blood concentrations.[4] Mild sedation can occur in the infant whose mother's blood alcohol concentration is 300 mg/dl. This is probably the highest alcohol concentration at which a mother would still be capable of nursing her infant. Furthermore, there is no evidence that occasional moderate ingestion of alcohol by the mother is harmful to the infant. For obvious reasons, intoxicated mothers should not breastfeed their babies, and chronic alcoholic mothers who will not stop drinking should be discouraged from breastfeeding.

Maternal ingestion of a single caffeinated beverage (35 to 336 mg) produces peak milk levels (2.09 to 7.17 mcg/ml) within 1 hour, and the average infant dose ingested is very small (0.57 mg).[21] However, if a breastfeeding mother drinks six to eight cups of caffeine-containing beverages, including coffee, tea, and colas, her infant is likely to show signs of caffeine stimulation such as hyperactivity and wakefulness.[22] It is therefore recommended that nursing mothers limit their intake of caffeine-containing beverages to one to two cups/day.

Nicotine can enter the milk and reach

relatively low levels (0.01 to 0.05 mg/dl) if 20 cigarettes are smoked per day.[9] Since nicotine is not readily absorbed by the infant's intestinal tract and is rather quickly metabolized, signs of nicotine intoxication are unlikely. If maternal smoking exceeds 20 to 30 cigarettes/day, milk yield may significantly decrease and may explain any symptoms of nausea, vomiting, abdominal cramping, and diarrhea in the infant.

ANALGESICS

Aspirin and nonsteroidal anti-inflammatory drugs (NSAIDs) are highly protein bound weak acids that do not favor passage into breast milk. Salicylate levels in milk are very low, but since infant elimination is slower than in adults, accumulation can occur with chronic exposure to high maternal doses. Some authors recommend monitoring infant prothrombin time if antiarthritic doses are required by the mother.[23] Metabolic acidosis has been reported in an infant whose mother was taking extremely large doses of aspirin.[24] Ibuprofen (Motrin) was not detectable in breast milk (by gas-liquid chromatography) of mothers taking 400 mg every 6 hours.[25,26] Small amounts of naproxen (Naprosen) were found in urine of an infant whose mother required 375 mg twice daily.[27]

Standard doses of acetominophen appear to have no harmful effects on infant. The estimated infant dose ingested in 100 ml of milk is 0.14 percent of a 10-grain maternal dose.[3]

Older studies of the excretion of narcotic analgesics into human breast milk were limited by inadequate sensitivity of the analytical methods employed. Amounts in milk were often reported to be nondetectable. These compounds are lipophilic weak bases and are expected to rapidly enter milk and achieve concentrations exceeding that of plasma. Recent studies on codeine in breast milk support this (M:P = 2.16), although the dose ingested by the nursing infant was calculated to be very small (0.07 mg) or 0.15 percent of a 60 mg maternal dose.[24] Infants of breastfeeding mothers on methadone maintenance (10 to 80 mg/day) reportedly do well[28] with the exception of the death of a five-week-old infant with multiple organ abnormalities found at autopsy and a blood methadone level of 0.04 mg/dl (toxic levels = 0.2 mg/dl) presumably ingested via breast milk.[29]

Antibiotics

Most antibiotics appear in breast milk, and their concentration in milk depends mainly upon the pKa of the drug, its lipid solubility, and protein-binding capabilities.

Sulfonamides appear in milk in varying concentrations according to their pKa values. Sulfapyridine readily passes into milk because it is a very weak acid (pKa 8.4) and is therefore unionized. Only rarely has an adverse reaction been reported from the presence of sulfas in milk. Hyperbilirubinemia and jaundice can occur in the early weeks of life due to displacement of protein-bound bilirubin.[30] One case of hemolytic anemia has been reported in a G6PD-deficient infant.[9]

Penicillins and cephalosporins are excreted in milk in relatively low concentrations with M:P ratios ranging from 0 to 0.2.[4] The risk of sensitization is possible, and an allergic reaction has been reported in an infant whose mother was being treated for syphilis with penicillin.[7] Cephalothin and cefazolin are not well absorbed into the systemic circulation when ingested orally through breast milk. Although the doses are pharmacologically insignificant, gut levels may be sufficient to disturb local flora and produce candidiasis, diarrhea, and thrush.

Tetracyclines appear in milk in concentrations ranging between 60 and 80 percent of the maternal plasma concentration, but are usually undetected in the infant's plasma.[4] The relative gastric achlorhydria of newborns may decrease solubility and absorption of tetracyclines.[4] Calcium and proteins bind tightly to tetracyclines, which limits the absorption of this group of drugs. The theoretical risks of teeth staining and delayed bone growth have not been reported during breastfeeding. Some authors still do not negate this possibility and recommend alternate therapy if possible.[31]

The aminoglycoside antibiotics are generally considered safe to use during lactation because of poor gastrointestinal absorption in the infant. If gastrointestinal inflammation or diarrhea exists in the infant, there may be increased absorption of aminoglycosides, and ototoxicity and nephrotoxicity become a greater risk. Infant plasma concentration should be monitored in such circumstances.

Chloramphenicol concentrations in milk are half that of the mother's plasma. Its use is contraindicated in the very early postpartum period because even small absorbed amounts can accumulate in the very young infant and cause bone marrow depression.[32]

Some antibiotics concentrate in the milk and their observed M:P ratios are greater than 1. These include erythromycin, metronidazole, isoniazid (INH), and trimethoprim.[4] Sources that state metronidazole (Flagyl) is contraindicated during breastfeeding base their advice on the compound's carcinogenic effect in rodents consuming high doses throughout their lives. Specific untoward effects have not been reported in infants. Short courses for parasitic infections for which metronidazole is the drug of choice (amebiasis, giardiasis, trichomoniasis) are probably not harmful to the infant. If a mother has active tuberculosis, breastfeeding is contraindicated. Both isoniazid (INH) and its metabolite acetylisoniazid, which is thought to be responsible for liver toxicity, are excreted in milk.[3] A breastfed infant could ingest significant quantities of both compounds while the mother is on chronic therapy. If treatment with INH is necessary, the infant should be monitored closely for signs of toxicity (vomiting, respiratory distress, and central nervous system depression).

Anticoagulants

The major anticoagulants are safe during breastfeeding. Heparin has a molecular weight of 17,000 and is too large to pass into breast milk. Warfarin is highly bound to plasma proteins, weakly acidic, and usually ionized, and therefore goes undetected in breast milk, even with very sensitive assays.[34,35] Dicumarol also appears to be safe for nursing mothers.[36] Bleeding problems and increases in the infant's prothrombin time have been associated with phenindione and ethylbiscoumacetate.[35]

Laxatives

It is believed that anthraquinone cathartics (senna, cascara sagrada, danthron, and casanthrol) may appear in breast milk. The exact form of the drug absorbed and the extent of absorption into the maternal circulation is unknown. Infant gastrointestinal effects such as diarrhea and colic when lactating mothers were given anthraquinone derivatives have been reported.[37] Another laxative, phenolphthalein, is seldom found in breast milk, and is therefore not often associated with diarrhea in the infant. Bisacodyl is not excreted in breast milk.[9] Anionic surfactants (dioctyl sodium sulfosuccinate) and bulk formers including bran, methylcellulose, and psyllium hydrophyllic mucilloid are the laxatives of choice for lactating mothers because they are not absorbed into the maternal circulation.

Oral Contraceptives

Controversy still exists regarding the use of oral contraceptives during lactation. Proliferation of vaginal epithelium in female nurslings has been ascribed to maternal contraceptive use,[38] while ingestion of the comparatively high sex steroid doses contained in earlier contraceptive preparations was reported to cause gynecomastia in one male infant.[39] If large amounts of estrogens and progestins are absorbed from the ingested milk into the baby's circulation, hyperbilirubinemia may result since the steroids compete for binding of glucuronic acid in the liver and displace bilirubin from plasma protein-binding sites.[15] However, adverse effects in the infant are rare and with less than 1 percent of the maternal dose appearing in milk, oral contraceptives containing 2.5 mg or less of a progestin (19-nortestosterone derivatives) and 50 mcg or less of ethinyl estradiol or 100 mcg or less of mestranol present no hazards to breastfeeding infants.[9] No adverse effects on the infant during the ensuing years in bone maturation, genital development, or impaired fertility have been substantiated.

The main controversy centers not on the hormone's direct effect on the infant, but on the effect of the contraceptive steroids on maternal milk composition and yield. Inhibition of lactation results from a direct suppressive effect of estrogen on the breast. Combination oral contraceptives used widely before 1966 contained higher doses of estrogens and progestogens and had a greater inhibitory effect on lactation than the present low dose preparations.[40] Products containing progestogens only have little or no effect on milk production.[41] Oral contraceptives have the most pronounced inhibitory effect on milk yield when started early in the puerperium before lactation is well established. Some studies have documented significantly lower infant weights during the first year when low dose oral contraceptives (ethinylestradiol 30 mcg, levonorgestrel 150 mcg) were instituted at 30 days postpartum,[42,43] while initiating the same low dose oral contraceptive at 90 days postpartum had only a moderate effect on lactation and no differences on infant weights at 1 year.[44] Other reviewers emphasize that the composition and volume of milk varies considerably in the absence of steroidal contraception and even though changes in these values occur with contraceptive use, they tend to be within normal ranges.[45,46] Numerous variables influence a woman's ability to breastfeed, and these factors are difficult to control during research. In Third World nations where maternal nutrition may be substandard and breast milk the sole source of nutrition in the infant, close monitoring of infant growth and development is advised when mothers use oral contraceptives for extended periods. When supplementation of the natural contraceptive effect of lactation is necessary in the early postpartum period, a progestin-only method (norethisterone 300 mcg, Depo-Provera injection) insures minimal effect on milk composition and yield.[40,41]

REFERENCES

1. Lawrence RA: Breast-Feeding: A Guide for Medical Profession. St. Louis, Mosby, 1980, pp 5–6
2. Jelliffee DB, Jelliffee EFP: "Breast is best": Modern meanings. N Engl J Med 297:912, 1977
3. Berlin CM Jr: Pharmacologic considerations of drug use in the lactating mother. Obstet Gynecol 58:195, 1981
4. Wilson JT, Brown RD, Cherek DR, et al.: Drug excretion in human breast milk, principles, pharmacokinetics, and projected consequences. Clin Pharmacokinet 5:1, 1980
5. Gaginella TS: Drugs and the nursing mother infant. US Pharmacist 3:39, 1978
6. Gross SJ, Geller J, Tomarelli RM: Composition of breast milk from mothers of preterm infants. Pediatrics 68:490, 1981
7. Catz CS, Giacoia GP: Drugs in breast milk (Symposium on pediatric pharmacology). Pediatr Clin North Am 19:151, 1972
8. Wilson JT: Determinants and consequences of drug excretion in breast milk. Drug Metabol Rev 14:619, 1983
9. Vorherr H: Drug excretion in breast milk. Postgrad Med 56:97, 1974
10. Giacoia GP, Catz CS: Drugs and pollutants in breast milk (Symposium on pharmacology). Clin Perinatol 6:181, 1979
11. Newton DW, Kluza RB: pKa values of medicinal compounds in pharmacy practice. Drug Intell Clin Pharmacol 12:546, 1978
12. Lien EJ, Kuwahara J, Koda RT: Diffusion of drugs into prostatic fluid and milk. Drug Intell Clin Pharm 8:470, 1974
13. Anderson PO: Drugs and breastfeeding. Semin Perinatol 3:271, 1979
14. Green TP Mirkin BL: Clinical Pharmacokinetics: Pediatric considerations. In Benet LZ, Massoud N, Gambertoglio JG (eds): Pharmacokinetic Basis for Drug Treatment. New York, Raven Press, 1984, pp 269–282
15. Wong YK, Wood BS: Breast-milk jaundice and oral contraceptives. Br Med J 4:403, 1971
16. Cole CH (ed.): The Harriet Lane Handbook ed 10. Chicago, Year Book Medical Publishers, 1984, p 214

17. Dickey RP: Drugs affecting lactation. Semin Perinatol 3:279, 1979
18. deGezelle H, Ooghe W, Thiery M: Metoclopramide and breast milk. Eur J Obstet Gynecol Reprod Biol 15:31, 1983
19. Sousa PL: Metoclopramide and breast-feeding. Br Med J 1:512, 1975
20. Bisdom CJW: Alcohol and nicotine poisoning in nurslings. Maandschr Kindergeneeskd 6:332, 1936
21. Berlin CM, Denson HM, Daniel CH, et al.: Disposition of dietary caffeine in milk, saliva, and plasma of lactating women. Pediatrics 73:59, 1984
22. Lawrence RA: Drugs in breast milk. In Breastfeeding: A Guide for the Medical Profession. St. Louis, Mosby, 1980, pp 157–170
23. Bleyer W, Brenkenridge RT: Studies on the detection of adverse drug reactions in the newborn: II. The effects of prenatal aspirin on newborn hemoatasis. JAMA 214:2049, 1970
24. Findlay JWA: The distribution of some commonly used drugs in human breast milk. Drug Metab Rev 14:653, 1983
25. Townsend RJ, Benedetti TJ, Erikson SH, et al.: Excretion of ibuprofen into breast milk. Am J Obstet Gynecol 149:184, 1984
26. Weibert RT, Townsend RJ, Kaiser DG, et al.: Lack of ibuprofen secretion into human milk. Clin Pharmacol 1:457, 1982
27. Jamali F, Tam YK, Stevens RD: Naproxen excretion in breast milk and its uptake by suckling infant. Drug Intell Clin Pharmacol 475, 1982
28. Ananth J: Side effects in the neonate from psychotropic agents excreted through breastfeeding. Am J Psychiatry 135:801, 1978
29. Smialek JE, Monforte JR, Aronow R, et al.: Methadone deaths in children. JAMA 238:2516, 1977
30. Forrest JM: Drugs in pregnancy and lactation. Med J Aust 2:138, 1976
31. Hervada AR, Feit E, Sagraves R: Drugs in breast milk. Perinatal Care 2:19, 1978
32. Abramowicz M (ed): Update: Drugs in breast milk. Med Lett Drug Ther 21:21, 1979
33. Bowes WA, Jr.: The effect of medications on the lactating mother and her infant. Clin Obstet Gynecol 23:1073, 1980
34. L'Orme M, Lewis PJ, DeSwiet M, et al.: May mothers given warfarin breastfeed their infants? Br Med J 1:1564, 1977
35. DeSwiet M, Lewis PJ: Excretion of anticoagulants in human milk. N Engl J Med 297:1471, 1977
36. Bambel CE, Hunter RE: Effect of dicoumarol on the nursing infant. Am J Obstet 59:1153, 1950
37. Knowles JA: Breast milk: A source of more than nutrition for the neonate. Clin Toxicol 7:69, 1974
38. Lauritzen C: On endocrine effects of oral contraceptives. Acta Endocrinol 124 (Suppl):87, 1967
39. Curtis EM: Oral contraceptives feminization of a normal male infant. Obstet Gynecol 23:295, 1964
40. Hull VJ: Research on the effects of hormonal contraceptives on lactation: Current findings, methadological considerations and future priorities. World Health Stat Q 36:168, 1983
41. Adey T, Brown JB: Norethisterone concentrations in milk of lactating women using a progestagen-only pill. J Obstet Gynaecol 3:112, 1982
42. Croxatto HB, Diaz S, Peralta O, et al.: Fertility regulation in nursing women. IV. Long term influences of a low-dose combined oral contraceptive initiated at day 30 postpartum upon lactation and infant growth. Contraception 27:13, 1983
43. Diaz S, Peralto O, Juez G, et al.: Fertility regulation in nursing women. III. Short term influences of a low-dose combined oral contraceptive initiated at day 30 postpartum upon lactation and infant growth. Contraception 27:13, 1983
44. Peralto O, Diaz S, Juez G, et al.: Fertility regulation in nursing women. V. Long term influences of a low-dose combined oral contraceptive initiated at day 90 postpartum upon lactation and infant growth. Contraception 27:27, 1983
45. Lonnerdal B, Forsum E, Hambraeus L: Effect of oral contraceptives on composition and volume of breast milk. Am J Clin Nutr 33:816, 1980
46. Segal S: Breastfeeding and contraception. Pediatrics 68:138, 1981
47. Anderson PO: Drugs and breastfeeding—A review. Drug Intell Clin Pharmacol II: 208, 1977
48. O'Brien TE: Excretion of drugs in human milk. Am J Hosp Pharmacol 31:844, 1974
49. Knowles JA: Excretion of drugs in milk—A review. J Pediatr 66:1068, 1965
50. Yoshioka H, Cho K, Takimoto M, et al.: Transfer of cefazolin into human milk. J Pediatr 94:151, 1979
51. Santo GH, Huch A: Passage of cefoxitin into breast milk. Infection 7(Suppl):90, 1979

52. Dresse A, Lambotte R, Dubois M, et al.: Transmammary passage of cefoxitin: Additional results. J Clin Pharmacol 23:438, 1983
53. Dubois M, Delapierre D, Chanteux L, et al.: A study of the transplacental transfer and the mammary excretion of cefoxitin in humans. J Clin Pharmacol 21:477, 1981
54. Snider DE, Powell KE: Should women taking antituberculosis drugs breastfeed? Arch Intern Med 14:589, 1984
55. Stoehr GP, Juhl RP, Veals J, et al.: The excretion of rosaramicin in breast milk. J Clin Pharmacol 25:89, 1985
56. Heisterburg L, Branebjerg PE: Blood and milk concentrations of metronidazole in mothers and infants. J Perinatol Med 11:114, 1983
57. Allgen LG, Holmberg G, Person B, et al.: Biological fate of methenamine in man. Acta Obstet Gynecol Scand 58:287, 1979
58. Miller RD, Keegan KA, Thrupp LD, et al.: Human breast milk concentration of moxalactam. Am J Obstet Gynecol 148:348, 1984
59. Kauffman RE, O'Brien C, Gilford P: Sulfisoxazole secretion into human milk. J Pediatr 97:839, 1980
60. Niebyl JR, Blake DA, Freeman JM, et al.: Carbamazepine levels in pregnancy and lactation. Obstet Gynecol 53:139, 1979
61. Kaneko S, Sata T, Suzuki K: The levels of anticonvulsants in breast milk. Br J Clin Pharmacol 7:624, 1979
62. Froescher W, Eichelbaum M, Niesen M, et al.: Carbamazepine levels in breast milk. Ther Drug Monitor 6:266, 1984
63. Rosenbloom D, Upton AR: Drug treatment of epilepsy: A review. Can Med Assoc J 128:261, 1983
64. Steen B, Rane A, Lonnerholm G, et al.: Phenytoin excretion in human breast milk and plasma levels in nursed infants. Ther Drug Monitor 4:331, 1982
65. Von Unruh GE, Froescher W, Hoffman F, et al.: Valproic acid in breast milk—How much is really there? Ther Drug Monitor 6:272, 1984
66. McKenna WJ: Amiodarone in pregnancy and lactation. Am J Cardiol 51:1231, 1983
67. White WB, Andreoli JW, Wong SH, et al.: Atenolol in human plasma and breast milk. Obstet Gynecol 63:42S, 1984
68. White WB: Management of hypertension during lactation. Hypertension 6:297, 1984
69. Levy M, Granit LB, Laufer N: Excretion of drugs in human milk. N Engl J Med 297:789, 1977
70. Hoskins JA, Holliday SB: Methyldopa in breast milk and its relation to maternal plasma levels. J Obstet Gynecol 3:109, 1982
71. Pittard WB, Glazier H: Procainamide excretion in human milk. J Pediatr 102:631, 1983
72. Baver JH, Pape B, Zajecek J, et al.: Propranolol in human plasma and breast milk. Am J Cardiol 43:860, 1979
73. Smith MT, Livingstone I, Hooper WD, et al.: Propranolol, propranolol glucuronide, and Naphthoxylactic acid in breast milk and plasma. Ther Drug Monitor 5:87, 1983
74. Joelsson I (ed): Drug use during pregnancy and breastfeeding. Acta Obstet Gynecol Scand Suppl 126:11, 1984
75. Fidler J, Smith V: Excretion of oxprenolol and timolol in breast milk. Br J Obstet Gynecol 90:961, 1983
76. Lustgarten JS, Podos SM: Topical timolol and the nursing mother. Arch Ophthalmol 101:1381, 1983
77. Anderson HJ: Excretion of verapamil in human milk. Eur J Clin Pharmacol 25:279, 1983
78. Miller ME, Cohn RD, Burghart PH: Hydrochlorothiazide disposition in a mother and her breastfed infant. J Pediatr 101:789, 1982
79. Kearns GL, McConnell RF, Trang JM, et al.: Appearance of ranitidine in breast milk following multiple dosing. Clin Pharmacol 4:322, 1985
80. Hayes AH, Novitch M, Nightingale S, et al. (eds): Advice on limiting intake of bonemeal. FDA Drug Bull 12:5, 1982
81. Sovner R, Orsulak PJ: Excretion of imipramine and desipramine in human breast milk. Am J Psychiatry 136:4A, 1979
82. Rey E, Giraux P, D'Athis PH, et al.: Pharmacokinetics of the placental transfer and distribution of clorazepate and its metabolite nordiazepam in the feto-placental unit and in the neonate. Eur J Clin Pharmacol 15:181, 1979
83. Linden S, Rich CL: The use of lithium during pregnancy and lactation. J Clin Psychiatry 44:358, 1983
84. Tegler L, Lindstron B: Antithyroid drugs in milk. Lancet 2:591, 1980
85. Lamberg BA, Skonen E, Osterlund K, et al.: Antithyroid treatment of maternal hyperthyroidism during lactation. Clin Endocrinol 21:81, 1984
86. Spak CJ, Hardell LI, deChateau P: Fluoride in human milk. Acta Paediatr Scand 72:699, 1983
87. Lindberg C, Boreus LD, deChateau P, et al.: Transfer of terbutaline into breast milk. Eur J Resp Dis 65:87, 1984

88. Yurchak AM, Jusko WJ: Theophylline secretion into breast milk. Pediatrics 57:518, 1976
89. Cruikshank DP, Varner MW, Pitkin RM: Breast milk magnesium and calcium concentrations following magnesium sulfate treatment. Am J Obstet Gynecol 143:685, 1982
90. Kim-Farley R, Brink E, Orenstein W, et al.: Vaccination and breastfeeding (letter). JAMA 248:2451, 1982
91. McKenma R, Cole ER, Vasan V: Is warfarin sodium contraindicated in the lactating mother? J Pediatr 103:325, 1983
92. Berlin CM, Yaffe SJ: Disposition of salicylazosulfapyridine (Azulfidine) and metabolites in human breast milk. Dev Pharmacol Ther 1:31, 1980

APPENDIX: DRUG OR CHEMICAL, QUANTITY EXCRETED IN BREAST MILK, AND NEONATAL EFFECTS (AT MATERNAL THERAPEUTIC DOSES)

Drug (Brand)	Quantity Excreted in Milk	Neonatal Effect at Maternal Therapeutic Doses	Reference(s)
Analgesics and Anti-Inflammatory Drugs			
Acetaminophen	M:P[†] = 0.76–0.92 less than 0.1% of a single 500-mg dose in 100 ml milk	NS* at usual doses. Estimated portion of one maternal dose delivered to infant is 0.14%.	8, 24
Aspirin	1–3 mg/dl when plasma level is 1–5 mg/dl; M:P = 0.05, 0.18–0.36% of maternal dose appears in milk	Transfer to milk not favored. At maternal dose of 12–16 tablets per day, no ill effects on infant. When mother requires high antiarthritic doses, monitor infant for bruisability. May interfere with infant's platelet function.	47, 24, 3
Codeine	M:P = 2.16	NS.	24
Flufenamic acid	M:P = 0.008	Passage into milk not favored due to compound's acidity.	24
Heroin	Variable amounts	Can cause addiction. Levels in milk not high enough to prevent withdrawal in addicted infants.	22, 47, 48
Ibuprofen (Motrin, Advil)	Not detectable (<1 mcg/ml) after 400 mg every 6h	NS.	25, 26
Indomethacin (Indocin)	Excreted	Case report of convulsions in breastfed infant. Used to close patent ductus arteriosus. Insufficient data on the effect on other vessels. May be nephrotoxic.	22
Mefenamic acid (Ponstel)	Negligible amounts	NS.	47, 48
Methadone (Dolophine)	Avg M:P = 0.83 (range 0.3–1.89)	Breastfeeding permissible during methadone maintenance. Up to 80 mg/day, no ill effects on infant.	24, 28
Meperidine (Demerol)	M:P = 1.1–1.2	NS.	24, 47
Morphine	Less than 6 mcg/ml	Amount excreted probably insignificant in clinical use, but may be ex-	22, 47, 48

(continued)

APPENDIX: (*Continued*)

Drug (Brand)	Quantity Excreted in Milk	Neonatal Effect at Maternal Therapeutic Doses	Reference(s)
		creted in higher amounts in addicts. Potential for accumulation. May be addicting to neonate.	
Naproxen (Naprosen)	176–237 mcg/dl; dose 375 mg bid	NS, total cumulative amount excreted in infant urine is 0.26% of maternal dose.	
Pentazocine (Talwin)	Not excreted	None.	5, 22, 49
Phenylbutazone (Butazolidin)	6.3 mcg/ml 1.5 hr after 750-mg IM dose; M:P = 0.13	Infant serum levels 3–20 mcg/ml after 750-mg IM dose. Risk to infant not well defined. May accumulate in infant. Caution due to possible idiosyncratic blood dyscrasias.	22, 47
Propoxyphene (Darvon, Darvocet)	0.4% of material dose (manufacturer states M:P = 0.5)	Only symptoms detectable would be failure to feed and drowsiness. If mother ingests maximum recommended dosage in a 24-hr period, the infant could receive 1 mg/day, a significant dose in a neonate.	22, 28
Oxyphenbutazone (Tandearil)	Not detectable in 53 of 55 subjects; 10–80% of material plasma level	No known effect. Oxyphenbutazone is a metabolite of phenylbutazone; caution is advised.	48
Antibiotics			
Amantadine (Symmetrel)	Excreted, not quantified	May cause vomiting, urinary retention, skin rash.	47, 48
Ampicillin	0.07 mcg/ml; M:P = 0.06–0.3	NS, possibility of allergic sensitization exists, can produce candidiasis and diarrhea in infant.	4, 47, 48
Carbenicillin (Geopen)	0.265 mcg/ml 1 hr after 1-g dose	NS.	48
Cefazolin (Ancef, Kefzol)	Peak level 1.51 mcg/ml 3 hr after 2-g IV dose; M:P = 0.023	NS, not absorbed well orally. 0.075% of maternal dose excreted in milk.	3, 50

APPENDIX: *(Continued)*

Drug (Brand)	Quantity Excreted in Milk	Neonatal Effect at Maternal Therapeutic Doses	Reference(s)
Cefoxitin (Mefoxin)	0.8–1.0 mcg/ml at maternal dosage of 3 g/day. Maximum milk concentration of 0.65 mcg/ml at 1 hr after 2 g IM dose	Infant could receive 0.7 mg/day, NS peak milk concentration occurs at 4–7 hr after IM injection in most subjects.	51, 52, 53
Cephalexin (Keflex)	Peak levels: 5 mcg/ml	Infant could receive up to 0.1 mg/oz of milk. This amount should have no deleterious effect.	4
Cephalothin (Keflin)	Has not yet been found in milk	NS.	22
Chloramphenicol (Chloromycetin)	15–25 mcg/ml; M:P = 0.5; 50% of drug in milk is inactive metabolite	Contraindicated due to possibility of bone marrow depression. Infant does not excrete drug well, may accumulate.	4, 9, 32, 47
Chloroquine (Aralen)	<2 mcg/ml	Reports to date have failed to consider chloroquin's 5-day half-life. Probably NS.	48
Clindamycin (Cleocin)	2.1–3.8 mcg/ml peak 2–4 hr after therapeutic dose	NS.	47
Colistin (Coly Mycin)	0.05–0.09 mg/100 ml	Not well absorbed orally. NS.	9
Cycloserine (Seromycin)	M:P = 0.3–1.18 (avg. 0.72); 6–19 mcg/ml after 250 mg PO four times daily	No adverse effects reported in infants. 0.6% of maternal dose excreted in milk.	47, 54
Demeclocycline (Declomycin)	Not detected at dose of 300 mg/day. 60 ng to 1.4 mcg/ml at doses > 600 mg/day. Avg. M:P = 0.7. Detectable for up to 3 days after last dose	Same precautions as tetracycline.	47
Doxycycline (Vibramycin)	Avg. 770 ng/ml 3 hr after second dose (200 mg × 1, 100 mg every 24 hr). 380 ng/ml 24 hr after second dose. M:P = 0.3–0.4	Same precautions as tetracycline.	47
Erythromycin	3–5 mcg/ml; M:P = 0.5–3.0. Milk concentration can be up to six times plasma	May concentrate in milk, although conflicting reports. Maternal plasma protein bind of 80%	4, 47, 48, 55

(continued)

APPENDIX: (*Continued*)

Drug (Brand)	Quantity Excreted in Milk	Neonatal Effect at Maternal Therapeutic Doses	Reference(s)
		should prevent high milk concentrations. Principally excreted in the liver. Infant's liver function is not fully developed. Risk of jaundice.	
Ethambutol	M:P = 1.0	No reports available.	54
Gentamicin (Garamycin)	Unknown	Not well absorbed from GI tract. May change gut flora. If GI inflammation or diarrhea exists, monitor infant's serum levels to avoid otoxicity and nephrotoxicity.	22
Isoniazid	Peak 16.6 mcg/ml; dose 300 mg 0.6–1.2 mg/100 ml after 10-mg/kg dose; M:P > 1 Metabolite acetyl-INH also excreted, peak 3.76 mcg/ml	Acetyl-INH thought to cause liver toxicity. Infant could ingest significant amounts (25% of maternal dose) if on chronic therapy.	3, 9, 49, 54
Kanamycin (Kantrex)	Peak 18.4 mcg/ml after 1-g IM dose. 0.05% of administered drug appears in the milk per day. M:P = 0.4–1.0	Probably NS. (Same precautions as Gentamicin.)	4, 48
Lincomycin (Lincocin)	0.5–2.4 mcg/ml; M:P = 0.15–2.25	NS.	4, 47, 48
Mandelic acid (Methenamine mandelate—Mandelamine is 50% mandelic acid)	300 mg every 24 hr after dose of 12 g/day	NS.	22, 48
Methacycline (Rondomycin)	50–260 mcg/100 ml; M:P = 0.5 after therapeutic dose	Same precautions as tetracycline.	9, 48
Methenamine hippurate (Hiprex)	71.4 μmol/L after 1-g dose; M:P = 1.08	Infant would receive 0.05–0.1 mg/kg. No untoward effects.	57
Metronidazole (Flagyl)	Up to 13.1 mcg/ml; after therapeutic doses of 600–1200 mg/day; M:P = 0.62–1.25 avg. M:P = 1.0; hydroxymetabolite M:P = 0.64–1.44	Several sources state contraindicated due to possibly carcinogenic effects in animal studies. Maximum calculated infant amount in-	

APPENDIX: (*Continued*)

Drug (Brand)	Quantity Excreted in Milk	Neonatal Effect at Maternal Therapeutic Doses	Reference(s)
		gested = 3.0 mg/kg. Infant plasma levels approach therapeutic concentrations. Short courses probably NS.	
Minocycline (Minocin)	0.8 mcg/ml after 200-mg dose	Same precautions as tetracycline.	4, 47
Moxalactam (Maxam)	1.56–3.24 mcg/ml after 2 g IV every 8h maternal dose	Infant could ingest 2 mg/day in 550 ml/milk. Theoretical risk of enterocolitis from altered GI flora.	58
Nalidixic acid (NegGram)	4 mcg/ml at dose of 1 g four times daily	NS. One case of hemolytic anemia in G6PD-deficient infant.	7, 47
Nitrofurantoin (Macrodantin)	Trace amount	NS, except in G6PD-deficient infants. No adverse effects reported in normal infants.	33, 47
Nystatin (Mycostatin)	Not found, not absorbed orally	None.	22
Oxacillin (Prostaphlin)	Not found	None.	48
Oxytetracycline (Terramycin)	2–3 mcg/ml	Same precautions as tetracycline.	4, 48
Para-aminosalicylic acid	Not found	None.	22
Penicillin, benzathine	10–12 units/100 ml	NS; possibility of allergic sensitization.	4, 9, 47, 48
Penicillin G	0.06–0.96 units/ml; M:P = 0.03–0.2	NS; possibility of allergic sensitization.	4, 9, 47, 48
Penicillin VK	0.05–0.3 units/ml	NS; possibility of allergic sensitization.	48
Pyrimethamine (Daraprim)	3.1–3.3 mcg/ml, peak at 6 hr after 50–75-mg dose, detectable up to 48 hr after single dose	Quantity excreted not sufficient to treat malaria in infants less than 6 months old, although there have been cases where this has been accomplished via drug in milk.	47
Quinine sulfate	0.4–1.6 mcg/ml, peak 1.5–6 hr after 600- to 1300-mg dose	Probably NS.	46
Rifampin	Peak 30 mcg/ml; M:P = 0.16–0.6	0.05% of maternal dose excreted in milk. Probably NS.	54

(*continued*)

APPENDIX: ***(Continued)***

Drug (Brand)	Quantity Excreted in Milk	Neonatal Effect at Maternal Therapeutic Doses	Reference(s)
Rosaramicin (investigational macrolide)	Mean M:P = 0.12 Peak milk concentrations 27.8–44.7 ng/ml occurred at 2–4 hr after 250-mg PO dose	Estimated infant dose ingested 30 mcg/day. Probably NS.	55
Streptomycin	M:P = 0.4–1.0, 1.1–1.3 mcg/ml 6 hr after 1-g IM dose	NS. (Same precautions as Gentamicin.) 0.5% of maternal dose excreted in milk.	4, 5, 48, 54
Sulfacetamide	M:P = 0.08	Probably NS. Neonatal jaundice due to displacement of bilirubin from protein-binding sites. Hemolytic anemia in G6PD-deficient infants. Rash.	5
Sulfadiazine	M:P = 0.21	Probably NS. (Same precautions as sulfacetamide.)	5
Sulfamethazine	M:P = 0.51	Same as sulfacetamide.	5
Sulfamethoxazole (Gantanol)	Excreted, not quantified	Caution during first 2 weeks of life. Same precautions as sulfacetamide.	48
Sulfanilamide	M:P = 1.0, 90 mcg/ml after dose of 2–4 g/day	Greater risk of hyperbilirubinemia encephalopathy because of high concentration in milk.	4, 5
Sulfapyridine	M:P = 0.85, 30–130 mcg/ml after dose of 3 g/day	Same as sulfanilamide.	5
Sulfathiazole	M:P = 0.43, 5 mcg/ml after dose of 3 g/day.	Probably NS. (Same precautions as sulfacetamide.)	5
Sulfisoxazole (Gantrisin)	Mean M:P = 0.06 for sulfisoxazole and M:P = 0.22 for N-acetyl metabolite, 0.45% of maternal dose recovered in milk	NS. Amount absorbed from milk too small to cause displacement of bilirubin from protein binding sites in healthy term neonate.	
Tetracycline (Sumycin)	0.5-2.6 mcg/ml after dose of 500 mg four times daily, M:P = 0.2-1.4 (avg. 0.7)	Infant serum levels less than lower limit of assay. Use not recommended due to possibility of mottling of teeth and delayed bone growth.	4, 31, 47

APPENDIX: (*Continued*)

Drug (Brand)	Quantity Excreted in Milk	Neonatal Effect at Maternal Therapeutic Doses	Reference(s)
Trimethoprim (Trimpex; also in combination with sulfamethoxazole in Bactrim and Septra)	1.2–5.5 mcg/ml; Avg. M:P = 3.7	Newborns absorb approximately 0.75–1.0 mg/day. May accumulate due to immature renal function. Toxicity includes vomiting, bone marrow depression, and thrombocytopenia.	13, 47
Anticoagulants			
Bishydroxycoumarin (Dicumarol)	0.2 mg/100 ml; M:P = 0.01–0.02	Usually NS. Monitor infant. Vitamin K may be given to infant if PT warrants or if infant to undergo surgery.	4, 9, 36
Ethyl Biscoumacetate (Tromexan)	0–0.17 mg/100 ml. No correlation with dosage, unidentified active metabolite found in milk	Avoid use due to reported episodes of hemorrhage of umbilical stump and cephalohematoma.	4, 9, 47
Heparin	Does not pass into milk	None.	4, 35, 47
Phenindione (Hedulin)	Secretion erratic. Levels less than 1 mcg/ml; M:P = 0.012–0.06	Case report of increased PT and PTT in infant, and incisional and scrotal hemorrhage after inguinal herniotomy.	4, 7, 9, 47
Warfarin (Coumadin)	Extensively, protein bound acidic. Not significantly excreted in milk. <25 ng/ml (lower limit of assay)	NS. May safely breastfeed.	34, 47, 91
Anticonvulsants			
Carbamazepine (Tegretol)	1.0–4.8 mcg/ml (mean 2.5 mcg/ml) M:P = 0.25–0.58 (mean 0.36). Epoxide metabolite M:P = 0.53. M:P = 0.4–0.7, 1.9 ± 1.6 mcg/ml; at maternal doses of 1000 mg/day	A 4-kg infant would receive approximately 0.5 mg/kg. Infant serum levels in range of 1.0 mcg/ml peak serum level of 4.7 mcg/ml reported in one infant. Long-term effects unknown. Monitor for poor sucking, sedation, and vomiting.	60, 61, 62
Ethosuximide (Zarontin)	21.3 ± 2.8 mcg/ml, M:P = 0.788 ± 0.328 at therapeutic dose	6% of maternal dose excreted in milk. Infant plasma levels may reach 25% of maternal	61, 63

(*continued*)

APPENDIX: ***(Continued)***

Drug (Brand)	Quantity Excreted in Milk	Neonatal Effect at Maternal Therapeutic Doses	Reference(s)
		plasma levels. Monitor infant closely.	
Phenobarbital	Marked individual variation due to pKa (7.2) near physiologic pH 10.4 ± 10.8 mcg/ml; M:P = 0.459 ± 0.249 at therapeutic dose	Maternal doses of 60–200 mg/day usually safe for infant. Infant may ingest up to 16.5 mg/day. May induce hepatic microsomal enzymes; drowsiness in some cases.	4, 28, 61
Phenytoin (Dilantin)	0.8 ± 0.3 mcg/ml; M:P = 0.181 ± 0.059.[38] When maternal plasma level = 4.5 ± 1.4 mcg/ml, M:P = 0.45.[3,7] One report of 6 mcg/ml in breast milk when maternal plasma level was 28 mcg/ml	Usually no effect at maternal doses of 300 mg/day. Calculated infant dose ingested 0.03–0.47 mg/kg/day. Infant phenytoin clearance usually high. In one study 2 infants had low but detectable plasma levels. None of the infants exhibited adverse effects. Possibility of enzyme induction. One case report of methemaglobinemia and cyanosis in infant whose mother was taking phenytoin and phenobarbital.	4, 9, 61, 64
Primidone (Mysoline)	2.3 ± 2.2 mcg/ml, M:P = 0.81 ± 0.176 at therapeutic doses	Drowsiness and decreased feeding. May cause bleeding due to hypoprothrombinemia. Avoid use during lactation.	5, 48, 61
Valproic acid (Depakene)	0.4–3.9 mcg/ml, mean 1.9 mcg/ml; dose 300–2400 mg/day M:P = 0.01–0.1	Amount of drug presented to infant via milk very small. Probably NS.	65
Antihistamines and Decongestants			
Dexbrompheniramine Maleate, 6 mg with *d*-isophedrine 120 mg (sustained release tablets) (Drixoral)	Excreted	One case report of irritability, excessive crying, and disturbed sleeping patterns of 5 days' duration. Avoid long-acting preparations.	4
Diphenhydramine (Benadryl)	Excreted	NS. May cause sedation, decreased feeding, or	4, 48

APPENDIX: (*Continued*)

Drug (Brand)	Quantity Excreted in Milk	Neonatal Effect at Maternal Therapeutic Doses	Reference(s)
		may produce stimulation and tachycardia.	
Trimeprazine (Temaril)	Excreted	NS. (Same precautions as diphenydramine.)	4, 48
Tripelennamine (Pyribenzamine)	Excreted	NS. (Same precautions as diphenhydramine.)	4, 48
Autonomic Drugs			
Atropine	0.1 mg/100 ml	Hyperthermia, atropine toxicity (infants especially sensitive). Inhibits lactation.	22, 48
Carisoprodol (Soma, Rela)	May be present at concentrations two to four times that of maternal plasma	CNS depression, GI effects.	48
Ergotamine (Cafergot)	Excreted, not quantified	Signs of ergotism; vomiting, diarrhea, weak pulse, and unstable blood pressure. Short courses probably NS. High doses inhibit prolactin.	22, 33
Menpenzolate bromide (Cantil)	Not excreted	None.	5, 48
Methocarbamol (Robaxin)	Trace amounts	NS.	48
Neostigmine	Not excreted	None.	22
Propantheline bromide (Probanthine)	Uncontrolled data indicate no measurable amounts	Drug is rapidly metabolized in maternal system to inactive metabolite. Avoid long-acting preparations.	22, 48
Scopolamine (Hyoscine)	Trace amounts	NS.	47
Cardiovascular Drugs			
Amiodarone	2.8–16.4 mg/L; desmethyl 1.1–6.5 mg/L	Estimated drug ingested by infant approximates a low maintenance dose. Not recommended during breastfeeding.	66
Atenolol (Tenormen)	Peak 1.3 mcg/ml; dose 50 mg peak. 1.8 mcg/ml; dose 100 mg M:P = 2.9–3.6	Concentrates in milk. No evidence of bradycardia.	67
Captopril (Capoten)	Peak 4.7 ng/ml; dose 100 mg tid M:P = 0.01	Quantity excreted not thought to be sufficient to cause adverse effects.	68

(*continued*)

APPENDIX: (*Continued*)

Drug (Brand)	Quantity Excreted in Milk	Neonatal Effect at Maternal Therapeutic Doses	Reference(s)
Clonidine (Catapres)	Peak 1.5 ng/ml; dose 150 mcg M:P = 1.5	No reports available.	68
Digoxin (Lanoxin)	0.5–1.0 ng/ml M:P = 0.45–1.0. 0.07–0.14% of maternal dose excreted in milk	Due to large volume of distribution the total daily excretion of digoxin in milk of mothers with therapeutic serum concentrations would not exceed 1–2 mcg, not sufficient to affect child.	3, 6
Dextrothyroxine (Choloxin)	Excreted, not quantified	NS.	40
Guanethidine (Ismelin)	Excreted, not quantified	No adverse effects noted; one infant breastfed by mother on chronic therapy.	68
Hydralazine (Apresoline)	Peak 0.76 mcg/ml; dose 50 mg tid M:P = 0.49	Calculated infant dose 0.013 mg/feeding.	68
Methyldopa (Aldomet)	Total (free ± O-sulfate) 0.8 mcg/ml M:P = 0.35	Infant dose less than 1 mg day. NS. No adverse effects in neonates reported.	71
Metoprolol (Lopressor)	Peak 1.69 mcg/ml; dose 200 mg Peak 1.56 mcg/ml/; dose 100 mg M:P = 3.0–3.7	Concentrates in milk.	68
Nadolol (Corgard)	Peak 357 ng/ml; dose 80 mg M:P = 4.6	Not reported.	68
Prazocin (Minipress)	No reports available	Unknown.	68
Procainamide (PA)	Peak PA 10.2 mcg/ml PA M:P = 4.3 ± 2.4 NAPA M:P = 3.8 ± 1.8	Amount consumed by infant <1.0% of maternal dose, probably NS.	71
Propranolol (Inderal)	Peak 160 ng/ml; dose 160 mg peak 75 ng/ml; chronic dose 1.2 mg/kg/day. Peak milk levels occur 2 hr after peak plasma levels. Avg. M:P = 0.64 (range 0.05–1.65)	Preferred β-blocker in breastfeeding maximum dose ingested by infant (21 mcg/day) less than 0.1% of maternal dose. No adverse effects in infants noted.	2, 6
Quinidine	Excreted, not quantified	Approximately 1% of maternal dose appears in milk.	22
Reserpine	Excreted, not quantified	May cause nasal stuffiness, lethargy, diarrhea,	4, 5

APPENDIX: (*Continued*)

Drug (Brand)	Quantity Excreted in Milk	Neonatal Effect at Maternal Therapeutic Doses	Reference(s)
		increased tracheobronchial secretions with difficulty breathing. Also reported to cause galactorrhea.	
Timolol	Peak 15.9 ng/ml; dose 5 mg tid. Avg. M:P = 0.8 (range 0.25–1.73). Milk levels after 0.5% solution ophthalmic drops OD bld (5.6 ng/ml) 5 × maternal plasma level	Calculated infant dose 2.4 mcg/kg/day when maternal dose 5 mg tid. Can accumulate in milk. Monitor infant for apnea, bradycardia.	75
Verapamil (Isoptin, Calan)	M:P = 0.23 after chronic maternal dose of 80 mg PO tid	Total drug excretion in milk <0.01% of maternal dose. Infant plasma level 2.1 mg/ml. Probably NS.	7
Chemotherapeutic Agents			
Cyclophosphamide (Cytoxan)	Excreted, not quantified	Contraindicated. One report of infant that developed neutropenia.	22, 33, 47
Methotrexate	Minor route of excretion, M:P = 0.08–1.0; 2.6 ng/ml at 10 hr after 22.5-mg dose	Infant could receive 0.26 mcg/100 ml, which researcher consider nontoxic for infant.	22
Diuretics			
Bendroflumethazide (Rauzide, Naturetin)	Excreted, not measured	Lactation suppressed.	47
Chlorthalidone (Hygroton)	0.36 mcg/ml M:P = 0.03–0.05	Baby may ingest 0.18 mg/day when maternal dose 50 mg/day. Effect on infant unknown. Caution due to long t½ (60 hr).	68, 74
Chlorthiazide (Diuril)	Less than 1 mcg/ml after 500-mg daily dose	Amount ingested by infant insignificant. May supress lactation due to dehydration of mother.	22, 74
Furosemide (Lasix)	Not found to be excreted	Possibility of reduced milk production. Effect on infant unknown.	22, 48, 68
Hydrochlorthiazide (Hydrodiuril)	Peak 120 ng/ml M:P = 0.25–0.43, maternal dose, 50 mg/day	Estimated dose ingested by infant 0.05 mg. Probably NS. Infant electrolytes normal.	68, 74, 78

(*continued*)

APPENDIX: (*Continued*)

Drug (Brand)	Quantity Excreted in Milk	Neonatal Effect at Maternal Therapeutic Doses	Reference(s)
Spironalactone (Aldactone)	Principal active metabolite, canrenone, 104 ng/ml M:P = 0.72 (one subject)	Electrolytes normal in infant. Approximately 0.2% of maternal dose transferred to infant.	68, 74
Environmental Agents			
Aldrin	Varies by location	Not a reason to wean. No need to test milk unless inordinate exposure.	22
Dieldrin	Varies by location	Not a reason to wean. Also, found in permanently mothproofed garments. Avoid.	22
DDT	Varies by location, highest in blacks in Mississippi and Arkansas. Avg. American 0.05–0.1 ppm	No need to test milk unless inordinate exposure.	22
Halothane	2 mcg/ml found in breast milk of anesthesiologists	Possibility of hepatic and renal damage. No reports of effects on infants.	10
Heptachlor epoxide	Varies by location	Not a reason to wean. No need to test milk unless inordinate exposure.	22
Hexachlorobenzene	Less than 8 ppb	Severe porphyria and some deaths occurred in nursing infants whose mothers had eaten wheat seed contaminated with hexachlorobenzene in Turkey in 1956.	10
Kepone	Varies by location, concentrates in milk	70 documented cases of poisoning of persons working with kepone. No need to test milk unless inordinate exposure.	10
Mercury	Excreted, varies by location	Several outbreaks of mercury poisoning have occurred in Japan, Iraq, Pakistan, and Guatemala. Poisoning of nursing infants has been documented.	10

APPENDIX: *(Continued)*

Drug (Brand)	Quantity Excreted in Milk	Neonatal Effect at Maternal Therapeutic Doses	Reference(s)
Polybrominated biphenyl (PBB)	Concentrated in milk. A high milk level is 92 ppm	PBB entered animal food chain when cattle feed was contaminated in Michigan; effects unknown.	8, 10
Polychlorinated biphenyl (PCB)	Concentrated in milk. Trace to 5.1 ppm on fat weight basis. Potentially dangerous level >2.3 ppm	If mother at high risk from environment or diet (usually contaminated fish), measure milk level. Breastfed infants of Japanese women who ingested PCBs in contaminated rice oil appeared enervated, expressionless, apathetic, hypotonic, and lacked endurance. Three presented with abnormalities 5 years later. Induction of microsomal liver enzymes.	8, 10
Texachlorethylene	Excreted	Obstructive jaundice.	10
Gastrointestinal Drugs			
Aloe (found in over-the-counter laxative combinations)	Detectable, not quantified	Possible diarrhea.	47
Bisacodyl (Dulcolax)	Not excreted	NS.	4, 9
Cimetidine (Tagamet)	4.88–6.0 mcg/ml after 1000 mg/day × 4 days. M:P = 4.6–11.76	The maximum amount of cimetidine an infant could ingest assuming 1 L/day and fed at times of peak levels, would be 6 mg (1.5 mg/kg for a 4-kg infant). Therefore, caution may be warranted. (Study included only one subject.)	79
Casanthrol (in combination with stool softener in Dialose Plus and PeriColace)	Excreted, not quantified	Possible diarrhea and colic. Usually NS.	4
Cascara sagrada	Excreted, amount not quantified	Possible diarrhea and colic.	4
Castor oil	Believed not to be excreted	NS.	4

(continued)

APPENDIX: (*Continued*)

Drug (Brand)	Quantity Excreted in Milk	Neonatal Effect at Maternal Therapeutic Doses	Reference(s)
Dioctyl sodium sulfosuocinate (Colace)	Not excreted	None.	4
Danthron (Modane, Doxidan)	Excreted, amount not quantified	Possible diarrhea and colic. Usually NS.	4
Magnesium citrate	Magnesium appearance in milk unknown	NS.	4
Milk of magnesia	Magnesium appearance in milk unknown	NS.	4, 47
Mineral oil	Not excreted	None.	4, 47
Phenolphthalein (Correctol, Ex-Lax, Feen-A-Mint)	<300 mg/ml	NS.	4, 47
Psyllium hydrophillic mucilloid (Metamucil)	Not excreted	None.	4
Ranitidine (Zantac)	722–2610 ng/ml after maternal dose of 150 mg every 12h × 5 doses; M:P = 6.8–23.8 (one subject)	Diffusion into milk promoted by low plasma protein binding (15%), weak base (pKa 8.2), and lipid solubility. Concentrates in milk. Peak milk concentration occurred prior to maternal dose.	79
Senna (Senokot)	Less than lower limit of assay (340 mg/ml)	Possible diarrhea and colic, Senokot appears to have no effect on infant.	4, 47
Heavy Metals			
Arsenic	Excreted	Can accumulate in infant's blood. Check level if there is reason to suspect exposure.	22
Copper	Excreted	Unknown.	22
Fluorine	Excreted	Monitor infant for excessive dose (excessive salivation and GI disturbances).	22
Gold thiomalate	0.022 mcg/ml when mother given 50 mg/week	No proteinuria or aminoaciduria observed. Hematologic aberrations, rashes, nephritis, and hepatitis theoretically may occur. No harmful effects have been reported.	10, 22

APPENDIX: (*Continued*)

Drug (Brand)	Quantity Excreted in Milk	Neonatal Effect at Maternal Therapeutic Doses	Reference(s)
Iron	Excreted	Intake of iron is beneficial to mother and infant.	22
Lead	Unknown	Nursing contraindicated if maternal serum 40 mcg/ml. Bone meal or dolomite in natural calcium/phosphorus supplements contains up to 20 ppm lead. Maximum recommended daily intake of lead for infants is 100 mcg/day.	22, 80
Mercury	Excreted	Hazardous to infant.	22
Hormones and Synthetic Substances			
Contraceptives	Less than 1% of dose	Reports of proliferation of vaginal epithelium in female nurslings and gynecomastia in male infants if daily dosage is greater than that recommended below. Diminished lactation if OC use instituted before fourth postpartum week.	9, 46, 42, 40, 43, 44
Ethinyl estradiol	Trace amount	Not significant if daily dose is 50 mcg or less.	9, 46
Mestranol	Trace amount	Not significant if daily dose is 100 or less.	9, 46, 40
Medroxyprogesterone (Depoprovera)	Excreted, not quantified	No significant effect on infant or milk yield.	40
Progestins (19-nortestosterone derivatives) Norethindrone Norgestrel Noresthindrone acetate Norethynodrel	Trace amount	Not significant if maternal daily dose is 2.5 mg or less. No effect on milk yield.	9, 41, 40
Corticotropin	Excreted, not quantified	Destroyed in infant's GI tract.	7, 47, 48
Cortisone	Excreted, not quantified	Corticosteroids have not been studied sufficiently to assess their potential for harm to the infant. One study in rats found deaths and retarded de-	7, 47, 48

(*continued*)

APPENDIX: (*Continued*)

Drug (Brand)	Quantity Excreted in Milk	Neonatal Effect at Maternal Therapeutic Doses	Reference(s)
		velopment after 20 mg/day of cortisone (a high dose in a rat) was given to mothers. Most sources advise against breastfeeding in women taking corticosteroids.	
Dihydrotachysterol (Hytakerol)	Excreted	May cause hypercalcemia. Need to monitor infant serum and urine calcium.	7
Epinephrine	Excreted	Destroyed in infant's GI tract.	7
Fluoxymesterone (Halotesin)	Excreted	Suppressed lactation. Masculinization.	47
Insulin	Unknown	Destroyed in infant's GI tract.	7
Prednisolone	Avg. 0.07-0.23% of dose/L of milk over 48 hr	Thought to be insignificant, but only a single-dose study.	47
Prednisone	2.67 mcg/dl prednisone and 0.61 mcg/dl prednisolone after a single 10-mg PO dose	Long-term effects unknown. When maternal dose 120 mg QD Infant ingests 47 mcg (<8% normal adrenal output). Probably NS.	4, 10, 22, 3
Psychoactive Substances			
Antidepressants			
Amitriptyline (Elavil, Endep)	Less then lower limit of assay (100 ng/ml) 4 and 12 hr after a single 25–50-mg dose	Probably NS, but long half-life not taken into consideration. Watch for depression or failure to feed.	28, 47, 48
Desipramine (Norpramin, Pertofrane)	Milk levels similar to plasma levels 17–35 ng/ml after 200 mg/day for 16 days of imipramine	NS at this level. Unknown at maternal therapeutic levels.	28, 81
Doxepin	M:P = 0.33 in one patient receiving 75 mg/day for 3 months	None known.	4
Imipramine (Tofranil)	Milk levels similar to plasma levels 12-29 ng/ml after 200 mg/day	NS at this level. Unknown at maternal therapeutic blood levels.	47, 48
Nortriptyline (Aventyl, Pamelor)	Not detectable after a 25-mg dose	Unknown at therapeutic levels.	47, 81

APPENDIX: (*Continued*)

Drug (Brand)	Quantity Excreted in Milk	Neonatal Effect at Maternal Therapeutic Doses	Reference(s)
Tranylcypromine (Parnate)	Trace amounts	NS. May inhibit lactation.	28
Alcohol	M:P = 0.9–1.0	Not significant in moderation. Lethargy and prolonged sleeping when mother consumes excessive amounts.	28
Barbiturates	Low levels	Usually NS. May induce liver microsomal enzymes.	28
Barbital	<40 mcg/ml after 325–650-mg dose	NS. One case of sedation.	5, 47
Butabarbital (Butisol)	0.37 mcg/ml 1.5 hr after seventh dose of 8 mg every 12 hr	NS.	4
Pentobarbital (Nembutal)	0.17 mcg/ml 19 hr after third dose of 100 mg/day	NS.	4
Phenobarbital (see Anticonvulsants)	M:P = 0.46 ± 0.25	2 of 11 infants became difficult to awaken and slept excessively after mother received hypnotic doses (90 mg) for 5 days. NS in maternal antiepileptic doses (60–200 mg/day). May induce liver microsomal enzymes.	4, 28, 47, 61
Secobarbital (Seconal)	Detectable 14 hr after unspecified dose	NS.	4, 47
Thiopental (Pentothal)	20 mcg/ml after IV dose of 1.125 g	NS.	4, 47
Benzodiazepines			
Chlordiazepoxide (Librium)	Excreted	Amount secreted usually insufficient to affect infant, although CNS depression has been reported.	28
Diazepam (Valium)	78 ng/ml after 10 mg three times daily for 6 days. Total benzodiazepines excreted at 50% of serum level	Reports of lethargy and weight loss. Infant most susceptible during first 4 days of life. Hyperbilirubinemia. Most sources do not advise its use during breast-	28

(*continued*)

APPENDIX: (*Continued*)

Drug (Brand)	Quantity Excreted in Milk	Neonatal Effect at Maternal Therapeutic Doses	Reference(s)
		feeding. Drug accumulation may occur.	
Chlorazepate (Tranxene)	M:P = 0.13–0.3 of chlorazepate and its metabolite nordiazepam	Drowsiness. Infant younger than 2 months may have prolonged drug half-life due to immaturity of drug-metabolizing enzymes. Possibility of accumulation on chronic administration. Caution because of long half-life.	82
N-Demethyldiazepam	Active metabolite of diazepam, excreted	Caution, due to long half-life.	28
Oxazepam (Serax)	Excreted, metabolite of diazepam M:P = 0.1	Approximately 0.1% of maternal dose excreted in milk.	8, 48, 74
Bromides	67 mcg/ml maximum after 1 g NaBr five times a day for 3 days	Drowsiness and rash. Possibility of allergic reactions.	5, 47
Caffeine	8.2 mcg/ml after 1 cup coffee (100 mg)	Accumulates when intake moderate and continual. Causes jitteriness, wakefulness, and irritability.	4, 22
Chloral hydrate (Noctec)	Chloral hydrate and its metabolite trichlorethanol reach 50–100% of blood levels	Sedation, usually not significant.	47
Chloroform	Excreted	Deep sleep.	4, 7
Dextroamphetamine (Dexedrine)	Excreted, not quantified	No effects on infants when given to 103 postpartum women for depression. Avoid long-acting preparations.	4, 28
Ether	Milk levels about equal to plasma levels for 8–10 hr after dose	Sedation.	47
Flurazepam (Dalmane)	Excreted	Some sedation, but usually not significant.	28
Glutethimide (Doriden)	Avg. peak of 270 ng/ml at 8–12 hr after 500-mg dose	Some sedation, usually not significant.	47
Haloperidol (Haldol)	Milk concentration similar to plasma level. M:P = 0.5–1.0	Unknown. Rabbit studies showed behavioral changes.	4, 28, 74

APPENDIX: (*Continued*)

Drug (Brand)	Quantity Excreted in Milk	Neonatal Effect at Maternal Therapeutic Doses	Reference(s)
Lithium	Avg. 0.6 mEq/L when maternal plasma level 1.5 mEq/L. M:P = 0.25–0.7 (avg. 0.5)	Measurable lithium in infant's serum. Infant kidney can clear lithium. Reports of cyanosis, hypothermia, poor muscle tone, and ECG changes in nursing infants.	4, 5, 22, 83
Marijuana	Excreted	Lipid-soluble, long t½, may be stored in milk; use not recommended.	3, 4, 22
Meprobamate	M:P = 2–4	Monitor infant for drug intoxication since drug accumulates in milk.	28, 48
Phenothiazines			
Chlorpromazine (Thorazine)	M:P = 0.3, not detectable at dose of 600 mg twice daily	NS at doses up to 1200 mg/day.	4, 28
Mesoridazine (Serentil)	Excreted, not quantified	None known.	28, 48
Perphenazine (Trilafon)	M:P = 1	None known.	4, 28
Piperacetazine (Quide)	Excreted, not quantified	None known.	28
Prochlorperazine (Compazine)	Excreted, not quantified	None known.	28, 48
Thioridazine (Mellaril)	Excreted, not quantified	None known.	28, 48
Trifluoperazine (Stelazine)	0.4–1.5 mg/100 ml in dogs after daily doses of 200 mg	None known.	28, 48
Radiopharmaceuticals and Diagnostic Materials			
Barium	Not excreted	None.	22
^{131}I	1.3–2.0 nCi/ml 24 hr after 100-mCi dose. Peak of 39 nCi/ml at 6 hr. Appears to concentrate in milk	Breastfeeding contraindicated after large therapeutic dose, and should be withheld for 24 hr minimum after smaller diagnostic doses. Check milk prior to resuming feeding.	47
[^{131}I] labeled macroaggregated albumin	4.2–28.0 nCi/ml after 200-mCi dose	Discontinue breastfeeding for 10–12 days. Extreme avidity for iodine by the thyroid of young infants. 1/10 of the International Commission on Radiological Protection (ICRP) for drinking	10, 47

(*continued*)

APPENDIX: (*Continued*)

Drug (Brand)	Quantity Excreted in Milk	Neonatal Effect at Maternal Therapeutic Doses	Reference(s)
		water reached 10 days after IV dose of 200 mCi.	
Iopanoic acid (Telepaque)	Peak iodide level at 5–19 hr; 3–11 mg iodide/feeding at this time	No adverse effects. Iodine excretion can cause rash. Probably no problem with just one dose.	22, 47, 48
Gallium citrate	70 nCi/ml 96 and 120 hr after 3-mCi dose	Discontinue nursing until 2 weeks. ^{69}Ga has cleared, usually.	10
^{90}Sr	M:P = 1.0	NS. Less than in cow's milk.	22
$^{99}TcO_4^-$	3.0–5.2 times plasma level at 17 and 20 hr, respectively	Breastfeeding contraindicated for 32–72 hr after 10-mCi dose. Breastfeeding can be resumed 24 hr after 2-mCi dose for lung scanning.	47, 48
Tuberculin test	Not excreted	Tuberculin-sensitive mothers can passively immunize their infants through breast milk. Immunity may last several years.	22
Thyroid Drugs			
Liothyronine (Cytomel)	Not excreted	None.	48
Methimazole (Tapazole)	Average M:P = 1.16 ± 0.12 Maternal dose 2.5 mg bid	Infant could receive 7–16% of maternal dose. Could interfere with thyroid function. Inhibits synthesis of thyroid hormone.	84
Potassium iodide	3 mg/100 ml	May alter thyroid function in infant. May cause goiter.	22, 48
Propylthiouracil (PTU)	M:P = 0.13–0.47	Infant could receive 0.5 mg/day at maternal dose of 600 mg/day. Maternal doses up to 150 mg/day not hazardous to infant. Infant could ingest 0.07% of mother's daily dose.	84, 85
Thyroid	Excreted	NS.	22

APPENDIX: (*Continued*)

Drug (Brand)	Quantity Excreted in Milk	Neonatal Effect at Maternal Therapeutic Doses	Reference(s)
Levo-Thyroxine (Synthroid)	4 ng/ml first week postpartum. Increases to 40 ng/ml by 2 months	May mask clinical symptoms of congenital hypothyroidism in nurslings. Improves milk supply in hypothyroid mothers. Not contraindicated.	10, 22, 74
Miscellaneous			
DPT Vaccine	Excreted in minimal amounts	Does not interfere with immunization schedule.	22
Ergonovine (Ergotrate)	Excreted, not quantified	Causes lowered prolactin levels in postpartum patients. Multiple doses may suppress lactation.	47
Fluoride	Milk from mothers living in 1-ppm area 0.37 μmol/L. Not significantly different from milk of mothers from 0.2-ppm areas	Fluoride intake 5–10 mcg/day in both 0.2-ppm and 1-ppm areas.	
Isoproterenol (Isoprel)	Not excreted	NS.	4
Sulfasalazine (Azulfidine)	Parent compound not found in milk, sulfapyridine M:P = 0.6; 5-aminosalicylate—not found in milk	Parent compound metabolized in gut to sulfapyridine and 5-aminosalicylate. When chronic maternal dose is 2 g/day infant ingests 2–4 mg/day (0.16% of maternal dose).	92
Magnesium sulfate	Milk level 6.4 mg/dl immediately after IV infusion of 1 g/hr discontinued (control levels 4.77 mg/dl). 24 hr postinfusion levels not significantly different from control subjects	Breastfed infant would receive only 1.5 mg more magnesium than nontreated mothers. NS. Milk calcium not affected.	89
Poliovirus vaccine	Not excreted	Live virus taken orally. Not necessary to withhold nursing 30 minutes before and after dose. Provide booster after infant no longer nursing.	22, 90
Rh antibodies	Excreted	Destroyed in GI tract.	22
Rubella virus vaccine	Minimal amounts	Will not confer passive immunity.	22

(*continued*)

APPENDIX: ***(Continued)***

Drug (Brand)	Quantity Excreted in Milk	Neonatal Effect at Maternal Therapeutic Doses	Reference(s)
Smallpox vaccine	Not excreted	Exposure is by direct contact. Live virus. Contraindicated when mother has infant under 1 year.	22
Terbutaline (Brethine, Bricanyl)	2.5–4.6 ng/ml; dose 2.5–5 mg tid M:P = 1.4–2.9	Estimated infant dose 0.4–0.6 mcg or 0.2–0.7% of maternal dose. Not detectable in infant plasma. No adverse effects reported.	
Theobromine	M:P = 0.82	No adverse effects observed in infants. 4 oz chocolate contains 240 mg theobromine.	3, 13
Theophylline	Avg. M:P = 0.7 with rapid equilibration; peak levels 1–3 hr after dose Peak milk levels 4 mcg/ml. Up to 4% of maternal dose appears in milk	Usually not significant. Some reports of irritability and insomnia in infant. Premature infants 3–15 days old have average half-lives of 30.2 hr. Maximum amount of theophylline that an infant could ingest is 8 mg/L milk per day. Avoid nursing at time of peak serum level.	4, 8, 24, 47, 88
Tolbutamide	Milk level is 9–40% of serum level, 3–18 mcg/ml 4 hr after 500-mg dose	Unknown.	47

* NS = Not significant in therapeutic dose to affect infant.

† M:P = Ratio of breast milk concentration to maternal plasma concentration.

Part II

GYNECOLOGY

19

Oral Contraceptives

Nichols Vorys

Since the Food and Drug Administration approved the marketing of the oral contraceptive in 1960, it has become the most popular reversible contraceptive method. An estimated 50 million women in developed and developing countries are taking "the Pill." The United States, Canada, the Netherlands, New Zealand, West Germany, and Australia report that 25 percent of women in the reproduction era take oral contraceptives, whereas 5 to 10 percent of the women in third world countries are using the pill.[1] Oral contraceptive use is more popular among women married less than five years (65 percent) than among women married longer.[2] Women intending to have future births have found the pill to be an effective temporary method of contraception. The oral contraceptive remains one of the most widely prescribed medications for the reproductive-age woman. This chapter is intended to review current information on the pharmacology, metabolic effects, and effectiveness of the various preparations, and to offer guidelines for oral contraceptive use.

PHARMACOLOGY

Each oral contraceptive combines a synthetic estrogen with a progestin component. These synthetic progestins and estrogens are discussed separately, as they differ from natural steroids in the normal menstrual cycle.

Synthetic Progestins

The synthetic progestins in combination oral contraceptives are formed by the removal of the 19-C atom from testosterone. They are called 19-nor compounds, and are shown in Figure 19–1. The effect of removing the 19-C atom is to remove nearly all the adrogenic and anabolic activity of testosterone. The progestational activity is enhanced by the addition of methyl (CH_3), ethinyl (C=CH), or acetate ($OCOCH_3$) groups at the 3-, 17-, or 18-β-positions. The 19-nor compounds (norethindrone, norethindrone acetate, and ethynodiol diacetate) differ only by the number of additional acetate groups at the 3- and 17-positions.

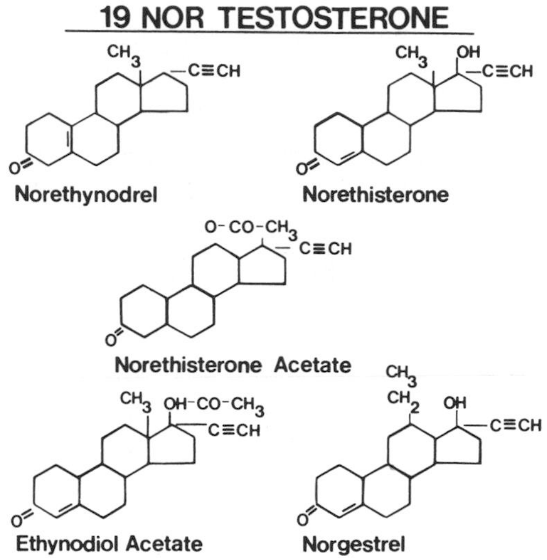

19 NOR TESTOSTERONE

Norethynodrel

Norethisterone

Norethisterone Acetate

Ethynodiol Acetate

Norgestrel

Figure 19–1. Synthetic progestins in oral contraceptives.

Molecular structural differences make some of these synthetic progestins act not only biologically as progesterone, but they also have inherent estrogen and androgen activity (Fig. 19–2). Two such compounds with estrogenic activity include norethynodrel and ethynodiol diacetate. Another oral progestin, norgestrel, has greater androgen activity and marked antiestrogen effect.

All oral contraceptives act on specific intracellular estrogen and progesterone receptors. Briggs has studied the protein receptor binding of synthetic progestins.[3] Norethynodrel, norethindrone acetate, norethindrone, and ethynodiol diacetate are metabolized to norethindrone in the liver before they are capable of receptor-binding. Norgestrel, the most potent available synthetic progestin, binds strongly to the progesterone receptor, which accounts for its potent biologic activity.[4,5]

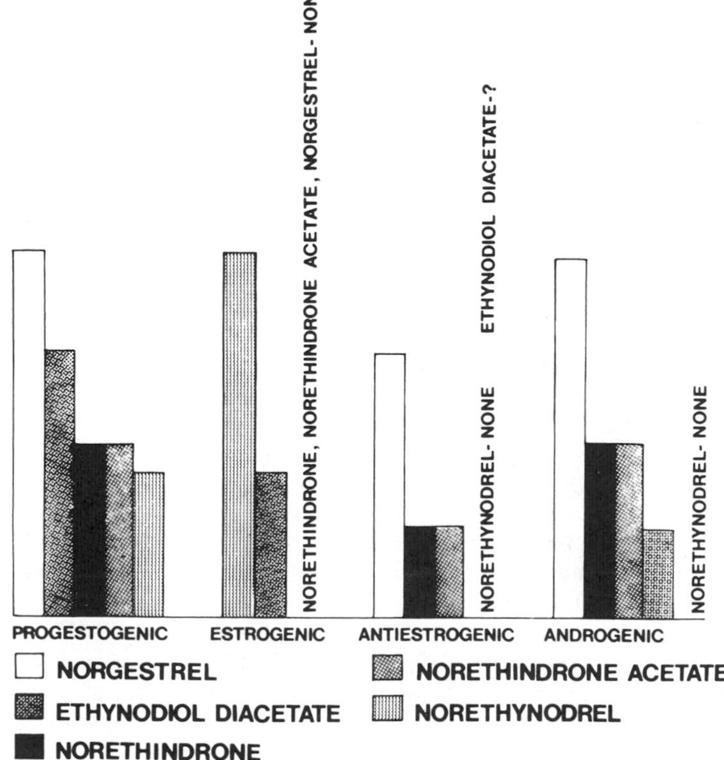

Figure 19–2. Inherent biologic effects of the synthetic progestins.

Synthetic Estrogens

Oral contraceptives contain one of the two synthetic estrogens, ethinyl estradiol and mestranol (Fig. 19–3).[6] Ethinyl estradiol is formed by adding an ethinyl group to estradiol, whereas a methyl ether group is added to estradiol to synthesize mestranol. Mestranol is converted in the body to ethinyl estradiol, and without this conversion, mestranol is inactive. Factors that influence potency include the rate of conversion and the rates of metabolism into inactive derivatives.[7] Ethinyl estradiol is the synthetic estrogen of choice, and has been estimated to be slightly more potent than the equivalent weight of mestranol.[8,9]

The structural difference, route of administration, dosage schedule, and metabolism between natural and synthetic estrogens are important factors when considering the intracellular biologic action of estrogen. The 17-ethinyl group in synthetic estrogens allows for oral administration and biologic potency. The metabolism of synthetic estrogens differs from estradiol 17-β in that ethinyl estradiol has a longer half-life, and there is a failure of ethinyl estradiol to have significant alternate pathways leading to such biologically weak metabolites as 2- and 16-hydroxy compounds as is seen with natural estradiol metabolism. The differences in biologic half-lives between the natural and synthetic estrogens relate to the different metabolic and conjugation processes and to the enterohepatic circulation.

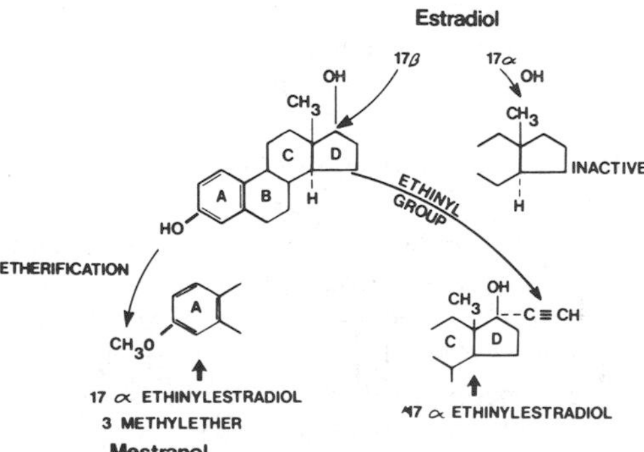

Figure 19–3. Mestranol and ethinyl estradiol, the two synthetic estrogens derived from estradiol and found in oral contraceptives.

The pharmacologic properties of the estrogen molecule determine the cellular response at the target organ. The sensitivity of the end organ is determined by the presence of cytosol receptor proteins within the cell.[10] The transport of natural or synthetic estrogen through the cell membrane has a mitigating effect on the concentration of estrogen within the cell. The intracellular concentrations of the hormone and the occupation of receptor sites are a function not only of estrogen dose and duration, but the presence of synthetic progestins.[11]

Dujovne measured cytosol receptor uptake of radiolabeled estrone and mestranol in monolayer tissue culture and found it altered by dose, duration of incubation, and the presence of the progestin, norethynodrel.[11] His experiments revealed that both estrone and mestranol have dose-related biologic effects on the liver cell. However, in the presence of norethynodrel, the uptake of mestranol was doubled. It was presumed that synthetic progestins such as norethynodrel and northindrone affect cell membrane permeability to estrogen. Therefore, the intracellular biologic activity of estrogen also depends on the progestin molecule with which it is administered, and the combination affects the intracellular pharmacodynamics at the end organ.

Oral Contraceptive Cycle Versus Natural Menstrual Cycle

For sex steroids to be biologically effective, one must consider the route of administration and the significance of the structure of the molecule. Oral contraceptives are absorbed into the intestinal wall, and pass through the portal circulation and liver prior to entering the general circulation. Ninety percent of oral contraceptives reach the liver in the active form, but only 20 percent of the administered dose is active at the target organs.[12] Conversely, estrogens produced in the ovary enter the vena cava and pass into the general circulation without having to first pass through the portal circulation. For orally administered sex steroids to achieve serum and tissue levels comparable to those of naturally secreted sex steroids, the liver must receive levels of steroids approximately five times as great as when the same steroid is derived from ovarian production.

Another important difference between oral contraceptive pill cycles and the normal menstrual cycle is that the synthetic estrogens and progestins are delivered concomitantly, and in a constant-dosage form. In the normal menstrual cycle, natural estrogen is secreted unopposed from day 7 to day 14 only, and with a mid-cycle peak. Natural progesterone is secreted only during the last 14 days of the menstrual cycle, and invariably in the presence of natural estrogen. The ratio of estrogen to progestin is constant in oral contraceptives, but varies according to the day of the normal menstrual cycle for sex steroids produced by the ovary. The ratio of synthetic estrogen to progestin ranges from 1:10 to 1:50 throughout the cycle in the various oral contraceptives, with the most frequently used range being 1:20. The ratio of estradiol and estrone to progesterone secreted by the ovary varies from 1:10 in the early proliferative phase, 1:1.2 in the late proliferative phase, and 1:60 in the luteal phase.

Thus, the differences between the oral contraceptive and the natural menstrual cycle are: (1) route of administration, which influences the pharmacologic impact on the liver; (2) difference in ratio of estrogen and progestin from the normal menstrual cycle; and (3) the administration of synthetic estrogen and progestin, which are administered concomitantly throughout the entire treatment cycle. These factors, and the metabolism of synthetic estrogen and progestins, undoubtedly account for some of the annoying clinical side effects (nausea, cyclic swelling, weight gain, breakthrough bleeding, etc.) and the metabolic adverse consequences, particularly as they involve the excretory function and protein synthesis by the liver.[13]

EFFECT ON REPRODUCTIVE ORGANS

The administration of a combined estrogen and progestin preparation interferes with fertility in many ways. The primary mechanism of action for contraception involves an inhibition of the hypothalamus and pituitary. This effect, along with the effects on other target tissues, such as the cervix and endometrium are dependent on the dose, progestin/estrogen ratio, and duration of therapy. Most changes are similar to changes during pregnancy, and are usually reversed by discontinuation of the preparation. It should be understood that these effects on reproductive organs were studied with moderate or higher dose pills rather than the newer but equally effective low-dose preparations.

Hypothalamus and Pituitary

Estrogen administered on a cyclic basis suppresses follicle-stimulating hormone (FSH) secretion. When mestranol is administered, this effect diminishes as the dose is decreased from 100 to 80 to 40.[14] The effect of estrogen on luteinizing hormone (LH) secretion is less consistent, but repeated cyclic administration of mestranol suppresses both FSH and LH excretion. Ethinyl estradiol, in daily doses of 50 given from day 5 through 24 of the cycle, can cause an abolition of the mid-cycle surge of serum FSH and LH.[5] Sporadic surges of LH may be seen even after 12 cycles of treatment, and low doses of mestranol (10) may add a stimulatory rather than a suppressive action on the excretion of both FSH and LH in the urine.[15]

Progestins act by suppressing the mid-cycle LH peak. Different progestin molecules have varying effects—norgestrel and ethyndiol diacetate being the more potent.[16] Those women receiving even microdoses of progestins exhibit suppression of the mid-cycle peak of LH.[17] Progestins alone do not lower the baseline level of either FSH or LH.[14]

Goldzieher et al. demonstrated that combination oral contraceptives suppress baseline plasma FSH to about 70 percent of control values, and LH to about 20 to 30 percent of control values, while eliminating the mid-cycle surge.[14] The differences between the follicular and luteal phase levels of FSH and LH were preserved. In addition, the combination oral contraceptives may have an effect on the pituitary gland by increasing prolactin release.[18] This was particularly obvious when thyroid-releasing hormone (TRH) and luteinizing hormone releasing factor (LHRF) were administered to combination oral contraceptive patients.[19]

The post-pill effect on reproduction has been studied at great length. After 3 months of discontinuation of combination oral contraceptives, plasma gonadotropin values should be in the range of normal cycles. Eighty-five percent of people discontinuing oral contraceptives are capable of becoming pregnant within 6 to 12 months.[20] There is, however, the possibility of post-pill amenorrhea continuing after 6 months, with the occurrence of this condition estimated to be between 2 and 2.6 percent.[21-23] If this figure were true in practice, 200,000 to 250,000 women currently using oral contraceptive pills would eventually require diagnosis and treatment for post-pill amenorrhea.

Post-pill amenorrhea is not a homogeneous entity. When such patients are compared with spontaneous amenorrhea patients, a number of subgroups become apparent. They have been identified by Jacobs et al. as (1) primary ovarian failure, (2) hyperprolactinemia, (3) clomiphene-responsive amenorrhea, (4) anorexia nervosa, and (5) amenorrhea associated with psychiatric disease and/or environmental stress.[22] Dickey and Stone identified three endocrine groups of post-pill amenorrhea patients related to serum, prolactin, LH, and estradiol levels.[21] Group 1 cases had high prolactin with low or normal LH values. In these, post-pill amenorrhea was due to increased prolactin, and such patients responded to bromergocriptine with ovulation. Group 2 cases had normal prolactin, low LH, and low estradiol values. These amenorrhea patients were thought to have a suppressed or immature hypothalamus, and required estrogen priming and clomiphene or human menopausal gonadotropin (hMG), followed by human chorionic gonadotropin (hCG). Group 3 cases had a normal prolactin level, with elevated LH and normal or elevated estradiol values. Such patients were thought to have persistent, uninterrupted estrogen stimulation, but responded to progesterone withdrawal, and invariably to clomiphene with ovulation.

Most normally ovulating and menstruating patients will respond with ovulatory cycles after oral contraceptive discontinuation. Those patients that have hypothalamic-pituitary—ovarian dysfunction prior to the initiation of oral contraceptives almost invariably revert to their pre-oral contraceptive treatment pattern after cessation of oral contraceptive therapy.[13] The incidence of secondary anovulation and/or amenorrhea, with or without galactorrhea, is higher in the latter type of patient than is found in the normal ovulating patient. Regardless of the prior menstrual history, women with post-pill amenorrhea are still capable of becoming pregnant.

There may be an overall association between prior oral contraceptive use and prolactinoma, but the degree of association is strongly related to the indication for such use. If the indication is for contraception, the risk of prolactinoma was increased to a small extent (relative risk 1.3). The risk was 7.7 times greater if used for menstrual regulation.[24]

Ovary

Steroidal contraceptives affect both ovarian morphology and function. The ovaries appear grossly small and inactive, and show no evidence of corpus lutea formation. Histologically, these ovaries have a thick collagenous capsule with no maturing follicles. Ryan estimated that the number of primordial follicles remained in the normal range in women treated for periods up to 2 years with norethynodrel.[25] Inactive cystic and atretic follicles are often present after oral contraceptive use, and there appears to be a focal condensation of stroma.

Along with these morphologic changes, ovarian steroidogenesis is profoundly affected by combination therapy. Estradiol 17-β and estrone synthesis is decreased markedly. Testosterone production is generally decreased by one-half or more, and androstenedione production is decreased by one-third. Less change in dehydroeprandosterone sulfate (DHEAS) is seen during oral contraceptive consumption.

Functional ovarian cyst formation is reduced with oral contraceptive use. However, the risk of developing other benign ovarian tumors or ovarian carcinoma is unrelated to oral contraceptive exposure. A lower risk of epithelial ovarian cancer associated with the use of oral contraceptives has been observed in older parous subjects and in women who had discontinued use more than 10 years previously.[26] The risk of ovarian cancer decreases with increasing duration of drug use and has remained low long after cessation of use.[27]

Oviducts

Ovarian hormones regulate segmental contraction of the oviduct and ciliogenesis of the endosalpinx, and control oviductal secretion and flow. These findings indicate that ovum transport and muscular activity of the oviduct are regulated by estrogen and progesterone, and a delicate balance is a prerequisite to normal function. Motility of the human oviduct is known to be influenced by combination oral contraceptives, which inhibit the spontaneous motility of the isolated human oviduct. With a scanning electron microscope, no alteration was seen of ciliary pattern of endosalpingeal epithelium in women receiving combination oral contraceptives.

Various protein substances, enzymes, and trace elements in the oviductal fluid also play a major role in fertilization and in early stages of differentiation and development of the embryo.[26] The alteration and their concentration as a result of hormonal changes may lead to the inhibition of fertilization and the cleavage process.

Current oral contraceptives are associated with a protective effect against pelvic inflammatory disease (PID).[28] This finding was restricted to women taking the pill for more than 12 months. Past oral contraceptive use does not exert a protective effect against PID.[28]

Uterus

Steroidal contraceptives affect the myometrium. The uterus becomes soft, cyanotic, and enlarged; and this effect is more pronounced when higher-dose oral contraceptives are used. Prolonged use produces either no change, or a slight decrease in the size of the uterus. Histologically, the myometrium shows some cellular hypertrophy, dilated sinusoids, and edema.

Hendricks, in 1977, recorded spontaneous uterine activity during oral contraceptive use.[29] The transport of spermatozoa through the uterus and oviduct depends, to a large extent, on myometrial and oviductal muscular activity. It was noted that estrogen administration was followed by uterine contractions, and sperm were found in the uterine cavity shortly after coitus. With the administration of an estrogen/progestin combination, alterations in myometrial motility patterns, sperm transport, and egg implantation have also been noted.

Ovarian hormones bring about well-recognized morphologic changes in the endometrium during the menstrual cycle. The effect of oral contraceptives on the endometrium depends on the preparation, the dosage, the duration of administration, and the ratio of estrogen to progestin. These effects consist of a rapid progression from proliferation to early secretory changes within a few days following the start of the compound. By 7 days, a mixed hormonal effect is observed. Thereafter the endometrium shows regressive changes, characterized by a compact stroma dotted with sparse atrophic glands, which are lined with cuboidal or flattened epithelium. Glandular secretory activity and tortuosity are either completely absent, or minimal.[27] Marked decidualization of the stroma is observed with most combination preparations. With prolonged use, the endometrium usually becomes progressively thin and inactive, but minimal cyclic changes occur even after long-term administration.[30] Withdrawal bleeding is often scanty, and shows no daily variation compared to normal menses. The lack of withdrawal bleeding is not to be taken lightly and is an indication for cessation of therapy or a change in preparation.

Reports indicate that adenomatous hyperplasia has never been observed during combination contraceptive therapy. A protective effect against endometrial cancer is thought to occur in women who had used oral contraceptives for at least 12 months.[32] It persisted for at least 10 years after cessation of use. A protective effect is most notable for nulliporous women. The development of endometrial carcinoma in users of sequential oral contraceptives has been reported, but no absolute cause-and-effect relationship between the sequential formulations and endometrial cancer has been demonstrated.[33] Some experimental and clinical data suggest that cyclic-combination oral contraceptive pills contain an adequate amount of progestin to prevent hyperplasia, and those with a low estrogen dosage may provide a certain degree of protection against endometrial cancer.[33]

Cervix

Like the myometrium, the cervix is extremely sensitive to estrogen and progestins. Changes in the composition and properties of cervical secretion have been used for many years as an in vivo biologic assay for sex steroids. The response of the cervix to oral contraceptives depends largely on the type of compound, dosage used, the potency, and specific activity of the progestin. The cervix often becomes moderately soft and bluish, and assumes an appearance similar to that during pregnancy. There is an increased incidence of cervical erosion, because of the advancement of the squamocolumnar junction, which is believed to be hormonally dependent.

The secretion of cervical mucus is regulated by ovarian hormones. Estrogen stimulates the production of large amounts of thin, watery, elastic, acellular cervical mucus with intense ferning, spinnbarkheit, and sperm receptivity. Progesterone and all synthetic oral progestins, alone or in combination with estrogen, inhibit the secretory activity of cervical epithelium, and produce a scanty, viscous, and cellular mucus with low spinnbarkheit and an absence of ferning. Spermatozoa are usually unable to penetrate this luteal-phase type of cervical mucus. The chemical constituents of cervical mucus show definite cyclic variations during the menstrual cycle, or with administration of estrogen/progestins. The extent of the physical and chemical alteration of the cervical mucus results from the administration of progestational agents, and depends on the preparation and dosage. Higher dosages of progestins add a more profound sustained effect than lower doses; but even microdose progestins have been shown to inhibit, or greatly reduce, sperm migration through the cervical mucus.

Cervical erosion and eversion are commonly observed in oral contraceptive users. A variety of expressions of mild atypia may be seen in the areas of epidermalization. These changes include nuclear disarray and hyperchromatism, cellular crowding, and variability in glandular cell size. An atypical endocervical hyperplastic pattern, which is reversible and benign, can be mistaken for adenocarcinoma in many women taking oral contraceptives.

Frederick has reported ultrastructural changes in the cervix following treatment with combination oral contraceptives.[34] The configuration of the cells and the distribution of their organelles were generally comparable to those of the normal menstrual cycle, and differences appeared to be only quantitative.

Pincus reported a decreased incidence of abnormal pap smears in users of oral contraceptives compared to controls.[35] Since these pioneer studies, many publications have confirmed no difference in the prevalence or incidence rate of abnormal cytology between oral contraceptive users and controls.[36,37] Cervical dysplasia is usually considered a precancerous lesion. Richard and Barron estimated that cervical dysplasia lesions progress to in situ cancer in about 12 to 86 months, depending on their severity.[38] Women diagnosed as having cervical dysplasia or carcinoma in situ, who received combination estrogen/progestin medication, showed no progressive changes of lesions. The prevalence of carcinoma in situ and cervical dysplasia in their study was higher, 2.64 percent in oral contraceptive users as compared to 1.5 percent in control users. Factors that seem of more relevance to the development of carcinoma of the cervix than the use of oral contraceptives are early age of sexual activity, multiple partners, and lower socioeconomic population, and have led some investigators to search for a transmissible disease as the etiologic cause.

Vagina

The cytologic response in the vagina to oral contraceptives depends on the type of estrogen/progestin, the relative and absolute amounts of estrogen/progestin, and the sensitivity of the vaginal mucosa to these steroids. Although one may occasionally encounter an appreciable number of superficial cells in the vaginal smears during oral contraceptive use, the usual pattern resembles more closely the late luteal phase, with intermediate cells predominating. Inflammatory cell patterns are occasionally observed. On rare occasions, parabasal cells, usually found in atrophic smears, are seen.

In contrast to the normal menstrual cycle, the vaginal cytology and karypknotic index in women treated with combination oral contraceptives do not exhibit a biphasic pattern in the relative number of superficial to intermediate or basal cells throughout the treatment cycle. Vaginal secretions of women receiving oral progestogens are scanty, multicellular, and contain large numbers of leukocytes and bacteria, and may account for inadequate lubrication during coitus.

Because of the heavy deposit of galactogen in vaginal mucosa and marked reduction of *Döderlein* bacilli produced by progestins, vaginal infections (particularly *Candida albicans*) are more likely to occur in women taking oral contraceptives.[39] Furthermore, it appears that there is progressive increase in this infection as the duration of oral contraceptive medication is increased. Whether oral contraceptives will increase the incidence of vulvo/vaginitis for each patient depends on her personal hygiene, life-style, and other factors, including dose and ratio of estrogen/progestin in the oral contraceptive.

Breast

Breast development is directed by genetic potential and sex steroid stimulation. Estrogen causes breast duct growth, and progesterone stimulates the development of the peripheral breast glands (lobule alveolus). Oral contraceptives may cause an increase in breast size (the same phenomena as seen in normal pregnancy), and some degree of breast tenderness has been associated with oral contraceptive use. The latter symptom is dose-related, and decreases with a lower-dose estrogen component.

Lactation is also, in part, controlled by sex steroids. Oral contraceptives have been shown to decrease the volume of milk, to shorten the duration of lactation, and sometimes to alter the constituents of milk. Primiparous women are affected more than multiparous women.[40] It is universally agreed that the estrogen component of the oral contraceptive is at fault, and the larger the dose, the greater the adverse effect on successful nursing. Low dose oral contraceptives are thought to be safe to prescribe during nursing.

Benign mammary disease (fibrocystic disease) is a relatively common disorder, and is associated with a higher risk of breast cancer development. These benign neoplasms appear to be the same or less in oral contraceptive users than in the general population.[41] The risk of fibrocystic disease of the breast in oral contraceptive users has been estimated to be 25 to 80 percent of that found in nonusers. In addition, long-term users of oral contraceptives seem to have less risk of benign breast dysplasia (fibrocystic disease) than short-term users. The progestin component of oral contraceptives is considered to be primarily responsible for this protection, especially if the progestin is less estrogenic (norgestrel in Ovral versus norethynodrel in Enovid). Oral contraceptive users in England were found to have significantly fewer benign breast tumors than patients using diaphragms and intrauterine devices (IUDs). There is no substantial information that would identify oral contraceptives as a causative factor in benign breast neoplasms.[42] However, oral contraceptives should not be administered to any patient with a single or multiple breast lump until carcinoma has been ruled out.

In monkeys, both estrogens and oral contraceptives have failed to elicit an observable increase in incidence in mammary tumors.[43] There appears to be neither a positive nor negative association with mammary cancer in short-term use (up to 4 years) of steroid contraceptives in human subjects. In agreement with the recommendations of its fertility and maternal Health Drugs Advisory Committee, the FDA has concluded that there appears to be no increased risk of breast cancer among oral contraceptive users. Recent studies by the Centers for Disease Control (CDC) and Steroid Hormone Study has revealed that oral contraceptive use before a woman's first pregnancy does not increase her risk of breast cancer significantly more than other methods of delaying her first pregnancy.[43,44] Despite these findings, any patient on oral contraceptives with a history of benign breast disease or a strong family history of breast cancer requires frequent examination.

Teratogenicity

The inadvertent use of oral contraceptives during early pregnancy has prompted much investigation to determine any teratogenic effects. Spontaneous abortion may represent a severe manifestation of a teratogen. The relationship of chromosome abnormalities in spontaneous abortion in women conceiving shortly after discontinuing or while on oral contraceptives is controversial. Carr reported on the types of chromosome abnormalities in spontaneously aborted conceptuses in which conception occurred after oral contraceptive use.[45] He found the percentage of chromosome anomalies in a control series to be 22 percent, whereas that in the post-oral contraceptive series was 48 percent. The striking difference between the control and study groups was in the incidence of polyploidy. Triploid abortuses were 4.5 times more common in the post-oral contraceptive group than in the control group. However, others have not confirmed this observation.

There are no good data to substantiate the increase of chromosome abnormalities in intrauterine pregnancies going to term in patients who have received oral contraception. In a well-done newborn study population, the observed control abnormality was 5.4/1000, and did not differ significantly from a rate of 6.9/1000 for post-oral contraceptive newborn patients.[46]

Janerich et al. published a report that linked oral contraceptives with congenital limb reduction defects.[47] These authors found that 15 of the 108 women with babies who have malformations were exposed to exogenous sex steroids at one time or another, as compared to 4 of 108 controls. There may also be some evidence to implicate exogenous estrogen/progestin exposure during pregnancy with congenital heart defects. These claims have not been established beyond reasonable doubt, or confirmed in depth by others.[48] A combination of anomalies involving the vertebrae, anal, cardiac, trachea, esophagus, and limbs was termed the "VACTERL" syndrome by Nora and Nora in 1973.[49] Although rare, this syndrome has been linked to sex steroid exposure in early pregnancy, but not substantiated.

EFFECTS ON OTHER ORGAN SYSTEMS AND METABOLISM

Effects on other organ systems and alterations in metabolism during oral contraceptive use were not fully realized at the time of initial marketing. After 20 years of use, many changes are now well appreciated. Although serious complications associated with oral contraceptive use are relatively rare, changes in laboratory test results may be caused by physiologic alterations. (These are listed in Table 19–1.) These test results usually remain within the normal range, and seldom reflect true pathologic changes. Most alterations result primarily from estrogen rather than progestin stimulation, and preparations containing less estrogen are less likely to influence laboratory tests.

Liver

Treatment of normal human subjects with large doses of estradiol does not produce any histologic or electronic microscopic alteration in the hepatic cell. However, treatment with regular-dose oral contraceptives is associated with canaliculi dilation, loss of canilicular microvilli, and a pericanalicular deposit of acid phosphatase.[50] Lactic dehydrogenase and transaminase values are not altered remarkably, but alkaline phosphatase may be increased.[51] Infusion of bromsulphalein (BSP) dye is invariably associated with BSP retention.[52,53] The observed decreased albumen/globulin ratio and serum cholinesterase are an early indication of derangement in hepatic protein synthesis of serum proteins and enzymes.[54]

Enterohepatic Circulation

The parenchymal cells of the liver have the capacity to take up and excrete into biliary channels organic anions of both endogenous and exogenous origin, at concentrations exceeding their plasma levels. The excretion of bilirubin and bile salts is a major hepatic function. The liver efficiently extracts bile acids from the portal blood, so that under normal circumstances the bile salt pool is confined largely to the enterohepatic cycle (liver–bile–intestine–portal blood–liver). In hepatobiliary disease, the liver often loses this high extraction efficiency, and increased amounts of circulating bile salts appear in peripheral plasma.

The capacity of the liver to excrete organic anions (bile salts or organic dyes) is consistently decreased by steroid hormones and pregnancy. Gross clinical tests, such as serum bilirubin concentration and the standard BSP test, do not detect these pregnancy-induced alterations in hepatic excretory function, but such studies are readily identified by kinetic studies. Like pregnancy, combination oral contraceptives appear to impair the final transport of bilirubin or BSP from the liver cell to the bile canaliliculi.

Mueller and Kappas described abnormal BSP metabolism in patients treated with the natural estrogens, estradiol and estriol.[53] Other natural steroids (progesterone, testosterone, and cortisol) do not alter BSP disposal by the liver,[55,56] but synthetic progestins and estrogens, given continuously, may be associated with jaundice, pruritus, and laboratory evidence of intrahepatic cholestasis, that is, elevated serum alkaline phosphatase, elevated bile salt levels, and liver biopsies revealing dilated bile canaliculi with bile plugs.[51,55,56] Patients demonstrating this sensitivity are also prone to jaundice of pregnancy.

TABLE 19–1. POSSIBLE EFFECTS OF ORAL CONTRACEPTIVES ON LABORATORY TESTS*

Laboratory Test	Effects	Probable Mechanism
Serum, Plasma, Blood		
Albumin	Slightly decreased	Decreased hepatic synthesis
Aldosterone	Increased	Activates renin-angiotensin system
Amylase	Slightly increased (common)	Not established
	Markedly increased (rare)	Pancreatitis
Antinuclear antibodies	Become detectable	Not established
Bilirubin	Increased (rare)	Reduced secretion into bile
Ceruloplasmin	Increased	Increased hepatic synthesis
Cholinesterase	Decreased	Decreased hepatic synthesis
Coagulation factors	Increased II, VII, IX, X	Increased synthesis
Cortisol	Increased	Increased cortisol-binding globulin
Fibrinogen	Increased	Increased hepatic synthesis
Folate	Decreased or no change	Decreased folate absorption
Glucose tolerance tests	Small decrease in tolerance	Several mechanisms proposed
γ-Glutamyl transpeptidase	Increased	Altered secretion in bile
Haptoglobin	Decreased	Decreased hepatic synthesis
HDL cholesterol	Increased with estrogens and decreased with progestins	Not established
Iron-binding capacity	Increased	Increased transferrin levels
Magnesium	Decreased or no change	Decreased bone resorption
Phosphatase, alkaline	Increased (rare)	Altered secretion in bile
Plasminogen	Increased	Increased hepatic synthesis
Platelets	Slightly increased	Not established
Prolactin	Increased	Not established
Renin activity	Increased	Increased synthesis of renin substrate
Thyroxine (total)	Increased	Increased thyroxine-binding globulin
Transaminases	Slightly increased	Not established
Transferrin	Increased	Increased hepatic synthesis
Triglycerides	Increased	Increased synthesis
Triiodothyronine resin uptake	Decreased	Increased thyroxine-binding globulin
Vitamin A	Increased	Increased retinol-binding protein
Vitamin B_{12}	Decreased	Not established
Zinc	Decreased	Shift of zinc into erythrocyte
Urine		
Δ-Aminolevulinic acid	Increased	Increased hepatic synthesis
Ascorbic acid	Decreased or no change	Not established
Bacteria	Increased incidence of bacteriuria	Not established
Calcium	Decreased	Decreased bone resorption
Cortisol (free)	Unchanged	
Porphyrins	Increased (may precipitate porphyria in susceptible patients)	Increased Δ-aminolevulinic acid synthetase
17-OHCS	Slightly decreased or no change	Increased binding proteins
17-KS	Slightly decreased or no change	Increased binding proteins

* These effects are thought to be dose-dependent and uncommon with use of low-dose preparations.

Estrogen and 17-alkylated progestins exert a general inhibitory effect on hepatic conjugation of bilirubin with glucuronic acid. The steroids that produce cholestasis inhibit the hepatic formation of the bile salt taurocholate, which provides the major osmotic force for bile flow.[57] 17-Aklylated progestins also produce a striking decrease in the 16-hydroxylation of estradiol, and thereby slow the metabolism of administered estradiol and its oxidative product, estrone. In addition, estrogens may cause a leak in the plasma membranes of the liver cell, causing a back diffusion from the bile canaliculi of conjugated bilirubin. Hence, the action of certain sex steroids on the liver are multiple, and may result in the development of intrahepatic cholestasis and, rarely, hyperbilirubinemia.

The enterohepatic circulation plays an important role in the metabolism of estrogen.[58] This circulation forms a second anatomic pool, from which estrogens are being continuously transported back and forth. Partial or complete interruption of the enterohepatic circulation of estrogens occurs in recurrent intrahepatic cholestatic jaundice of pregnancy and, to a degree, in patients on oral contraceptives. Accordingly, there may be a retention of estrogens in the liver following conjugation; these steroids are transported back to the blood instead of being secreted into the bile. Because the synthetic estrogens are excreted via the bile, they exert a greater effect in the liver when cholestasis and partial failure of excretory function occur. In frank or occult liver disease, the hepatic uptake of estrogen is increased and protein synthesis activities of the liver are altered.

Gallstone Formation

Bile excretion may also be impeded by progestin effects on ductal motility. The composition of bile may also contain a higher concentration of cholesterol because of a reduced cholesterol clearance, initiated by exogenous estrogen and progestins. The incidence of cholelithiasis has been reported to double in patients taking oral contraceptives,[59] but the actual number of patients is less than 0.1 percent per year among oral contraceptive users. Progestins not only contribute to bile stasis and cholelithiasis, but have also been implicated in the hepatic metabolism of certain drugs. Progestins have been shown to have an effect on the smooth endoplasmic reticulum, whose microsomal fraction plays an important role in enzyme induction for drug metabolism (Table 19–2).[55,56]

Hepatic Tumors

Another serious oral contraceptive related disorder is the development of benign tumors of the liver (estimates are 5 per 1 million users). This hepatoma tends to involve the right lobe, but may also appear in the left lobe. It is usually superficial and solitary, but may be multiple. Intrahepatic or intraperitoneal hemorrhage is the presenting clinical complaint one-half the time. The suspicion from palpation of a liver mass requires radiographic confirmation or liver biopsy. Tumor growth is likely steroid related, but it is virtually impossible to predict which users of synthetic sex steroids will develop these tumors. Baum et al. first suggested the association in 1973.[60] Mays and co-workers,[61] at the University of Louisville, and Nissen and Kent,[62] at the University of California, Irvine, have established tumor registries. Fechner recently reported a critical analysis of the Anglo-American literature in benign hepatic tumors between 1940 and 1976.[63] Prior to 1960, the incidence of liver tumor had no association with oral contraceptives, and such cases served as a control group. Approximately 300 instances of benign liver tumors have been reported since 1973 in oral contraceptive users, but the actual incidence remains unknown.[64]

In the late 1950s, Edmonson and Henderson clearly defined and separated the two most common forms, focal nodular hyperplasia and liver cell adenomas, by gross and

TABLE 19-2. DEVIATION OF THE PLASMA PROTEIN CONCENTRATION FROM THE NORMAL MEAN DURING LATE PREGNANCY COMPARED WITH THAT DURING USE OF MEGESTROL-MESTRANOL

	Mean Change in Concentration	
Serum Proteins	***During Use of Contraceptive Steroids (%)***	***During Late Pregnancy (%)***
Haptoglobin	−25	0
Albumin	−12	−10
Immunoglobulins	(0)	(0)
α_2-Macroglobulin	+7	+40
Lipoproteins	+15	+45
Transferrin	+26	+40
Plasminogen	+47	+50
α_1-Antitryspin	+51	+100
Thyroxine-binding globulin	+65	+65
Ceruloplasmin	+188	+200

microscopic pathology.[65] This has practical application, since the risk of potential hemorrhage is much greater with liver cell adenomas. Focal nodular hyperplasia (FNH) is characterized by one or more visible nodules in an otherwise normal liver, with bile ductules concentrated at the edge of the nodules. In contrast to FNH, liver cell adenoma was an extremely rare lesion prior to 1960.[64] Young women are the most likely group to develop this liver tumor. Adenomas may be single or multiple, and tend to be sharply circumscribed with a thin capsule and no nodularity. Small adenomas often have no capsule, and are confluent with normal cells. The possibility of malignant transformation must be viewed with extreme caution. Hepatocellular carcinoma is reported in both young and old, but its association with oral contraceptives appears highly unlikely.

The most reliable information on the clinical occurrence of liver tumors and oral contraceptive use emanates from the hepatic registries. The University of Louisville registry was established in 1973, and its clinical data were published in 1974.[61] Forty-four tumors were classified as focal nodular hyperplasia, 40 as hepatocellular adenoma, and 13 as hepatocellular carcinomas. Of the 101 tumors, 81 occurred in oral contraceptive users (the majority had taken large-dose oral contraceptives for a long period of time), three were long-term users of estrogen, one had a thecoma, and six were either pregnant or immediately postpartum. The average age of onset was 29, but most of the benign liver tumors, either pill-associated or spontaneous, were found during the reproductive years. Nissen and Kent found 85 percent of liver tumors from their registry were in patients under 35 years of age.[62] Eighty-five percent of those patients in which the association of pill and tumor was present had been on oral contraceptives over 4 years. The actual risk of long-term estrogen exposure in the presence of synthetic 17-alkylated progestins for increased mitosis and cell replication (which progresses to hepatic cell adenoma) is unknown.

Protein Synthesis

Many plasma proteins are synthesized by the hepatocyte.[66] Estrogen can influence the synthesis, distribution, degradation, and function of RNA, which has a central role in the control of protein synthesis.[67] Estrogen may activate genes and allow transcription of new species of mRNA, which then code the synthesis of specific plasma proteins by the hepatocyte.[68,69]

A change in the serum concentrations of a broad variety of proteins synthesized within the liver is seen during oral contraceptive use.[68,69,70] Table 19–2 lists these changes, and shows how such alterations are similar to those seen during late pregnancy. Ramcharan, Honger and co-workers have demonstrated a decrease in serum albumin levels, as well as a number of other specific serum proteins.[66,71] There is a known relationship between the hepatic production of albumin and serum cholinesterase, both of which are significantly decreased during oral contraceptive use. The α_1-, α_2-, and β-protein globulins are increased, and the albumin/globulin ratio is further decreased. Oral contraceptives play a role in the increased synthesis of many carrier proteins (thyroxine-binding globulin, corticosteroid-binding globulin, pre-β and β-lipoprotein, testosterone–estrogen-binding globulin, transferrin, casuloplasmin) and vitamin K-dependent coagulation factors (II, V, VII, IX, X, and plasminogen). Of all the serum proteins, cortisol-binding globulin (CBG) shows the best correlation of estrogen dose to hepatocyte protein synthesis, because estrogen is the only factor known to increase CBG.[72]

Haptoglobin, cholinesterase, orosomucoid, antithrombin III, and γ-globulin show a decrease. Subgroups of the immunoglobulins IgG, IgA, IgM have been studied, and changes resulting during oral contraceptive use have been small and are not considered statistically significant or clinically pertinent.

Thyroid Function

Despite the increased hepatic synthesis of thyroid-binding globulin (TBG), oral contraceptives do not adversely affect thyroid function.[54] The evaluation of thyroid status by determination of free thyroxine and radioiodine tests suggest normal thyroid function. Total thyroxine (T_4) is elevated, and indirect tests of thyroid function, like resin uptake of [^{131}I], triodothyronine (T_3), are decreased. The latter test reflects an alteration secondary to the increase in TBG.

Carbohydrate Metabolism

The data in glucocorticoid metabolism and its endocrine effect in patients who are chronically administered oral contraceptives are more complex than for the thyroid gland. Plasma 17-hydroxycorticosteroids (17-OHCS) are higher, and urinary 17-OHCS are unchanged or slightly decreased.[73] Cortical secretions are not increased, but the metabolic clearance rate (MCR) is decreased because the biologic half-life is prolonged from increased binding to increased CBG levels. The tissue concentrations of cortisol are not increased in patients treated with long-term and high doses of estrogen, and these patients do not appear cushinoid.

A blunting of the adrenocorticotropic hormone (ACTH) response to the metapyrone challenge test has been observed. This may be caused by the increased reservoir of bound cortisol or by the decreased pituitary reserves of ACTH. The latter seems unlikely, since the pituitary—adrenal response to stress is normal. In patients treated with oral contraceptives, the two constant features are an elevated CBG, which is dose-dependent with estrogen, and an elevated total serum cortisol, which are both reversed when the oral contraceptives are discontinued.

Although signs of hyperadrenocorticism are not clinically evident with oral contraceptive use, there are certain metabolic findings in pill users that are similar to glucocorticoid-like activity. Wynn has suggested that the persistently decreased tolerance to a glucose challenge and the resultant transient hyperinsulinemia during oral contraceptive use are similar to glucocorticoid-induced diabetes.[74] More specifically, he considered the metabolic picture to be similar to that found after the prolonged daily administration of 5 mg of prednisone. This may produce an excess in glucocorticoid metabolic activity without showing obvious symptoms of Cushing's syndrome. Others have found glycosuria in female patients challenged with low-dose oral glucocorticoids coupled with oral contraceptives.[75,76] Glucocorticoids promote liver gluconeogenesis and glycogenolysis, in contrast to hyperinsulinemia, which stimulates both the conversion of glucose to glycogen and its metabolism by glycolysis. Estrogens are thought to elevate glucose levels, whereas progestins may cause a hyperinsulinemia state. Glucagon concentrations are not thought to change or play a role in any glucose metabolic changes. The estrogen/progestin ratio is, therefore, important to consider. Changes in glucose tolerance tests performed by Spellacy et al. are thought to be negligible and reversible, especially with low dose oral contraceptives. As a measure of carbohydrate metabolism, the oral glucose tolerance test is preferred over the intravenous test.[75,76]

A chronic stress to pancreatic β-cell production is strongly implied in long-term oral contraceptive users. This appears to be dose-dependent, that is, less in low-dose combination. Clinically, those patients who may have relative islet cell insufficiency (gestational diabetes, women with large babies, stillborns, obesity, and family history of diabetes) do not appear to be good candidates for high- or intermediate-dose combination oral contraceptives.

Lipid Metabolism

Whereas carbohydrate metabolic changes seem to be related to exogenous estrogen and progestin, alterations of lipid metabolism are influenced by estrogen. Wynn, in 1968, observed an increase in low-density lipoprotein levels with combination oral contraceptives, particularly those whose progestin had inherent estrogen activity.[74] Others have demonstrated elevated β-lipoproteins and pre-β-lipoproteins, both synthesized in the liver and increased by exogenous estrogen. It is now generally agreed that very low-density lipoproteins (VLDL) and their binding with triglyceride (TG) are greater. High-density lipoproteins (HDLP) levels increase from estrogen stimulation. There seems to be a worrisome increase in triglycerides, a commensurate rise in phospholipids, a questionable elevation of cholesterol, and an alteration in HDL structure and metabolism which could be related to the risk of development of atherosclerosis.[77]

The coincidental appearance of Fredrickson class II or IV hyperlipemia has been associated with combination oral contraceptives. Class IV patients with elevated pre-β-lipoproteinemia and trigylcerides are a clinical concern, because of the association with eruptive xanthoma and early or accelerated atherosclerosis (with or without a propensity for coronary artery disease).

Hypertension

Weir et al., in a carefully monitored study, found systolic and diastolic blood pressure to increase 13.5 mm and 6.2 mm, respectively, in all combination oral contraceptive users.[78] Laragh et al. suggest that angiotensinogen synthesis is augmented by estrogen which invariably increases levels of angiotensin II.[79] This potent vasopressor and stimulator of aldosterone may eventually cause sodium retention, an increased blood volume, and hypertension.

The exact changes in renin-substrate, plasma renin, and angiotensin II concentration are not universally agreed upon. Combination oral contraceptives consistently raise circulating levels of renin-substrate. Plasma renin activity is also usually increased, even though plasma renin concentration is not increased, and may fall. An impaired feedback mechanism has been suggested to explain the normal or reduced plasma renin concentration and augmented renin activity.

A combination pill with a low dose of estrogen (0.05 mg or less) is recommended. The mean systolic and diastolic blood pressures in women with a past history of elevated blood pressures are not thought to rise with low-dose oral contraceptive use.[80] Discontinuation of an oral contraceptive should reverse any blood pressure elevation within the first 3 months. Periodic blood pressure determinations are necessary in oral contraceptive users, particularly whenever there has been a history of pregnancy-induced hypertension.

Vitamin and Mineral Metabolism

The literature on oral contraceptives and their effect on vitamins and minerals is moderate. When a tryptophane load is administered, vitamin B_6 (pyridoxine) deficient subjects have an increased excretion of xanthurenic acid (XA). This phenomenon may be seen in pregnancy or in oral contraceptive users, and is reversed by giving 30 mg of pyridoxine hydrochloride each day.[81] The need for riboflavin may be greater when increased amounts of pyridoxine are required for tryptophane metabolism. Folic acid deficiency in oral contraceptive users has been documented by decreased serum folate and red blood cell folate levels.[82,83] It is generally accepted that there is a reduced gastrointestinal absorption of folate from foods during oral contraceptive use. Serum vitamin B_{12} levels decrease, and the binding capacity increases during pregnancy and with oral contraceptive use.[84] The increased ceruloplasmin levels catalyze the oxidation of ascorbic acid (vitamin C), and vitamin C levels fall during pregnancy and oral contraceptive use. Therefore, there is a general consensus that selective vitamin replacement during oral contraceptive therapy is theoretically justifiable.

Along with vitamin metabolism, minerals undergo rather profound changes with oral contraceptive use. Marked elevation of serum copper has occurred, because of the increased copper absorption and the increase in serum ceruloplasmin. Serum iodine and iron are also elevated, because of increased TBG and transferrin levels. Persistent findings of iron metabolism in patients on oral contraceptives reveal an increased serum iron, total iron-binding capacity, and red blood cell volume.[83] Because albumin levels are decreased, less calcium, magnesium, and phosphorous are bound, and levels are decreased with oral contraceptive use.[85]

Coagulation Changes and Thromboembolism

Most of the serious complications reported in association with oral contraception involve problems of the vascular system, the vast majority occurring as a result of inappropriate coagulation.[59,86–90] Blood platelets may be slightly increased, and certain vitamin K-dependent coagulation factors (II, V, VII, IX, X) that are manufactured in the liver are increased. There is endothelial proliferation and thickening of the interna in medium-sized arteries of women receiving oral contraceptives. Fibrinogen, which is important to blood clot formation, increases 50 percent in oral contraceptive users. Blood-clotting factor V is elevated in 25 percent of users, factors II and IX are elevated in 75 percent; and factor XII is increased in almost all users. Other investigators have found that blood clot lysis was found to decrease significantly. Such changes are reversible after oral contraception therapy is terminated.

These changes in the clotting mechanisms are associated with an increased incidence of thrombosis in the pelvis and lower extremity, as well as pulmonary embolism in the lung. In April 1979, two companion articles published in the *British Medical Journal* reported that women taking oral contraception have a higher incidence of thrombophlebitis and pulmonary embolus.[87,88] Other factors found to influence the incidence rates of thrombophlebitis were obesity, genetics (three times as common in mothers and sisters), major surgery, blood group (lower incidence in group O patients, higher in blood group A), chronic disease, and immobility. In a prospective study, The Royal College of General Practice found deep-vein thrombosis to be 5.6 times greater in oral contraceptive users.[90] The risk of deep-vein thrombosis was dose-dependent—the greater the estrogen dose, the greater the risk of thrombosis.[87,89] An increase of a variety of coagulation factors is appreciable only above a dose of 0.5 mcg of ethinyl estradiol.[88] Smaller amounts are less effective or not at all active. Use of a low-dose (35 mcg ethinyl estradiol or 0.4 mg norethindrone) pill is not associated with an increased procoagulant risk and do not significantly enhance coagulation.

- 50 mcg estrogen pill: 81 cases of blood clots per 100,000 users
- 100 mcg estrogen pill: 111 cases of blood clots per 100,000 users

Whenever thrombosis is evident, the oral contraceptive should be immediately discontinued and not restarted after successful therapy. An alternate method of birth control is also recommended in the presence of appreciable varicose veins or superficial thrombophlebitis.

Cardiovascular Disease

British data reveal a fourfold increase in the relative chance of developing a cerebrovascular accident in women taking oral contraceptives.[91] This risk is related to the dosages of estrogen and progestin components. The pill is contraindicated if there is a strong family history of stroke, or is to be discontinued if persistent migraine-like headaches or hemiparesis occurs.

The risk of myocardial infarction is significantly altered in women taking oral contraceptives and who have hypertension, hypercholesterolemia, are smokers; this risk increases with age. The relative risk of a cardiovascular accident among oral contraceptive users who smoke is shown below:

Oral contraceptive + smoker + age 27 to 39 = 1 cardiovascular accident per 8400 patients annually

Oral contraceptive + smoker + age 40 to 45 = 1 cardiovascular accident per 250 patients annually

Goldzieher emphasized the inexactness of "anecdotal" reports and retrospective case/control studies in his investigation, and concluded.[48]

1. Women aged 40 to 44 are at no greater risk from pill use than younger women.
2. Smoking, and particularly heavy smoking, is a much more important risk factor (as is obesity) than pill use.
3. There appears to be an additive effect between smoking and pill use, especially in heavy smokers over the age of 35.

Conversely, Jick et al. concluded that it is advisable not to prescribe oral contraceptives to women older than 37 years with conditions predisposing to heart attacks, such as hypertension, diabetes, hyperlipoproteinemia (type II hyperlipoproteinemia), obesity, and smoking.[92] Regardless of the estrogen dose, oral contraceptives are not recommended in patients over 35 years of age who smoke or have other risk factors.[93] Certainly smokers should be advised that they are subject to greater risk, and oral contraceptives should not be prescribed for smokers over the age of 40 (Fig. 19–4). Finally, oral contraception should be discontinued 4 weeks prior to elective major surgery. It is important to realize, however, that many of the cardiovascular concerns are based on estrogen and progestin doses higher than those found in low dose oral contraceptives currently available in the United States.[93] Currently, there is not thought to be a positive association between present oral contraceptives and stroke or myocardial infarction.[94]

PREPARATIONS

Combination Oral Contraceptives

In 1985, 32 oral contraceptive products were marketed by a number of pharmaceutical firms, and prescribed to 10 million domestic users. These preparations contain 20 to 150 mcg of ethinyl estradiol or mestranol, and usually 1 mg or less of a progestin, in varying

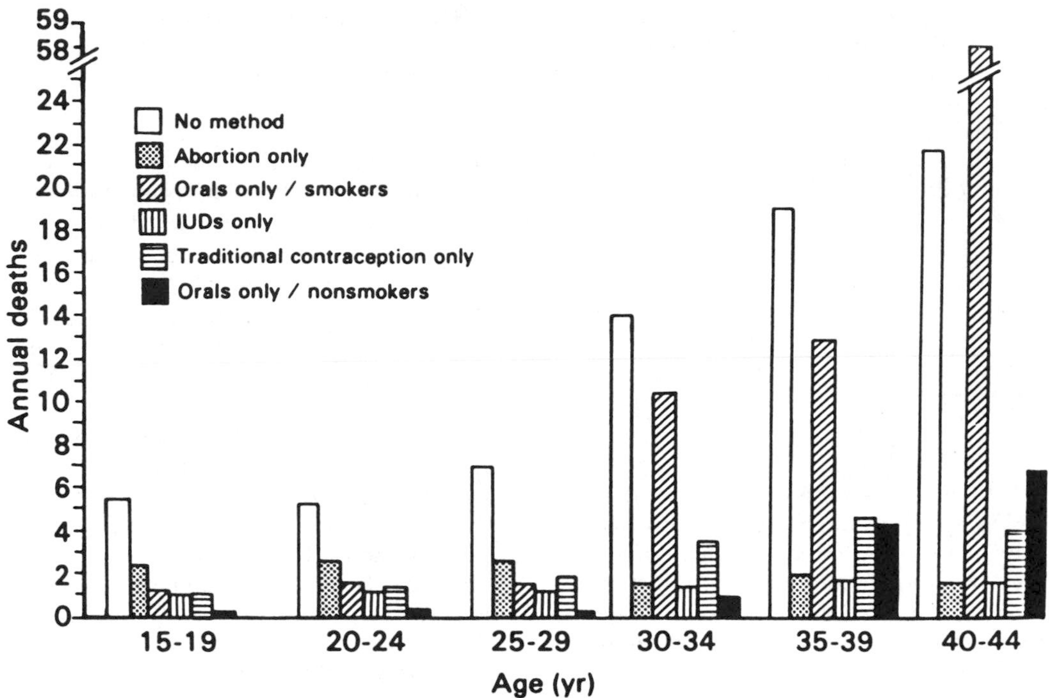

Figure 19–4. Mortality associated with fertility control. Note low mortality levels with all major reversible methods including oral contraceptives, compared to risk of death from pregnancy and childbirth when no fertility control is used, except for women who use oral contraceptives and also smoke. *(Modified from Tietze C: Family Planning Perspectives 9:74, 1977, with permission.)*

ratios. Table 19–3 lists those preparations which are currently available. Each active tablet contains a specific concentration of each steroid, and is to be taken daily for 21 days each month. The tablets are packaged in calendar-like containers, which aid the user in counting the days. The containers holding 28 tablets have an additional 7 inactive tablets, which permit the patient to take 1 pill daily throughout the menstrual cycle.

The effectiveness of these combined estrogen and progestin preparations is nearly 100 percent when taken properly, and is better than any other nonpermanent method of contraception. Even preparations containing 20 mcg of ethinyl estradiol are associated with a pregnancy rate of less than 0.2 percent per 100 women. The differences in effectiveness between the various preparations is, therefore, too small to recommend a higher-containing estrogen formulation.

An alternate regimen to high- and intermediate-dose combination estrogen/progestin was made possible by the synthesis of the potent progestin, norgestrel. This progestin molecule permitted the formulation of a low-dose combination estrogen/progestin. In this instance, the synthetic estrogen was reduced to 20 mcg. Similarly, the progestin was reduced when estrogen was given in combination with norgestrel, and it became possible to use 0.3 mg of progestin (Lo Ovral). Other weaker progestins, such as norethindrone and norethindrone acetate, have been used with low-dose estrogen in a combination pill (Table 19–3). The reported incidence of breakthrough bleeding using Loestrin (1.5/30) is 20 percent, while using Norinyl 1 + 35 is 12 percent. Most reproduction endocrinologists prefer these low-dose estrogen/progestin preparations to their higher-dose counterparts for oral contraception.[28,93–95]

Alternate Formulations for Oral Contraceptives

In 1967 an alternative formulation to combination oral contraception was proposed and marketed. Estrogen-progestin sequential preparations provided for 15 days of unop-

TABLE 19–3. COMPOSITION AND DOSES OF SOME ORAL CONTRACEPTIVES

Mcg-Estrogen	Mg-Progestin		Trade Name
1. Combination Oral Contraceptives			
Less than 50 mcg			
20 Ethinyl estradiol	1	Norethindrone	Loestrin 1/20; Zorane 1/20
30 Ethinyl estradiol	0.3	Norgestrel	Lo/Ovral
30 Ethinyl estradiol	1.5	Norethindrone	Loestrin 1.5/30; Zorane 1.5/3
35 Ethinyl estradiol	0.4	Norethindrone	Ovcon-35
35 Ethinyl estradiol	0.5	Norethindrone	Brevicon; Modicon
35 Ethinyl estradiol	1	Norethindrone	Norinyl 1 + 35, Ortho-Novum 1/35
35 Ethinyl estradiol	1	Ethynodiol diacetate	Demulin 35
50 mcg			
50 Mestranol	1	Norethindrone	Norinyl 1 + 50; Ortho-Novum 1/50
50 Ethinyl estradiol	0.5	Norgestrel	Ovral
50 Ethinyl estradiol	1	Ethynodiol diacetate	Demulen
50 Ethinyl estradiol	1	Norethindrone	Ovcon-50; Zoranel 1/50
50 Ethinyl estradiol	1	Norethindrone acetate	Norlestrin, 1
50 Ethinyl estradiol	2.5	Norethindrone acetate	Norlestrin, 2.5
More than 50 mcg			
75 Mestranol	5	Norethynodrel	Enovid 5 mg
80 Mestranol	1	Norethindrone	Norinyl 1 + 80; Ortho-Novum 1/80
100 Mestranol	1	Ethynodiol diacetate	Ovulen
100 Mestranol	2	Norethindrone	Norinyl, 2 mg; Ortho-Novum, 2 mg
100 Mestranol	2.5	Norethyndrel	Enovid-E
150 Mestranol	9.85	Norethynodrel	Enovid 10 mg
2. Progestin-Only Oral Contraceptives			
	0.35	Norethindrone	Micronor, Nor-Q.D.
	0.075	Norgestrel	Ovrette
3. Biphasic Combination Oral Contraceptives			
35 Ethinyl Estradiol	0.05	Norethindrone (days 1–10)	Ortho-Novum 10/11
35 Ethinyl Estradiol	1	Norethindrone (days 11–21)	
4. Triphastic Combination Oral Contraceptives			
30 Ethinyl Estradiol	0.05	Norgestrel (days 1–6)	
40 Ethinyl Estradiol	0.075	Norgestrel (days 7–11)	Triphasic
30 Ethinyl Estradiol	0.125	Norgestrel (days 12–22)	
35 Ethinyl Estradiol	0.5	Norethindrone (days 1–7)	
35 Ethinyl Estradiol	0.75	Norethindrone (days 8–14)	Ortho-Novum 7, 7, 7
35 Ethinyl Estradiol	1	Norethindrone (days 15–21)	

posed estrogen, and 6 days of estrogen/progestin. This formulation was adopted and marketed by several pharmaceutical companies. It was accompanied by clinical and metabolic side effects from large doses of exogenous, unopposed estrogen, which included leukorrhea, fluid retention, weight gain, escape ovulation, and unexpected pregnancies. The sequential preparation was also associated with an abnormal histologic appearance to the endometrium, suggesting a premalignant lesion, or carcinoma of the endometrium.[11] Such formulations were removed from the market for these reasons.

Subsequently, in an attempt to reduce the amount of exogenous estrogen, progestin alone was administered as an oral contraceptive. Norethindrone 0.35 and Norgestrel 0.075 were marketed. The clinical data has indicated a high incidence of breakthrough bleeding, with 30 percent of patients becoming anovulatory and 30 percent having an inadequate corpeus luteum. The progestin only formulation has been associated with clinically unacceptable menstrual dysfunction.

In 1983 biphasic combination oral contraceptives were introduced in a further attempt to reduce the dose of exogenous estrogen and minimize breakthrough bleeding. Triphasic combination ethinyl estradiol and norethindrone are being used in a 7, 7, 7 formulation with the progestin being increased from 0.05 to 0.075, to 1 mg. The later formulation provides minimal side effects and breakthrough bleeding. The most recent triphasic, Triphasel, contains ethinyl estradiol 30 mcg (6 days), 40 mcg (5 days), and 10 days of 30 mcg administered with Levonorgestrel 0.05 mg, 0.075 mg, and 0.125 mg. There is no reason to doubt the effectiveness of the biphasic and triphasic preparations, but available data have not established any advantage over older formulators.[96,97]

There have been various "after the fact" oral contraceptive formulations discussed in the oral contraception literature for 15 years. The data base suggests that oral synthetic estrogens (Stelbuterol 5 mg or ethinyl estradiol 0.05) tid or qid po for 7 days postexposure interferes with embryo transfer and implantation consistently with a very low failure rate.

GUIDELINES FOR ORAL CONTRACEPTIVE USE

Patient Selection

Oral contraception selection requires an interested patient and an informed physician or physician's assistant. Pertinent clinical information is necessary before an oral contraceptive may be prescribed. A knowledge of the patient's menstrual history, growth and secondary sex characteristics, and general medical and social background is necessary. The menstrual history should include the patient's age at menarche, the presence or absence of regular menstrual cycles during adolescence, any current history of irregular or infrequent periods, and the presence or absence of dysmenorrhea. The presence or history of certain medical complications (breast disease, phlebitis, liver disease, hypertension, diabetes, epilepsy, estrogen-sensitive tumor) must be sought. Questions dealing with coital exposure, pregnancy plans, and any desire for sterilization are also informative. The general physicial examination should assess the patient's growth and secondary sexual development. Along with height and weight determinations, signs of hyperandrogenism (acne, inappropriate hair growth) and a thorough breast and pelvic examination are recommended.

The cost of contraception is an important factor affecting the choice of birth control method. These costs can be considerable. The methods associated with the lowest failure rates—sterilization, the pill, and IUD—are the most expensive (Table 19–4).[98]

After the pertinent clinical information is gathered, it must be decided whether the patient is a suitable candidate for oral contraceptive use. Table 19–5 lists those conditions in which oral contraceptives are either

TABLE 19-4. ESTIMATED FIRST-YEAR COSTS OF VARIOUS CONTRACEPTIVE METHODS

Method	Total	Medical Care	Supplies
Prescription			
Pill	$ 172	$ 65	$170
Diaphragm	160	65	95
IUD	131	65	66
Nonprescription			
Foam	50	NA	50
Condom	30	NA	30
Rhythm	NA	NA	NA
Withdrawal	NA	NA	NA
Sterilization			
Tubal ligation	1180	1180	NA
Vasectomy	241	241	NA

NA = not applicable.
From Torres A, Forrest JD, 1983.[98]

relatively or absolutely contraindicated. Another temporary method of contraception (IUD, diaphragm) or permanent method (vasectomy, tubal ligation) of contraception may be preferred.

Oral Contraceptive Selection

It is important to remember that women using oral contraception are not receiving this medication because they are ill, but for family planning purposes. Therefore, the medication should fulfill the following criteria: (1) not initiate any medical problems, (2) not aggravate any preexisting medical problems, (3) successfully eliminate unwanted pregnancies, and (4) not be associated with any danger to an inadvertent pregnancy or interfere with future pregnancies. Oral contraceptives fulfill criteria 3 and 4, but selection must be carefully individualized for criteria 1 and 2.

Table 19-6 provides guidelines to combination oral contraceptive selection. It is preferable to begin with a low-dose preparation (less than 50 mcg of estrogen, 1 mg or less of progestin). A change to an intermediate dose or, eventually, a high dose is necessary if undesired side effects persist. The adolescent desiring oral contraceptives or the patient who is in between pregnancies requires special attention (Tables 19-7 and 19-8). The prior menstrual history and signs of secondary sex characteristics and hyperandrogenism are important to consider when choosing the appropriate preparation.

Oral contraceptives are routinely started on the fifth day of menses. The effectiveness of the agent should be apparent within the first 2 to 3 days. Women with irregular menses may begin the pill anytime, but a barrier method (condoms, diaphragm) is recommended during the first few weeks.

Following pregnancy, it is encouraged that oral contraceptives be avoided during the initial postpartum period to minimize any risk of thromboembolic formation. Instead, the pill may be safely started at the initial postpartum visit, unless a medical complication (hypertension, poorly controlled diabetes, liver disease) remains present. Persons past spontaneous or induced abortion may safely begin taking oral contraceptives within the first week.

Side Effects

Side effects during oral contraceptive use in otherwise healthy patients are many and variable in nature. Table 19-9 lists undesired effects expressed by the patient, and describes the likely ethiology and recommended management. It is known that the majority of side effects occur in the first 3 months, and that 66 percent of users discontinue the pill in 1 year. All oral contraceptive users should be seen 3 months after beginning oral contraceptive therapy, and have a yearly office visit for blood pressure, breast exam, pelvic, Pap smear, and follow-up clinical history.

Many physiologic changes may be managed by reassurance alone (especially during the initial three cycles) or by changing the preparation to a different estrogen and/or progestin component. An increase in the estrogen component to more than 50 mcg is rarely necessary. The activity of these syn-

TABLE 19-5. ABSOLUTE (A) AND RELATIVE (R) CONTRAINDICATIONS TO ORAL CONTRACEPTIVE USE

Vascular

A 1. Phlebitis—leg vein, pelvic blood clots (i.e. thrombosis)
A 2. Pulmonary embolus—blood clots in lung
A 3. Cerebral vascular accident—stroke
A 4. Coronary occlusion—heart attack
A 5. Blood dyscrasias—leukemia, sickle cell anemia, polycythemia are associated with intravascular blood clotting

Liver

A 1. Jaundice—chronic or recurrent
A 2. Hepatitis—with decreased liver function
A 3. Recurrent pruritis of pregnancy
A 4. Cirrhosis with decreased liver function
A 5. Hepatic prophyria
A 6. Hepatic tumor

Metabolic

R 1. Predisposition to diabetes mellitus
 a. Family history
 b. Family history and obesity
 c. History of large babies (9 lb+)
A 2. Hypertension
 a. Blood pressure 140/90
 b. Previous history of high blood pressure
 c. Black, with family history of high blood pressure
A 3. Lipids
 a. Increased triglycerides
 b. Age 38 and over

Obstetrics and Gynecology (OB-GYN) Reproduction

A 1. Pregnancy
R 2. Lactation—i.e., nursing
A 3. First-degree amenorrhea—i.e., no previous menstrual period
A 4. Second-degree amenorrhea—i.e., history of repeated cessation of menstrual periods for 3 or more months *or* chronic infrequent periods
R 5. Second-degree amenorrhea and/or lactation while on OCs—i.e., cessation of menstrual periods and/or breast discharge
R 6. Chronic breakthrough bleeding on OCs—i.e., unpredictable bleeding while on OCs
A 7. Chronic cystic mastitis in smoker and/or a heavy caffeine user

Miscellaneous Concurrent Diseases

A 1. Epilepsy
R 2. Migraine headache
A 3. Porphyria
R 4. Fibroid tumors of uterus
R 5. Benign breast tumors
R 6. Varicose veins—severe
R 7. Gallstones or chronic biliary symptoms
A 9. Hyperthyroidism
R 10. Diabetes Mellitus

Associated Side Effects and Symptoms

R 1. Chronic weight gain
R 2. Chronic fluid retention
R 3. Chronic gastrointestinal symptoms—nausea, vomiting, dyspepsia
R 4. Chronic premenstrual symptoms—nervous, irritable, depressed, headache, fatigue, lassitude
R 5. Chronic unmanageable leg cramps
R 6. Recurrent vaginal monilla (fungus) infection

thetic steroids at receptor tissues may be either greater or less than the activity of the patient's own natural ovarian steroids. Effects similar to those seen premenstrually (nausea, nervousness, irritability, edema, headaches) are likely from estrogen excess, whereas symptoms similar to those occurring during pregnancy (fatigue, lassitude, depression, increased appetite, weight gain) are primarily from progestin excess. An organic etiology must always be considered, especially when symptoms are severe or persist after the appropriate change or discontinuation of the preparation.

Interaction with Other Drugs

Oral contraceptives may interact with other drugs to alter absorption or affect metabolic pathways. Microsomal enzymes within the liver may be inhibited or induced and thereby affect drug metabolism and clear-

TABLE 19-6. GUIDELINES TO "COMBINATION PILL" SELECTION

Estrogenic Combination		Intermediate		Androgenic Combination	
A	Low Dose—First Choice Demulen 1/35	B	Brevicon, modicon, Norinyl 1 + 35 Loestrin 1/20 Triphase EE 0.35 Noreth 0.5 EE 0.35 Noreth 0.75 EE 0.35 Noreth 1 mg	C	Lo-Ovral Triphasic EE 0.30 LNorgestrel 0.05 mg EE 0.40 LNorgestrel 0.075 mg EE 0.30 LNorgestrel 0.125 mg
D	Intermediate Dose—Alternate Choice Cemulen				
G	High Dose—Final Choice Ovulen				
K	Provera 10 mg (day 15–25) with barrier contraception	E	Ortho-Novum 1/50 mcg Norinyl 1 + 50 mcg Ortho-Novum 10/11 EE 0.35 Noreth/mg EE 0.50 Noreth/mg	F	Ovral
L, J	Follicular estrogen (Premarin 1.25 day 1–15) with luteal, estrogen/progestin (Premarin 1.25 plus Provera 10 mg day 15–25 day) with barrier contraception	H	Ortho-Novum 2 mg Norinyl 2 mg Norlestrin 2.5 mg	I	Ovral 1/80

ance. Because of this interaction, the desired effect of each drug may be antagonized or potentiated, and undesired side effects from oral contraceptive use may occur. Another form of contraception may therefore be necessary when interaction from chronic exposure is thought to either reduce the efficacy of the contraceptive or modify the activity of the other drug(s). Table 19–10 lists those known drugs with which oral contraceptives may interact and describes the presumed mechanism of action and recommended management.

THE FUTURE

The exploding world population frequently brings the medical profession face to face with the contemporary geopolitical and sociologic problems of our times. (Figure 19–5 displays those contraceptive methods used among married women.) The year 2,000 will see 8 billion people on this earth, with grave doubts about the ability to sustain ourselves. The oral contraceptive, IUD, and other temporary forms of contraception have made little progress in thwarting this specter.

TABLE 19-7. GUIDELINES TO "COMBINATION PILL" SELECTION: PUBERTY AND ADOLESCENCE (AGE 11–18)

A, B, C	1. Contraception—mature second degree sex characteristics
A, B, C	2. Contraception—regular menstrual periods
D, E, G	3. (±) Hyperandrogenism—acne, hirsutism
D, E, F, G	4. (±) Dysmenorrhea—cramps with menstrual periods
K, L	5. Amenorrhea
K	6. Infrequent menstrual periods (2–8 per year)
D, E	7. Infrequent menstrual periods (2–8 per year), with evidence of transient or early hyperandrogenism, premenstrual acne, acne, or hirsutism*
D, E, F, G*	8. Irregular menstrual periods†

* An option is C or F day 15–25 of treatment cycle.
† An option is C, D, E, F, G day 15–25 of treatment cycle.

TABLE 19-8. GUIDELINES TO "COMBINATION PILL" SELECTION: REPRODUCTION YEARS (AGE 15–35); AND PREGNANCY SPACING

A, B, C	1. Contraception—regular menstrual periods
C, F	2. Contraception—(±) hyperandrogenism (acne, hirsutism)*
D, E, G	3. Contraception—(±) dysmenorrhea (cramps with menstrual period)†
D, E, F, G	4. Contraception—with or without irregular menstrual periods
D, E, F	5. Contraception—with or without infrequent menstrual periods (3–6 years)‡
A, B, C, I, J	6. Contraception—with cessation of menstrual periods
D, E, F, G, H	7. Alternate choice for breakthrough bleeding (BTB)
A, B, C	8. Alternate choice for weight gain, nausea, headache, fatigue, lassitude
A, B, C	9. Alternate choice for recurrent vaginitis
A, B, C	10. After 38 years, only as a final option

* An option is day 15–25 of treatment cycle, with barrier contraception.
† With antiprostaglandins: (1) Motrin, (2) Ponstel.
‡ Administer day 5–25, or day 15–25, the latter with barrier contraception.

Any new contraceptive agent should, in part, possess as restricted and specific mechanisms of action as possible. Although extremely effective in most instances, all oral contraceptives utilized to date have exhibited ancillary side effects. Alterations of the cardiovascular system and coagulation mechanisms with the use of combination oral contraceptives have been well documented. Antispermatogenic compounds, GnRH antagonists and agonists, and even vasectomies have been linked with changes in hepatic function, libido, and lipogenesis.

Specific immunologic intervention of such reproductive processes as gametogenesis, fertilization, and embryo development has been proposed, as well as investigated, for many years as potential contraceptive mechanisms. The development and eventual widespread clinical use of these concepts, however, depends on the satisfactory completion of several requirements: safety, specificity, efficacy, teratogenecity or cytotoxicity to offspring in case of failure, ease of distribution and administration, and reversibility. To date, no immunization techniques have adequately fulfilled all of these standards.

Methods designed to evoke a response

TABLE 19-9. PATIENT CONCERNS

Problem	Etiology	Recommendations
Hyperandrogenism Acne Hirsutism Weight gain	1. Ovral steroid decreases hormone-binding globulin and serum albumin 2. Norgestrel in Ovral is anabolic and androgenic 3. Norethindrone and Norethindrone acetate are anabolic at 1 mg+ dose 4. Estrogen promotes fluid retention	1. For acne and hirsutism, cycle with Ovulen, Norinyl 2 mg or Demulin, which increases steroid hormone-binding globulin 2. For weight gain, minimize estrogen/progestin (i.e., Ovcon −35, Norinyl 1 + 35)
Breast Mastodynia Cystitis-mastitis Enlarged breasts	1. Estrogens increase ductal proliferation 2. Progestins increase alveolar proliferation	1. Use lower dose estrogen/progestin (progestin should be androgenic, i.e., LoOvral or Ovral)

TABLE 19–9. (*Continued*)

Problem	Etiology	Recommendations
Amenorrhea	1. Inadequate priming of endometrium 2. Excess progestin/estrogen ratio	1. Rule out pregnancy 2. Discontinue OCs for 3 months 3. Recycle with higher-dose estrogen component
Post-Pill Amenorrhea	1. Hypothalamic-pituitary dysfunction 2. Hypoestrogenism 3. Elevated prolactin 4. Hyperandrogenism	1. Hormone profile 2. Cycle with natural estrogen (Premarin 1.25 mcg) day 1–25, and Provera 10 mg day 15–25 3. Ovulation stimulation after hormone profile if pregnancy desired
Amenorrhea-Galactorrhea Post-Pill Galactorrhea	1. Hypothalamic-pituitary dysfunction 2. Elevated prolactin	1. Serum prolactin 2. Rule out pituitary tumor 3. Pap smear of any unilateral breast discharge 4. Discontinue OCs if annoying
Premenstrual Tension-like Symptoms Fluid retention Nervous Irritable Headache	1. Estrogen associated with fluid retention 2. Estrogen/progestins have an unknown effect on the renin-angiotensin-aldosterone system 3. Estrogen/progestin associated with pelvic congestion and cerebral edema, and lowered albumin/globulin ratio affecting osmolarity	1. Use minimal-dose estrogen/progestin 2. Sodium restricted diet 3. Minimize use of diuretics
Breakthrough Bleeding (BTB)	1. Inadequate estrogen priming 2. Inadequate progestin 3. Insufficient estrogen/progestin ratio	1. Higher dose estrogen/progestin preparation 2. If BTB continues, discontinue OCs
Chloasma	1. Estrogen stimulates melanocyte-stimulating hormone secretion (?)	1. Use minimal-dose estrogen/progestin 2. Avoid exposure to sunlight
CNS Syndrome Fatigue Lassitude Decreased libido Mild depression	1. Similar to first and second trimester pregnancy changes 2. Vitamin B_{12} alteration 3. Relative pyridoxine deficiency	1. Use low-dose estrogen/progestin 2. Multiple vitamin replacement 3. Pyridoxine 30 mg QID
GI Disturbances Nausea Vomiting Epigastric distress Bloating Pruritis	1. Pregnancy-like GI symptoms 2. Oral synthetic estrogen induces cholestasis 3. Progestin relaxes smooth muscle and GI motility 4. Cholelithiasis and pancreatitis	1. Low-dose estrogen/progestin 2. Pruritis associated with BSP retention and occasional peripheral bile salts; treat with oral cholestyramine and discontinue OC
Monilial Vaginitis	1. More glycogen in vagina 2. Alter vaginal pH, flora	1. Monilial treatment (Chap. 23)

TABLE 19–10. DRUGS THAT INTERACT WITH ORAL CONTRACEPTIVES

Class of Compound	Drug	Supposed Method of Action	Suggested Management
Drugs that May Reduce the Efficacy of Oral Contraceptives			
Anticonvulsant drugs	Barbiturates: phenobarbital, primidone, phenytoin, ethosuximide	Induction of microsomal liver enzymes Fluid retention caused by OCs may precipitate seizures	20–35 mcg combination OCs or progestin-only pills or another method
Cholesterol-lowering agents	Clofibrate	Reduce elevated serum triglycerides and cholesterol; this reduces OC efficacy	Use another method
Phenylbutazone and allied drugs	Phenylbutazone, indomethacin, ibuprofen	Hepatic microsomal enzyme induction	Use alternate method
Antibiotics	Rifampicin, penicillin V	Enzyme induction: rapid breakdown of estrogen in liver; intestinal motility increased with penicillins	Higher-dose OCs during short course of antibiotics or additional contraceptives. For long course, use another method
Sedatives and hypnotics	Benzodiazepines, barbiturates, chloral hydrate	Enzyme induction, increased estrogen metabolism	Alternative method
Modification of Other Drug Activity by Oral Contraceptives			
Anticoagulants	All	Efficacy impaired, as OCs increase clotting factors	Do not use OCs with anticoagulant therapy
Antidiabetic agents	Insulin and oral hypoglycemic agents	High-dose estrogen pills cause impaired glucose tolerance	Use 20–35 mcg OCs or progestin only. Consider other methods
Antihypertensive agents	Guanethidine and occasionally methyldopa	Estrogen component involved with Na^{++} retention and increased angiotensenogen	Use progestin-only pill or another method
Phenothiazine	All phenothiazides: Reserpine, tricyclic antidepressants	Serum prolactin alters, while combination OCs are associated with increased response to serum prolactin to TRH	Use alternative method
Mild analgesics	Acetaminophen	Stimulates liver metabolism of drug	None; increase dose of analgesic if insufficient pain relief

against self-antigens (i.e., zona pellucida, spermatazoa, and placental antigens) are limited because of tolerance, thereby making it difficult to elicit a uniform and predictable response. Immunologic recognition of foreign antigens (i.e., sperm antigens in the woman), although easier to initiate, has the problem of being able to immobilize or neutralize millions of spermatazoa within minutes. This type of absolute effectiveness over significant periods of time has eluded successful development. Active immunization

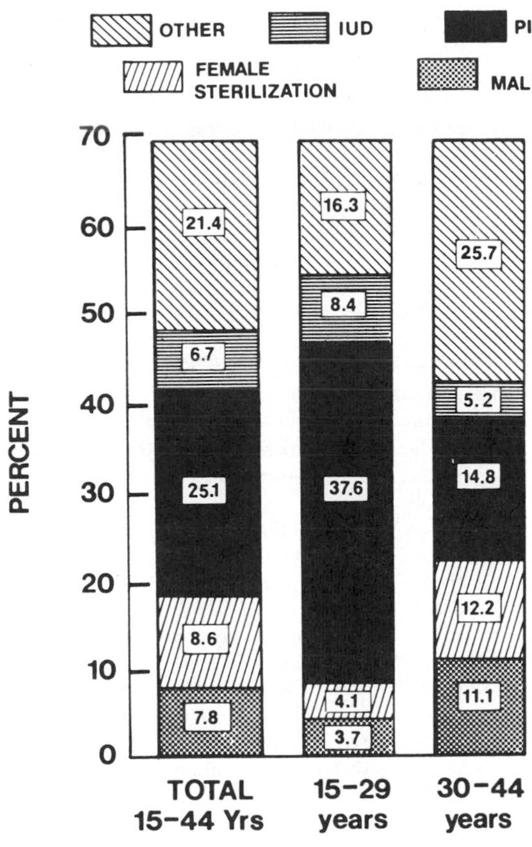

Figure 19–5. Contraception methods used by currently married women in the United States, 1973. *(From Ford K: Contraception utilization among currently married women 15–44 years of age: United States, 1973. Monthly Vital Statistics Report 25 [no 7 Suppl], Oct 1976, with permission.)*

against hCG, although extremely promising and well advanced in clinical studies, also possesses the inherent problems of overcoming tolerance, hormone and tissue specificity, individual responsiveness, and reversibility. Immunologic contraception, although still holding much promise for the future, continues to be an active area of research, with eventual clinical acceptability being a part of future expectations.

The use of sex steroid treatment in preventing contraception is becoming more therapeutically acceptable as the estrogen dose is reduced. Low dose estrogen/progestin will also be delivered as biphasics and triphasics to climateric women and in the menopause. The original high dose combination oral contraceptive formulations with ethinyl estradiol and mestranol over 0.5 mg are pharmacologically inappropriate, especially when adverse pathophysiology to the liver and coagulation system is considered. However, newer low dose estrogen/progestin preparations with tricyclic formulations, and new and novel delivery systems, such as biodegradable contraceptive capsules, promise to reduce estrogen to almost physiologic levels.[96,97,99] Clearly, synthetic estrogen/progestin will be used in the future with few, if any, serious adverse consequences.

REFERENCES

1. Arrata WSM: Oral contraceptives: General considerations. In Hafez ESE, et al. (eds): Human Reproduction: Conception and Contraception, ed. 2. New York, Harper & Row, 1980, pp 509–520
2. Rock J, Garcia CR, Pinkus G: Oral contraception. Recent Progr Horm Res 13:323, 1957

3. Briggs M: Biochemical effects of oral contraceptives. Adv Steroid Biochem Pharmacol 5:65, 1976
4. Dickey RP, Stone SC: Progestational potency of oral contraceptives. Obstet Gynecol 47:106, 1976
5. Edgren RA: Relative potency of oral contraceptives. In Moghissi KS (ed): Controversies in Contraception. Baltimore, Williams & Wilkins, 1979, p 1
6. Chihal HJW, Peppler RD, Dickey RP: Estrogen potency of oral contraceptive pills. Am J Obstet Gynecol 212:75, 1975
7. Reed MJ, Fotherby K, Steel SJ, Addison J: In vivo and in vitro metabolism of ethynlestradiol. Proc Soc Endocrinol 53:28, 1972
8. Goldzieher JW, DeLaPena A, Chenault CB, et al.: Comparative studies of the ethinyl estrogens used in oral contraception: II. Antiovulatory potency. Am J Obstet Gynecol 122:619, 1975
9. Goldzieher JW, DeLaPena A, Chenault CB et al.: Comparative studies of the ethinyl estrogens used in oral contraception: III. Effect on plasma gonadotropins. Am J Obstet Gynecol 122:625, 1975
10. Chen L, O'Malley BW: Mechanism of action of the sex steroid hormones, N Engl J Med 294:1322, 1976
11. Dujovne CA: Cytotoxic interactions between estrogens and progestins on liver cell cultures. Unpublished data, 1976
12. Vorys N: The effect of sex steroids on the liver. In Givens JR (ed): Clinical Use of Sex Steroids. Chicago, Year Book Medical Publishers, 1980, pp 184–206
13. Editorial: Metabolic effects of oral contraceptives. Lancet 2:783, 1969
14. Goldzieher JW, Maqueo M, Ricand L, et al.: Effect of combination oral contraceptives on pituitary gonadotropins. Am J Obstet Gynecol 96:1078, 1966
15. Vorys N, Stevens V: the effect of varying progestogen–estrogen ratios on pituitary gonadotropins (Proceedings of a symposium). Clin Trails J (Lond), Jan 1966, pp 73–75
16. Diczfalusy E: Mode of action of contraceptive drugs. Am J Obstet Gynecol 100:136, 1968
17. Krog W, Aktories K, Jurgensen O, et al.: Contrasting effects of combined and sequential oral contraceptives on LH–RH stimulated release of LH and FSH as compared to minipills. Acta Endocrinol (KBH) 32(Suppl):21, 1975
18. Dickey RP: The pill: Physiology, pharmacology, and clinical use. In Typer LB, Isenman AW (eds): American College of Obstetrics and Gynecology Seminar in Family Planning. Chicago, Knox, 1974, pp 24–37
19. Israel R, March CM, Kletzkz O: Post-pill amenorrhea: Investigative and therapeutic response. In Crosignami PG, Mishell DR Jr (eds): Ovulation in the Human. London, Academic, 1976, p 181
20. Mishell DR Jr: The effects of contraceptive steroids on hypothalamic-pituitary function. Am J Obstet Gynecol 128:60, 1977
21. Dickey RP, Stone SC: Effect of bromergocryptine on serum in PRL, HLH, FSH, and estradiol 17B in women with galactorrhea-amenorrhea. Obstet Gynecol 48:84, 1976
22. Jacobs HS, Franks SM, Murray MAF, et al.: Clinical and endocrine features of hyperprolactinemic amenorrhea. Clin Endocrinol 5:439, 1976
23. Tyson JE: Neuroendocrine dysfunction in galactorrhea–amenorrhea after oral contraceptive use. Obstet Gynecol 46:1, 1975
24. Shy KK, McTiernan AM, Daling JR: Oral contraceptive use and the occurrence of pituitary prolactinoma. J Am Med Assoc 249:2204, 1983
25. Ryan KJ; Estrogens and atherosclerosis. Clin Obstet Gynecol 19:805, 1976
26. Cramer DW, Hutchison GB, Welch WR: Factors affecting the association of oral contraceptives and ovarian cancer. N Engl J Med 307:1047, 1982
27. Oral contraceptive use and the risk of ovarian cancer. The Centers for Disease Control Cancer and Steroid Hormone Study. JAMA 249:1596, 1983
28. Rubin GL, Ory HW, Layde PM: Oral contraceptives and pelvic inflammatory disease. Am J Obstet Gynecol 144:630, 1982
29. Hendricks CH: Inherent motility patterns and response characteristics of the nonpregnant human uterus. Am J Obstet Gynecol 96:824, 1966
30. Maques M, Becerra C, Mungria H, et al.: Endometrial changes in women using hormonal contraceptives for periods up to 10 years. Conception 1:115, 1970
31. Kaufman RH, Reeves KO, Daugherty CM: Severe atypical endometrial changes and sequential contraceptive use. JAMA 236:923, 1976
32. Oral contraceptive use and the risk of endometrial cancer: The Centers for Disease Control Cancer and Steroid Hormone Study. JAMA 249:1600, 1983
33. Grusberg SB: The histogenesis of endometrial cancer. Obstet Gynecol 30:287, 1967

34. Frederick ER: The effect of oral contraceptives on the cytology of the secretory cells of the cervix. In Blandau R, Moghissi KS (eds): Biology of the Cervix. Chicago, Univ Chicago Press, 1977, p 102
35. Pincus G: The Control of Fertility. New York, Academic, 1977 pp 240–255
36. Weid GL, Davis E, Frank R et al.: Statistical evaluation of the effect of hormonal contraceptives on the cytologic smear pattern. Obstet Gynecol 27:327, 1966
37. Bibbo M, Bartils DH, Weid GI: Abnormal cytologic and cervical neoplasia in users of oral contraceptives and IUD's. In Moghissi KS (ed): Controversies in Contraception. Baltimore, Williams & Wilkins, 1979, p 151
38. Richard RM, Barron BA: A followup study of patients with cervical dysplasia. Am J Obstet Gynecol 105:386, 1969
39. Spellacy WN, Azias N, Buhi WC, et al.: Vaginal yeast growth and contraceptive practice. Obstet Gynecol 38:342, 1971
40. Barsivala VM, Vikar RD: The effect of oral contraceptives on concentrations of various components of human milk. Contraception 7:307, 1973
41. Franceschi S, La Vecchia C, Parazzini F: Oral contraceptives and benign breast disease: A case-control study. Am J Obstet Gynecol 149:602, 1984
42. Goldrath MH: Contraception and endometrial, cervical, and breast cancers. In Hafez ESE (ed): Human Reproduction. New York, Harper & Row, 1980, pp 312–331
43. Stadel B, Rubin G, Webster L, et al.: Oral contraceptives and breast cancer in young women. Lancet ii:970, 1985
44. Long-term oral contraceptive use and the risk of breast cancer: The Centers for Disease Control Cancer and Steroid Hormone Study. JAMA 249:1591, 1983
45. Carr DH: Chromosomes after oral contraception. Lancet 2:830, 1967
46. Klinger HP, Glasser M, Glebatis DM: Contraceptives and the conceptus: I. Chromosome abnormalities of the fetus and neonate related to maternal contraceptive history. Obstet Gynecol 48:40, 1976
47. Janeruh RF, Piper JM, Glebatis DM: Oral contraceptives and congenital limb reduction defects. N Engl J Med 291:597, 1974
48. Goldzieher JW: In defense of the pill. J Contin Educ Obstet Gynecol, Oct 1978, p 15
49. Nora AH, Nora JJ: A syndrome of multiple congenital anomalies associated with teratogenic exposure. Arch Environ Health 30:17, 1975
50. Schaffner F, Popper H: Electron microscopic study of cholestasis. Proc Soc Exp Biol Med 101:777, 1959
51. Hecker RW: the liver toxicity of oral contraceptives: A critical review of the literature. Med J Aust 2:682, 1968
52. Combes B, Shibata H, Adams R, et al.: Alteration in BSP removal mechanism from blood during normal pregnancy. J Clin Invest 42:1431, 1963
53. Mueller MN, Kappas A: Estrogen pharmacology: the influences of estradiol and estriol on hepatic disposal of sulfa bromophthalein. J Clin Invest 43:1903, 1964
54. Mishell DR Jr, Colodyn SZ, Swanson LA: The effect of an oral contraceptive on tests of thyroid function. Fertil Steril 20:339, 1969
55. Jones AL, Emans JB: The effects of progesterone on hepatic endoplasmic reticulum: An electron microscopic and biochemical study. In Salhanick HA, Kipnis DM, Vande Wiele RL (eds): Metabolic Effects of Gonadal Hormones and Contraceptive Steroids. New York, Plenum, 1969, pp 68–85
56. Bianchetti JA, Prestine PE: Effect of contraceptive agents on drug metabolism. Eur J Pharmacol 7:196, 1969
57. Forker EL: the effect of estrogen on bile formation in the rat. J Clin Invest 48:654, 1969
58. Addlercreutz H, Luukkainen T: Biochemical and clinical aspects of the enterohepatic circulation of estrogens. Acta Endocrinol 124 (Suppl):101, 1967
59. Boston Collaborative Drug Surveillance Program: Oral contraceptives and venous thromboembolic disease, surgically confirmed gallbladder disease, and breast tumors. Lancet 1:1399, 1973
60. Baum JK, Holtz F, Bookstein JJ, et al.: Possible association between benign hepatomas and oral contraceptives. Lancet 2:926, 1973
61. Mays ET, Christopherson WM, Barrows GH: Focal nodular hyperplasia of the liver: Possible relationship of oral contraception. Am J Clin Pathol 61:735, 1974
62. Nissen ED, Kent DR: Liver tumors and oral contraceptives. Obstet Gynecol 46:460, 1975
63. Fechner RE: Pathologic aspects of tumors and tumor-like lesions in women taking oral contraceptives. In Silvergerg SG, Mayor FJ (eds): Estrogen and Cancer. New York, Wiley, 1978, pp 111–123
64. Sturtevant FM: Oral contraceptives and liver

tumors. In Moghissi SK (ed): Controversies in Contraception. Baltimore, Williams & Wilkins, 1979, p 93
65. Edmondson HA, Henderson BB: Liver cell adenomas associated with the use of oral contraceptives. N Engl J Med 294:470, 1976
66. Ramcharan S, Sponzelli E. Wingerd MA: Serum protein fractions. Obstet Gynecol 48:211, 1976
67. Jensen E, Brecher PE, Mobla S, et al.: Receptor transformation in estrogenic action—molecular events in hormone action. Acta Endocrinol 191(Suppl):159, 1974
68. Doe RP, Mellinger GT, Swain WR, Seal US: Estrogen dosage effects on serum proteins: A longitudinal study. J Clin Endocrinol 27:1081, 1967
69. Musa BU, Doe RP, Seal US: Serum protein alterations produced in women by synthetic estrogens. J Clin Endocrinol Metab 27:1463, 1967
70. Laurell CB, Kullander S, Thorell J: Effect of administration of a combined estrogen–progestin contraceptive on the level of individual plasma proteins. Scand J Clin Lab Invest 21:337, 1967
71. Honger PE, Rossing N: Albumin metabolism and oral contraception. Clin Sci 36:41, 1969
72. Robertson ME, Stiefel M, Landlaw, JC: The influence of estrogens on the secretory disposition and biologic activity of cortisol. J Clin Endocrinol Metab 19:1381, 1959
73. Pulkkinen MO: The levels of 17-hydroxycorticosteroids in the plasma of users of oral contraception. Acta Endocrinol (KBH) 119(Suppl):156, 1967
74. Wynn V: Some metabolic effects of oral contraceptives. Proceedings of a symposium. Clin Trails J (Lond) Jan 1966, pp 171–180
75. Spellacy WN: A review of carbohydrate metabolism and the oral contraceptives. Am J Obstet Gynecol 104:448, 1969
76. Spellacy WN, Buhi WC, Birk SA: Carbohydrate metabolism studies in women using Brevicon, a low-estrogen type of oral contraceptive, for one year. Am J Obstet Gynecol 142:105, 1982
77. Krauss RM, Roy S, Mishell DR: Effects of two low-dose oral contraceptives on serum lipids and lipoproteins: Differential changes in high-density lipoprotein subclasses. Am J Obstet Gynecol 145:446, 1983
78. Weir RJ, Briggs E, Mack A, et al.: Blood pressure in women taking oral contraceptives. Br Med J 1:535, 1974
79. Laragh JH, Sealey JE, Ledingham JG, Newton MA: Oral contraception: Renin aldosterone and high blood pressure. JAMA 201:918, 1967
80. Tsai CC, Williamson HO, Kirkland BH: Low-dose oral contraception and blood pressure in women with a past history of elevated blood pressure. Am J Obstet Gynecol 151:28, 1985
81. Wachstein M, Gudaitis A: The disturbance of vitamin B_6 metabolism in pregnancy. J Lab Clin Med 42:99, 1953
82. McLean R, Heine MW, Held B, Streiff B: Relationship between the oral contraceptive and folic acid metabolism. Am J Obstet Gynecol 104:745, 1969
83. Mandell J. Symmons C, Zilva JF: Comparison of the effects of oral contraceptives and pregnancy on iron metabolism. J Clin Endocrinol 29:1489, 1969
84. Bianchine JR, Bonnlander B, Placido VJ, et al.: Serum vitamin B_{12} binding capacity and oral contraceptive hormones. J Clin Endocrinol Metab 29:1425, 1969
85. Young MM, Jasani C, Smith DA, et al.: Some effects of ethinyl estradiol on calcium and phosphorous metabolism in osteoporosis. Clin Sci 34:411, 1968
86. Walters WAW, Linn YL: Haemodynamic changes in women taking oral contraception. J Obstet Gynecol Br Commonw 77:1007, 1970
87. Inman WH, Vessey MP, Westerholm B, Engelund A: Thromboembolic disease and steroidal content of oral contraceptives: A report to the Committee for Safety of Drugs. Br Med J 2:203, 1970
88. Beller F, Ebert C: Effects of oral contraceptives on blood coagulation: A review. Obstet Gynecol Survey 40:425, 1985
89. Sartwell PE, Masi AT, Arthes FG, et al.: Thromboembolism and oral contraceptives: An epidemiology case-control study. Am J Epidemiol 90:365, 1969
90. The Royal College of General Practitioners: Oral Contraceptives and Health. New York, Pitman; 1974
91. Inman WH, Mann JI: Oral contraceptives and death from myocardial infarction. Br Med J 2:245, 1975
92. Jick H, Duran B, Rothman KJ: Oral contraception and nonfatal myocardial infarction. JAMA 239:1403, 1978
93. Oral contraceptives and the risk of cardiovascular disease. Medical Letter 25:69, 1983
94. Porter J, Hunter J, Jick H, et al.: Oral contra-

ceptives and nonfatal vascular disease. Obstet Gynecol 66:1, 1985
95. Preston SN: A report of a collaborative dose-response clinical study using decreasing doses of combination oral contraceptives. Contraception 6:17, 1972
96. Ortho-Novum 10/11—A new "bi-phasic" oral contraceptive: Medical Letter 24:93, 1982
97. Tri-norinyl and ortho-novum 7/7/7—Two tri-phasic oral contraceptives. Medical Letter 26:93, 1984
98. Torres A, Forrest JD: The costs of contraception. Family Planning Perspectives 15:70, 1983
99. Ory SJ, Hammond CB, Yancy SG: The effect of a biodegradable contraceptive capsule (Capronor) containing levonorgestrel on gonadotropin, estrogen, and progesterone levels. Am J Obstet Gynecol 145:600, 1983

20

Estrogen and Progestin Therapy

Chad I. Friedman and L. L. Penney

The intent of this chapter is to review the uses of estrogens and progestins in clinical practice excluding their use as contraceptives. The magnitude of this task is reflected by the fact that almost every American woman has utilized an estrogen or progestational compound during some period in her life. Use of estrogens and progestins has been a matter of controversy producing a massive collection of conflicting recommendations and warnings. A complete review of the literature surrounding their use is beyond the scope of this text, which attempts only to acquaint the reader with the present status of therapy with estrogens and progestins.

ESTROGENS

Chemistry and Metabolism

Based on their chemical structure, estrogens may be divided into two groups, steroid and nonsteroid compounds. Although their biologic properties are similar, the metabolic fate of the steroid estrogens is quite different from the nonsteroid compounds.

Steroid Estrogens

NATURAL ESTROGEN. The naturally occurring estrogens include estradiol, estrone, estriol, equelin, and equilenin. The steroid structure consists of 18 carbons. All contain an unsaturated A-ring, a methyl group at C-13, a phenolic hydroxyl group at C-3, and a ketone or hydroxy group at C-17, as shown in Figure 20–1. Natural estrogens circulating in the blood are bound to albumin and testosterone–estradiol-binding globulin (sex hormone-binding globulin) with only a small fraction being free steroid. They are distributed throughout most body tissues with high concentrations occurring in fat deposits.

Estradiol 17-β is the major estrogen secreted from the maturing follicle and corpus luteum in ovulatory women. Among the naturally occurring estrogens it has the greatest biologic potency and the highest affinity for the estrogen receptor in target tissues.

Estrone is formed extensively in extraglandular tissue sites by the aromatization of androstenedione, which is produced primarily in the adrenal cortex and in the ovary.[1]

NATURAL ESTROGENS

H3C OH

HO

ESTRADIOL

H3C O

HO

ESTRONE

H3C OH

OH

HO

ESTRIOL

SYNTHETIC STEROIDAL ESTROGENS

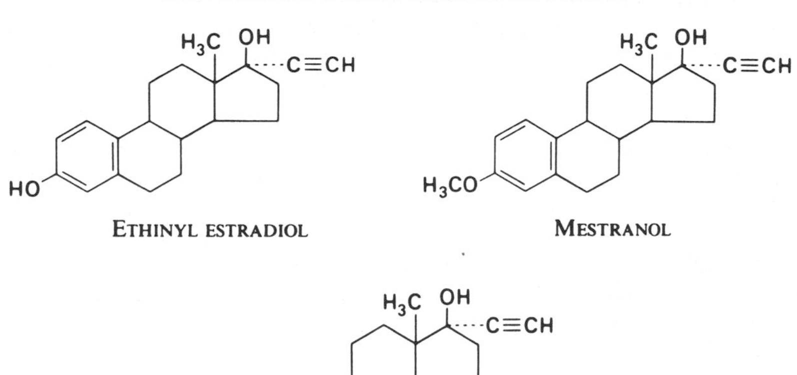

H3C OH

C≡CH

O

QUINESTROL

NONSTEROIDAL ESTROGENS

C2H5

HO

C=C

OH

C2H5

DIETHYLSTILBESTROL (Stilbestrol)

H3CO

OCH3

C=C

H3CO

Cl

CHLOROTRIANISENE (Tace)

Figure 20–1. Chemical structure of natural estrogens, synthetic steroidal estrogens, and nonsteroidal estrogens. *(From Csáky, TZ: Cutting's Handbook of Pharmacology: The Actions and Uses of Drugs, ed. 7. Norwalk, Connecticut, Appleton-Century-Crofts, 1984, pp 429–431, with permission.)*

After menopause, depletion of the follicles occurs and peripheral conversion of androstenedione becomes the primary source of estrogen. Extraglandular aromatization occurs in liver, brain, kidney, and adipose tissue. Production is noncyclic though not necessarily static. Ovarian disease states may result in increased production of androstenedione. Also, metabolic processes associated with an increased capacity for aromatization may result in increased estrone production. This has been observed to occur with obesity, hepatic disease, hyperthyroidism, compensated congestive heart failure, and starvation.

Estriol is formed by 16-α-hydroxylation and reduction of the ketone at C-17. It is a major metabolite of estradiol and estrone and is readily excreted in the urine.

Equelin and equilenin are found in the urine of pregnant mares and cannot be produced by humans.

The metabolic pathways of estrogen have not been fully elucidated. 17-β-Hydroxysteroid dehydrogenase is considered a key enzyme in estrogen metabolism allowing for the conversion of estradiol to estrone. It is present in most tissues, including the gut and target tissues.

Estrone serves as a substrate for the hydroxylating enzymes (estrogen-2-hydroxylase and estrogen-16-α-hydroxylase), and is oxidized to form the 2-hydroxy (catechol) estrogens and other hydroxylated metabolites (i.e., estriol). Polyhydroxylated estrogens are polar and water soluble, and may be excreted in the urine. Other, more lipid-soluble forms must be conjugated with glucuronic or sulfuric acid as a prerequisite for their excretion via urine or bile. Conjugation may occur in kidney tissue and intestinal mucosa as well as in the liver. The conjugated estrogens excreted in bile may be hydrolyzed by bacteria present in the gut, permitting reabsorption via the enterohepatic pathway. One conjugate, estrone-3-sulfate, may represent a storage form of estradiol. Its plasma levels exceed those of estradiol and it may be reconverted in the liver and other organs, including the uterus, to estrone and estradiol.[2]

SYNTHETIC STEROID ESTROGENS. Naturally occurring estrogens given orally are metabolized in a "first-pass effect" through the liver and are thus relatively ineffective. When natural estrogens are given intramuscularly (IM), metabolism is rapid. Synthetic forms have been developed to improve absorption and slow inactivation. Changes in the steroid structure, which do not cause loss of estrogenic activity, include interconversion of the hydroxy and ketone groups and the addition of various side chains at C-3 and C-17.

The addition of an ethinyl group to the C-17 position of estradiol produces ethinyl estradiol, the most biologically active of the synthetic steroid estrogens. Its prolonged activity is due to slower elimination from the circulation, as compared to estradiol. From a quantitative viewpoint, the major metabolic pathway for ethinyl estradiol is aromatic hydroxylation, as it is for the natural estrogens.[2] Due to the substitution at C-17, the production of estriol analogue is reduced, accounting for the slower inactivation. However, some deethinylation does occur. Controversy exists in the literature regarding the quantitative extent of this reaction. Ethinyl estradiol-sulfate is the principal circulating form of ethinyl estradiol. This may represent a storage form with functions comparable to those of estrone sulfate.[3] Unlike estradiol, substantial amounts of ethinyl estradiol are excreted in the feces with the ratio of excretion being 4:6 for feces and urine.[2]

Mestranol differs from ethinyl estradiol by the addition of a methoxy group at C-3. About 54 percent of this compound is demethylated in the liver to ethinyl estradiol. Because demethylation is not complete, more mestranol must be administered at low doses to achieve an equal therapeutic effect to ethinyl estradiol. The 3-methoxy group of mestranol causes it to be more lipophilic than ethinyl estradiol.

Quinestrol is another synthetic estrogen having a high affinity for adipose tissue, where it is stored in a chemically unaltered form and slowly released over a period of days. The unstored portion is rapidly metabolized, mainly to ethinyl estradiol. Excretion occurs mostly in urine and bile. Slow release results in an extended biologic half-life which has been reported to be 120 ± 7 hours.[4]

Longer-acting parenteral forms of synthetic estrogens have also been developed. Esterfication or polymerization of the natural estrogens slows absorption from the injection site and prolongs the action so that a single dose may be effective for days to weeks.

Nonsteroid Estrogens

Nonsteroid compounds have also been developed to overcome the problems encountered with natural estrogens. These are synthetic substances closely related structurally to stilbene. Metabolic pathways are not fully determined.

Like steroid estrogens, diethylstilbesterol (DES) and its metabolites undergo enterohepatic circulation. Metabolic pathways include: (1) aromatic ring hydroxylation and methylation of the catechol, (2) hydroxylation at one of the ethyl side chains, and (3) oxidation at the stilbene double bond. This latter pathway leads to the formation of dienestrol.[2]

Chlorotrianisene (Tace) is derived from DES. It has weak estrogenic properties but is metabolized to a more active compound. It is stored in fat tissues with a slow release resulting in prolonged action.

Mechanism of Action

In contrast to protein hormones, which interact with cell membrane receptors, estrogens enter target cells by passive diffusion. Estrogen concentrates within the cell by binding to a high-capacity, low-affinity protein conceptually similar to the steroid-binding globulin in serum. The estrogen receptor is a protein with high affinity for estrogen compounds and is essential for transport of estrogen into the nucleus. Saturation of the estrogen receptors is readily achieved due to the limited number of receptors and the ability to bind only a single estrogen molecule per receptor. Alterations in structure occur during this process, accounting for a change in sedimentation rate.

Once inside the nucleus the steroid receptor complex interacts with DNA, resulting in RNA and protein synthesis. Transport of estrogen into the nucleus results in both short- and long-acting effects.[5] Short-acting effects have a rapid on-and-off mechanism and involve the majority of nuclear receptors. Biologic effect appears to correlate well with the number of receptors occupied. Fluid imbibition in the uterus is perhaps the best-studied short-acting effect of estrogen. Teleologically, the short-acting effects could be involved in feedback mechanisms, although this has not been shown.

Long-acting effects of estrogen include cellular growth and division. They have been better studied because of suspected relationships to neoplastic changes. Long-acting effects involve a limited number of nuclear receptors which are readily saturated. Biologic effect requires nuclear retention of the steroid receptor complex for a prolonged period of time. Given similar steroid receptor complex concentrations, the "biologically weaker" estrogens (i.e., estriol) can be shown to disappear from the nucleus at a more rapid rate than biologically more potent estrogens (i.e., estradiol).[6] Differences in dissociation between the estrogens and the nuclear receptors may be compensated for by persistent reassociation. The differences in biologic potency demonstrated by bolus injection studies become inapparent when the ligand is provided in a steady state at the low concentrations required for saturation.[7]

Replenishment of the cytosol receptor, as well as continued ligand receptor transport into the nucleus, appears necessary for continued cellular stimulation. Some estrogens are unable to stimulate receptor replenishment despite prolonged nuclear retention. This appears to be one of the major mechanisms for the antiestrogens used in clinical practice.[5]

Estrogens may also have actions not mediated by cytosol receptors (i.e., inhibition of bone resorption and vascular permeability).

The means by which estrogens work in these situations are not well understood.

Pharmacologic Actions

Some of the major pharmacologic actions of estrogens are shown in Table 20–1. Many other drug interactions[8] and alterations in laboratory values[9] are known.

TABLE 20–1. PHARMACOLOGIC ACTIONS OF ESTROGENS

Genital Tract
- Stimulation of endometrial glandular and stromal compartment
- Stimulation of myometrium
- Proliferation of vaginal and urethral epithelium
- Increase in vascular flow to genital tract
- Increase in cervical gland secretions
- Stimulation of production of receptors for progesterone and luteinizing hormone

Breast
- Stimulation of ductular growth

Skin
- Increase in content of hyaluronic acid and water
- Reduction in breakdown of collagen
- Decrease in sebum production
- Decrease in epithelial proliferation

Bone
- Decrease in bone resorption
- Increase in parathyroid hormone concentrations

Liver
- Stimulation of production of multiple binding globulins (i.e., steroid-binding globulin, cortisol-binding globulin, thyroid-binding globulin)
- Increase in concentration of bile salts

Pituitary–Hypothalamus
- Suppression of vasomotor symptoms
- Suppression and stimulation of gonadotropin secretion
- Increase in prolactin secretion

Coagulation
- Stimulation of factor VII, VIII, IX, X, and prothrombin
- Depression of antithrombin III
- Increase in platelet adhesiveness

Lipids
- Increase HDL cholesterol

Clinical Use

It is appropriate for estrogens to be used in the lowest effective dose. Some individuals require higher doses than others to achieve a therapeutic response. Most patients are given estrogens on a cyclic basis: 21 days on, 7 days off, or for the first 25 days of each month. There are few data to support this regimen for the prevention of endometrial carcinoma, although it appears to be more physiologic and may be used to establish the need for estrogens in patients being treated for relief of vasomotor symptoms. Prior to starting estrogen in postmenopausal patients, a thorough breast exam and pelvic examination are performed. A Pap smear is obtained and an endometrial biopsy may be taken.

Progestational compounds should be used for at least 10 days each month in all patients with a uterus receiving estrogen replacement. In patients without a uterus, progestins are seldom used, although consideration should be given for their use if data suggesting beneficial effects on the incidence of breast carcinoma are substantiated.[10]

Throughout this chapter, doses of estrogens are expressed predominantly as the equivalent of conjugated estrogens, because these are the most commonly used preparations. The most frequently used preparation, Premarin, is a mixture of at least nine different estrogens. Serum and urinary concentrations of the administered estrogens are of little value in assessing dose equivalents. Estrogen production rates vary widely between patients and the hormones are subject to rapid interconversion and metabolism. Attempts to determine the estrogenic activity of various preparations have not been uniformly in agreement.[11] Some comparative dosages of different estrogens are given in Table 20–2.

Clinical Use After the Reproductive Years

Despite continuing controversy, the most common indications for estrogens are noted after menopause.

TABLE 20–2. COMPARATIVE DOSAGES OF VARIOUS ESTROGENS (mg)

Ethinyl estradiol	0.015
Mestranol	0.02
Conjugated estrogens	0.625
Diethylstilbestrol	0.25

VASOMOTOR SYMPTOMS. The "hot flush" is the best known symptom of the menopausal syndrome. Following a physiologic menopause it is noted in over 70 percent of women.[12] Only 15 percent of these women seek medical treatment for the symptoms, although 50 percent of reproductive-age women undergoing castration may request treatment. Clinically, there is no reasonable means to follow the response to treatment other than subjective symptomatic improvement. Using double-blind crossover studies, estrogens have been shown to be effective in reducing the frequency of vasomotor symptoms. Such studies are necessary not only to eliminate a considerable placebo effect but to correct for the spontaneous abatement of symptoms which occurs with time. In the absence of other indications, doses for replacement therapy should be individualized to the lowest dosage required to achieve a reasonable clinical response and should be reevaluated every 6 months. Short-acting estrogen compounds given for 21 to 25 days per month will allow for assessment of the spontaneous reduction in vasomotor symptoms. Reduced symptomatology during the drug-free period is frequently found within 2 years of the menopause. An example of the proposed treatment regimen is shown in Figure 20–2. Al-

Baseline evaluation: No historical contraindications for estrogen use. Pelvic exam, cytology, breast exam and endometrial biopsy, if indicated benign.

Begin estrogen therapy at lowest available dose from days 1–25 of each month. An oral progestin, medroxyprogesterone, 10 mg/day, or norethindrone acetate, 5 mg/day, is given from day 16–25.

↓ 4 weeks

If vasomotor symptoms are intolerable, increase to a higher estrogen dosage, continue progestin therapy day 16–25.

↓ 4 weeks

If symptoms are tolerable, continue present regimen.

↓ 6 months

If symptoms are tolerable with fewer flushes noted while off medication, reduce daily estrogen dosage.

↓ 6 months

If symptoms are tolerable but still bothersome during the drug-free period, continue present regimen and perform endometrial sampling for any abnormal uterine bleeding.

↓ 6 months

If symptoms are tolerable with minimal symptoms during the drug-free period, attempt to terminate estrogen treatment.

Figure 20–2. Treatment of vasomotor symptoms. The lowest effective dose of estrogen is determined based on the patient's symptomatic response. Patients with an intact uterus are given progestin for 10 days during each cycle. The drug-free period is used to assess the natural course of the climacteric.

ternate medications suggested for the relief of vasomotor symptoms include medroxyprogesterone[13] and clonidine.[14]

VAGINAL ATROPHY. Vaginal dryness or discharge, irritation and dyspareunia are common complaints associated with vaginal atrophy. Although estrogens do not increase vaginal depth or caliber, the resulting increase in vascularity and epithelial proliferation allow greater lubrication, increased protection from vaginitis, and reduced vaginal trauma with coitus. The resultant change in genital tract flora could be associated with increased posthysterectomy infection rates but organisms unusual for the genital tract have not been isolated in estrogen users.[15] Restoration of vaginal tissue function requires 18 to 24 months and explains why dyspareunia may persist in the early months of replacement therapy despite hormonal and cytologic return to premenopausal values.

Dosages of estrogen equivalent to 1.25 mg of conjugated estrogens are given initially to produce a rapid response. Once this is achieved, the dose may be decreased or given at less frequent intervals and intermittent progesterone therapy implemented. Local treatment has not been shown to be more effective than systemic administration, and estrogens administered via the vaginal route are well absorbed for systemic distribution.[16,17] If this is the sole indication and no counterindications develop, treatment should continue at least until the patient is no longer sexually active. Lubricants have been used as alternatives to estrogens. but their inability to stimulate the vaginal mucosa has limited their utility.

DYSURIA. Dysuria is classically a symptom of a urinary tract infection, although estrogen depletion may be a cause of it. The distal vagina and urethra are derived from similar embryologic structure and both are sensitive to estrogen stimulation and depletion. Prior to attempts at treatment with estrogen, an infectious etiology must be ruled out. Estrogen therapy similar to that for vaginal atrophy is appropriate. Maintenance dosages should again be as low as necessary to achieve the desired clinical response.

The increased vascularity resulting from estrogen therapy is associated with increased blood flow through the periurethral venous plexus. This or other mechanisms may result in small increases in periurethral pressures, occasionally sufficient to correct urinary stress incontinence in some postmenopausal subjects.

OSTEOPOROSIS. Multiple studies have demonstrated that estrogens are effective in decreasing the rate of bone resorption.[19–21] In contrast to treatment of vasomotor symptoms, estrogen therapy for a minimum of 6 years appears necessary to maintain the beneficial effects.[22] Accelerated bone loss is found after discontinuation of estrogen replacement. Although the classic patient who develops osteoporosis is slender and an inactive Caucasian, the present clinical use of estrogen for prophylaxis has not been selective enough to demonstrate value when evaluated by cost-benefit analysis. The addition of a progestin improves the cost–benefit analysis.[23] Special consideration for treatment should be given to patients who develop ovarian failure prior to the age of 40.

The majority of studies evaluating the ability of estrogen to prevent accelerated bone loss have dealt with high dosages of estrogens (i.e., 1.25 to 2.5 mg of conjugated estrogens). Mestranol in a dose of 20 mcg/day has been shown effective in preventing bone loss and capable of increasing bone density in subjects 3 to 6 years following castration.[24] Equivalent potency doses of conjugated estrogens and ethinyl estradiol are also effective in preventing postmenopausal bone loss (see Table 20–2).[25,26] Conjugated estrogens at a dose of 0.625 mg/day appear effective in reducing the incidence of subsequent fractures during a prolonged study period.[22] It has been suggested that the use of supplemental calcium prior to discontinuing estrogen replacement may prevent accelerated bone loss after estrogen withdrawal.[20] Further long-term studies to determine the lowest effective dose of estrogen, the value of calcium supplementation,[19] and the roles of body weight, calcitonin,[20] vitamin D, fluoride,[20,27] and possibly exercise are necessary to determine optimal treatment of osteoporosis.

Estrogen is used in the treatment of established osteoporosis. Although few studies have shown that estrogens started beyond 3 years after menopause can increase bone mass, estrogens alone or in conjunction with other agents (vitamin D and calcium) can decrease the incidence of new fractures.[28,29] Equivalents of conjugated estrogens in excess of 0.625 mg/day were used in most reports.

PSYCHOLOGICAL ASPECT. Estrogens may be of benefit in improving the sense of well-being in normal menopausal subjects at a daily dose of 0.625 mg of conjugated estrogens.[30] One mechanism of accomplishing this is to reduce the incidence of vasomotor symptoms. Others have suggested that estrogen can increase the duration of time spent in REM sleep and reduce the sleep-latency period, thereby causing an elevation in mood.[31] The data, however, are not consistent and appear dependent on population as well as testing modalities.[31] It is of interest that while estrogens are effective in reducing vaginal atrophy they have not been shown to improve libido. Estrogens are not approved nor are they reliable as psychotherapeutic agents.

Clinical Uses During the Reproductive Years

DYSFUNCTIONAL UTERINE BLEEDING. Abnormal, heavy uterine bleeding in a reproductive-age woman is most commonly caused by anovulation. Due to the absence of progesterone, the endometrium overgrows its blood supply and rests tenuously on an unstable matrix. Bleeding follows breakdown and sloughing of the endometrium without the normal hemostatic controls induced by progesterone. If treated early, progesterone alone is usually effective in stabilizing the endometrium and controlling the bleeding. If extensive endometrial sloughing has occurred, as is seen following a prolonged course of bleeding, exogenous estrogens (i.e., conjugated estrogen 5 mg/day for 14 to 21 days) may be required to induce proliferation and stabilization of the now denuded endometrium. Except in adolescents an endometrial biopsy is recommended prior to treatment. Concurrently, the exogenous estrogens will stimulate production of progesterone receptors, making the endometrium more responsive to the effects of exogenous progestins, such as medroxyprogesterone 10 mg/day for the last 7 to 10 days of treatment.

Treatment regimens have included intravenous (IV) administration of estrogens (25 mg of conjugated estrogen) every 4 hours until the bleeding stabilizes, for a maximum of six doses.[32] This form of treatment is reserved for patients requiring a rapid response. In these cases, once the patient is stabilized, oral contraceptives with intermediate-strength progestin may be administered for 21 days, and a synchronized planned withdrawal bleed will then result. Failure to stabilize with IV estrogens should in most cases necessitate a diagnostic curettage. Adolescent patients are also usually an exception to this policy. Bleeding resulting from the prolonged use of progestin or progestin-dominant oral contraceptives may be treated by the addition of 1.25 to 2.5 mg/day of conjugated estrogens for 2 weeks.

Although estrogens are extremely useful and effective in cases of dysfunctional uterine bleeding, an examination must rule out the presence of a pregnancy, cervical lesion, traumatic vaginal lesion, or a coagulopathy.

In cases of bleeding secondary to anovulation, a progestin administered each month or every 2 months following the last menstrual period will prevent such a recurrence. Attempts should be made to determine the cause of the anovulation.

DYSMUCORRHEA. In infertility patients with scanty or poor-quality cervical mucus at the presumed time of ovulation, exogenous estrogens have been used to improve the quality of the cervical mucus. Estrogen administration to hypogonadal females causes changes in the water content, pH, electrolytes, and protein concentrations of cervical mucus. These are clinically demonstrated by increased volume, transparency, ferning, spinnbarkeit, and sperm penetration. A dose of 0.3 to 0.625 mg of conjugated estrogens can be given daily during the mid- to late-follicular phase, days 8 through 14. The mechanism whereby estrogens are effective in patients with dysmucorrhea is not known. Patients with dysmucorrhea have not been shown to be hypoestrogenic. Estriol has been promoted as an estrogen with preferential actions on cervical mucus and vaginal epithelium, although recent clinical studies have failed to support this suggestion.[33] Higher dosages of estrogens have been used effectively to counteract the antiestrogen effects of clomiphene citrate on cervical mucus. It is important to discontinue the use of exogenous estrogens following ovulation to reduce the chance of any teratogenic effect. The use of estrogens in excess of 0.625 mg of conjugated estrogens may delay ovulation.

INTERCEPTION. High doses of estrogens have been used to prevent pregnancy following unprotected intercourse. Diethylstilbesterol 25 mg twice a day or conjugated estrogens 30 mg/day for 5 days may be used within 72 hours of coitus to prevent pregnancy. A failure rate of 0.5 percent has been reported.[34] Treatment should be limited to unpredictable and potentially conceptual exposures (e.g., rape, mechanical contraceptive defects). Treatment is associated with significant nausea, possible vomiting, and an increased incidence of ectopic pregnancy in failed treatments.[34] Alternate drugs and dosages have been used to decrease side effects but preliminary reports indicate higher failure rates.[35] The patient must be fully counseled concerning potential teratogenic effects of high-dose estrogens if a pregnancy is already established or treatment is ineffective.

Uses During Adolescence

HYPOGONADAL STATES. Exogenous estrogens may be utilized to stimulate sexual development in hypogonadal female individuals. A thorough investigation should precede any such treatment. Failure to diagnose a brain tumor, sex chromosomal anomaly with a Y chromosome, other endocrinologic disorders, or systemic disorders associated with certain hypogonadal states (e.g., cardiac and renal abnormalities) could be extremely detrimental to the patient.

Cyclic administration of a daily dose of estrogen equivalent to 1.25 to 2.5 mg of conjugated estrogens for 3 weeks out of 4 is usually sufficient to maximally stimulate development of secondary sex characteristics. Lower dosages should be used initially to maximize growth.[36] After a plateau in breast development is achieved, the dose may be readjusted again. A progestational compound should be added for the last 10 days of estrogen therapy each month. Menstruation, a desired response in young individuals, should occur with these dosages. Long-acting oral estrogens may also be used for maintenance therapy. The cyclic administration of a progestin will still be required each month. Oral contraceptives are not appropriate substitutes for replacement therapy as the dosage of estrogen in oral contraceptives necessary to induce secondary sex characteristics and maintain menstrual function exceeds that required in substitutional therapy.

TREATMENT OF TALL STATURE. Administration of estrogens prior to attainment of peak growth velocity is capable of prematurely closing epiphyses and thereby reducing a subject's potential height. Although the indication remains controversial, considerable experience has been gained.[37] Dose equivalents of 2.5 to 20 mg/day of conjugated estrogens have been used with success. Predicted heights are calculated from available charts after obtaining films to assess the present bone age. Treatment should be started at a bone age around 11 years to assure a reliable response. Following initiation of treatment a relative increase in growth velocity is noted, as well as accelerated maturation of the bone age. After achieving a bone age of 15 to 16 years, treatment is discontinued. Minimal further growth may be expected beyond this point. The long-term effects of such treatment are not known. It is essential that the patient, her parents, and the physician feel such treatment is justified prior to commencing therapy. The addition of a progestational agent for 10 days each month is advised.

Adverse Effect of Estrogen Therapy

ENDOMETRIAL CARCINOMA. The incidence of low-grade endometrial carcinoma is increased by the use of unopposed estrogen therapy. Estimated increases in relative risk vary between 1.7- and 15-fold.[38,39] Dose and duration of therapy positively correlate with the occurrence of endometrial carcinoma. Cyclic therapy has not been shown to reduce the occurrence of endometrial carcinoma. Therefore, the indications and duration of therapy have been reassessed. In-depth reviews continue to appear.[40] The addition of a progestational compound is now strongly encouraged during estrogen replacement when the uterus is present. Some authors have suggested that 10 days of a progestational compound each month reduce the incidence of endometrial carcinoma to or below that found in an untreated population.[41,42] A further discussion of the use of progestins in replacement therapy is presented later in this chapter.

BREAST CARCINOMA. An increased incidence of breast cancer associated with estrogen replacement has been reported.[43] Statistical significance is noted only if oophorectomized patients are eliminated from the study population. The majority of studies have been unable to confirm an increased risk in postmenopausal women taking estrogen therapy.[10,44–47] Progestational therapy may be effective in reducing the incidence of breast carcinoma in estrogen users.[10]

THROMBOPHLEBITIS. In contrast to the findings with oral contraceptives, menopausal estrogen therapy has not been associated with an increased incidence of idiopathic thrombophlebitis.[46] The lower dosages of estrogens used in replacement therapy may in part explain the failure of association. As opposed to most oral contraceptives usually prescribed doses of conjugated estrogens and medroxyprogesterone acetate have been reported not to adversely affect coagulation parameters.[48] The use of estrogens in patients with a previous history of thrombophlebitis or in situations predisposing to thrombophlebitis (i.e., surgery) is generally contraindicated.

CORONARY VASCULAR DISEASE. Although the use of oral contraceptives in older-age women is associated with an increased risk of coronary vascular disease, few data are available to support this association with menopausal estrogen replacement. Several studies have found no increased risk.[49,50] One group reported a reduced incidence of expected myocardial infarctions in hysterectomized patients started on estrogens and followed for 5 to 28 years.[51] Furthermore, an overall lower risk of mortality is present in estrogen users as opposed to nonusers which is probably in part accounted for by increased levels of high density lipoprotein cholesterol in users.[52]

CEREBRAL VASCULAR DISEASE AND HYPERTENSION. In contrast to oral contraceptives, replacement therapy has not been found to increase the likelihood of a stroke nor is there a strong association with hypertension.[50]

GALLBLADDER DISEASE. The Boston Collaborative study reported a 2.5-fold increase in gallbladder disease during estrogen replacement therapy.[46] This finding is supported by reports of higher concentrations of cholesterol found in bile after estrogen treatment. Oral administration of estrogens, causing the liver to be exposed to high concentrations of estrogens, may in part explain these findings despite the relatively low doses used. Parenteral administration of estrogens potentially may reduce this complication. Vaginal administration in equivalent doses has similar effects to oral administration.

GLUCOSE INTOLERANCE. The detrimental effect of estrogens on glucose tolerance is a dose-related phenomenon. Menopausal replacement dosages exert little influence on fasting glucose concentrations. The alteration in glucose tolerance must be considered in the treatment of borderline diabetics and patients receiving hypoglycemic agents.

LEIOMYOMATA. Stimulation of leiomyomata may be found following estrogen therapy. The growth, however, is probably dose-related. Using estrogen therapy equivalent to 0.625 mg of conjugated estrogen or less, this complication is unlikely.

POSTMENOPAUSAL BLEEDING. Using a dose of estrogen capable of suppressing vasomotor symptoms and a progestational compound, most postmenopausal subjects with intact uteri will be expected to bleed during the withdrawal phase. The use of estrogens without progestins increases the occurrence of unexpected postmenopausal bleeding. Histologic correlates and additional rationale for the use of progestins in estrogen users have recently been published.[54] Bleeding at times other than the drug-free interval is an indication for endometrial sampling.

TERATOGENIC EFFECTS. The effects of large doses of estrogen administered during early pregnancy have been extensively studied in DES progeny. The inadvertent use of replacement doses of estrogens has not been proven to be teratogenic. In potentially fertile subjects estrogen therapy should be limited to the preconception period.

Estrogen Dose Forms

For most patients, short-acting oral estrogens are the preferred agents allowing for cyclic therapy and ease in dose adjustments. Whether natural or synthetic estrogens are more clinically beneficial has not been established. Well-designed studies documenting therapeutic superiority of either form are lacking. The proven carcinogenic effect of DES, along with the availability of equally effective steroid estrogens, suggests that DES and its cogeners should be used cautiously.

Oral Preparations

See Table 20–3.

Oral Combination Preparations

Oral dosage forms are available from various manufacturers; these combine estrogen with antianxiety agents (Melprin, Menrium). Use of these products is not rational for most patients. As with any fixed-combination preparation, doses of individual drugs cannot be adjusted without altering the dose of other components. The recommended dose schedule is 1 tablet three times daily for 21 days followed by a 1-week, drug-free period. This schedule is irrational both for the estrogen and the antianxiety components, and is not recommended.

Parenteral Preparations

Many estrogen preparations are available for parenteral use. Due to the inconvenience and cost, short-acting forms are seldom utilized. Longer-acting estrogens and subcutaneous implants offer the advantage of infrequent administration and are not presented to the liver as a large bolus, as is found with oral preparations. As stated earlier, this may obviate many hepatic side effects.[55,56] It may also allow concomitant administration of testosterone.[57,58] Variability in absorption, difficulties in individualizing the dosage, and the increased cost continue to limit utility (Table 20–4).

Vaginal Preparations

For postmenopausal patients, when vulvovaginitis or urethritis are the only symptoms, use of vaginally applied estrogens may be indicated. Both estradiol and estrone are rapidly absorbed by the vaginal epithelium with plasma levels peaking in 3 to 4 hours after application.[16] Recommended doses have been shown to produce high blood levels of estrogen. Plasma levels may exceed those normally found in reproductive-age women. Because vaginal absorption may give levels similar to those achieved by oral dosing regimens, dosing schedules currently recommended by manufacturers of vaginal creams and suppositories may be higher than needed. The recommended daily dose of 2 to 4 g of conjugated estrogen creams contains

TABLE 20-3. ESTROGEN PREPARATIONS AND TABLET STRENGTHS

Preparation	Tablet Strength
Steroidal	
Conjugated estrogens (Premarin, Menotab, Ovest, and others): 50–60% sodium estrone sulfate and 20–35% sodium equilin sulfate	0.3, 0.625, 0.9, 1.25, and 2.5 mg
Esterfied estrogens (Menest, Femogen, Estratabs and others): 75–85% sodium estrone sulfate and 6–15% sodium equilin sulfate	0.3, 0.625, 1.25, and 2.5 mg
Piperazine estrone sulfate (Ogen): Crystalline estrone solubilized as the sulfate and stabilized with piperazine	0.625, 1.25, 2.5, and 5 mg
Combined estrogen (Hormonin)	
Hormonin #1: 0.135 mg estriol, 0.7 mg estrone, and 0.3 mg estradiol	
Hormonin #2: 0.27 mg estriol, 1.4 mg estrone, and 0.6 mg estradiol	
Ethinyl estradiol (Estinyl, Feminone, and others)	0.02, 0.05, and 0.5 mg
Estradiol-17β (Estrace)	1 and 2 mg
Quinestrol (Estrovis)	100 mcg
Nonsteroidal	
Diethylstilbestrol (various): Also available as enteric-coated tablets	0.1, 0.25, 0.5, 1, and 5 mg

1.25 to 2.5 mg of estrogens. A more conservative dose of 1.25 mg daily of conjugated estrogens (or estrogen equivalent) used intravaginally for 1 week should be tried. After initial stimulation of the vaginal mucosa, administration of 1 g once or twice weekly may control symptoms.

Vaginal Products

- Creams
  - Conjugated estrogens 0.625 mg/g (Premarin)
  - Piperazine estrone sulfate 1.5 mg/g (Ogen)
  - Dienestrol 0.01 percent (DV, Estraguard, others)
  - Micronized estradiol 0.1 mg/g (Estrace)
- Suppositories
  - Diethylstilbestrol 0.1 mg, 0.5 mg, 0.7 mg (various)
  - Estrone 0.2 mg (ATV, Prinn-VS)
  - Estradiol 0.5 mg, and testosterone 5 mg (test-Estrin)

TABLE 20-4. ESTROGENS FOR PARENTERAL USE

Available Parenteral Estrogens	Manufacturer's Recommended Dosage (mg)	Approximate Frequency of Administration
Estrone aqueous or oil suspensions	0.5–2	Once a week
Estradiol aqueous or oil suspension	0.2–1.5	Once a week
Estradiol cypronate	1–5	Once every 3–4 weeks
Estradiol valerate	10–20	Once every 4 weeks
Estradiol subcutaneous pellets	25	Once every 3 months

PROGESTERONE AND PROGESTINS

The terms progestins and gestagens are used to describe the compounds with progesterone-like activity. One bioassay of progestin activity involves the ability of a compound to convert an estrogen-primed endometrium into a histologically luteal phase endometrium (Clauberg test in rabbits, Kaufman test in humans). Another assay tests the ability to support a pregnancy in an ovariectomized pregnant rat. The Greenblatt test evaluates the capacity of the drug to prolong the luteal phase after spontaneous ovulation. The Kaufman test comes closest to evaluating the physiologic phenomena as required in clinical practice. The test relies on descriptive characteristics, but the dosage of estrogen required for priming has not been standardized.

Chemistry and Metabolism

Progesterone, as shown in Figure 20–3, is secreted primarily by the corpus luteum but also by the placenta and adrenal glands. It is synthesized from cholesterol, which is converted to pregnenolone. This immediate precursor is converted to progesterone by a combined dehydrogenase and isomerase reaction.

Exogenous progesterone from any route is rapidly absorbed. Because progesterone is almost completely metabolized in one passage through the intestinal mucosa and liver, low doses administered orally are ineffective. In the bloodstream progesterone shows a high affinity for cortisol-binding globulin and albumin and is 88.9 percent protein bound. A small amount is stored in body fat. The half-life of IV administered progesterone has been reported to range from 3 to 90 minutes.[59] Once-daily dosing regimens are usually effective, indicating a more prolonged action upon body tissues. Progesterone is metabolized in the liver, the endometrium, and the myometrium. Liver metabolism, which accounts for about two-thirds of all metabolic pathways, converts progesterone to pregnanediol. This and other metabolites are conjugated in the liver with glucuronic acid. Following injection of labeled progesterone, 50 to 60 percent of the metabolites are excreted via the kidney and 10 percent in the bile and feces.

Progesterone is most effective by parenteral administration. In equal doses, oral administration is about one-twelfth as effective, buccal about one-eighth as effective, and intravaginal one-fifth as effective.[59] Buccal and intravaginal routes give variable absorption. Progesterone in oil (25 mg) given IM will achieve plasma levels equivalent to the concentrations seen during the midluteal phase.[60]

Synthetic progestins have been developed to overcome limitations of the naturally occurring hormone.[61] Products are available that are orally effective, longer acting, and cause less irritation at injection sites.

C-19 and 19-Nor Progestins

These compounds are derived from testosterone. Addition of an ethinyl group at C-17 on the steroid ring reduces the androgenicity of the parent compound, increases its oral activity, and elicits progestational characteristics. Removal of the methyl group (C-19) attached at C-10 (thus, 19-nor testosterone) further enhances progestational activity and reduces the androgenic activity of the parent compound. These two modifications of testosterone are reponsible for the potent oral progestin, norethindrone (17-α ethinyl-19-nortestosterone). In attempting to prolong the half-life of norethindrone, an acetate group may be added at C-17, forming norethindrone acetate. In humans, the acetate on norethindrone acetate is readily cleaved, accounting for the relatively equal potency of norethindrone and norethindrone acetate.

Norethindrone has a half-life approaching 8 hours. Excretion is predominantly via the urinary system as conjugated metabolites. The C-19 progestins are metabolized similarly to progesterone, undergoing reduction of the 4-ene-3-one group in ring A. The C-17 ethinyl group is not cleaved during in vivo metabolism and is believed to be responsible for preventing conversion of the C-19 progestins to ethinyl estradiol.

PROGESTERONE

HYDROXYPROGESTERONE CAPROATE (Delalutin)

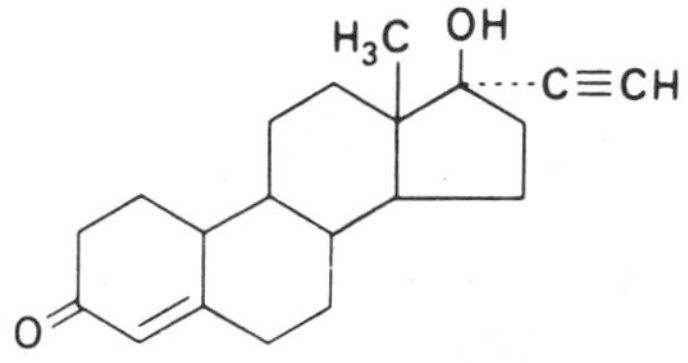

MEDROXYPROGESTERONE ACETATE (Provera)

MEGESTROL ACETATE (Megase)

NORETHINDRONE

Figure 20–3. Chemical structure of progestins and natural progesterone. *(From Csáky, TZ: Cutting's Handbook of Pharmacology: The Actions and Uses of Drugs, ed. 7. Norwalk, Connecticut, Appleton-Century-Crofts, 1984, pp 433, 437, 438, 440, with permission.)*

Progesterone-like Synthetic Progestins (C-21)

Adding a hydroxyl group at C-17 of progesterone in the α-position dramatically reduces progestational activity. Esterification with a relatively long alkyl group at this position produces modestly potent but long-acting progestins. This is the case for 17-α hydroxyprogesterone caproate, shown in Figure 20–3, an effective, parenteral progestational agent. Methylation at C-6 of 17-α hydroxyprogesterone acetate produces medroxyprogesterone acetate with increased progestational activity permitting oral as well as parenteral administration. The addition of a double bond between C-6 and C-7 of medroxyprogesterone acetate still further increases the progestational activity (megestrol).

Changing the methyl group on C-19 of progesterone from the β-position to the α-position (dydrogesterone) increases the progestational activity on the endometrium following oral administration. This change in spatial configuration appears to result in loss of hypothalamic activity (i.e., thermogenic changes and suppression of ovulation.).

The metabolism of these progestins is similar to the parent compound. Metabolism occurs predominantly in the liver involving hydroxylation and conjugation. The majority of metabolites are excreted in the urine.

Mechanism of Action

Progesterone appears to function intracellularly in a manner similar to estrogen. Entry into the cell is by passive diffusion. The high-affinity, low-capacity binding protein differs from the estrogen receptor; it consists of two subunits and binds two molecules of progesterone per complex.[62] Bound to the receptor, progesterone enters the nucleus and interacts in some fashion with DNA.

In contrast to the estrogen receptor, progesterone, rather than stimulating an overall replenishment of cytosol receptors, actually decreases the number of progesterone receptors. Progesterone not only decreases its own receptors but also those of estrogen. This is one mechanism to explain inhibition of estrogen activity by progesterone. Progesterone is capable of inducing estradiol-17β dehydrogenase, an enzyme responsible for conversion of estradiol to estrone. Reducing the tissue concentration of estradiol, progesterone further antagonizes the action of estrogens. The antagonism of estrogen by progesterone is a consistent finding in the myometrium and the epithelial component of the endometrium. Some authors have suggested that when estrogen and progesterone are administered, the stromal compartment fails to recognize the suppressive action of progesterone.[63,64] Progesterone may not be uniformly suppressive on the effects of estrogen; it does not decrease the efficacy of estrogen in reducing bone reabsorption.

Progesterone also functions as an antagonist for aldosterone. It is presumed to act as a competitive inhibitor, although further investigation is needed to clarify its mechanism of action.

Pharmacologic Actions

The majority of actions of progesterone require the concurrent or prior administration of estrogen. A list of progesterone actions is given in Table 20–5.

Clinical Uses During the Menopausal Years

In the first portion of this chapter the use of a progestin during estrogen replacement was advised in patients with an intact uterus. Although the value of progestins in reducing the occurrence of endometrial carcinoma has not been uniformly accepted, recommendations to prolong progestational treatment to at least 10 days each month have become standard.[20–23] A study by Jick[65] is the most commonly quoted epidemiologic study failing to show beneficial effects of progesterone. There is published data suggesting that less than 10 days of progestins are not protective of the endometrium in patients using estro-

TABLE 20–5. PHYSIOLOGIC EFFECTS OF PROGESTERONE

Genital Tract
- Endometrial glandular epithelium
  - Reduces mitotic activity
  - Increases glandular secretions
  - Suppresses estrogen stimulation
- Endometrial stroma
  - Increases mitotic activity in response to estrogen
  - Causes vascular tortuosity
- Myometrium
  - Reduces myometrial activity
- Cervix
  - Reduces glandular secretions
  - Inhibits ferning of cervical mucus
  - Decreases elasticity of mucus

Breast
- Stimulates alveolar growth

Skin
- Reduces hair follicle responsiveness to androgens (inhibits 5-α-reductase)

Bone
- Decreases bone resorption

Kidney
- Inhibits aldosterone activity

Coagulation
- No effect

Lipids
- Decreases serum concentrations of high-density lipoproteins

gen continuously.[66] Gambrell et al.[67] have previously shown that 10 mg of medroxyprogesterone or 5 mg norethindrone acetate for 7 to 10 days each month is effective in treating various degrees of endometrial hyperplasia. Megestrol acetate, 40 mg per day, for 9 to 10 months has been reported to be an effective alternate drug.[68] In a prospective study from Wilford Hall[42] the protective influence of progestins in preventing endometrial carcinoma was demonstrated. A prospective study from Great Britain[41] and a retrospective study by Hammond and coworkers[69] further emphasized the protective influence of progestins in preventing endometrial carcinoma. All these authors suggested that the greatest benefit may be seen if progestins are used for 10 or more days each month. There continues to be no scientific support for an increased incidence of breast, uterine, or ovarian cancer from medroxyprogesterone use in humans.[70]

Progestins may be effective in relieving vasomotor symptoms and preventing bone mineral loss. Intramuscular medroxyprogesterone acetate in doses of 150 mg monthly relieves vasomotor symptoms in most treated patients.[13,71] Oral administration also appears to be of benefit.[72] Temporary depression has been associated with the use of progestins as well as worsening of vaginal atrophic changes. Low-dose combined estrogen and progestin therapy may reduce the side effects of each medication while preserving its benefits.[73] The effects of progestins on osteoporosis require further study.

Clinical Uses During the Reproductive Years

ENDOMETRIAL HYPERPLASIA. Endometrial hyperplasia has been suggested as a precursor of endometrial carcinoma. With increasing degrees of atypia, better correlations exist between hyperplasia and carcinoma. Progestational agents have been shown to be effective in treating endometrial hyperplasia and are therefore believed to be effective in reducing the likelihood of progression to endometrial carcinoma. Oral regimens have varied from continuous administration of C-21 progestational compounds (i.e., megesterol 20 to 40 mg twice a day) to a 10- to 14-day/month treatment protocol with medroxyprogesterone acetate 10 mg/day or norethindrone acetate 5 mg/day for 3 to 6 months. Parenteral administration may also be used on a continuous basis for a 3- to 6-month period (medroxyprogesterone acetate suspension 400 mg IM every 2 weeks).[74] Continuous therapy is based on a rationale similar to that for endometrial carcinoma. Treatment may be complicated by bleeding from the atrophic endometrium. This may mandate further endometrial sampling to exclude the possibility of a focus of endometrial carcinoma not found during the first endometrial sampling. Once the appropriate diagnostic steps have been taken, discontinuation of the medication for 2 weeks or the addition of a 1-week course of estrogen are sufficient to stop the bleeding and allow for completion of the planned treatment regimen. The intermittent therapy relies on induction of progesterone receptors during the nontreatment portion of the cycle to promote a greater response. In addition, the superficial and intermediate layers of the endometrium are sloughed. Use of C-19 progestational compounds should cause endometrial atrophy by their androgenic characteristics as well as their progestational activity.

All patients being treated for endometrial hyperplasia should undergo a thorough endometrial biopsy the month after discontinuing progestational treatment. If intermittent therapy is to be utilized for a prolonged period, a biopsy should be repeated at 3 months after the initial diagnosis while off progestin therapy. Routine endometrial sampling should be performed as part of follow-up at 6-month to 1-year intervals in subjects at risk.

ANOVULATORY BLEEDING. The administration of progestins is effective in the control of bleeding resulting from unopposed estrogen. Progestins stabilize the endometrium and, on withdrawal, cause a synchronous shedding of the endometrium. Various 5 to 7 day treatment regimens have been used; medroxyprogesterone acetate 10 mg/day, norethindrone acetate 5 mg/day, and progestin-dominant oral contraceptives 4 tablets/day. Progesterone in oil (50 to 100 mg IM) has also been utilized. During the course of therapy bleeding should stop and should be followed by withdrawal bleeding 2 to 7 days after discontinuing therapy. The patient must be made aware that the ensuing bleeding is to be expected.

In patients with prolonged bleeding where the endometrium may be exhausted, estrogen therapy followed by a progestin is often more effective. With either treatment, after the expected withdrawal bleeding an investigation should be made to determine the cause of anovulation. Plans should be established to prevent recurrences either by correcting the cause of anovulation or establishing a monthly (or alternate month) course of exogenous progestins for a duration of 10 days. Clinical parameters (i.e., cervical mucus) should be used to evaluate the presence of unopposed estrogen and reduce the possibilities of an undiagnosed pregnancy prior to administration of prophylactic progestins. The alternate monthly use of progestins is advantageous in observing for spontaneous ovulation and reducing the number of physician visits. If spontaneous ovulation and menses occur, treatment need not be considered unless the patient fails to bleed within another 60 days. Premenstrual symptoms and temperature charts are useful in differentiating ovulatory from anovulatory bleeding.

If contraception is required, oral contraceptives may be used rather than progestins alone to prevent anovulatory, irregular bleeding. The patient should be informed that anovulation is likely to persist after discontinuation of the oral contraceptives.

As noted previously in most patients, an office curettage should be performed prior to initiating therapy.

ENDOMETRIOSIS, CONTRACEPTION. For a discussion of this topic, see Chapters 19 and 26.

DYSMENORRHEA. Progestins have been used during the luteal phase to prevent dysmenorrhea. More effective agents are now available (Chap. 26).

DIAGNOSTIC AGENT IN AMENORRHEA. The most common cause of amenorrhea during the reproductive years is pregnancy. Progestin should not be used as a pregnancy test. If pregnancy is ruled out by human chorionic gonadotropin determination and physical examination, progesterone or a progestin may be used. Withdrawal bleeding documents the presence of an intact, responsive, estrogen-primed endometrium. Progesterone in oil, 50 to 100 mg in a single injection, or an oral progestin for 5 to 7 days (i.e., medroxyprogesterone acetate 10 mg/day) may be used.

INADEQUATE LUTEAL PHASE. Natural progesterone is used in the treatment of an inadequate luteal phase resulting in infertility or habitual abortion.[75] Documentation classically relies on endometrial histologic studies showing a lag of 2 or preferably more days in secretory changes of the endometrium. The etiology is believed to be inadequate follicle-stimulating hormone production during the follicular phase, hyperprolactinemia, an inadequate luteinizing hormone surge at mid-cycle, decreased progesterone receptors, or an unknown luteolytic factor. Gonadotropin therapy is an alternative treatment regimen to progestins. The inadequate luteal phase may respond to clomiphene citrate use. It may also develop during clomiphene citrate use, in which case higher dose luteal phase progesterone therapy or gonatropins are again alternatives.

Progesterone therapy is best accomplished by using vaginal suppositories containing 25 mg of progesterone twice a day.[75] Therapy is begun 2 days following a thermogenic rise in basal body temperature and continued until menstrual bleeding occurs or for 8 to 10 weeks in the absence of menstrual bleeding. Progesterone in oil 12.5 mg/day IM may be substituted for the vaginal preparation. The serum progesterone concentrations obtained following either route of administration approximate those found during the normal luteal phase.[60] Term pregnancy rates of 46 to 91 percent have been reported.[76-78] Use of synthetic progestins is strongly discouraged.

Progesterone as a fertility agent is not

approved by the Food and Drug Administration. The patient should be advised of the possible teratogenic risks involved with such treatment and the indications for its use. Treatment beyond 8 to 10 weeks after conception should not be necessary as the placenta becomes the major source of progesterone synthesis.

PREMENSTRUAL SPOTTING. Progestins have been recommended for the treatment of recurrent premenstrual spotting. A progestin is administered orally for the last 7 days of the luteal phase. It was initally conceived as treatment for a recurrent inadequate luteal phase. Premenstrual spotting is reportedly associated more often with endometriosis.[79] Treatment is occasionally effective, although the mechanism is not clear. Precautions should be taken to prevent the occurrence of conception during treatment. For these reasons treatment with full, cyclic combination oral contraceptives is preferred.

THREATENED ABORTION. Genetic abnormalities account for 60 percent of all abortions. Recognizing the high percentage of threatened abortions that proceed normally to term, the empiric use of progestins in this situation is strongly discouraged. Use of progestins with threatened abortion may result in an increased incidence of missed abortions.

PREVENTION OF PREMATURE LABOR. Progesterone has been shown to decrease uterine activity. A randomized study by Johnston et al.[80] reported that 17-α hydroxyprogesterone caproate 250 mg/week IM administered after the first trimester resulted in prolongation of the gestational period in patients with a history of premature labor. The study population was small, although statistical significance was obtained. Many other agents are available for the acute treatment of premature labor. If 17-α hydroxyprogesterone caproate is to be used, treatment should not be initiated until 16 weeks, following major embryologic development.

Treatment Prior to Reproductive Age

Medroxyprogesterone acetate has been used in the treatment of precocious puberty. It appears to have little beneficial effect upon the rate of growth and ultimate height. Its use has been recommended to reduce breast development and produce an amenorrheic state. Except in extreme situations, counseling appears safer and more logical. Long-term follow-up may prove LHRH analogues to be the treatment of choice.[81] An amenorrheic state may be obtained using doses of medroxyprogesterone acetate 150 mg IM every 3 to 6 months if the patient is felt to be incapable of managing menstrual bleeding in the opinion of the physician and her guardians. A thorough evaluation of the cause of precocious puberty is necessary prior to any treatment. Table 20–6 lists progestin products available for clinical use.

Complications Associated with Progestin Use

BLEEDING. During prolonged use of progestins uterine bleeding may occur. In using medroxyprogesterone acetate suspension as a contraceptive approximately 10 percent of subjects will discontinue the medication due to persistent abnormal uterine bleeding. Estrogen is usually effective in correcting this complication.

HYPERTENSION. Most studies have failed to show a change in blood pressure with prolonged use of oral progestins.[82] Medroxyprogesterone acetate in high dosages, for the treatment of precocious puberty, has been reported to cause hypertension and other symptoms similar to Cushing's syndrome.[83]

WEIGHT GAIN. An increase in weight has been found following progestin therapy. The increase in weight is secondary both to water retention and residual anabolic activity in some of the synthetic progestins.

WATER RETENTION. Progesterone is a diuretic due to its inhibition of aldosterone. The body, however, readily compensates for this diuretic activity by increased production of aldosterone. Water retention during progestin therapy possibly results from fluctuating progestin concentrations with excessive compensatory increases in aldosterone production. The use of megesterol has been reported to produce a carpal tunnel-like syndrome.[84] This complication is believed to result from

TABLE 20–6. PROGESTIN PRODUCTS AVAILABLE

Product	Trade Name	Route	Strength Supplied
Progesterone Inj USP	Femotrone, Progelan, and others	IM	In oil and aqueous* 25, 50, and 100 mg/ml
17-Hydroxyprogesterone caproate in oil	Delalutin, Gesterol LA, Hylutin, and others	IM	125 and 250 mg/ml
Medroxyprogesterone acetate	Depo Provera	IM	100 and 400 mg/ml†
Megestrol acetate	Megace	PO	20 and 40 mg
	Amen, Curretab, Provera	PO	2.5 and 10 mg
Norethindrone	Norlutin	PO	5 mg
Norethindrone acetate	Norlutate	PO	5 mg
Dydrogesterone	Duphaston, Gynorest	PO	5 and 10 mg

* Progesterone suppositories are not commercially available but may be prepared from the progesterone suspension. See Ref. 82.

† Indicated only for advanced metastatic endometrial carcinoma.

increased water retention in the collagen matrix of the aponeurosis, as may occur during pregnancy.

PROLONGED AMENORRHEA. The use of medroxyprogesterone acetate suspension may result in prolonged amenorrhea. The absorption and duration of action of this compound is exceedingly variable.

TERATOGENICITY. Although speculation exists, there are few reports to support teratogenic effects resulting from the clinical use of natural progesterone. Controversy exists on the teratogenic actions of synthetic progestins. Administration of progestins during early pregnancy is reported to increase, by over eightfold, the incidence of the VACTERL syndrome.[76] VACTERL is an acronym for a complex of anomalies involving the vertebral, anal, cardiac, tracheal, esophageal, renal, or limb structures. Cardiac anomalies are the most commonly found abnormalities of the syndrome. In the Collaborative Perinatal Project[85] a relative increased risk of 1.8 was found for cardiac anomalies when progestins were used during early gestation. No other statistically significant increase in anomalies was found with the use of progestins. At least one reviewer of data available through 1979 concluded that the evidence was insufficient to incriminate progestins with the possible exception of medroxyprogesterone.[86] Other experts continue to challenge the existence of a causal relationship between birth defects and maternal use of progestins.[87,88] Their use during pregnancy should be restricted unless a specific indication necessitates their use.

REFERENCES

1. Siiteri PK, MacDonald PC: Role of extraglandular estrogen in human endocrinology. In Geiger SR, Astwood EB, Greep RO (eds.): Handbook of Physiology. Section of Endocrinology, Washington, DC, American Physiology Society, 1973, pp 615–629
2. Bolt HM: Metabolism of estrogens—Natural and synthetic. Pharmacol Ther 4:155, 1979
3. Newburger J, Castracane VD, Moore PH Jr, et al.: The pharmacokinetics and metabolism of ethinyl estradiol and its three sulfates in the baboon. Am J Obstet Gynecol 146:80, 1983
4. Physician's Desk Reference, ed 39. Oradell, New Jersey, Medical Economics Co, 1985
5. Clark JH, Peck EJ: Nuclear binding and biological response. In Gross F, Grumbach M, Labhart A, et al. (eds): Female Sex Steroid. New York, Springer-Verlag, 1979, pp 70–97
6. Clark JH, Paszko Z, Peck EJ Jr: Nuclear binding and retention of the estrogen receptor complex: Relation to the agonist and antagonist properties of estriol. Endocrinology 100:91, 1977
7. Martucci C, Fishman J: Direction of estradiol

metabolism as a control of its hormonal action—Uterotrophic activity of estradiol metabolites. Endocrinology 101:1709, 1977
8. Hansten PD: Hormone interactions. In Hansten PD (ed): Drug Interactions. Philadelphia, Lea and Febiger, 1975, p 165
9. Givens JR (ed): Clinical Use of Sex Steroids. Chicago, Yearbook, 1980, pp 257–346
10. Gambrell RD Jr, Maier RC, Sanders BI: Decreased incidence of breast cancer in postmenopausal estrogen-progestogen users. Obstet Gynecol 62:435, 1983
11. Mashchak CA, Lobo RA, Dozono-Takano R, et al.: Comparison of pharmacodynamic properties of various estrogen formulations. Am J Obstet Gynecol 144:511, 1982
12. Utiam WH: Current status of the menopausal and postmenopausal therapy. Obstet Gynecol Surv 32:193, 1977
13. Bullock JL, Massey FM, Gambrell RD Jr: Use of progesterone medroxy acetate to prevent menopausal symptoms. Obstet Gynecol 46:165, 1975
14. Clayden JR, Bell JW, Pollard P: Menopausal flushing: Double blind trial of a nonhormonal medication. Br J Med 4:409, 1974
15. Larsen B, Goplerud C, Petzold R, et al.: Effect of estrogen treatment on the genital tract flora of postmenopausal women. Obstet Gynecol 60:20, 1982
16. Rigg LA, Hermann H, Yen SSC: Absorption of estrogens from vaginal creams. N Engl J Med 298:195, 1978
17. Martin PL, Greaney MO, Burnier AM, et al.: Estradiol, estrone, and gonadotropin levels after use of vaginal estradiol. Obstet Gynecol 63:441, 1984
18. Hilton P, Stanton SL: The use of intravaginal oestrogen cream in genuine stress incontinence. Br J Gynaecol 90:940, 1983
19. Recker RR, Saville PD, Heaney RP: Effects of oestrogens and calcium carbonate on bone loss in postmenopausal women. Ann Intern Med 87:649, 1977
20. Nordin BE, Peacock M, Aaron J, et al.: Osteoporosis and osteomalacia. Clin Endocrinol Metab 9:177, 1980
21. Jensen GF, Christiansen C, Tranbol IB: Fracture frequency and bone preservation in postmenopausal women treated with estrogen. Obstet Gynecol 60:493, 1982
22. Weiss NS, Ure CL, Ballard JH, et al.: Decreased risk of fractures of the hip and lower forearm with postmenopausal use of estrogens. N Engl J Med 303:1195, 1980
23. Weinstien MC: Estrogen use in postmenopausal women—Costs, risks, and benefits. N Engl J Med 303:308, 1980
24. Aitken JM: Osteoporosis and its relation to estrogen deficiency. In Campbell S (ed): The Management of the Menopause and Post-Menopausal Years. Lancaster, England, MTP Press, 1976
25. Lindsay R, Hart DM, Clark DM: The minimum effective dose of estrogen for prevention of postmenopausal bone loss. Obstet Gynecol 63:759, 1984
26. Horsman A, Jones M, Francis R, Nordin C: The effect of estrogen dose on postmenopausal bone loss. N Engl J Med 309:1405, 1983
27. Riggs BL, Seeman E, Hodgson SF, et al.: Effect of the fluoride/calcium regimen on vertebral fracture occurrence in postmenopausal osteoporosis. N Engl J Med 306:446, 1982
28. Nordin BE, Horsman A, Crilly RG, et al.: Treatment of spinal osteoporosis in postmenopausal women. Br Med J 280:451, 1980
29. Heany RP, Recker RR, Saville PD: Menopausal changes in calcium balance. J Lab Clin Med 92:953, 1978
30. Scheider MA, Brotherton PL, Hailes J: The effect of exogenous estrogens on depression in menopausal women. Med J Aust 2:162, 1977
31. Schiff I, Ryan KJ: Benefits of estrogen replacement. Obstet Gynecol Surv 35:400, 1980
32. Speroff L: Dysfunctional uterine bleeding. In Speroff L, Glass RH, Kase NG (eds): Clinical Gynecologic Endocrinology and Infertility. Baltimore, Williams & Wilkins, 1983, p 225
33. Rezai P, Dmowski WP, Auletta F, Scommegna A: Effect of oral estriol on cervical secretions and on ovulatory response in infertile women. Fertil Steril 31:627, 1979
34. Morris JM, VanWagenen G: Interception: The use of postovulatory estrogens to prevent implantation. Am J Obstet Gynecol 115:101, 1973
35. Hoffman KOK: International Federation of Fertility Societies, 11th World Congress on Fertility and Sterility, Dublin, 26 June–1 July 1983
36. Ross JL, Cassorla FG, Skerda MC, et al.: A preliminary study of the effect of estrogen dose on growth in Turner's syndrome. N Engl J Med 309:1104, 1983
37. Kuhn N, Blunek W, Stahnke N, et al.: Estrogen treatment in tall girls. Acta Paediatr Scand 66:161, 1977
38. Horowitz RI, Feinstein AR: Alternative analytic methods for case control studies of estro-

gens and endometrial carcinoma. N Engl J Med 299:1089, 1978
39. Antunes CM, Stolley PD, Rosenhein NB, et al.: Endometrial cancer and estrogen use. N Engl J Med 300:9, 1979
40. Gambrell RD, Bagnell CA, Greenblatt RB: Role of estrogens and progesterone in the etiology and prevention of endometrial cancer: Review. Am J Obstet Gynecol 146:696, 1983
41. Patterson ME, Wade-Evans T, Sturdee DW, et al.: Endometrial disease after treatment with oestrogens and progestogens in the climacteric. Br Med J 279:822, 1980
42. Gambrell RD, Massey FM, Castaneda TA, et al.: Use of the progestogen challenge test to reduce the risk of endometrial carcinoma. Obstet Gynecol 55:732, 1980
43. Ross RK, Pagonini Hill A, Gerkins VR, et al.: A case control study of menopausal estrogen therapy and breast cancer. JAMA 243:1635, 1980
44. Gambrell RD, Massey FM, Castaneda TA, et al.: Estrogen therapy and breast cancer in postmenopausal women. Obstet Gynecol 23:265, 1974
45. Hoover R, Gray LA, Cole P, et al.: Menopausal estrogens and breast cancer. N Engl J Med 295:401, 1976
46. Surgically confirmed gallbladder disease, venous thromboembolism, and breast tumors in relation to postmenopausal estrogen therapy: A report from the Boston Collaborative Drug Surveillance Program, Boston University Medical Center. N Engl J Med 290:15, 1974
47. Kaufman DW, Miller DR, Rosenberg L, et al.: Noncontraceptive estrogen use and the risk of breast cancer. JAMA 252:63, 1984
48. Notelovitz M, Kitchens C, Ware M, et al.: Combination estrogen and progestogen replacement therapy does not adversely affect coagulation. Obstet Gynecol 62:596, 1983
49. Rosenberg L, Armstrong B, Jick H: Myocardial infarction and estrogen therapy in postmenopausal women. N Engl J Med 299:1256, 1976
50. Hammond CB, Jelovsek FR, Lee K, et al.: Effects of long-term estrogen therapy. Am J Obstet Gyencol 133:525, 1979
51. Burch JC, Byrd BF, Vaughn WK: The effect of long-term estrogen on hysterectomized women. Am J Obstet Gynecol 118:778, 1974
52. Bush TL, Cowan LD, Barrett-Connor E, et al.: Estrogen use and all-cause mortality. JAMA 249:903, 1983
53. Goebelsmann U, Mashchak CA, Mishell DR: Vaginal administration of ethinylestradiol (EE) does not selectively reduce its hepatic effects in post-menopausal women. Washington DC, Society of Gynecol Invest, 1983
54. Flowers CE, Wilborn WH, Hyde BM: Mechanisms of uterine bleeding in postmenopausal patients receiving estrogen alone or with a progestin. Obstet Gynecol 61:135, 1983
55. Holst J, Cajander JH, Carlstrom K, et al.: A comparison of liver protein induction in postmenopausal women during oral and percutaneous oestrogen replacement therapy. Br J Obstet Gynaecol 90:355, 1983
56. Laufer LR, DeFazio JL, Lu JKH, et al.: Estrogen replacement therapy by transdermal estradiol administration. Am J Obstet Gynecol 146:533, 1983
57. Cardozo L, Gibb DM, Studd JW, et al.: The use of hormone implants for climacteric symptoms. Am J Obstet Gynecol 149:336, 1984
58. Brincat M, Magos A, Studd JWW, et al.: Subcutaneous hormone implants for the control of climacteric symptoms. Lancet, Jan 7, 1984. p 16
59. Aufrere MB, Benson H: Progesterone: An overview and recent advances. J Pharm Sci 65:783, 1976
60. Johansson ED: Plasma levels of progesterone achieved by different routes of administration. Acta Obstet Gynecol Scand 19(Suppl):17, 1972
61. Edgren RA: Progestogens. In Givens JR (ed): Clinical Use of Sex Steroids. Chicago, Yearbook, 1980, pp 1–30
62. Grady WW, Schader WT, O'Malley BA: Activation, transformation, and subunit structure of steroid hormone receptors. Endocr Rev 3:141, 1982
63. Tachi C, Tachi S, Lindner HR: Modification by progesterone of estradiol-induced cell proliferation, RNA synthesis and estradiol distribution in the rat uterus. J Reprod Fertil 31:59, 1972
64. Tchernitchin A: Effects of progesterone on the in vivo binding of estrogens by uterine cells. Experientia 32:1069, 1976
65. Jick H, Watkins RN, Hunter JR, et al.: Replacement estrogens and endometrial cancer. N Engl J Med 299:1089, 1978
66. Whitehead MI, Townsend PT, Pryse-Davies J, et al.: Effects of estrogens and progestins on the biochemistry and morphology of the postmenopausal endometrium. N Engl J Med 305:1599, 1981

67. Gambrell RD, Massey FM, Castaneda TA, et al.: Reduced incidence of endometrial cancer amongst women treated with progestogens. J Am Geriatr Soc 27:389, 1979
68. Gal D, Edman CD, Vellios F, Forney JP: Long-term effect of megestrol acetate in the treatment of endometrial hyperplasia. Am J Obstet Gynecol 146:316, 1983
69. Hammond CB, Jelovsek FR, Lee K, et al.: Effects of long-term estrogen replacement: Neoplasia. Am J Obstet Gynecol 133:537, 1979
70. Liang AP, Levenson AG, Layde PM, et al.: Risk of breast, uterine corpus, and ovarian cancer in women receiving medroxyprogesterone injections. JAMA 249:2909, 1983
71. Lobo RA, McCormick W, Singer F, Roy S: Depo-medroxyprogesterone acetate compared with conjugated estrogens for the treatment of postmenopausal women. Obstet Gynecol 63:1, 1984
72. Aslaksen K, Frankendal B: Effect of oral medroxyprogesterone acetate on menopausal symptoms in patients with endometrial carcinoma. Acta Obstet Gynecol Scand 61:423, 1982
73. Ylostalo P, Kauppila A, Kivinen S, et al.: Endocrine and metablic effects of low-dose estrogen-progestin treatment in climacteric women. Obstet Gynecol 62:682, 1983
74. DiSaia PJ, Creasman WT: Endometrial hyperplasia. In DiSaia PJ, Creasman WT (eds): Clinical Gynecologic Oncology. St. Louis, CV Mosby, 1984, pp 142–143
75. Jones GS: The luteal phase defect. Fertil Steril 27:351, 1976
76. Chez RA: Proceedings of the symposium: Progesterone, progestins, and fetal development. Fertil Steril 30:16, 1978
77. Soules MR, Wiebe RH, Aksel S, et al.: The diagnosis and therapy of luteal phase deficiencies. Fertil Steril 28:1033, 1977
78. Tho PT, Byrd J, McDonough PG: Etiologies and subsequent reproductive performance of 100 couples with recurrent abortion. Fertil Steril 32:389, 1978
79. Wentz AC: Premenstrual spotting: Its association with endometriosis but not luteal phase inadequacy. Fertil Steril 33:605, 1980
80. Johnston JWC, Austin KL, Jones GS, et al.: Efficacy of 17 hydroxyprogesterone caproate in the prevention of premature labor. N Engl J Med 293:675, 1975
81. Crowley WF, Cornite F, Vale W, et al.: Therapeutic use of pituitary desensitization with a long-acting LHRH agonist: A potential new treatment for idiopathic precocious puberty. J Clin Endocrin Metab 52:370, 1981
82. Hall WD, Douglas BM, Blumenstein BA, Hatcher RA: Blood pressure and oral progestational agents. Am J Obstet Gynecol 136:34, 1980
83. Richman RA, Underwood LE, French FS, Van Wyk JJ: Adverse effects of large doses of medroxyprogesterone in idiopathic isosexual precocity. J Pediatr 79:963, 1971
84. Disaia PJ, Morrow CP: Unusual side effect of megesterol acetate. Am J Obstet Gynecol 129:460, 1977
85. Heinonen OP, Slone D, Monson RR, et al.: Cardiovascular birth defects and antenatal exposure to female sex hormones. N Engl J Med 196:67, 1977
86. Blake DA: Teratogenic effects of sex steroids. In Gwen JR (ed): Clinical Uses of Sex Steroids. Chicago, Yearbook, 1980, pp 339–346
87. Wilson JG, Brent RL: Are female sex hormones teratogenic? Am J Obstet Gynecol 141:567, 1981
88. Katz Z, Lancet M, Skornik J, et al.: Teratogenicity of progestogens given during the first trimester of pregnancy. Obstet Gynecol 65:775, 1985

21

Induction of Ovulation

Grant Schmidt, Sherif G. Awadalla, and Chad I. Friedman

Treatment of oligo-ovulation and anovulation is one of the most rewarding endeavors in the treatment of infertility. The number of drugs available for ovulation induction has expanded considerably in the past 5 years, in part due to the increased understanding of follicular development from experience in in vitro fertilization (IVF) programs. While relatively safe and effective, each drug has specific indications and mechanism(s) of action, and requires varying degrees of clinical monitoring. This chapter reviews the more commonly used drugs for the induction of ovulation.

A working diagnosis of the cause of the ovulatory disorder should be established prior to commencement of treatment. Ovulatory dysfunction may be a presenting sign of several major disease entities, including hypothalamic disorders, pituitary adenomas, adrenal and ovarian tumors, and systemic diseases such as diabetes or systemic lupus erythematosis (SLE). In addition, functional disorders, such as polycystic ovarian disease, hyperprolactinemia, and hyperandrogenism, may lead to an oligo- or anovulatory state. A thorough medical history and physical examination followed by the judicious use of laboratory studies provides a good baseline evaluation. The selection of an ovulatory agent will often be based on these findings. Several texts are available for consultation on the evaluation of ovulatory disorders.[1,2]

CLOMIPHENE CITRATE

Chemistry and Physiology

Clomiphene citrate (Clomid—Merrill Dow Pharmaceuticals; Serophene—Serono Laboratories) is a triphenylethylene compound (Fig. 21–1) structurally related to diethylstilbestrol and chlorotrianisene (Tace). It is a racemic mixture of the isomers enclomiphene and zuclomiphene citrates, which has been demonstrated to exhibit both estrogenic and antiestrogenic effects,[3] with the isomer zuclomiphene displaying primarily estrogenic actions. Early studies by Greenblatt et al.[4] evaluated its potential use for induction of ovulation in patients with secondary amen-

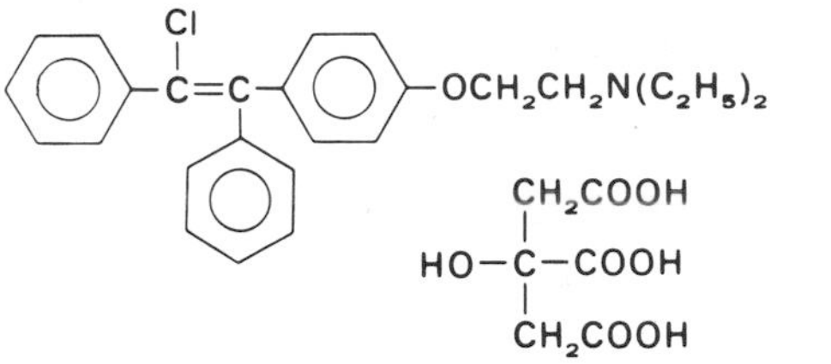

Figure 21–1. Chemical structure of clomiphene citrate. *(From Csáky, TZ: Cutting's Handbook of Pharmacology: The Actions and Uses of Drugs, ed. 7. Norwalk, Connecticut, Appleton-Century-Crofts, 1984, p 444, with permission.)*

orrhea and in 1968 it was approved for clinical use. To this day, the widespread clinical usefulness of clomiphene citrate makes it the mainstay of therapy for ovulatory disorders.

Clomiphene citrate binds readily to the cytoplasmic estrogen receptor, undergoes nuclear transport, and is retained within the nucleus. In contrast to natural estrogens, it fails to induce cytosol receptor replenishment.[5] In postmenopausal women, clomiphene citrate acts as an estrogen agonist, suppressing the release of luteinizing hormone (LH) and follicle-stimulating hormone (FSH) by the pituitary,[6] while in premenopausal women it may induce hot flashes,[7] and antagonize various estrogen-dependent functions including cervical mucus production, uterine histology, and vaginal cytology,[8,9] clearly antiestrogenic functions. Therefore, clomiphene citrate demonstrates both agonist and antagonist properties, and it now appears that both mechanisms may be important in its activity.[10]

Clomiphene citrate is most effective in inducing ovulation in individuals with endogenous estrogen production. Based on current evidence, it appears the site of action involves the hypothalamus, the pituitary, and the ovary. While the antiestrogenic properties are important at the level of the hypothalamus, the majority of reports suggest primarily an estrogenic effect at the pituitary and ovarian levels.[10] Functionally, following clomiphene citrate administration, an increased secretion of gonadotropin-releasing hormone (GnRH) acting on sensitized gonadotrophs in the pituitary leads to an increased secretion of gonadotropins. This rise in turn recruits or stimulates several ovarian follicular units from quiescence or early maturation into maturing follicles. Once properly primed, the follicles continue to mature, and through continued stimulation and feedback inhibition the hypothalamic–pituitary–ovarian axis results in the appearance of a dominant follicle and a subsequent midcycle gonadotropin surge. It is apparent that in cases of severe pituitary or hypothalamic dysfunction, clomiphene citrate is ineffective. In hypoestrogenic subjects, its antiestrogenic activity is of little benefit in producing increased gonadotropin secretion. Figure 21–2 is an example of the expected changes in gonadotropins and steroids seen in a patient with polycystic ovarian disease (PCO) treated with clomiphene citrate.

Clomiphene citrate is readily absorbed after oral administration. Up to 50 percent of the compound will be excreted within 5 days. Despite its relatively long half-life, less than 5 percent of the administered dose appears to be stored in fat.[11] It is excreted predominantly in feces, and traces may be found in feces 6 weeks after administration. A preliminary report suggests a differential elimination of the two clomiphene isomers, with zuclomiphene easily quantitated in plasma 28 days after a single oral 50 mg tablet.[12]

Clinical Use

The primary use of clomiphene citrate should be for the induction of ovulation in the anovulatory patient who desires pregnancy. Because of the mechanism of action discussed above, clomiphene citrate is most useful as an ovulatory agent in patients with normal or increased endogenous estrogen production. Demonstration of withdrawal bleeding in response to an exogenous progestin helps to assess the likelihood of an ovulatory response to clomiphene citrate. Lack of bleed-

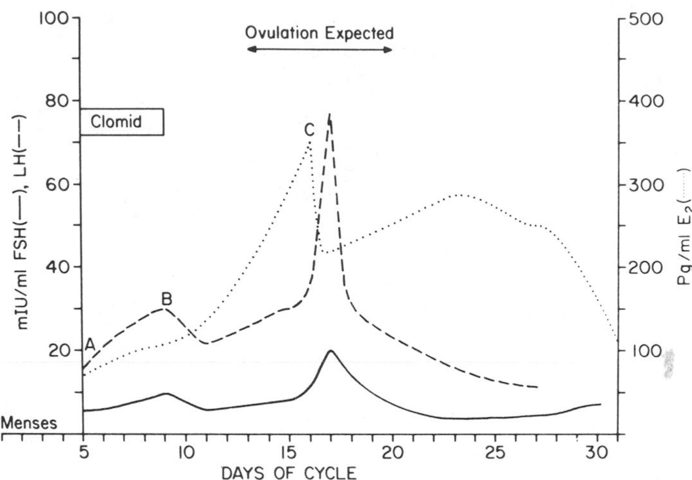

Figure 21–2. This is an idealized response of gonadotropins and estradiol to clomiphene citrate. A and B are labeled to draw attention to the persistent abnormal LH:FSH ratio in patients with PCO despite an ovulatory response. C represents the approximate time when human chorionic gonadotropins (hCG) may be administered in a clomiphene citrate–hCG regimen. A determination of serum estradiol would be helpful in determining follicular maturation in response to clomid at this point.

ing after progestin administration reduces the likelihood of ovulatory response to therapy.

Ovulation can be induced with clomiphene citrate in greater than 80 percent of patients depending on the cause of anovulation.[13] Pregnancy rates during six treatment cycles vary between 50 and 80 percent of the individuals ovulating successfully.[13,14] As the goal of treatment is pregnancy, a semen analysis and (postcoital) sperm test should be performed before treatment is initiated. While it has been our practice to obtain a hysterosalpingogram before or within the first treatment cycle, others have advised deferring this diagnostic test until three ovulatory cycles have failed to result in pregnancy.[15] Laparoscopy is not performed until pregnancy has failed to occur despite six or more ovulatory cycles, unless the history or abnormal physical findings warrant intraperitoneal evaluation. Within three ovulatory cycles, the majority of clomiphene-related pregnancies will occur.[16] Beyond six ovulatory cycles, only a small percentage of pregnancies may be expected unless other causes of infertility are found and corrected. Pregnancies have been reported as late as the 29th ovulatory cycle[17] and the patient and physician must be cognizant of the diminishing benefit of continued treatment beyond six cycles.

Clomiphene citrate treatment is usually started at a dose of 50 mg/day for 5 days. If anovulatory, menstrual bleeding is usually induced with a progestational agent, such as medroxyprogesterone, and clomiphene citrate begun on the third to fifth day of bleeding. Progestin administration before treatment has not been shown to alter either the ovulation or pregnancy rate, but the benefit of this regimen is a reduction in the likelihood of anovulatory bleeding during the course of treatment and the establishment of a uniform cyclic pattern of treatment.

Ovulation is expected to occur 5 to 11 days following discontinuation of clomiphene citrate. The daily dose of clomiphene citrate may be raised by 50-mg increments during each treatment cycle until ovulation is achieved or a total dose of 200 to 250 mg/day is reached.[16] A positive correlation exists between the weight of the patient and the dose of clomiphene citrate required to achieve ovulation.[18] Clomiphene citrate in doses higher than required to achieve ovulation and a normal luteal phase will not increase the conception rate and is more likely to result in hyperstimulation.[19] While clomiphene citrate has no benefit for regularly ovulating women, it can be used in patients who have an oligo-ovulatory pattern. The clinical definition of oligo-ovulation must be restricted to menstrual cycles in excess of 35 days to justify the risks and side effects associated with clomiphene citrate. Due to a relatively uniform response in repetitive cycles, clomiphene citrate may also be utilized for regulation of ovulation when artificial insemination is required.[20]

Monitoring During Treatment

As documentation of ovulation is essential, one must by some means assess the presence of a functioning corpus luteum following treatment with clomiphene citrate. The basal body temperature recording has traditionally been used to document progesterone production from the corpus luteum. While assuring neither ovulation nor the adequacy of progesterone production, the basal body temperature graph is an inexpensive means of monitoring the response to treatment. In up to 20 percent of patients, however, the temperature charts may be uninterpretable, and another means to assess ovulatory function is necessary. The occurrence of menstruation following clomiphene citrate treatment is supportive of ovulation but insufficient for documentation.

Since up to 80 percent of all conceptions during treatment with clomiphene citrate occur within the first three ovulatory cycles,[16] an assessment for the etiology of a failure to conceive should be performed during the fourth cycle. More precise evaluations of the adequacy of the ovulatory cycle include midluteal serum progesterone values, ultrasonic assessment of follicular growth, and timed endometrial biopsies.[21] A midluteal progesterone less than 15 ng/ml, poor follicle growth without evidence of rupture, or histology more than 2 days discrepant from the subsequent menses will indicate inadequate clomiphene dosages. A repeat postcoital sperm survival test should also be repeated within a day or two prior to the presumed day of ovulation since clomiphene citrate may preferentially exert a prolonged antiestrogenic effect on the cervical mucus.

The incidence of ovarian enlargement during treatment with clomiphene citrate should be below 10 percent and without significant complications except for mild discomfort. To minimize hyperstimulation, ovarian size is determined before initiating a subsequent treatment cycle. If ovarian enlargement is noted, treatment should be withheld until resolution of the mass is noted. An intermediate dose between the preceding dose and that resulting in hyperstimulation should then be used.

Adverse Reactions

Hyperstimulation

MacGregor et al.[13] have reported a 13.6 percent incidence of ovarian enlargement following treatment with clomiphene citrate. While moderate and severe ovarian hyperstimulation has been reported with this agent, it is extremely rare. Monthly monitoring of ovarian size should be sufficient to prevent an advanced form of hyperstimulation. Future courses of induction of ovulation may proceed after regression of the cyst, with slightly reduced dosages.

Multiple Gestation

The occurrence of multiple gestations following clomiphene citrate induction of ovulation is reported between 4 and 9 percent.[13-16] Patients with polycystic ovarian disease appear to be at increased risk. Ninety percent of the clomiphene citrate-induced multiple gestations are dizygotic twins. Multiple gestations account for only a small percentage of the increased abortion rate associated with the use of clomiphene citrate. The incidence of multiple gestations in excess of two concepti is less than 1 percent of all pregnancies occurring after clomiphene citrate.[13]

Luteal Phase Defect

This potential cause of ovulatory infertility or reproductive wastage is found with increased frequency when clomiphene citrate is required for induction of ovulation.[22,23] Whether this complication results from the direct effects of clomiphene on the ovary, the endometrium, or at another site, or from nonphysiologic circulating gonadotropin/estradiol levels is not known. While increased doses of clomiphene citrate may[24] or may not[22] correct this abnormality, other options including human chorionic gonadotropin (hCG)[23] and progesterone supplementation[23] have been used to correct this abnormality.

Abortion

Clinically diagnosed abortion rates are higher in patients treated for infertility. This general statement is especially true for patients receiving clomiphene citrate. A 20 percent incidence of clinically diagnosed abortions may be found with clomiphene citrate treatment.[6] The causes of the increased abortion rate appear to be heterogenous.

Dysmucorrhea

The use of clomiphene citrate may, in certain individuals, result in failure to produce periovulatory type cervical mucus despite appropriate endogenous estrogen concentrations.[23] It has been suggested that this adverse reaction may be dependent upon an increased sensitivity of the endocervical glands to the antiestrogen activity of clomiphene citrate.

Teratology

The incidence of congenital anomalies in pregnancies following the use of clomiphene citrate appears to be no different from the findings in an infertility population being treated by other modalities or for other causes.[25] In the case of inadvertent administration of clomiphene citrate following conception, a 5.1 percent incidence of major congenital anomalies has been reported.[26] While the structure of clomiphene citrate is quite similar to diethylstilbestrol, no specific anomalies related to clomiphene citrate are known.

Other Reactions

Vasomotor symptoms (10 percent), bloating (approximately 5 percent), and nausea and vomiting (approximately 2 percent) are the most common symptomatic complaints associated with clomiphene citrate.[13]

Adjuvants to Clomiphene Citrate Therapy

Treatment with gonadotropins is an appropriate alternative in subjects failing to ovulate in response to clomiphene citrate. Because of the expense, the limitation of facilities for appropriate treatment with gonadotropins, and the greater inconvenience involved, combination therapies of clomiphene citrate and other agents are often tried before proceeding to treatment with gonadotropins. Patients ovulating with clomiphene citrate but failing to become pregnant have in the past been treated with gonadotropins. While in many cases this would appear to be irrational, some of the causes of infertility found with the use of clomiphene citrate may have been avoided by the use of gonadotropins. Consideration of combined regimens in many of these cases may have diminished the need to use gonadotropins.[23] Table 21–1 is a summary of some combination regimens.

GONADOTROPIN THERAPY

Human menopausal gonadotropins (Pergonal—Serono Laboratories, Inc., Braintree, Massachusetts) is the only commercial preparation of LH and FSH available for induction of ovulation in the United States. Although isolation of pregnant mare serum gonadotropins (PMSG) in 1930 led to their successful use for ovulation induction in the human,[27] antigenic difficulties precluded clinical use. More than 12 years later, gonadotropins extracted from the human pituitary (hPG) were used for induction of ovulation.[28] Unfortunately, this made the FSH/LH preparation's availability an extremely limiting factor. In 1962, Lunenfeld and co-workers[29] reported a successful induction of ovulation with a gonadotropin preparation derived from human menopausal urine. Human menopausal gonadotropin (hMG) is a preparation of LH and FSH extracted from human menopausal ur-

TABLE 21-1. DRUGS UTILIZED CONCURRENTLY WITH CLOMIPHENE CITRATE

Adjuvant Agent	Indication	Regimen	Source(s)
Estrogen	Dysmucorrhea	Conjugated estrogens 0.3–0.625 mg or ethinyl estradiol 0.1 mg for 6–10 days prior to ovulation	1
Glucocorticoids	Hyperandrogenism preventing adequate follicular maturation	Dexamethasone 0.5 mg q.h.s.	94
Human chorionic gonadotropin (hCG)	Anovulation in estrogen-primed individual despite high doses of clomid; hyperprolactinemic subjects; inadequate luteal phase	10,000 IU IM on day 6 following discontinuance of clomiphene citrate	19
		5000 IU IM on days 3 and 6 following ovulation	95
Luteinizing hormone-releasing factor	Anovulation in estrogen-primed individual despite high doses of clomid	Preparations presently not commercially available	96,97
Progesterone suppositories	Inadequate luteal phase	25 mg two times a day vaginally starting on second day of basal body temperature rise	98
Human menopausal gonadotropin (+hCG)	Anovulation in estrogen-primed subject resistant to maximum doses of clomiphene citrate; hyperprolactinemic patients	HMG is begun after discontinuing clomiphene citrate. Monitoring is necessary	99

ine. It is currently available only as a 1:1 ratio (75 IU:75 IU) of LH and FSH.

The availability of hCG predates that of hMG. HCG is known to possess potent LH-like activity. The combination of hMG for follicular maturation and hCG as the ovulatory stimulus results in a reliable means of inducing ovulation in subjects devoid of pituitary function. While it is conceptually a relatively simple and effective means of treating anovulation, its expense, significant side effects, and demand for careful monitoring have limited its use and appropriately delegated it as a secondary form of treatment.

Chemistry and Physiology

LH, FSH, and hCG are all glycoproteins and consist of two subunits. The α-subunit is identical for all three hormones. The β-subunits have minor amino acid alterations capable of imparting very different biologic effects between LH, hCG, and FSH. Also differing among these three glycoproteins is the carbohydrate content. The β-subunit of LH consists of only one oligosaccharide, FSH has two, and hCG has five oligosaccharide chains. Increasing oligosaccharide content not only alters the configuration of the molecule but positively correlates with the half-life of the hormone. The average half-life of endogenous LH in plasma is about 30 minutes, while for hCG it is about 6 hours. The longer functional activity and greater availability of hCG makes it the agent of choice to recreate the physiologic LH surge.

Little is known about the metabolism of gonadotropins. Of administered gonadotropins, 10 to 20 percent may be recovered in the urine. Gonadotropin preparations are effective only with parenteral administration because of their size and potential for degradation in the gastrointestinal tract.

The biologic activity of gonadotropins is mediated through membrane receptors and activation of the adenylate cyclase system which generates intracellular cyclic adenosine 5′-monophosphate (cAMP). FSH stimulation of the follicular unit results in steroid production and follicular maturation. Within the follicular unit, FSH and estrogen are necessary to induce LH receptors. LH actions are synergistic with FSH, causing increased production of estrogen precursors. An LH or LH-like surge is necessary for reinitiation of meiotic division within the ovum and for the release of the ovum from the ovary.

It is important to recognize that the follicular units exert considerable local control on their own development. Studies in rhesus monkeys have shown that high doses of gonadotropins early in follicular maturation may cause multiple follicles to reach a stage capable of ovulation. Later in follicular maturation, however, increased dosages of gonadotropins appear unable to rescue follicles destined for atresia or to recruit new follicles into the process of maturation.[30] The mechanism by which the ovaries limit the follicular units eventually reaching maturation remains speculative but may involve FSH receptor numbers and sensitivity, follicular hormone levels, inhibin, other follicular proteins, or peritoneal factors. This concept of production of a dominant follicle[31] is important in the understanding of several empiric regimens for administering gonadotropins. Many of the concepts of induction of ovulation with gonadotropins were originally derived from experiments in animals that are naturally multiovulators. A complete reassessment of the ovulatory process has taken place as a result of the experience derived from IVF programs.

Clinical Use

The primary indication for hMG therapy is the failure to ovulate in response to other appropriate treatment regimens, i.e., clomiphene citrate, bromocriptine, or glucocorticoids. Gonadotropins have been used in patients ovulating in response to clomiphene citrate but failing to become pregnant after 6 to 12 months of continuous treatment. Pregnancy rates exceeding 50 percent have been reported in this group.[32] It also has direct application in those patients with hypogonadotropic anovulation and for the controlled ovarian hyperstimulation in IVF programs.

Patients requiring gonadotropin treatment may be divided into two categories: group 1 has primary or secondary amenorrhea with serum gonadotropins below the normal range and clinically demonstrable signs of estrogen deficiency; group 2 has normal levels of gonadotropins and evidence of endogenous estrogen production.[33]

Clinically, these two groups of patients can be differentiated by response to a progesterone challenge. Serum concentrations of FSH in patients failing to have withdrawal bleeding to progesterone are essential to confirm the presence of intact follicular units in the ovary. Markedly elevated levels of FSH imply primary ovarian failure or gonadotropin-resistant ovaries (Savage's syndrome). Little benefit would be anticipated from gonadotropin therapy in these cases, although some exceptions exist.[34,35]

Most patients in group 1 with low gonadotropins are totally dependent on exogenous gonadotropins for follicular maturation and ovulation. While longer treatment cycles and larger amounts of gonadotropins are required, fewer complications are seen in these patients. In group 2 patients, treatment is begun at various stages of follicular maturation, and unplanned ovulations may occur.[32] The combination of endogenous ovarian stimulation and exogenous gonadotropin therapy may result in higher complication rates.[33]

Treatment Regimens

The ideal treatment regimen has (1) a high rate of ovulation and pregnancy, (2) a low incidence of hyperstimulation and multiple gestations, (3) a low incidence of abortion, and

(4) relative economy. Numerous treatment regimens have been designed for induction of ovulation with gonadotropins. A daily individualized dosage regimen incorporating frequent monitoring techniques has been most widely accepted. The term "individualized" is perhaps deceiving, since proponents of different individualized treatment protocols advise strict adherence to specific predetermined dose schedules. Variation in ovarian responses to a set dose of gonadotropins during consecutive treatment cycles readily clarifies this apparent dilemma. Two treatment regimens and means of monitoring are presented. Other regimens and references are shown in Table 21–2.

March[36] reported his results in 108 treatment cycles with hMG. A basal body temperature chart, daily palpation of the ovaries, and daily inspection of cervical mucus were used concurrently with daily determinations of total serum estrogen. Two ampules of hMG were administered daily for 3 or 4 days. If serum estrogens were noted to gradually increase, this daily dose was continued. The dose of gonadotropins was increased by 50 percent if serum estrogen concentrations did not increase. After 3 days more of therapy,

TABLE 21–2. COMBINED hMG AND hCG TREATMENT REGIMENS AND MEANS OF MONITORING

Administration hMG	Administration hCG	Overall Pregnancy Rate (%)	Incidence of Hyperstimulation	Monitoring	Source
Individualized dosing regimen with or without clomiphene citrate pretreatment	10,000 IU 24–36 hr following optimal E_2 concentration, then 3000 IU on days 4 and 8 after first dose	51	7% mild hyperstimulation, 0% severe hyperstimulation	Serum estrogens daily: opt. 500–1000 pg/ml, max. 1000 pg/ml	36
HMG 3–8 ampules on days 1, 3, 5 (group II patients only)	10,000 IU on day 8 with optional boost 5000 IU on day 15	32	None; withheld hCG in 8% of treatment cycles	Serum estrogens; opt. range day 8 300–1500 pg/ml, max. 2000 pg/ml	100
Individualized dosing regimen with stepdown	8000 IU administered 2–3 days after 3+ ferning is noted	57	14% moderate hyperstimulation, 5% severe hyperstimulation	No chemical monitoring	101
Individualized dosing regimen with possible stepdown	8000 IU following optimal 24-hr urinary estrogen concentration	54	8% moderate hyperstimulation, 0% severe hyperstimulation	Urinary estrogens; 100–200 mcg/24 hr, max. 200 mcg/24 hr	101
Individualized dosing regimen	10,000 IU hCG at time of optimal serum estrogen	55	4.1% moderate hyperstimulation, 0% severe hyperstimulation; withheld dose in 12% of cycles	Serum estradiol: opt. 100–2000 pg/ml, max. 2000 pg/ml; sample obtained 12–15 hr after last injection	102

consideration for a higher dosage was again made. Once a serum concentration of total estrogens of 200 pg/ml was obtained, the patient was seen twice daily. The patient was examined each morning, and the serum level of estrogen was measured. Based on the findings from the morning specimen, treatment was administered or withheld that afternoon. When serum estrogens were between 500 and 1000 pg/ml, with normal-sized, nontender ovaries, administration of hCG was planned. Twenty-four to 36 hours after the last hMG injection, 10,000 IU of hCG was administered. If the ovaries were not enlarged, a booster injection of hCG was given 4 and 8 days following the initial hCG injection to support the corpus luteum. In repeated cycles, treatment was initiated with the lowest dose of hMG that was capable of initiating adequate follicular steroidogenesis. In patients with endogenous ovarian estrogen production, a similar regimen was recommended but immediately preceded by a 5-day course of 200 mg/day of clomiphene citrate.

If ovarian enlargement or serum concentrations of estrogen beyond 1000 pg/ml were encountered, hCG was withheld. In this series, no cases of severe hyperstimulation were reported, the ovulation rate exceeded 98 percent, the multiple pregnancy rate was 5 percent, and the overall pregnancy rate was 51 percent. A conceptualized treatment scheme is shown in Figure 21–3.

Oesler et al.[33] reported on over 1800 treatment cycles using a regimen similar to March's protocol for patients failing to have withdrawal bleeding to progesterone. However, reliance was placed on a cervical mucus scoring system rather than estrogen assays until good quality mucus was obtained. Urinary estrogen concentrations were then used to assess the adequacy of the follicular maturation for an ovulatory response. They began with a lower initial dose (1 ampule of hMG/day) with changes in dosages being made on a weekly basis. In patients with endogenous estrogen production, early frequent determinations of urinary estrogens were advised. Follicular rupture was induced with 5000 IU of hCG followed by similar daily injections for 3 to 4 days, provided that the ovaries were not enlarged and urinary estrogen concentrations did not exceed 150 mcg/

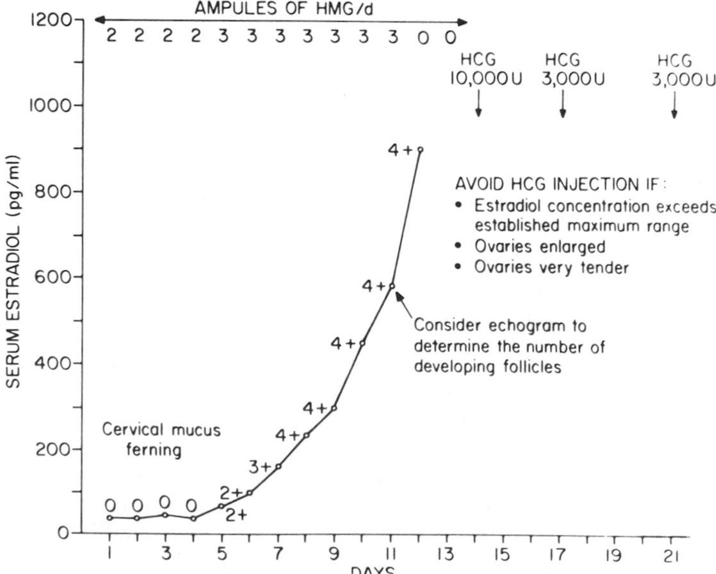

Figure 21–3. This diagram represents an ideal response to an individualized dosage regimen. Note that cervical mucus becomes an invalid monitor when estradiol serum concentrations exceed 200 pg/ml.

24 hours. In this series, the incidence of severe hyperstimulation was 0.36 percent, the multiple pregnancy rate was 32.5 percent (78 percent being twins), and an overall pregnancy rate of 54.5 percent was achieved. The report stretches over 15 years with several refinements during recent years.

A pure FSH (Metrodin—Serono Laboratories) preparation containing 75 IU of FSH and less than 0.11 IU of LH is also available. Data utilizing pure FSH for ovulation induction are limited, early studies suggest equivalent results with that of the LH/FSH preparations.[37-39] Dosage, administration, cycle monitoring, and the use of hCG are essentially identical with that of hMG therapy.

Monitoring of Treatment Effects

The capacity for daily monitoring of serum or urinary estradiol levels is essential for treatment with gonadotropins. The point in therapy where daily measurements are initiated is, however, controversial. Generally, group 2 patients require hormonal monitoring immediately after initiating treatment. In group 1 patients, cervical mucus is frequently used during the early part of therapy until good quality mucus is obtained. This usually correlates with levels of serum estrogens between 150 and 200 pg/ml. Daily hormonal monitoring is then begun. With appropriate clinical experience, this form of monitoring is associated with few complications, although hCG treatment may be withheld in more treatment cycles using this monitoring regimen.

The ideal response to gonadotropin therapy is a cycle with gradually increasing estrogen production. Incremental rises of serum estradiol should approximate a 100 percent rise over the value of the previous day during active follicular maturation. Too rapid a rise may be associated with the stimulation of multiple follicles or be an indicator of subsequent hyperstimulation. If too rapid a rise is noted, a reduction in dose of hMG may be contemplated with consideration for withholding hCG if the preovulatory range of estrogens is exceeded.

The optimal range for administration of hCG varies in different laboratories. The serum concentration or urinary concentration of estradiol chosen as an endpoint is considerably in excess of the values found during the normal preovulatory period. These values are chosen to maximize the ovulation rate while maintaining an acceptable rate of multiple gestation and complications. The reader may refer to Table 21-2 to review these values in different treatment regimens.

Luteal function is confirmed by a serum concentration of progesterone approximately 7 to 10 days following the initial hCG injection. Pregnancy may be implied from a persistent thermogenic rise on the basal body temperature chart exceeding 14 days. A serum hCG (β-subunit) level may be used to confirm a pregnancy at that time.

Ultrasound has also been utilized as a means for monitoring follicular maturation. While it appears unlikely to completely replace hormonal monitoring, consideration should be given for its use as means of determining whether multiple follicles have reached the preovulatory stage. Withholding hCG in these situations would reduce the incidence of multiple gestations.

Complications of Gonadotropin Treatment

Ovarian Hyperstimulation Syndrome (OHSS)

The use of estrogen monitoring and nonoverlapping administration of hCG have helped to reduce the occurrence of the hyperstimulation syndrome. The syndrome is characterized by ovarian enlargement, excessive ovarian hormone production, abdominal discomfort, and in severe cases, by dehydration, increased capillary permeability, ascites, and hypercoagulability.

The initial signs of hyperstimulation generally manifest 3 to 6 days following the administration of hCG. Hyperstimulation in the absence of hCG administration generally results from spontaneous ovulation and is a rare phenomenon. Worsening of this complication may result if pregnancy was achieved during the cycle. Management of mild or moderate OHSS consists of observation and rest. Severe cases of OHSS mandate hospitalization, hydration, and careful monitoring of fluids, electrolytes, and coagulation factors. Benefit has been reported with the use of an antiprostaglandin agent, i.e., indomethecin,[40] antihistamines,[41] and plasma expanders like low-molecular-weight dextran.[40] Surgical intervention should be avoided, although it is occasionally required for ovarian torsion, ovarian hemorrhage, or the occurrence of a simultaneous ectopic pregnancy.

Multiple Gestations

An incidence of multiple gestations approaching 25 percent is to be expected with the use of gonadotropins, despite careful monitoring during treatment. Multiple gestations exceeding twins can be limited by careful estrogen monitoring. Determining the number of preovulatory follicles by ultrasound before administering hCG may further reduce the incidence of multiple gestations.

Abortion

Abortion rates of 20 to 25 percent are found in subjects who conceived during gonadotropin treatment. While it is significantly greater than the incidence reported in a normal population, intermediate values are frequently reported in an infertility population. Multiple gestations account for a significant proportion of the reported abortions.

Ectopic Pregnancy

The occurrence of ectopic pregnancies has been reported in association with the hyperstimulation syndrome.[42] While uncommon, it must be considered in the differential diagnosis of abdominal pain and hypotension following treatment with gonadotropins.

Rapid Growth of Pituitary Adenomas

Neurologic complications from rapidly enlarging pituitary tumors have been reported.[43] While not resulting from hMG therapy but rather from the ensuing pregnancy, the differential diagnosis preceding therapy must consider the possibility of a space-occupying lesion as the cause of severe pituitary dysfunction.

Hypersensitivity

Early use of gonadotropin preparations were associated with occasionally severe allergic reactions. Febrile reactions to hMG therapy have also been reported.[44]

GONADOTROPIN-RELEASING HORMONE (GnRH)

Early experimentation with pituitary stalk resection and with pituitary transplantation to extrasellar sites demonstrated that the hypothalamus controlled pituitary secretions of gonadotropins. The exact controlling substance, however, was unknown until 1971 when Schally and Guillemin characterized the structure of gonadotropin-releasing hormone (GnRH).[45,46] Initial use of GnRH to induce ovulation was unsuccessful until Knobil[47] demonstrated in hypothalamically lesioned Rhesus monkeys that pulsatile administration was necessary for appropriate secretion of LH and FSH. It was initially hoped that pulsatile administration of GnRH could be used to induce ovulation in a physiologic manner. Such use could avoid complications of conventional therapy including hyperstimulation and multiple birth. Although initial trials were disappointing, subsequent experience with GnRH use has been very promising.

Chemistry and Physiology

GnRH is a decapeptide which is synthesized in the medial basal region of the hypothalamus and secreted in a pulsatile fashion into the hypothalamic–pituitary–portal system.[48] It is transported via the portal system to the anterior pituitary where it binds to specific GnRH receptors on the gonadotropes and results in the pulsatile release of LH and to a lesser extent FSH. The number of GnRH receptors is known to increase with intermittent exposure to GnRH and decrease with constant exposure (down regulation).[49,50] Thus intermittent intravenous (IV) administration of GnRH results in gonadotropin secretion by the pituitary whereas continuous chronic IV administration results in a hypogonadotropic state. FSH and LH bind to receptors in the ovary and stimulate orderly development of follicles, ovulation, and steroidogenesis. GnRH is thought to play a permissive role in controlling gonadotropin secretions. The natural periodicity of its pulsatile secretion is approximately 90 minutes except in the luteal phase when it changes to approximately 3 to 4 hours.

In 1983, the Food and Drug Administration (FDA) approved Factrel (synthetic GnRH—Ayerst Laboratories) for use as an agent for diagnostic purposes. Prior to that time, GnRH was not available commercially in the United States. While approved only for diagnostic purposes, the clinician has the option of utilizing Factrel for therapeutic purposes such as ovulation induction. Such therapeutic uses are now widespread both in the United States and in Europe and it can no longer be considered an experimental agent for this purpose. Factrel is a synthetic decapeptide that appears to be identical to the naturally occurring GnRH. Factrel is available as a white powder in vials of 100 mcg and 500 mcg to be used for diagnostic and therapeutic purposes respectively.

GnRH is ineffective after oral administration due to rapid degradation of its polypeptide structure within the intestinal tract. Administration is therefore generally by IV or subcutaneous (SQ) routes. The half-life of GnRH is approximately 4 minutes reflecting rapid breakdown into its basic amino acid sequence. In normal women, a 100 mcg IV bolus dose results in a rapid rise in LH (within 5 minutes) with peak levels occurring within 30 minutes. Maximal LH response occurs after administration of a 100 mcg dose in women. Doses as small as 0.025 mcg/kg repeatedly have resulted in LH release.[51] Studies in mammals with radioactively tagged GnRH demonstrate that activity rapidly disappears from the serum and concentrates in the pituitary gland, pineal gland, kidneys, and liver. The latter two organs are probably the main sites of inactivation and excretion of GnRH.

Clinical Use

Generally accepted guidelines for ovulation induction with GnRH do not yet exist. This is primarily due to the fact that the agent is new and experience with its use is limited. It is therefore recommended that institutions utilizing this agent for therapeutic purposes do so under a standardized protocol.

Ideal candidates are patients with hypothalamic amenorrhea who display no withdrawal bleeding after progesterone administration. Although these individuals generally do not respond well to clomiphene citrate, this should be attempted in gradually increasing dosages since this represents simpler, less expensive therapy, and some successes are known to occur.[52] For patients who fail clomiphene citrate therapy and have no other correctable abnormality, e.g., hyperprolactinemia, the two available options are hMG or GnRH therapy. The advantages and disadvantages of hMG therapy have been previously discussed. GnRH therapy offers the advantage of lower cost, a more physiologic ovulation with less chance of hyperstimulation, and less time-consuming monitoring. Because of these advantages we do not feel that such therapy should be reserved purely for patients who have failed hMG; it can be used as an alternative to hMG therapy.

Additional uses of GnRH have included treatment of luteal phase defects and disordered folliculogenesis resistant to other therapy. In males with Kallman's syndrome, pulsatile administration of GnRH has resulted in initiation of spermatogenesis and pubertal changes. Intraveneous GnRH in high doses has also been utilized for controlled ovarian hyperstimulation for IVF and embryo transfer. GnRH in doses of 100 mcg SQ or IV can also be used to differentiate between hypothalamic and pituitary causes of hypogonadotropic hypogonadism.

Gonadotropin response to a 100 mcg IV bolus of GnRH was originally proposed as a screening test to identify patients who are deficient in FSH and LH and would therefore be unlikely to benefit from pulsatile GnRH therapy. The response to a single dose of GnRH, however, is not predictive of response to chronic pulsatile administration because such chronic administration results in increased numbers of pituitary GnRH receptors (up regulation).[49] Therefore, we do not currently require a formal GnRH stimulation test prior to instituting GnRH pump therapy. The cost per cycle including medication, pump usage fee, and monitoring is estimated to be $500 to $600 at our institution.

Ovulation induction can be successfully accomplished by either IV or SQ routes of administration. Currently controversy exists as to the most preferable route. The IV route is generally more predictable in inducing ovulation, requires less drug usage and is therefore less expensive, and probably more closely resembles the normal physiologic situation. However, it has the distinct disadvantage of requiring prolonged IV access which is likely to become more difficult in subsequent cycles. Potential IV site complications include infiltration with interruption of drug delivery and superficial thrombophlebitis. Due to the low infusion volumes, IV administration requires the addition of 1000 units heparin/ml in order to avoid clotting at the catheter tip. Subcutaneous administration is generally by a 26-gauge needle designed for use in the lower abdomen where it can be taped securely in place. Heparin should not be added to the solution as this has been reported to result in hematoma formation and subsequently poor absorption of GnRH from the SQ region. The SQ site can be easily changed every 3 to 5 days. Higher doses of GnRH are generally required. We prefer IV administration in certain patients such as those with polycystic ovary syndrome where interruption of the tonically elevated LH secretion appears critical to restoring normal folliculogenesis. For patients who are concerned about having an indwelling IV catheter or for those individuals for whom IV access is difficult, the SQ is chosen. For all other patients either route is acceptable and probably equally effective.

Dosage and Pulse Frequency

Based on the information available from numerous recent [53-64] published series, the most common successfully used interpulse time intervals are 60 to 120 minutes with 90 minutes being the most common. This pulse frequency approximates the normal physiologic follicular phase pulse frequency. Although there is no clear evidence that any one particular pulse interval is optimal, there is initial information to suggest that patients with polycystic ovaries respond better to the 120-minute pulse interval.[65] Also, with SQ administration there is concern that pulse intervals less than 90 minutes in duration may result in chronically elevated GnRH levels and pituitary down regulation. We therefore initiate IV therapy with a pulse interval of 90 minutes and initiate SQ therapy with a pulse interval of 120 minutes.

Ovulation has been successfully achieved with dosages from 1 mcg per pulse to 25 mcg per pulse. Most investigators use a dose of 5 to 15 mcg per pulse. For IV therapy a starting dose of 2.5 to 5 mcg per pulse is useful. Increments of approximately 5 mcg can then be used if response is inadequate. For SQ therapy most patients will ultimately require 10 to 20 mcg per pulse with few patients ovulating at doses less than 15 mcg per pulse.[56] A starting dose of 5 to 10 mcg per pulse is therefore recommended.

Pulsatile administration is accomplished

using a portable, battery-operated pump. Several types are available with a cost ranging from $1000 to $1500. It is ideal for the pump to be able to vary both pulse frequency as well as volume infused per pulse. One such pump which we have used without difficulty is the Autosyringe (Auto Syringe, Inc., Hookset, New Hampshire). The device is small and can be carried in its case attached to the belt and hidden from view.

Monitoring

There is no general agreement as to the level of monitoring necessary with pulsatile infusion of GnRH. Since the incidence of hyperstimulation and multiple ovulation is much lower than with hMG, however, it is felt that the monitoring can be less intensive without incurring adverse effects. We have adopted a protocol of monitoring initially every 3 days. At each visit the site of infusion and pump settings are checked. IV sites are changed routinely every 5 days and SQ sites every 3 days. Serum estradiol is determined at each visit until a value of 250 pg/ml is reached. If the serum estradiol displays insufficient increase over a 6-day period, we first increase the dosage by 5 mcg increments until a dose of 20 mcg per pulse is reached. If insufficient stimulation still exists the pulse interval is decreased serially by 30 minutes until 60 minutes is reached.

When the estradiol is approximately 250 pg/ml, pelvic ultrasound every other day is accomplished until the leading follicle is 20 mm or ovulation has occurred. When the leading follicle reaches 20 mm, 5000 units of hCG is administered IM to induce ovulation. When there is a clear elevation of the basal body temperature for greater than 48 hours, the pump is then discontinued. Three thousand units of hCG is then administered 5 days and 10 days after the initial dose for luteal phase support. Alternative means of luteal phase support include continuing the pump until conception is documented or use of progesterone vaginal suppositories (25 mg twice daily). There appears to be no evidence that one method of luteal phase support is superior. However, there is clear evidence that discontinuance of the pump after ovulation without luteal phase support results in a luteal phase defect.[58]

The actual reported incidence of ovulation and pregnancy varies with the particular center reporting, route of administration, dosage, and pulse frequency. A total of 389 cycles recently reported in the literature[53–65] were well described in terms of the incidence of ovulation, pregnancy, and drug dosage as well as pulse intervals. One hundred ninety-three SQ administration cycles showed an overall ovulation rate of 88 percent. The pregnancy rate per cycle was 29 percent and 25 percent of the pregnancies terminated in spontaneous abortion. The dosage range was 10 to 20 mcg per pulse and the pulse interval varied from 90 to 120 minutes. In 196 IV cycles the ovulation rate was 95 percent and the rate of pregnancy per cycle was 30 percent. The incidence of spontaneous abortion was also 25 percent. These initial results are indeed promising and compare favorably with results observed with hMG therapy.

Complications of GnRH Therapy

Hyperstimulation

It was initially hoped that due to the physiologic nature of pulsatile GnRH administration, hyperstimulation would not occur. While this has been predominantly the experience, several cases of mild hyperstimulation have been reported. Insufficient experience currently exists to accurately estimate the incidence of hyperstimulation but it appears to be much lower than the incidence of hyperstimulation syndrome with either clomiphene citrate or human menopausal gonadotropins.

Multiple Gestations

The incidence of multiple gestations is also not well known at the present time. Isolated cases of triplets and quadruplets after pulsatile GnRH therapy have been reported.[66,67] It is felt that the administration of ovulatory doses of hCG may override natural feedback mechanisms and result in multiple ovulations and increased potential for multiple pregnancies.[66] Initial experience suggests, however, that multiple pregnancy will be less frequent than the 20 to 30 percent incidence observed with hMG therapy.

Other Effects

Nonspecific side effects such as dizziness, nausea, and flushing are occasionally seen after administration of the 100-mcg test dose IV. However, at the relatively lower doses used for ovulation induction these side effects have not been reported. In nonhuman primates, no toxic effects were noted from the administration of 0.5 mg GnRH daily for 1 month.

BROMOCRIPTINE

Bromocriptine, 2-bromo-ergocriptine mesylate (Parlodel—Sandoz Pharmaceuticals, East Hanover, New Jersey) is an ergot derivative with potent dopamine receptor agonist activity (Fig. 21–4). It is approved for use in the treatment of infertility or amenorrhea associated with hyperprolactinemia once a pituitary tumor has been excluded. It is not currently approved either for normoprolactinemic individuals or those with documented micro- or macroadenomas. However, considerable data have been obtained on its use in all of these circumstances. Bromocriptine is extremely effective as an ovulatory agent in most patients with hyperprolactinemia whether from a nontumorous source or from a neoplastic source.[68,69] The potential for rapid enlargement of pituitary tumors during pregnancy, however, makes an evaluation of the cause of hyperprolactinemia mandatory before utilizing bromocriptine in patients desiring pregnancy.

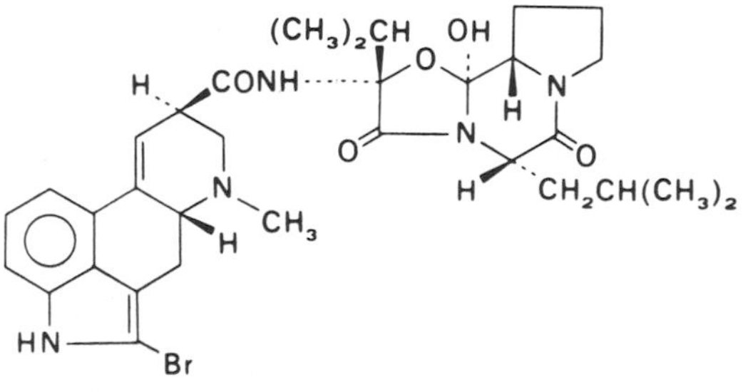

$(CH_3)_2CH$ OH CONH O N H N O O H H $CH_2CH(CH_3)_2$ N CH_3 H HN Br

Figure 21–4. Chemical structure of bromocriptine. *(From Csáky, TZ: Cutting's Handbook of Pharmacology: The Actions and Uses of Drugs, ed. 7. Norwalk, Connecticut, Appleton-Century-Crofts, 1984, p. 301, with permission.)*

Chemistry and Physiology

Bromocriptine is a semisynthetic ergot alkaloid that is rapidly and extensively absorbed from the gastrointestinal tract. Its peak plasma concentrations occur 2 to 3 hours following ingestion.[70] A single dose of bromocriptine will suppress prolactin for 8 to 12 hours.[69] Excretion is primarily accomplished through the biliary system and traces of the drug may be found up to 5 days after a single dose. Metabolism is extensive and varied, primarily involving the lysergic acid portion of the molecule.

Dopamine is an endogenous catecholamine believed to be the major inhibiting factor for the release and synthesis of prolactin. Dopamine agonists decrease while dopamine antagonists elevate prolactin levels. Thus bromocriptine, as a dopamine agonist, is believed to interact at the dopamine receptors in prolactin-secreting lactotrophs to inhibit prolactin secretion. While extremely potent in its ability to suppress prolactin, bromocriptine exerts little influence on motor functions dependent on dopamine. Available evidence suggests the existence of multiple receptors for dopamine. Bromocriptine exerts its actions preferentially at the dopamine D_2 receptor, as defined by Kebabian and Calne.[71]

By suppressing central and peripheral concentrations of prolactin, bromocriptine allows for restitution of ovulation function; it has demonstrable effects throughout the hypothalamic–pituitary–ovarian axis. Of interest is the absence of control of the decidual secretion of prolactin.[72]

Clinical Use for Induction of Ovulation

The use of bromocriptine for lactation suppression has already been discussed in Chapter 17. A preliminary work-up in a patient with hyperprolactinemia should involve a thyroid evaluation including a thyroid-stimulating hormone (TSH) level and most likely a computed tomography (CT) scan since pregnancy is being contemplated. With the availability of radioimmunoassays for prolactin, a large proportion of anovulation (3 to 20 percent) has been found in association with hyperprolactinemia.[73] Anovulation may result from inhibition of hypothalamic tonic and cyclic secretion of gonadotropin-releasing factor, direct pituitary suppression, ovarian follicular disruption, or disturbances in catecholamine regulation. If iatrogenic causes of hyperprolactinemia are eliminated, microadenomas (less than 10 mm) or macroadenomas (greater than 10 mm) may be found in up to 45 percent of hyperprolactinemic amenorrheic subjects.[73] Bromocriptine is capable of suppressing pituitary prolactin secretion from almost all causes. With a return of prolactin levels to normal, an ovulatory rate of 80 percent may be achieved in previously anovulatory subjects.[68]

The dose of bromocriptine required for treatment of hyperprolactinemia is generally determined by the clinical response. There are several benefits to be achieved by using the lowest effective dose. High dosages reduce the specificity of bromocriptine for the D_2 receptor and may result in hypotensive episodes, excessive nausea, and motor dysfunction. Hypotension may be minimized by administering the drug at bedtime, the time of greatest prolactin secretion in idiopathic hyperprolactinemia. Nausea is reduced by using gradually increasing doses. Motor dysfunction is associated almost exclusively with very high doses of bromocriptine. In addition to these side effects, excessive suppression of prolactin by bromocriptine may result in decreased progesterone synthesis from the corpus luteum.[74]

To determine the lowest effective dose, treatment is begun with one tablet (2.5 mg) at bedtime. The administered dose may be raised by 2.5-mg increments every 2 weeks, until ovulation occurs or a prolactin level within the normal range is obtained. The basal body temperature chart is used to monitor an ovulatory response. The average interval from achieving a euprolactinemic state to ovulation is 3 to 4 weeks.[43]

Once the dose required to achieve ovulation has been determined, treatment is continued at that level until pregnancy is confirmed. Because of nausea, some patients will require starting at the 2.5 mg/day dose, increasing daily until the dosage required for ovulation is achieved. Most patients will respond to a dose of 5 to 7.5 mg/day.

Treatment with bromocriptine is effective in inducing ovulation only during the cycles in which it is used. Induction of ovulation with bromocriptine is of limited value unless attempts at pregnancy are contemplated. While there have been reports of continued euprolactinemia following prolonged continuous treatment with bromocriptine, most patients return to their pretreatment level of hyperprolactinemia following discontinuation of the medication.[75]

Bromocriptine has been reported to be effective in euprolactinemic amenorrhea,[76] but controlled studies have not substantiated this claim.[77] Midcycle prolactin elevation which was detected only by serial prolactin values was postulated to be the explanation of successfully treating "euprolactinemic" women in one study.[78] Circadian fluctuation in prolactin offers another possible explanation.

Bromocriptine is presently approved for the treatment of anovulation in the United States. Other treatments that have been used for hyperprolactinemic amenorrhea include clomiphene citrate, hMG–hCG, transphenoidal excision of microadenomas, and radiation therapy. In amenorrhea–galactorrhea, clomiphene citrate has been reported to successfully induce ovulation in up to 42 percent of patients with a pregnancy rate of only 16 percent.[5] Successful induction of ovulation in hypoestrogenic hyperprolactinemia subjects is rare. Gonadotropin therapy in patients with amenorrhea and galactorrhea desiring pregnancy is relatively effective. Pregnancy rates greater than 75 percent are reported.[33] The high cost and potential complications associated with gonadotropin therapy make this form of treatment less than ideal. Pregnancies following transphenoidal surgery alone in most series occur in less than 40 percent of patients.[79] Radiation therapy involves a long lag phase before normal prolactin levels are achieved and often results in subsequent hypogonadotropism. To achieve pregnancy, exogenous gonadotropins are frequently required following radiation therapy.

Bromocriptine, when used in the treatment of infertility from anovulation and hyperprolactinemia, has resulted in a pregnancy rate of greater than 60 percent.[80,81] The abortion rate is less than that found with gonadotropin therapy and similar to the normal population.[80,82] Its ease of administration and relatively minor side effects makes it currently the best agent available for the medical management of infertility resulting from hyperprolactinemia. While not currently FDA approved for this indication, the vast majority of studies clearly show the safety and efficacy of bromocriptine when used in cases of microadenoma as well.[82,83] Few neurologic complications are found in pregnancies occurring in patients with pituitary microadenomas.[82] The ability to manage neurologic complications during pregnancy with bromocriptine or with surgery without significant pemanent sequelae is further support for the use of bromocriptine, even in cases of macroadenomas.[82,83]

The finding of hyperprolactinemia and polycystic ovarian disease has been reported in several series.[84] Treatment for anovulation in these cases should initially utilize the approved agent, clomiphene citrate. Failure to induce withdrawal bleeding with progesterone implies the need for bromocriptine. If ovulation fails to occur in response to bromocriptine and euprolactinemia, the addition of clomiphene citrate may be of value if progesterone-induced withdrawal bleeding can now be demonstrated.

Adverse Reactions

During initial therapy, a high incidence of nausea (52 percent), headaches (18 percent), orthostatic hypotension (6 percent), dizziness (16 percent), and vomiting (5 percent) may be encountered.[68] Stepwise increases in dosages and nocturnal administration appear to reduce these occurrences.

Alterations in awareness and behavior have been reported in 1 percent of patients.[69] Hallucinations have also been reported but are rare with the dosages utilized for hormonal control. Bromocriptine should not be used in patients with mental disturbances, coronary vascular disease, or peripheral vascular disease.

An abortion rate similar to the normal population is found when bromocriptine is used continuously[85] or in a cyclic fasion, as described previously. Among 1113 infants born to mothers exposed to bromocriptine during pregnancy, there were 37 cases of congenital anomalies, 9 of which were considered major. The total incidence (3.3 percent) is not statistically significant.[86]

OTHER AGENTS FOR INDUCTION OF OVULATION

Tamoxifen

Tamoxifen citrate (Nolvadex—Stuart Pharmaceuticals) is another triphenylethylene compound, the trans isomer of 2(4-(1,2-diphenyl-1-butenyl)phenoxy)-N,N-dimethylethanamine. It is a nonsteroidal antiestrogen which is primarily marketed in the United

States for treatment of breast cancer. It has been used quite successfully both for ovulation induction and correction of luteal phase defects.[86-89] There appears to be at least three distinct advantages to the use of tamoxifen instead of clomiphene citrate for ovulation induction: There seems to be the lack of any antiestrogenic effect on the cervical mucus, there is an absence of a hyperstimulation syndrome, and the cost is one-third to one-half that of clomiphene.

Dosage should be started on 10 mg/day for 5 days beginning either day 3 or 5 of the cycle. This may be increased to 40 mg/day if an inadequate response occurs. No toxicity has been reported at these concentrations, although hot flashes may be more prevalent than with clomiphene citrate.

Glucocorticoids

Glucocorticoids, i.e., dexamethasone, prednisone, have been used with success in hyperandrogenic anovulatory patients. Resumption of regular ovulatory cycles are reported to occur in up to 60 percent of such patients.[90] By reducing the adrenal contribution to the excessive androgen pool, ovulation may resume. Doses utilized have varied with the patient's weight. Using 0.5 mg of dexamethasone at bedtime in patients over 150 lb, serum levels of dehydroepiandrosterone sulfate are effectively suppressed.

With the exception of hyperandrogenism and anovulation resulting from adrenal hyperactivity, i.e., congenital adrenal hyperplasia, glucocorticoids should not be used as a primary agent for induction of ovulation. They are less reliable than clomiphene citrate, require daily administration, and have the potential for significant complications when used for long periods of time and during periods of stress.

Estrogens

Parenteral injection of estradiol has been used alone[91] or in combination with clomiphene citrate[92] for induction of ovulation. The treatment assumes that a mature follicle will respond to a LH surge induced by a bolus injection of estradiol. This is not a reliable means of inducing ovulation.

Epimestrol

Epimestrol, a methylated form of the natural estrogen 17β-epiestriol, has been tested as an agent for induction of ovulation. It is presently not available in the United States for clinical use, and little data exist on its efficacy. Its actions are probably similar to clomiphene citrate, but antiestrogen effects on the cervical mucus are reported to be less frequent.[93]

Combination Therapy

Clomiphene Citrate Plus hMG

In subjects capable of demonstrating withdrawal bleeding, March has reported that the use of clomiphene citrate immediately prior to hMG therapy reduces the amount of hMG required by 50 percent.[36] HCG is administered based on hormone monitoring. Although large series are not available to compare the incidence of multiple gestation or hyperstimulation, this reduction in time commitment and cost appears to be beneficial. Daily hormonal monitoring is required once gonadotropins are begun in these patients.

hMG-hCG and Bromocriptine

In infertile patients with hyperprolactinemia failing to ovulate on bromocriptine alone or in combination with clomiphene citrate, hMG–hCG may be utilized.[94] The amount of gonadotropins required may be reduced if bromocriptine is utilized concurrently with hMG administration. Prior to such treatment, a thorough diagnostic evaluation should have been performed, with consideration for surgical treatment if a prolactin-producing tumor of the pituitary is present.

Bromocriptine has been suggested to reduce the requirement for hMG in euprolactinemic subjects.[94] Considering the present indications for the use of bromocriptine, this tenuous finding appears to be of little value in clinical practice.

REFERENCES

1. Speroff L, Glass RH, Kase NG (eds): Anovulation. In Clinical Gynecologic Endocrinology and Infertility. Baltimore, Williams and Wilkins, 1983, p 185
2. Yen SSC: Chronic anovulation due to CNS-hypothalamic-pituitary dysfunction. In Yen SSC, Jaffe RB (eds): Reproductive Endocrinology. Philadelphia, Saunders, 1986, p 500
3. Clark JH, Markaverich BM: The agonistic-antagonistic properties of clomiphene: A review. Pharmacol Ther 15:467, 1982
4. Greenblatt RB, Varfield WE, Junget EC, Roy AW: Induction of ovulation with MRL-41. JAMA 178:101, 1961
5. Clark JH, Peck EJ, Anderson JN: Oestrogen receptors and antogonisms of steroid hormone action. Nature 251:446, 1974
6. Hashimoto T, Miyai K, Izumi K, Kumahara Y: Effect of clomiphene citrate on basal and LRH-induced gonadotropin secretion in postmenopausal women. J Clin Endocrinol Metab 42:593, 1976
7. Jones GS, de Moraes-Ruehsen M: Induction of ovulation with human gonadotropins and with clomiphene. Fertil Steril 16:461, 1965
8. Riley GM, Evans TM: Effects of clomiphene citrate on anovulatory ovarian function. Am J Obstet Gynecol 89:97, 1964
9. Van Compenhout J, Simard R, Leduc B: Antiestrogenic effect of clomiphene in the human being. Fertil Steril 19:700, 1968
10. Adashi EY: Clomiphene citrate: Mechanism(s) and site(s) of action—A hypothesis revisited. Fertil Steril 42:331, 1984
11. Schreiber E, Johnson JE, Protz EJ, et al.: Studies with ^{14}C-labeled clomiphene citrate. Clin Res 14:287, 1966
12. Mikkelson TJ, Baustian CL, Cameron WJ: Preliminary report of the disposition of clomiphene in healthy human subjects (abst). Fertil Steril 41:395, 1984
13. MacGregor AH, Johnson JE, Bunde CE: Further clinical experience with clomiphene citrate. Fertil Steril 19:616, 1968
14. Mishell DR, March CM: Induction of ovulation. In Mishell DR, Davajan V (eds): Reproductive Endocrinology Infertility and Contraception. Philadelphia, Davis, 1979, p 317
15. Drake TS, Tredway DR, Buchanan GC: Continued clinical experience with an increasing dosage regimen of clomiphene citrate administration. Fertil Steril 30:274, 1978
16. Ruse LA, Israel R, Mishell DR: An individualized graduated therapeutic regimen for clomiphene citrate. Am J Obstet Gynecol 120:785, 1974
17. March CM, Israel R, Mishell DR: Pregnancy following 29 cycles of clomiphene citrate therapy: A case report. Am J Obstet Gynecol 124:209, 1976
18. Shepard M, Balmaceda JP, Leija CG: Relationship of weight to successful induction of ovulation with clomiphene citrate. Fertil Steril 32:641, 1979
19. Hupper LC: Induction of ovulation with clomiphene citrate. Fertil Steril 31:1, 1979
20. Beck WW Jr, Barrett ATM: Adjunctive therapy to the women in couples undergoing artificial insemination (abst). Fertil Steril 29:254, 1978
21. Hammond MG: Monitoring techniques for improved pregnancy rates during clomiphene ovulation induction. Fertil Steril 42:499, 1984
22. Cook CL, Schroeder JA, Yussman MA, et al.: Induction of luteal phase defect with clomiphene citrate. Am J Obstet Gynecol 149:613, 1984
23. Wu CH: Monitoring of ovulation induction. Fertil Steril 30:617, 1978
24. Quagliarello J, Weiss G: Clomiphene citrate in the management of infertility associated with shortened luteal phase. Fertil Steril 31:373, 1979
25. Adashi EY, Rock JA, Sapp KC, et al.: Gestational outcome of clomiphene-related conceptions. Fertil Steril 31:620, 1979
26. Merrell-National Laboratories: Product Information 1972. Division of Richardson Merrell Inc., Cincinnati, Ohio 43215
27. Hamblen EC, Davis CD: Treatment of hypoovarianism by the sequential and cyclic administration of equine and chorionic gonadotropins. Am J Obstet Gynecol 50:137, 1945
28. Gemzell CA, Diczfalusy E, Tillinger KG: Clinical effect of human pituitary follicle stimulating hormone. J Clin Endocrinol Metab 18:1333, 1958

29. Lunenfeld B, Sulimovici S, Rabau E, Eshkol A: L'induction de l'ovulation dans les amenorrhea hypophysaires par un traitement combaine de gonadotropines urinaires menopausique et de gonadotropines chorioniques. CR Soc Fr Gynecol 35:346, 1962
30. DiZerega GS, Hodgen GD: The primate ovarian cycle: Suppression of human menopausal gonadotropin-induced follicular growth in the presence of the dominant follicle. J Clin Endocrinol Metab 50:819, 1980
31. DiZerega GS, Hodgen GD: Luteal phase dysfunction infertility: A sequel to aberrant folliculogenesis. Fertil Steril 35:489, 1981
32. Wang CF, Gemzell C: Use of human gonadotropin for the induction of ovulation in women with polycystic ovarian disease. Fertil Steril 33:479, 1980
33. Oesler G, Serr DM, Mashiach S, et al.: The study of induction of ovulation with menotropins, analysis of results of 1897 treatment cycles. Fertil Steril 30:538, 1978
34. Johnson TR, Peterson EP: Gonadotropin-induced pregnancy following "premature ovarian failure." Fertil Steril 31:351, 1979
35. Zourlas P, Mantzaevinos T: Primary amenorrhea with normally developed secondary sex characteristics. Fertil Steril 34:112, 1980
36. March CM: Therapeutic regimens and monitoring techniques for human menopausal gonadotropin administration. J Repro Med 21:198, 1978
37. Venturoli S, Paradisi R, Fabbri R, et al.: Comparison between human urinary follicle stimulating hormone and human menopausal gonadotropin treatment in polycystic ovary. Obstet Gynecol 63:6, 1984
38. Hoffman DI, Lobo RA, Campeau JD, et al.: Ovulation induction in clomiphene-resistant anovulatory women: Different follicular response to purified urinary follicle-stimulating hormone (FSH) versus purified urinary FSH and luteinizing hormone. J Clin Endocrinol Metab 60:922, 1985
39. Jones GS, Acosta AA, Garcia JE, et al.: The effect of follicle-stimulating hormone without additional luteinizing hormone on follicular stimulation and oocyte development in normal ovulatory women. Fertil Steril 43:696, 1985
40. Schenker J, Weinstein D: Ovarian hyperstimulation syndrome: A current survey. Fertil Steril 30:255, 1978
41. Gergeley RZ, Paldi E, Erlik Y, Makler A: Treatment of ovarian hyperstimulation syndrome by antihistamine. Obstet Gynecol 47:883, 1976
42. Evans JH, McBain JC, Pepperell RJ, et al.: An increased ectopic pregnancy rate on gonadotropin therapy (abstr #444). Melbourne, Australia, Sixth International Congress of Endocrinology, 1980
43. Gemzell C: Induction of ovulation in infertile women with pituitary adenomas. Am J Obstet Gynecol 121:311, 1975
44. Physicians' Desk Reference, ed 39. Oradell, New Jersey, Medical Economics Co, 1985
45. Matsuo H, Baba Y, Nair RMG, et al.: Structure of the porcine LH and FSH releasing hormone: I. The proposed amino acid sequence. Biochem Biophys Res Comm 43:1334, 1971
46. Burgus R, Butcher M, Amoss N, et al.: Primary structure of the hypothalamic luteinizing hormone-releasing factor (LRF) of ovine origin. Proc Natl Acad Sci USA 69:278, 1972
47. Knobil E: The neuroendocrine control of the menstrual cycle. Recent Prog Horm Res 36:53, 1980
48. Santen RJ, Bardin CW: Episodic luteinizing secretion in man. Pulse analysis clinical interpretation, physiological mechanism. J Clin Invest 52:2617, 1973
49. Frager MS, Pieper DR, Tonetta S, et al.: Pituitary gonadotropin-releasing hormone (GnRH) receptors: Effects of castration, steroid replacement and the role of GnRH in modulating receptors in the rat. J Clin Invest 67:615, 1981
50. Clayton RN, Catt KJ: Gonadotropin-releasing hormone receptors: Characterization, physiological regulation and relationship to reproductive function. Endocrinol Rev 2:186, 1981
51. Marshall JC, Kelch RP: Low dose pulsatile gonadotropin-releasing hormone in anorexia nervosa: A model of human pubertal development. J Clin Endocrinol Metab 49:712, 1979
52. Rust LA, Israel R, Mishell DR: An individualized graduated therapeutic regime for clomiphene citrate. Am J Obstet Gynecol 120:785, 1974
53. Zacur HA: Ovulation induction with gonadotropin-releasing hormone. Fertil Steril 44:435, 1985
54. Leyendecker G, Wildt L, Hansmann M: Pregnancies following chronic intermittent (pulsatile) administration of GnRH by means of a portable pump (Zyklomat): A new approach

in the treatment of infertility in hypothalamic amenorrhea. J Clin Endocrinol Metab 51:1214, 1980
55. Schoemaker J, Simons AHM, von Osnabrugge GJC, et al.: Pregnancy after prolonged pulsatile administration of luteinizing hormone-releasing hormone in a patient with clomiphene-resistant secondary amenorrhea. J Clin Endocrinol Metab 52:882, 1981
56. Mason P, Adams J, Morris DV, et al.: Induction of ovulation using pulsatile luteinizing hormone-releasing hormone. Br Med J 288:181, 1984
57. Goerzen J, Corenblum B, Wisemand DA, Taylor PJ: Ovulation induction and pregnancy in hypothalamic amenorrhea using self-administered intravenous gonadotropin-releasing hormone. Fertil Steril 41:319, 1984
58. Weinstein FG, Seibel MM, Taymor ML: Ovulation induction with subcutaneous pulsatile gonadotropin-releasing hormone: The role of supplemental human chorionic gonadotropin in the luteal phase. Fertil Steril 41:546, 1984
59. Miller DS, Reid RL, Cetel NS, et al.: Pulsatile administration of low-dose gonadotropin-releasing hormone. JAMA 250:2937, 1983
60. Hurley DM, Brian R, Outch K, et al.: Induction of ovulation and fertility in amenorrheic women by pulsatile low-dose gonadotropin-releasing hormone. N Engl J Med 310:1069, 1984
61. Leyendecker G: Induction of ovulation with pulsatile LH-RH in hypothalamic amenorrhea. Upsala J Med Sci 89:19, 1984
62. Skarin G, Nillius SJ, Wide L: Pulsatile subcutaneous low-dose gonadotropin-releasing hormone treatment of anovulatory infertility. Fertil Steril 40:455, 1983
63. Menon V, Butt WR, Clayton RN, et al.: Pulsatile treatment of hypogonadotrophic hypogonadism. Clin Endocrinol 21:223, 1984
64. Liu JH, Durfee R, Muse K, Yens S: Induction of multiple ovulation by pulsatile administration of gonadotropin-releasing hormone. Fertil Steril 40:18, 1983
65. Bringer J, Hedon B, Jaffiol C, et al.: Influence of the frequency of gonadotropin-releasing hormone (GnRH) administration on ovulatory responses in women with anovulation. Fertil Steril 44:42, 1985
66. Boghelmann D, Lappohn RE, Janssens J: Triplet pregnancy after pulsatile administration of gonadotropin releasing hormone. Lancet 2:45, 1982
67. Heineman MJ, Bouckaert PXJM, Schellenkens LA: A quadruplet pregnancy following ovulation induction with pulsatile luteinizing hormone-releasing hormone. Fertil Steril 42:300, 1984
68. Cuellar FG: Bromocriptine mesylate (Parlodel) in the management of amenorrhea/galactorrhea associated with hyperprolactinemia. Obstet Gynecol 55:278, 1980
69. Parkes D: Bromocriptine. N Engl J Med 301:873, 1979
70. Mehta AE, Tolis G: Pharmacology of bromocriptine in health and disease. Drugs 17:313, 1979
71. Kebabian JW, Calne DB: Multiple receptors for dopamine. Nature 277:93, 1979
72. Riddick DH, Kusnik WF: Decidua: A possible source of amniotic fluid PRL. Am J Obstet Gynecol 127:187, 1977
73. Greer ME, Moraczewski T, Rakoff J: Prevalence of hyperprolactinemia in anovulatory women. Obstet Gynecol 56:65, 1980
74. Schulz KD, Geiger W, del Pozo E, et al.: Pattern of sexual steroids, prolactin, and gonadotropic hormones during prolactin inhibition in normally cycling women. Am J Obstet Gynecol 132:561, 1978
75. Herjan JT, Bennink C: Intermittent bromocriptine treatment for induction of ovulation in hyperprolactinemic patients. Fertil Steril 31:267, 1979
76. Corenblum B, Taylor P: A rationale for the use of bromocriptine in patients with amenorrhea and normoprolactinemia. Fertil Steril 34:239, 1980
77. Crosignani PG, Reschini E, Lombrosco GC, et al.: Comparison of placebo and bromocriptine in the treatment of patients with normoprolactinemic amenorrhea. Br J Obstet Gynecol 85:773, 1978
78. Ben-David M, Schenker JG: Transient hyperprolactinemia: A correctable cause of idiopathic female fertility. J Clin Endocrinol Metab 57:442, 1983
79. Gomez F, Reyes FI, Faiman C: Nonpuerperal galactorrhea and hyperprolactinemia: Clinical findings, endocrine features and therapeutic response in 56 cases. Am J Med 62:648, 1977
80. Zarate A, Canales E, Forsbach G, Fernandez-Lazala R: Bromocriptine: Clinical experience in the initiation of pregnancy in amenorrhea galactorrhea syndrome. Obstet Gynecol 52:442, 1978

81. Friesen HG, Tolis G: The use of bromocriptine in the galactorrhea amenorrhea syndrome: The Canadian cooperative study. Clin Endocrinol 6(Suppl):91s, 1977
82. Gemzell C, Wang CF: Outcome of pregnancy in women with pituitary adenomas. Fertil Steril 31:363, 1979
83. Comales E, Garcia IC, Ruiz JE, Zarate A: Bromocriptine as prophylactic therapy in prolactinomas during pregnancy. Fertil Steril 36:524, 1981
84. Futterweit W, Kreiger DT: Pituitary tumors associated with hyperprolactinemia and polycystic ovarian disease. Fertil Steril 31:608, 1979
85. Griffith RW, Turkalj I, Braun P: Outcome of pregnancy in mothers given bromocriptine. Br J Clin Pharmacol 5:277, 1978
86. Turkalj I, Braun P, Krupp P: Surveillance of bromocriptine in pregnancy. J Am Med Assoc 247:1589, 1982
87. Groom GV, Griffiths K: Effect of the antiestrogen tamoxifen on plasma levels of luteinizing hormone, follicle stimulating hormone, prolactin, oestradiol and progesterone in normal premenopausal women. J Endocrinol 70:421, 1976
88. Roumen FJME, Doesburg WH, Rolland R: Treatment of infertile women with a deficient post-coital test with two antiestrogens: Clomiphene and tamoxifen. Fertil Steril 41:237, 1984
89. Tajima C: Endocrine profiles in tamoxifen-induced conception cycles. Fertil Steril 42:548, 1984
90. Abraham GE, Maroulis GB, Boyers SP, et al.: Dexamethasone suppression test in the management of hyperandrogenic patients. Obstet Gynecol 57:158, 1981
91. Weiss G, Nachtigall L, Ganguly M: Induction of an LH surge with estradiol benzoate. Obstet Gynecol 47:415, 1976
92. Canales ES, Cabezas A, Vasquez-Matute L, Zarate A: Induction of ovulation with clomiphene and estradiol benzoate in anovulatory women refractory to clomiphene citrate. Fertil Steril 29:496, 1978
93. Schmidt-Elmendorf H, Kammerling R: Vergleichende klinishe untersuchungen von clomiphen, cyclofenil und epimestrol. Geburtshilfe Frauenhelikd 37:531, 1977
94. Chang RJ, Abraham GE: Effect of dexamethasone and clomiphene citrate on peripheral steroid levels in a hirsute amenorrheic patient. Fertil Steril 27:640, 1976
95. Radwanska E, McGarrigle HH, Little V, et al.: Induction of ovulation in women with hyperprolactinemic amenorrhea using clomiphene and human chorionic gonadotropins or bromocriptine. Fertil Steril 32:187, 1979
96. Phansey SA, Barnes MA, Williamson HO, et al.: Combined use of clomiphene and intranasal luteinizing hormone-releasing hormone for induction of ovulation in chronically anovulatory women. Fertil Steril 34:448, 1980
97. Huang KE: The induction of ovulation in amenorrheic patients with synthetic luteinizing hormone-releasing hormone: The significance of pituitary responsiveness. Fertil Steril 27:65, 1976
98. Jones GS: The luteal phase defect. Fertil Steril 27:351, 1976
99. March CM, Tredway DR, Mishell DR: Effect of clomiphene citrate on amount and duration of human menopausal gonadotropin therapy. Am J Obstet Gynecol 125:699, 1976
100. Radwanska E, Hammond J, Hammond M, Smith P: Current experience with a standardized method of human menopausal gonadotropins/human chorionic gonadotropin administration. Fertil Steril 33:510, 1980
101. Taymor ML: Induction of ovulation with gonadotropins. Clin Obstet Gynecol 16:201, 1973
102. Haning R, Levin R, Behrman HR, et al.: Plasma estradiol window and urinary estriol glucuronide determinations for monitoring menotropin induction of ovulation. Obstet Gynecol 54:442, 1979

22

Over-the-Counter Drugs for Gynecologic Use

Paul E. Hafner

Over-the-counter (OTC) drugs can provide safe, convenient, and effective treatment for a variety of gynecologic disorders. Because OTC drugs may be purchased in various retail settings, including grocery stores, the patient may not come in contact with a health professional to provide guidance in product selection and use. Furthermore, much of the information the patient receives about OTCs comes from often misleading commercial advertisements or family members and friends. Present laws do not require manufacturers of OTC products to list the concentration or quantity of each ingredient. Therefore, this information is often unavailable and can only be guessed at. This chapter attempts to fill this information gap by discussing current knowledge about vaginal contraceptives, vaginal cleansing and deodorant products, menstrual preparations, and topical antipruritics or anesthetics.

VAGINAL CONTRACEPTIVES

Vaginal contraceptives, alone or in combination with a condom or diaphragm, are attractive alternatives for patients not desiring sterilization or adverse effects from either oral contraceptives or intrauterine devices. All nonprescription vaginal contraceptives work primarily as spermicides and as mechanical barriers to prevent sperm from entering the cervix and uterine cavity. The spermicide in most products is nonoxynol-9, a surfactant or detergent, which solubilizes cell membranes and thus immobilizes the spermatozoa.[1] The extent of spermicidal activity in these alkylphenol compounds is influenced by the number of polyoxyethylene groups (5 to 15) in the side chain (Fig. 22–1). Nonoxynol-9 has nine groups in its side chain (n-9) and has been shown to be the most effective of the nonionic surfactants used in spermicidal contraceptives.[2]

Certain vaginal contraceptives contain acidic agents (boric acid, phenylmercuric acid), which lower the vaginal pH. A pH of less than 3.5 is considered to be spermicidal, and greater effectiveness is theoretically obtained as the pH is lowered. Phenylmercuric compounds are effective but may be absorbed systemically. Because of the possible adverse effects from mercury and the availability of other effective and less potentially harmful spermicides, mercury-containing

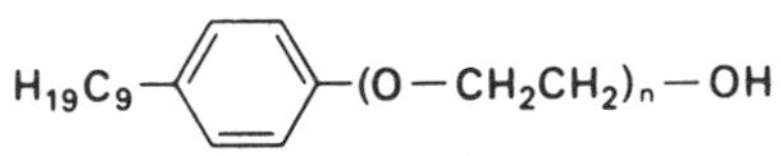

$$H_{19}C_9-C_6H_4-(O-CH_2CH_2)_n-OH$$

Figure 22–1. Chemical structure of nonoxynol-9. *(From Csáky TZ, Barnes BA: Cutting's Handbook of Pharmacology: The Actions and Uses of Drugs, ed. 7. New York, Appleton-Century-Crofts, 1984, p 156, with permission.)*

vaginal contraceptives are not recommended.

Preparations

The major difference in vaginal spermicides is how the dose is delivered. Most preparations deliver 50 to 100 mg of nonoxynol-9 per dose, since human testing indicates a minimum of 50 mg of free nonoxynol-9 must be present in the vaginal vault to inhibit all spermatozoa.[3] No advantage has been shown among products with different nonoxynol-9 concentrations,[4] although spermicides designed to be used with a diaphragm are less concentrated and are in a base which has different diffusion or mechanical barrier characteristics. Vaginal spermicides come in cream, jelly, foam, vaginal sponge, and suppository or tablet form (Table 22–1). Jellies and creams are the least expensive, while convenience packages of prefilled applicators (foam or cream) and tablets or suppositories are the most expensive per dose.

Creams and jellies are applied near the cervix using an applicator at least 10 minutes but no longer than 1 hour before intercourse. Creams are more lubricating, but jellies are water soluble which enhances vaginal distribution and easy removal.

Foams are creams packaged in an aerosol form. Foams are also applied using an applicator which is filled from a dispenser. They should be applied no longer than 1 hour before intercourse and should remain in the vagina for at least 9 hours. For convenience, certain newer products allow one to prefill the applicator up to 7 days before use. Foams do not provide the lubrication of creams and jellies but tend to be less noticeable to the partners. They adhere well to vaginal surfaces and only a small amount of leakage usually occurs during and after intercourse.

The vaginal sponge is permeated with a spermicide that is released during intercourse. The sponge also blocks the cervix and absorbs semen. It is effective up to 24 hours, even after multiple intercourse. It must remain in place for 6 hours after intercourse and is recommended for 1-day use only.[5,6]

Vaginal tablets and suppositories are easily inserted and deliver a consistent dose of spermicide in a base that melts, dissolves, or effervesces. Noneffervescent preparations should be inserted at least 20 minutes before intercourse to allow complete liquefaction and distribution. The manufacturers of effervescent forms recommend a wait of only 10 minutes before intercourse, but one recent study found the Encare suppository was still almost intact 15 minutes after insertion in 9 of 20 patients.[7]

Effervescence and dispersion are influenced by the amount of vaginal fluid and the freshness of the tablet. Tablet freshness can be tested by moistening it with a drop of water prior to insertion. If bubbling begins, the tablet may be inserted. Effervescent tablets should be stored in a cool dry location and used within 6 months after purchase. Tablets and suppositories provide no lubrication. A warm or sometimes burning sensation for both partners is occasionally produced with effervescent preparations and can be relieved with discontinuation.

One manufacturer combines a spermicide with a condom by adding 5 percent nonoxynol-9 to the condom lubricant.

Effectiveness

If used properly, all vaginal spermicides are equally effective. Patient preference affects compliance and ultimately product effectiveness. When vaginal spermicides are used with barrier methods, such as condoms or diaphragms, the combined effectiveness is greater than either method alone (Table 22–

TABLE 22–1. VAGINAL SPERMICIDES

- Creams
  - Contraceptrol Birth Control (Ortho)
    - Nonoxynol-9, 5% in an oil-in-water emulsion
- Gels
  - Contraceptrol Contraceptive Gel (Ortho)
    - Nonoxynol-9, 4%
  - Contraceptrol Disposable Contraceptive Jelly (Ortho)
    - Nonoxynol-9, 4%
  - Koromex Jelly (Holland-Rantos)
    - Nonoxynol-9, 3%; purified water; propylene glycol; cellulose gum; boric acid; sorbitol; starch; simethicone; fragrance
  - Ramses Jelly (Schmid)
    - Dodecaethyleneglycol monolaurate, 5%; glycerin; tragacanth; carboxymethylcellulose; preservatives
- Foams
  - Delfen (Ortho)
    - Nonoxynol-9, 12/5%; oil-in-water emulsion
  - Emko Because Contraceptor (Emko-Schering)
    - Nonoxynol-9, 8%; oil-in-water emulsion
  - Emko & Emko Pre-Fil (Emko-Schering)
    - Nonoxynol-9, 8%; benzethonium chloride, 0.2%; oil-in-water emulsion; stearic acid; triethanolamine; glyceryl monostearate; poloxamer 188; PEG-600; substituted adamantane; dichlorodifluoro methane; dichlorotetrafluoroethane
  - Koromex (Holland-Rantos)
    - Nonoxynol-9, 8%; water; propylene glycol; propellant 114; isopropyl alcohol; laureth-4; cetyl alcohol; propellant 12; PEG-50; fragrance

Products Used in Conjunction with Vaginal Diaphragm

- Gels
  - Gynol II (Ortho)
    - Nonoxynol-9, 2%; unscented, colorless, stainless, greaseless, aqueous jelly
  - Koromex Contraceptive Crystal Clear Gel (Holland-Rantos)
    - Nonoxynol-9, 2%; purified water; propylene glycol; cellulose gum; boric acid; sorbitol; simethicone
  - Ortho-Gynol (Ortho)
    - p-diisobutylphenoxypolyethoxyethanol, 1%; water dispersible jelly
  - Shur-Seal Gel (Milex)
    - Nonoxynol-9, 2%
- Creams
  - Koromex Cream (Holland-Rantos)
    - Octoxynol 3%, water, propylene glycol, stearic acid, sorbitan stearate, polysorbate 60, boric acid, fragrance,[b] buffered to pH 4.5
  - Ortho-Creme (Ortho)
    - Nonoxynol-9, 2%, in nonfatty acid cream base
- Suppositories/Inserts
  - Encare Oval (Thompson Medical)
    - Nonoxynol-9, 2.27%; effervescent water-soluble base. Most widely used nonprescription spermicide.
  - Intercept (Ortho)
    - Nonoxynol-9, 5.56%; effervescent water-soluble base
  - Semicid (Whitehall)
    - Nonoxynol-9, 100 mg; polyethyleneglycol base
- Sponge
  - Today (VLI)
    - 1 g nonoxynol 9; citric, sorbic, benzoic acid; sodium dihydrogen; citrate; sodium metabisulfite; polyurethane foam sponge

TABLE 22–2. COMPARATIVE EFFECTIVENESS OF CONTRACEPTIVE METHODS

Method	% Effective Theoretical Use (100% Compliance)	% Effective Actual Use (U.S. Women not Wanting More Children)
Abortion	100	100
Tubal ligation	99.96	99.96
Vasectomy	99.85	99.85
Progestin-only pill	99	97.5
Combined oral contraceptive	99.66	90.96
Condom plus spermicide	99	95
IUD	98.5	96
Condom	98	90
Diaphragm plus spermicide	98	90
Contraceptive sponge*	97	78
Spermicide only	95–98	85
Coitus interruptus	84	77
Rhythm (calendar)	90–98	70–80
Lactation for 23 months	75	60
Chance (sexually active)	10	10

* From Vernon Laboratories, Inc. dispensing literature.
From Hatcher RA et al.: 1 Contraceptive technology. New York, Irvington, 1982.

2). One large-scale study indicates a first-year failure rate of 15 percent* for foams, creams and jellies, compared with 2 percent for oral contraceptives, 4 percent for intrauterine devices, 10 percent for condoms, 13 percent for diaphragms, and 19 percent for the rhythm method.[8] One appplication provides protection for one act of intercourse and repeated intercourse requires repeated applications. A recent study has revealed that the contraceptive sponge is a safe and acceptable method with an effectiveness rate in the range of that for other vaginal contraceptives.[6]

* Failure rate relates to the number of pregnancies per 100 woman years of use.

Precautions

Spermicidal agents are considered nontoxic and usually cause no allergic reactions. Inflammatory changes in the vaginal epithelium of rabbits and rats from nonoxynol-9 exposure have been demonstrated and are related to the concentration and duration of use.[9] Ingredients such as fragrance additives may cause local burning or irritation, allergic reactions, or vaginal discharge. A change in or discontinuation of products should solve this problem.

Postcoital douching is inadequate for vaginal contraception. Active spermatozoa have been isolated in the endocervix within 1.5 to 3 minutes after coitus and have been recovered from the fallopian tubes within 5 minutes after insemination, which is well before douching could be completed. Furthermore, douching should be avoided for at least 9 hours after intercourse when a vaginal spermicide is used, since douching will dilute the spermicide to ineffective levels and remove the mechanical barrier provided by the product base. Any increased risk of abortion or specific anomalies associated with vaginal contraceptive use is tentative in humans and not apparent in rat models.[10,11]

One report suggested a possible increase in congenital anomalies and spontaneous abortions in women using spermicidal agents,[10] but other studies have failed to confirm these findings.[12,13]

As with virtually any absorbant material retained in the vagina, a few users of vaginal sponges have reported toxic shock syndrome.[14] The short-term presence of a vaginal contraceptive does not diminish the sensitivity of endocervical culture for the diagnosis of gonorrhea.[15] Preliminary information has suggested that there may be a protective effect of vaginal spermicides against gonorrhea and other venereal diseases.[18]

VAGINAL CLEANSING AND DEODORANT PRODUCTS

Vaginal Cleansers

The routine use of vaginal douches and deodorants by healthy women is controversial. The products listed in Table 22–3 are promoted as general vaginal and perineal cleansers that produce a refreshed feeling, relieve itching and burning, remove vaginal discharges, and deodorize. The benefits of their use appear to be minimal and offer no great advantage over perineal cleansing with mild soap and water or infrequent douching with 1 teaspoonful of white vinegar in 1 quart of warm water. Nevertheless, it is important for the physician to become familiar with the names and ingredients of the products that their patients may use. Furthermore, it is necessary to determine whether tampons are used with vaginal cleansers, since recurrent vaginal and cervical ulcers are associated with tampon use.[17,18]

If commercial products are used, the concentrates and stock bottle sizes of powder or solution are the most economical, while disposable and premeasured packages are least economical per dose. When used as directed, vaginal cleansers are not likely to be hazardous. Mixing with hot water, instillation with excessive pressure, and overuse are examples of improper self-administration. In addition, many ingredients in douche preparations may produce direct mucosal or dermal irritation or an allergic reaction.

Few OTC douches are medicinal and the user may delay seeking proper treatment. Povidone-iodine products (Betadine, Pharmadine) serve as adjunctive antimicrobial therapy in selected cases of vaginitis by cleansing the vaginal vault or altering the vaginal pH (Chap. 23).

Their multiple uses reflect the array of ingredients found in these products. With the exception of povidone-iodine and boric acid, the antimicrobials (benzalkonium chloride, cetylpyridinium chloride, and benzethonium chloride) are merely preservatives. Acids (lactic, citric) and bases (sodium bicarbonate, perborate, citrate, lactate) alone or in combination with buffers (sodium phosphate, EDTA)

TABLE 22–3. VAGINAL DOUCHE PRODUCTS

Betadine (Purdue Frederick)
Solution: povidone-iodine, fragrance

Betadine Medicated Disposable Douche (Purdue Frederick)
Solution: 5.2 ml povidone-iodine in 177 ml water which yields a 0.25% solution in 180-ml and 180-ml twin-packs

Biochemic Tissue Salts (NuAge)
Schuessler homeopathic ingredients as the recommended triturated tablet in the required lactose base per USHP

Dismiss Disposable (Schering)
Solution: sodium chloride, sodium citrate, citric acid, cetearyl octoate, ceteareth-27, fragrance

Femidine Douche (AVP)
Solution: povidone iodine. In 240-ml pack.

Feminique Disposable Douche (Schmid)
Solution: sodium benzoate, sorbic acid, lactic acid and octoxynol-9, baby powder or wild flower scents. In 150-ml twin-packs

Feminique Disposable Douche (Schmid)
Solution: vinegar and water. In 150-ml twin-packs

Gentle Spring disposable (Block Drug)
Powder: sodium edetate, sodium lauryl sulfate, sodium phosphate

TABLE 22–3. (*Continued*)

Massengill Disposables (Beecham)
Solution: water, alcohol, lactic acid, sodium lactate, octoxynol-9, cetylpyridinium chloride, imidazolidinyl urea, disodium EDTA, fragrance, color

Massengill (Beecham)
Liquid concentrate: lactic acid, water, sodium lactate, methylsalicylate, eucalyptol, menthol, thymol, octoxynol-9, color, alcohol

Massengill Disposable (Beecham)
Liquid: vinegar, water

Massengill (Beecham)
Powder: sodium chloride, ammonium alum, PEG-8, methylsalicylate, eucalyptus oil, menthol, thymol, phenol, color

Massengill (Beecham)
Floral powder: sodium chloride, ammonium alum, octoxynol-9, alcohol, fragrance, color

Massengill Medicated Disposable Douche with Cepticin (Beecham)
Solution: 5 ml povidone-iodine in 180 ml water which yields a 0.23% solution. In 180-ml and 180-ml twin-packs

New Freshness (Personal Laboratories)
Concentrate: vinegar, water
Disposable: vinegar, water

Nylmerate II (Holland-Rantos)
Solution concentrate: SD alcohol, 50%, water; acetic acid; boric acid; polysorbate 20; nonoxynol-9, sodium acetate; FD&C blue #1; D&C yellow #10

Povi-Douche (Parmed)
Povidone-iodine 7.5%

Sorbex Douche (Holloway)
Granules: potassium and 4-hexadienoate. In 40 and 100-g pack

Stomaseptine (Berlex)
Powder: sodium perborate, sodium bicarbonate, sodium chloride, sodium borate, fragrance

Summer's Eve Disposable Douche (Fleet)
Solution: vinegar and water. In 135-ml and 135-ml twin-packs

Summer's Eve Disposable (Fleet)
Solution, regular: sodium citrate, citric acid, quaternarium-15 solution, herbal scented: sodium citrate, citric acid, EDTA, octoxynol-9, quaternium-15, tartrazine

Summer's Eve Medicated Disposable (Fleet)
Solution: povidone-iodine. In 135-ml and 135-ml twin-packs

Trichotine (Reed & Carnrick)
Liquid: sodium lauryl sulfate, sodium borate, ethyl alcohol 8%, aromatics
Powder: sodium lauryl sulfate, sodium perborate, sodium chloride, aromatics

Trivia (Boyle)
Powder: oxyquinoline sulfate, 2%, alkylaryl sulfonate, 35%; EDTA, 0.33%; sodium sulfate, 52.5%, lactose, 9.67% disodium ethylene hydrated silica, 0.5%

Vagisec (Schmid)
Liquid: polyoxyethylene nonylphenol, sodium edetate, docusate sodium, 5% ethyl alcohol

Vanite Douche (Halsey)
Powder: boric acid, potassium alum, carbolic acid, menthol, thymol, eucalyptol and methyl salicylate. In 120-g pack

Zonite Douche (Norcliff Thayer)
Solution concentrate: 0.1% benzalkonium chloride, propylene glycol, menthol, and thymol. In 240 and 360-ml packs

are added to alter or maintain a stable pH. Because of the short exposure time in the vaginal vault, the douche solution causes no sustained pH changes.

Phenol, menthol, and eucalyptol are included for their unproven antipruritic effect. Phenol has some local anesthetic effects but can cause irritation. Menthol produces a cooling effect that may temporarily relieve itching. Eucalyptol also provides a fragrance.

Astringents (ammonium alum, potassium alum, and zinc sulfate) may reduce inflammation, local edema, and exudation. Menthol, methyl salicylate, and thymol have some counterirritant effect. Various surfactants are sometimes included to help spread the douche into the mucosal folds and rugae to aid in cleansing.

Feminine Deodorant Sprays

These products are deodorants and have no medicinal or therapeutic properties. The Food and Drug Administration has classified such sprays as cosmetic rather than "hygiene" products. Ingredients include perfumes to mask odor, antimicrobials to preserve the product, emollients to soothe the skin, and propellants to deliver the ingredients. Irritation is the most common adverse effect and is caused by overuse, application to previously inflamed surfaces, and holding the spray too close upon application.

MENSTRUAL DISCOMFORT PRODUCTS

OTC menstrual products are promoted to relieve premenstrual tension and edema along with menstrual pain and discomfort. Ingredients include analgesics, diuretics, antihistamines, stimulants, and antispasmodics (Table 22–4). With the exception of the analgesics, these ingredients are of questionable value. The cost of multiple ingredient products is two to three times greater than brand name ones and as much as 10 times greater than generic aspirin or acetaminophen tablets.

Acetaminophen, followed by aspirin, is the analgesic most often included in these preparations. Both are effective in relieving mild pain. Aspirin has an additional anti-inflammatory action. Acetaminophen is generally thought to be "safer than aspirin" by the public, since it does not cause gastrointestinal irritation. However, acetaminophen has been reported to cause hepatotoxicity in excessive doses,[19] and patients should be advised not to exceed recommended maximum daily doses.

Ibuprofen, previously available only by prescription, is felt by many practitioners to be more effective than either aspirin or acetaminophen in treating dysmenorrhea. For mild to moderate pain, 200 mg is felt to be as effective as 650 mg of aspirin. Ibuprofen is safer than either aspirin or acetaminophen in overdosage but is not free of adverse effects. Like aspirin, it can cause gastrointestinal irritation and bleeding. Menstrual delays, dysfunctional uterine bleeding, sodium retention, and cross sensitivity to aspirin and other nonsteroidal anti-inflammatory drugs have been reported.[20]

The value of diuretics is questionable because of subtherapeutic doses or unsubstantiated effectiveness. Ingredients in these products that are thought to add diuretic effects include pamabrom, ammonium chloride, caffeine, and vegetable extracts.

Antihistamines may provide sedative effects to relieve tension, irritability, and nervousness. The doses used are less than recommended to produce sedation but may produce drowsiness. A drowsy patient is not necessarily less tense, irritable, or nervous. Pyrilamine maleate is the most common antihistamine in these compounds.

The stimulant caffeine is traditionally combined with OTC analgesics, but its relation to pain relief is unknown. Caffeine is now being used less often, although it may improve the analgesic properties of aspirin and acetaminophen. One product contains ephedrine sulfate, which is a stimulant and a β-adrenergic receptor agonist on uterine smooth muscle. The effectiveness of ephedrine, cinnamedrine, and atropine in relieving muscle cramps is not well documented.

TABLE 22–4. OTC MENSTRUAL DISCOMFORT PRODUCTS

Advil (Whitehall)
Ibuprofen 200 mg

Ammonium Chloride USP (various)
Tablets: plain or enteric coated Ammonium chloride 5 grains and 7½ grains

Aqua-Ban (Thompson Medical)
Ammonium chloride, 325 mg; caffeine, 100 mg

Aqua-Ban Plus (Thompson Medical)
Ammonium chloride, 650 mg; caffeine, 200 mg; bran, 6 mg

Femcaps (Otis Clapp/Buffington)
Acetaminophen, 324 mg; caffeine, 32 mg; ephedrine sulfate, 8 mg; atropine sulfate, 0.0325 mg

Maximum Cramp Relief Formula Pamprin (Chattem)
Acetominophen 500 mg, pamabrom 25 mg, pyrilamine maleate 15 mg

Maximum Strength Aqua-Ban Plus Enteric Coated (Thompson Medical)
Ammonium chloride 650 mg, caffeine 200 mg, ferrous sulfate 6 mg

Midol (Glenbrook)
Aspirin 454 mg, caffeine 32.4 mg, cinnamedrine HCl 14.9 mg

Nuprin (Bristol-Myers)
Ibuprofen 200 mg

Ordrinil (Fox)
Powdered extract of buchu, powdered extract of uva ursi, powdered extract of corn silk, powdered extract of juniper, caffeine

Pamprin (Chattem)
Acetaminophen 325 mg, pamabrom 50 mg, pyricamine maleate 25 mg

Premesyn PMS (Chattem)
Acetaminophen 500 mg, pamabrom 25 mg, pyrilamine maleate 15 mg

Pursettes Premenstral (Jeffrey Martin)
Acetaminophen 500 mg, pamabrom 25 mg, pyrilamine maleate 15 mg

Sunril Premenstrual Capsules (Schering)
Acetaminophen 300 mg, pamabrom 50 mg, pyrilamine maleate 25 mg

Tender Menstrual Relief Tablets (Whitehall)
Acetaminophen, 325 mg; pamabrom, 25 mg

Tri-Aqua (Pfeiffer)
Extracts of buchu, uva ursi, triticum; zea; caffeine 100 mg

Water Pill (Natures Bounty)
Bochu leaf powder 50 mg, uva ursi leaf powder 50 mg, parsley leaf powder 50 mg, juniper berries powder 10 mg, potassium 20 mg

OTHER GYNECOLOGIC PRODUCTS

Topical Antipruritics and Anesthetics

A variety of products is available which contain local anesthetics, antihistamines, astringents, antimicrobials, and hydrocortisone. Their usefulness in relieving vulvar pruritis is limited and treatment for a serious underlying disorder may be delayed. The preparations are safe, but allergic reactions may occur and require discontinuation. Table 22–5 lists some topical antipruritic and anesthetic products currently available. Topical anesthetics may also be found on the surfaces of certain condoms that may aid in delaying orgasm and ejaculation.

TABLE 22–5. TOPICAL ANTIPRURITICS AND ANESTHETICS FOR GYNECOLOGIC USE

- Antihistamines
  - Benadryl Cream (P-D)
    - Diphenhydramine HCl 2% in water-miscible ointment base
  - PBZ (Geigy)
    - Tripelennamine HCl 2%
      - Cream: water-washable base
      - Ointment: petrolatum base
  - Ziradryl Lotion (P-D)
    - Diphenhydramine HCl 2%, ZnO 2%, alcohol 2%, camphor, chlorophylline sodium, glycerin, methocel, polysorbate 40, purified water, fragrance
- Anesthetics
  - Benzocaine (various)
    - Benzocaine 10% or 20%; cream, ointment base
  - Butesin Picrate (Abbott)
    - Butamben picrate 1%; ointment base
  - Dibucaine Ointment USP (various)
    - Dibucaine 1%; ointment base
  - Mercurochrome II (Becton Dickinson)
    - Anesthetic liquid, spray, lidocaine HCl, menthol, benzalkonium Cl, isopropyl alcohol 5%. Does not sting or irritate injured skin.
  - Nupercainal Anesthetic Ointment (CIBA)*
    - Dibucaine 1%; lubricant base
  - Nupercainal Pain Relief Cream (CIBA)*
    - Dibucaine 0.5%; water soluble base
  - Pontocaine (Breon)
    - Cream: Tetracaine HCl 1%; water-miscible base
    - Ointment: Tetracaine HCl 0.5% and menthol in white petrolatum and white wax base
  - Proctofoam (Reed & Carnrick)—nonsteroidal
    - Foam: pramoxine HCl 1%
  - Quotane (Menly & James)
    - Dimethisoquin HCl 0.5%, thimerosal 1:50,000, water-miscible base
  - Surfacaine (Lilly)
    - Cream: cyclomethycaine sulfate 0.5%; vanishing cream base
    - Ointment: cyclomethycaine sulfate 1%
  - Tronolane Cream (Ross)
    - Pramoxine HCl 1%; water-miscible base
  - Xylocaine Ointment (Astra)
    - Lidocaine 2.5%; water-miscible base (PEG and PG)
- Corticosteroids
  - Cortaid (Upjohn)
    - Cream, ointment, lotion: HC acetate equivalent to 0.5% HC Spray: 0.5% HC in nonaerosol vanishing liquid; 46% alcohol
  - Cortef Cream (Upjohn)
    - HC acetate equivalent to 0.5% HC in vanishing cream base
  - Delacort (Mericon)
    - 0.5% HC cream (vaginal/perianal allergy relief)
  - Dermolate Anti-Itch (Schering)
    - HC 0.5% cream, spray, ointment, lotion
  - Gynecort Antipruritic (Combe)
    - HC acetate equivalent to 0.5% HC in highly emollient white vanishing cream. Hypoallergenic
  - Hytone Cream (Dermik)
    - HC 0.5%

TABLE 22–5. *(Continued)*

Lanacort Anti-Itch (Combe)
Cream and Ointment: HC 0.5% as acetate with aloe moisturizer
Resticort Cream (Mentholatum Co.)
HC acetate 0.5% in cream base

Combination Products
Aerotherm Spray (Aeroceuticals)
Benzocaine 13.6%, benzyl alcohol 22.7%
Balneol Perianal Cleansing Lotion (Rowell)
Water, mineral oil, PG, glyceryl stearate, PEG-100 stearate, PEG-40 stearate, PEG-4 dilaurate, lanolin oil, Na acetate, carbomed 934, triethanolamine, methylparabin, dioctyl Na sulfasuccinate, fragrance, acetic acid
Bicozene Cream (Creighton)
Benzocaine 6%, resorcinol 1.67%
Dermamedicane Ointment (Medicane)
Benzocaine 2%, 8-hydroxyquinoline SO_4 1.05%, menthol 0.48%, ichthammol 1%, ZnO 13.7%, petrolatum, lanolin, perfume
Dermoplast (Ayerst)
Spray: benzocaine 20%, menthol 0.5%, water-miscible base
Diperodon (Various)
Diperodon 1%, petrolatum, PG, sorbitan sesquioleate: oxyquinoline benzoate 0.1%
Foille (Blistex)
Aerosol, liquid, ointment: Benzocaine 5%, chloroxylenol 0.1%, vegetable oil base, benzyl alcohol
Foille Plus Aerosol (Blistex)
Benzocaine 5%, chloroxylenol 0.6%, benzyl alcohol 82.6% w/w
Lanacane Medicated Cream (Combe)
Benzocaine, Resorcinol
Lily of the Desert (Vera)
Aloe vera gel 97% (counterirritant)
Lobana Derm-Ade Cream (Ulmer)
Vitamin A, Vitamin D, Vitamin E in vanishing cream, moisturizers, emollients, silicone; also available in perianal cleanser with mild sudsing base
Massengill Powder (Beecham)
NaCl, ammonium alum, PEG-8, phenolmethyl salicylate, eucalyptus oil, menthol, thymol, FD&C yellow 6 and 10
Medicane Dressing Cream (Medicane)
Benzocaine 0.5%, 8-hydroxy quinoline SO_4, 0.5%, cod liver oil 12.5%, menthol 0.18%, petrolatum, talcum, lanolin, paraffin, perfume
Medicated Cleansing Pads (Whitehall)
Witch hazel 50% W/V, water, glycerin 10% W/V, methylparaben, octoxynol-9, alcohol 7.4%
Mediconet Medicated Wipes (Medicane)
Benzalkonium Cl 0.02%, ethoxylated lanolin 0.5%, methylparaben 0.15%, hamamelis water 50%, glycerin 10%, purified water, perfume
Pontocaine (Breon)
Tetracaine 0.5%, menthol 0.5%, white petrolatum, white wax
Tucks (P.D.)
Cream and ointment: witch hazel 50%
Premoistened pads: witch hazel 50%, glycerin 10%, water methyl paraben 0.1%, benzethonium Cl 0.003#
Vaginex (Schmid)
Benzocaine, resorcinol
Vagisil Feminine Itching Medication (Combe)
Benzocaine 5%, resorcinol 2%

*Indicated for hemorrhoids and perianal inflammation and itching.

Lubricants

Lubricants are useful when treating dyspareunia from excessive dryness. A lack of estrogen support of vaginal mucosa must be considered when prolonged dryness is evident. A water-soluble lubricant can be safely applied to the introitus or penis prior to intercourse. The least expensive but effective products are H-R Lubricating Jelly or K-Y Jelly. Lubrin, available as a premeasured vaginal insert, is a colorless, unscented, and water-soluble lubricant. It is inserted 5 to 10 minutes before intercourse with complete liquefaction within 30 minutes. Transi-Lube, a more exotic product, is promoted as a sexual-foaming lubricant, because it is packaged as an aerosol foam and has a mild strawberry flavor and aroma.

REFERENCES

1. Helenius A, Simons K: Solubilization of membranes by detergents. Biochem Biophys Acta 415:29, 1975
2. Chvapil M, Droegemueller W, Owen J, et al.: Studies on nonoxynol-9 III: Effect on Fibroblast and spermatozoa. Fertil Steril 33(5):521, May 1980
3. Chantler E, Duncan GW, Gallegos AJ, et al.: Vaginal rings capable of constant release rate of spermicides. In Sciarra JJ, Zatuchni GI, Speidel JJ (eds): Risks, Benefits and Controversies in Fertility Control. New York, Harper & Row, 1977, p 2
4. Topical spermacides for contraception. Med Lett 22(21):91, 1977
5. A vaginal contraceptive sponge. Med Lett 25(642):78–80, 1983
6. Edelman D, McIntyre S, Harper J: A comparative trial of the Today contraceptive sponge and diaphragm. Am J Obstet Gynecol 150:869, 1984
7. Stone SC, Cardinale F: Evaluation of a new vaginal contraceptive. Am J Obstet Gynecol 133:635, 1979
8. Vaughan B, Trussell J, Menken J, et al.: Contraceptive failure among married women in the United States, 1970–1973. Fam Plan Perspect 9:251, 1977
9. Chvapil M, Droegenueller W, Owen J, et al.: Studies on nonoxynol-9: I. The effect on the vaginas of rabbits and rats. Fertil Steril 33(4):445, April 1980
10. Jick H, Walker A, Rothman K, et al.: Vaginal spermacides and congenital disorders. JAMA 245:1329, 1981
11. Abrutyn D, McKenzie B, Nadaskay N: Teratology study of intravaginally administered nonoxynol-9-containing contraceptive cream in rats. Fertil Steril 37:113, 1982
12. Cordero JF, Layde PM: Vaginal spermicides, chromosome abnormalities, and limb reduction defects. Am J Hum Genet 33:74A, 1981
13. Shapiro S, Slone D, Heinonen OP, et al.: Birth defects and vaginal spermicides. JAMA 247:2381, 1982
14. Toxic-shock syndrome and the vaginal contraceptive sponge. MMWR 33(4):43, 1984
15. Livengood CH, Addison WA, Voeller B: Effect of a topical contraceptive on endocervical culture for Neisseria Gonnorhea. Am J Obstet Gynecol 150(3):319–320, 1984
16. Jick H, Hannan M, Stergachis A, et al.: Vaginal spermicides and gonorrhea. JAMA 248:1619, 1982
17. Danielson RW: Vaginal ulcers caused by tampons. Am J Obstet Gynecol 146(5):547–549, 1983
18. Weissbert SM, Dodson MG: Recurrent vaginal and cervical ulcers associated with tampon use. JAMA 250:1430, 1983
19. Peterson RG, Rumack B: Toxicity of acetaminophen overdose. J Am Coll Emerg Phys 7:202, 1978
20. Ibuprofen without a prescription. Med Lett 26(665):63–65, 1984

23

Vulvovaginal Infections

James K. Crane and Richard C. Bump

Vulvovaginal symptoms are probably the most common problems encountered in the practice of general gynecology. It has been estimated that 5 to 10 percent of all gynecologic office visits in the United States are for the evaluation of symptomatic vaginal discharge. Yet as Friedrich insightfully observed a decade ago: "The diagnosis of vulvovaginal disease does not command prime time in most medical school curricula. Even postgraduate training programs are apt to bypass this subject, expecting the resident to somehow acquire this information by a process of self-instruction."[1] More recently another authority in this area, David Eschenbach, has pointed out that a lack of proficiency in dealing with vaginal discharge complaints not only has dramatic adverse effects on patient cure rates, but also on the individual physician's practice by undermining patient and consulting physician confidence in his ability as a specialist and consultant.[2]

While there have been many recent advances in the therapy of vulvovaginal infection, thoughtful assessment and accurate diagnosis are still the most important steps in assuring cure. Failure to make a specific diagnosis leads to the majority of therapeutic failures. Most cases of infectious vaginitis result from *Candida albicans, Trichomonas vaginalis,* or *Gardnerella vaginalis.* Cervicitis, caused principally by *Neisseria gonorrhoeae, Chlamydia trachomatis,* and herpes simplex virus,[3] and physiologic vaginal secretions are responsible for most patient complaints of excessive vaginal discharge when infectious vaginitis is not present. These entities are responsible for 98 percent of vaginal discharge complaints and can usually be diagnosed accurately at a single brief office visit.

In this chapter, the pharmacologic agents currently used in the management of these infections are discussed. Also considered are the common viral infections of the vulva as well as the peculiar problems that affect the anestrogenic vulva and vagina prepubertally and postmenopausally.

VULVOVAGINAL CANDIDIASIS

Candida albicans is a fungus found on many areas of the body. Differentiating the colonization of *Candida* from true infection becomes difficult, since the organism has been recovered in 25 to 50 percent of women who were considered free of vaginal disease.[4,5]

The diagnosis is based on a thorough medical history and physical examination with confirming laboratory studies. The patient most frequently complains of moderately intense vulvar pruritis but also may complain of dyspareunia, dysuria, or a mild to moderate curdy-white discharge. The onset is usually abrupt and often occurs in the luteal phase of the menstrual cycle just prior to menstruation. Like normal vaginal secretions, the discharge is usually not noted at the introitus and typically is white, highly viscous and floccular, and has a pH ≤4.5. Unlike normal secretions, however, it is frequently adherent in patches to the vaginal walls rather than pooled in the dependent posterior fornix.[2] Diagnosis solely on the physical appearance of the discharge is unwarrented, however, since microscopic confirmation of the diagnosis is simple, inexpensive, and accurate.

Microscopic examination of the vaginal discharge is imperative for proper diagnosis, with the wet mount having a sensitivity of 40 to 80 percent in detecting *Candida.*[6,7] This sensitivity is improved by adding a drop of 10 percent potassium hydroxide to the wet mount allowing the characteristic branching mycelia to be easily identified with 100× magnification once adherent epithelial cells and leukocytes are lysed. Mycelia may be clumped irregularly on the slide so it is important to scan the entire slide and carefully evaluate any cellular areas after KOH (potassium hydroxide) application. The organism may also be seen on Gram stain as gram-positive ovoid bodies with pseudohyphae with a sensitivity reported to be from 70 to nearly 100 percent.[6] The Papanicolau smear has only a 20 to 46 percent positive rate in culture-positive patients.[6,7] Culture may be done on Nickerson or Sabourand medium, but a positive growth is not an indication of disease, and culture is seldom necessary for diagnosis.

There is a strong correlation between symptomatic vulvovaginal candidiasis (VVC) and the presence of germinated, filamentous *Candida,* possibly due to the germinated organism's enhanced adherence to epithelial cells.[8,9] This fact has clinical implications for therapy since the azole antifungal agents are most effective against the hyphae and mycelia of *Candida* and inhibit germination at very low concentrations. It also explains the lack of predictive value of culture isolation of yeast in asymptomatic patients with nongerminated *Candida.*

Predisposing factors in *Candida* vulvovaginitis include diabetes, broad-spectrum antibiotics, including metronidazole, and depressed cell-mediated immunity[10] due to pregnancy or immunosuppressive drug therapy. Although there is a twofold increase in the incidence of positive *Candida* culture in women on oral contraceptives, there is no increase in the symptoms and signs of infection.[5]

Recurrent vaginal infections are a clinical dilemma. Miles et al.[11] reported a virtual 100 percent correlation between the anorectal candidiasis and VVC. Patients without vulvovaginal involvement had negative anorectal cultures. This would seem to indicate that a "cure" in a certain number of patients is impossible due to persistent rectal colonization. This rectal reservoir theory of recurrent VVC has been challenged recently by Van Slyke et al.[12] Their data suggest that most positive rectal cultures for *Candida* are due to perianal skin contamination and show that successful therapy of vaginal candidiasis with boric acid eliminates most positive "stool" cultures.

Nystatin

Nystatin (Nilstat, Mycostatin) is a polyene antibiotic produced by a strain of *Streptomyces noursei* and acts by interfering with preformed cell membrane ergosterol in the fungus.[13] The cell permeability is thus altered, allowing lethal leakage of intracellular contents. Nystatin exhibits no appreciable activity against bacteria.

Nystatin comes as a vaginal suppository or cream. The suppository contains 100,000 units and is inserted in the deep vaginal vault twice daily for 14 days. Treatment must be continuous, regardless of menstruation. Nystatin cream should be used on the vulva and the skin of the male partner if he shows any signs of the disease. The combination of oral and topical therapy may be considered for recurrent VVC if a rectal reservoir is suspected. It should be reemphasized, however, that the role that the rectal reservoir plays in reinfection has been exaggerated. In addition, many authorities question the ability of oral nystatin to either reduce the concentration of *Candida* in the stool[2] or reduce recurrence rates.[8] Vaginal reinoculation via sexual transmission of the organism due to symptomatic or asymptomatic penile yeast carriage can likely occur, although Sobel concludes that this is a relatively rare cause for reinfection and that routine topical penile therapy is unwarranted.[8] Although all of these factors are recognized as possibly contributing to recurrent infection with *Candida,* the majority of women with recurrences have none of these commonly cited predisposing factors, including diabetes or general immunosuppression.[8]

A *Candida*-specific defect in cellular immune response, mediated by *Candida*-specific supressor lymphocytes that block the cellular immune response only to that organism, has been proposed by Witkin et al. as contributing to recurrent candidiasis in some women.[14] They have proposed using various adjunctive immunotherapeutic agents, including the prostaglandin inhibitor ibuprofen, to reverse poor lymphocyte response to *Candida* and prevent recurrent infection.[15] It has also been suggested that many persistent symptomatic yeast infections are due to *Candida tropicalis* rather than *C. albicans,* the former being difficult to eradicate due to an apparent lack of susceptibility of the cell membrane to the commonly used polyene and azole classes of antifungal agents.[13]

The agents that have proved most useful in the treatment of VVC will now be considered. While nystatin was the first easily self-administered antifungal agent, more active agents are now available. Both of the available azole antifungal agents as well as boric acid capsules have proved more effective than nystatin in the therapy of VVC, and particularly in the therapy of recurrent infection. Eschenbach[16] has reviewed 11 studies comparing these antifungal agents and found nystatin effective in 33 to 65 percent of patients compared to 60 to 90 percent for miconazole, clotrimazole, or boric acid. Whereas the latter agents maintained similar ranges of efficacy with retreatment, nystatin was effective in only 10 to 30 percent of retreated patients. Thus, nystatin has been replaced by these other agents as the antifungal agent of choice.[16]

Topical Azole Antifungal Agents

The azole compounds include clotrimazole (Gyne-Lotrimin, Mycelex-G) and miconazole (Monistat). Like nystatin, these compounds affect cell wall ergosterol composition, but at an earlier stage during sterol synthesis and cell membrane formation.[13] This may explain their greater efficiency and their ability to inhibit germination at very low concentrations.[8,9] Both clotrimazole and miconazole are available in vaginal tablet or suppository as well as cream and lotion form. Both compounds are used in similar dosages and in similar treatment schedules. It does appear that neither agent is more effective than the other nor does any treatment schedule seem superior.[16] Cure rates are essentially the same with 100 mg once daily for 7 days, 100 mg twice daily for 3½ days, and 200 mg once daily for 3 days with either agent.[17-19] There appears to be no benefit to prolonging therapy beyond 7 days. Recently multiple studies have shown that a single 500-mg vaginal tablet of clotrimazole is as effective as 200 mg daily for 3 days[20,21] or 100 mg daily for 6 days.[22] This single-dose regimen has obvious advantages with respect to patient convenience and compliance. Short (one-dose) prophylactic courses of these agents on a scheduled basis may be a valuable tactic to prevent frequent symptomatic recurrences perhaps by preventing germination.[23]

The tablet and suppository forms of the medications are somewhat more convenient to use vaginally although the creams allow simultaneous cutaneous application and better control of vulvar symptoms and infection. The lotion forms can also be used on the skin of the vulva and penis when indicated. Perianal application of the cream or lotion forms may be more promising than ineffective oral nystatin administration in controlling cases where recurrent VVC is the result of recolonization from the rectal reservoir.[23]

It is generally most convenient to use all vaginal medications in the evening just before lying down. This maximizes the time the medication is in contact with the organisms and minimizes drainage of medication due to gravity. We recommend sexual abstinence for the duration of therapy and until symptoms are relieved, both to minimize the risk of reinoculation and to minimize traumatic irritation to the already irritated vulvovaginal epithelium. Patients should feel better with initiation of therapy and any woman who has acute worsening of symptoms should be considered sensitive to the vehicle in the antifungal preparation she has been prescribed, and should be changed to an agent containing a different vehicle.[2]

Boric Acid Capsules

Two reports have supported the efficacy of boric acid in the treatment of VVC. Swate and Weed reported a 100 percent rate of immediate symptomatic relief with a 5 percent recurrence rate at 30 days treating 40 cases of confirmed vaginal candidiasis with the insertion of 600-mg boric acid capsules vaginally once daily for 14 days.[24] Van Slyke et al. compared the effectiveness of 600-mg boric acid capsules vaginally once daily for 14 days to 100,000 units of nystatin vaginally once daily for the same duration in a double-blind study of 108 patients.[12] Boric acid had a 7- to 10-day posttreatment cure rate of 92 percent versus 64 percent for nystatin. Thirty-day cure rates also favored boric acid, 72 percent to 50 percent. Both of these differences proved statistically significant. Furthermore, the boric acid regimen proved effective in 9 out of 10 nystatin failures.

The mechanism of boric acid's fungistatic activity is not defined. Its usefulness in treating *C. tropicalis* infection resistant to the polyene and azole antimycotics has not been reported. While toxic reactions and poisonings can occur with boric acid, the boron blood levels following vaginal administration as described are far below even the most conservative estimates of toxic boron levels.[12] Although the safety of boric acid therapy in pregnancy has been alluded to,[24] Eschenbach has advised against its use in pregnancy until more is known about its vaginal absorption.[16]

Boric acid capsules are not commercially marketed. They can be produced extremely inexpensively using size 0 gelatin capsules and 600 mg of boric acid powder.[12] Five percent boric acid ointment (Borofax) is available for topical cutaneous administration.

Gentian Violet

Gentian violet (hexamethylpararosanilin) has long been used as an extremely effective antifungal agent. While Friedrich considers it the primary drug of choice for VVC,[1] other authorities feel that the newer, more active agents (azole compounds and boric acid) have replaced gentian violet as the first-line antifungals.[16,25] Gentian violet's chief limitations are rare (1 percent) but severe allergic reactions[25] and the need for relatively expensive and time consuming office visits for application of the agent at least twice at 72-hour intervals and often at subsequent weekly intervals. While the agent's messiness is often cited as a significant limitation, this is rarely an issue so long as the application technique described by Friedrich[1] is followed and the patient is forwarned to wear older underwear and provided with a perineal pad after application. A 1 percent aqueous solution of the dye should be carefully applied to the cervical, vaginal, introital, and inner vulvar surfaces and allowed to completely dry. Gentian violet still has a place in the antifungal armamentarium, especially in selected cases of resistant or recurrent VVC.

Ketoconazole

Ketoconazole (Nizoral) is an orally absorbable imidazole antimycotic that has been effective in treating fungal skin infections unresponsive to topical therapy. While the agent is effective in treating VVC, it has not been used as a first-line agent due to concerns over potential toxicity and the high efficacy of topical azole compounds. A role for ketoconazole has been proposed for the therapy of persistent and recurrent VVC, however. Eschenbach et al.[26] observed a highly significant reduction in signs and symptoms in 42 patients with recurrent VVC (mean number of episodes per year = 5.7) 7 days after ketoconazole given either 200 mg/day for 3 days or 400 mg/day for 5 days. The high recurrence rate by 28 days (75 percent) led them to conclude that these short regimens were not effective in permanently managing recurrent disease. Sobel proposed a regimen employing more prolonged initial therapy followed by intermitent prophylaxis in an open prospective uncontrolled study of 40 women with severe recurrent VVC.[27] Patients were treated with 400 mg/day for 14 days, followed by 400 mg/day for 5 days with the onset of menses for three menstrual cycles. One hundred percent and 97.4 percent of subjects had symptomatic and microbiologic cures at the end of the 14-day course and at 1 month, respectively. The symptomatic and culture cure rates fell to 75.7 percent and 64.9 percent, respectively, by the end of the 3-month prophylaxis, to 43.2 percent and 35.2 percent, respectively, at 6 months, and to 37.5 percent and 24.3 percent, respectively, at 1 year. While it is obvious that the majority of patients had recurrences, 14 of 40 patients who had been highly refractory to traditional therapy were free of signs and symptoms for a full year. This approach may hold some promise for selected patients with recurrent or persistent VVC.

Side effects of oral ketoconazole are not frequent. Fifteen percent of patients in Sobel's study experienced nausea not requiring discontinuation of the drug. The most significant complication of therapy is hepatic toxicity, primarily of the hepatocellular type. The incidence of mild nonprogressive serum transaminase elevation during ketoconazole therapy is 5 to 10 percent.[26,27] Symptomatic liver injury is estimated to occur in 1 in 10,000 to 15,000 recipients and is usually reversible upon discontinuation of the drug. It is recommended that patients on long term therapy have monthly bilirubin and transaminase determinations with discontinuation of therapy for persistent or progressive elevations. There has also been a single instance of reversible adrenal insufficiency induced by high dose (800 mg/day) ketoconazole therapy.[28] This was felt to be a result of the drug's recognized ability to block testicular and adrenal steroid synthesis in a dose and time-dependent manner.

Table 23–1 summarizes current treatment schedules for VVC.

TRICHOMONAS VAGINALIS

Trichomoniasis is one of the most frequently occurring sexually acquired diseases. Of those patients with symptomatic vaginitis, 15 to 20 percent harbor this anaerobic, flagellated protozoan. The organism is capable of infecting the vagina, urethra, vas deferens, seminal vesicles and prostate. Catteral and Nicol[29] reported that all female partners of 56 men with trichomonal urethritis harbored the organism, thus substantiating the venereal nature of the disease.[29] Only 12 percent of male consorts with *Trichomonas* will have symptoms.[29]

The peak incidence of trichomoniasis occurs between the ages of 16 and 35, which coincides with peak sexual activity. There is a high incidence of other venereal diseases,

TABLE 23-1. DRUGS USED IN THE TREATMENT OF VULVOVAGINAL CANDIDIASIS

Drug Name	Doses	Comments
Gentian violet	Paint vulvo-vaginal area—repeat 72 hr and weekly prn	Severe allergy (1%); office procedure; messy
Nystatin (Mycostatin, Nilstat)	100,000 units vaginally qd-bid × 14 days	Least active antifungal; poor for recurrent infection; oral ineffective to eliminate rectal reservoir
Clotrimazole (Gynelotrimin, Mycelex)	100 mg/day vaginally × 7 days 200 mg/day vaginally × 3 days 500 mg vaginally × 1 day	Suppository, tablet, cream, lotion forms; worsening symptoms suggest vehicle sensitivity
Miconazole (Monistat)	100 mg/day vaginally × 7 days	
	200 mg/day vaginally × 3 days	Same as clotrimazole
Boric acid capsules	600 mg vaginally qd-bid × 14 days	Inexpensive; must be made; topical ointment (Borofax) available
Ketoconazole (Nizoril)	200 mg/day PO × 3 days	
	400 mg/day PO × 3 days 400 mg/day PO × 5 days 400 mg/day PO × 14 days	
	400 mg/day PO × 5 days each month (intermittent prophylaxis)	For selected recurrent–persistent cases; hepatotoxic potential

and about half of the women in a British study presenting with gonorrhea were found to have trichomoniasis as well.[30]

Up to 50 percent of women with trichomoniasis will be asymptomatic. When present, symptoms can be protean owing to variations in inflammatory response to the organism. Symptoms vary from a simple increase in discharge to intense vulvovaginal discomfort. When most severe, trichomoniasis is manifested by a profuse, malodorous, irritating discharge, pruritis or pain, dyspareunia, excoriations, intermenstrual or postcoital spotting, internal or external dysurea, and a sense of vulvovaginal fullness.

The discharge of trichomoniasis differs from normal vaginal secretions in that it is homogeneous, of low viscosity, adherent to the vaginal walls, and present at the introitus. Color varies from white to the classic gray, green, or yellow. While the discharge is typically described as frothy, this is neither the rule nor so common as with bacterial vaginosis. Like the latter, the discharge of trichomoniasis typically has a fishy odor (though less intense than with bacterial vaginosis) and an elevated pH > 4.5.[2] While small subepithelial hemorrhages and a typical double capillary punctate pattern are nearly always seen colposcopically on the cervix and vagina in patients with trichomoniasis, the classic grossly visible strawberry cervix is an infrequent finding.

As with all the vaginitis syndromes, the diagnosis should be confirmed microscopically. A portion of the vaginal discharge should be mixed with several drops of fresh normal saline solution and promptly examined microscopically. Trichomonads are identified as motile, flagellated organisms slightly larger than a white blood cell with 100× magnification or by a beating flagellar motion with 400× magnification if motility is not obvious. There is usually an intense leukocytic reaction noted and white blood cells may clump around the trichomonads, inhibiting gross movement. A carefully performed wet mount is capable of establishing a diagnosis in 80 to 90 percent of symptomatic patients, but its accuracy drops considerably in asymptomatic patients.[16,31] While *Trichomonas* culture is relatively easy to peform with Diamond's media, its clinical applicability is limited by the need for fresh media and the infrequent need for culture confirmation.[16] Pap smears have poor sensitivity (63 percent), specificity (56 percent), and predicitive values (64 percent when abnormal, 55 percent when normal) for trichomoniasis and should not be relied upon to establish or rule out the diagnosis.[32] In addition, *Trichomonas* can cause an atypical Pap smear and vascular changes colposcopically which are actually an indication of inflammatory changes and unrelated to the malignant change.

Metronidazole

The current treatment of trichomoniasis is metronidazole, an imidazole derivative. Metronidazole is directly trichomonacidal, although the mechanism is unknown. The drug is well absorbed after oral administration. Durel et al. found that oral doses of the drug imparted trichomonacidal activity to semen and urine, and showed that high cure rates could be obtained in both male and female patients.[33] Both unchanged metronidazole and several metabolites are excreted in various proportions in urine after oral administration and may lead to a brownish discoloration of the urine. Low concentrations of metronidazole also appear in the saliva and in the breast milk during treatment. There are drugs similar to metronidazole used in Europe, including tinidazole which is undergoing testing in the United States.

The recommended dose of metronidazole has changed. The prior recommendation was one 250-mg tablet three times a day for 7 days. Morton (1972), Dykers (1975), and Fleury et al. (1977) found a single 2-g dose of metronidazole to be as effective in treating vaginal trichomoniasis[34–36] as the traditional 7-day regimen. Lossick demonstrated that the single 2-g dose cure rate was 97 percent in 237 female prison inmates not at risk for sexual exposure and reinfection.[37] In addition, the single-dose regimen has a higher compliance rate, lower cost, and lower posttreatment incidence of candidiasis.[31]

The vast majority of treatment failures are probably due to reinfection, although reports of resistance have emerged.[38,39] Poor gastrointestinal absorption or too rapid metabolic transformation may also explain treatment failure.[40,41] The coincidental use of drugs such as phenobarbital or phenytoin appear to enhance liver metabolism of metronidazole, and may explain some instances of resistance to usual dosage regimens.[42]

Concurrent single-dose therapy of the patient and male sexual partners is recommended as the initial therapeutic response to persistence after the 2-g dose. If this fails, 500 mg orally twice per day for a week may be effective.[16] In the unusual circumstance where these regimens fail, Eschenbach recommends 1 g of metronidazole orally with 500 mg vaginally every 12 hours as long as the organism is not resistant to the drug.[16]

The rate of metronidazole resistence is estimated to be less than 1 in 6000 to 10,000 individuals,[43] and thus represent a small minority of recurrent or persistent trichomoniasis. If true resistance is suspected, the use of tube dilutional assays to determine minimum lethal concentrations is recommended (but not widely available) to determine the dose and duration of metronidazole therapy needed to eradicate the organism.[43] Parenteral therapy with up to 6 g of metronidazole daily for 7 to 8 days, doses that not uncommonly result in peripheral neuropathy, may be necessary to eliminate the trichomonad.[43]

Side effects from metronidazole include gastrointestinal disturbances such as nausea, anorexia, diarrhea, epigastric distress, abdominal cramping, and vomiting. A metallic taste and a furry tongue are not uncommon. The consumption of alcohol with metronidazole can produce nausea, vomiting, abdominal cramps, headaches, and flushing. Alcohol intake should be avoided during therapy and for 24 hours after the last dose. A sudden overgrowth of *Candida* may occur in the vagina. Neutropenia has been reported, and low neutrophil counts returned to normal in all cases after the course of medication was completed. The manufacturer recommends a total and differential leukocyte count before and after treatment, but most clinicians reserve this for retreatment. Dizziness, vertigo, incoordination, ataxia, and convulsive seizures have also been reported. Confusion, irritability, depression, weakness, insomnia, mild erythematous eruptions, and peripheral neuropathy characterized mainly by numbness or parasthesia of an extremity have been described. Metronidazole is contraindicated in patients with evidence or history of a blood dyscrasia, active organic disease of the central nervous system, first trimester of pregnancy, and prior sensitization to metronidazole.

Metronidazole has not been shown to be teratogenic in either animal or human studies, but has been reported to be mutagenic in bacteria.[44-46] The drug has been shown to be tumorogenic in rodents, and the manufacturer suggests that treatment in the second and third trimesters be limited to those in whom local palliative treatment has been inadequate in controlling symptoms.[47] There is, however, no consistently effective local treatment. The understandable concern for the theoretical risk to the fetus can be countered by a strong theoretical argument for metronidazole therapy in pregnancy based on the role trichomoniasis and its concurrent anaerobic bacterial overgrowth may play in premature rupture of membranes and postpartum endometritis.[31] Similar concerns with respect to infectious morbidity following gynecologic surgical procedures makes preoperative therapy of trichomoniasis a reasonable consideration.

BACTERIAL VAGINOSIS (NONSPECIFIC VAGINITIS, *GARDNERELLA VAGINALIS* VAGINITIS)

The term *bacterial vaginosis* has been adopted as the preferred designation for the entity formerly designated nonspecific vaginitis. The new term emphasizes the facts that (1) both *Gardnerella vaginalis* (formerly *Corynebacterium vaginale* and earlier *Hemophilus vaginalis* and anaerobic bacterial overgrowth characterize the entity bacteriologically, and (2) a lack of host inflammatory response is evident clinically. Gardner and Dukes[48] and Gardner et al.'s[49] classic studies in the mid-1950s first implicated the small nonmotile, nonencapsulated, pleopmorphic, gram-negative rod now designated *G. vaginalis* as the overwhelmingly predominant organism and etiologic agent in most cases of what was then called nonspecific vaginitis. While some still maintain that *G. vaginalis* is never indigenous, never commensal, and always induces a recognizable vaginal disease,[50] there is considerable evidence that this is not the case. *G. vaginalis* can be isolated from 10 to 40 percent of asymptomatic women[51-60] and even from 10 percent of asymptomatic women with no evidence of bacterial vaginosis when carefully assessed for signs of the disease.[52,61] This does not mean that *G. vaginalis* does not play an important role in the genesis of bacterial vaginosis, but does emphasize that the isolation of *G. vaginalis* on culture does not define the clinical entity. The concept that a symbiotic relationship between *G. vaginalis* and anaerobic bacterial flora overgrowth in the vagina is responsible for the signs and symptoms of bacterial vaginosis has been demonstrated in a series of articles from the University of Washington.[62,65] Amine by-products of the anaerobic proliferation, chiefly cadaverine and putrescine, are responsible for the "fishy" vaginal odor that characterizes the syndrome.[63] Patients with signs and symptoms of bacterial vaginosis have organic acid chromatographic patterns characteristic for anaerobic overgrowth that normalize after successful therapy.[64] An understanding of these fundamental microbiologic and chemical alterations aid in both the diagnosis and effective therapy of bacterial vaginosis.

Patients with bacterial vaginosis rarely complain of the irritation or pruritis that characterizes candidiasis and trichomoniasis. Rather their most consistent complaints are an increase in the volume of their vaginal secretions and, most significantly, malodor. The patient will usually describe the odor as fishy or musty and often mentions that it is accentuated postcoitally and menstrually. This is because the amines are volatilized and thus more odorous in the alkalinized vagina. It is not unusual for some patients not to volunteer the complaint of the malodorous discharge out of embarrassment. Thus, it is important to ask the patient if she is bothered by this symptom if her examination reveals discharge consistent with bacterial vaginosis.

The discharge of bacterial vaginosis is typically copious, gray, homogeneous, of low viscosity, present at the introitus and adherent to the vaginal walls. It usually has a pH > 4.5, is often frothy, and always has the characteristic fishy amine odor.[65] The diagnosis is confirmed microscopically on saline wet prep by identifying clue cells, vaginal epithelial cells with indistinct cell borders obscured by the large number of attached organisms[65] and by noting the intensification of the amine odor upon alkalinization of the secretions with 10 percent potassium hydroxide[62] (the sniff test). The wet prep characteristically shows a lack of lactobacilli and white blood cells. When white blood cells are seen in a patient suspected of having bacterial vaginosis, coexistent trichomoniasis or endocervicitis should be suspected. Clue cells can also be demonstrated on Papanicolaou smears or with Gram staining, but this is not usually necessary. Cultures play no role in the diagnosis since both *G. vaginalis* and anaerobic bacteria are commonly found in the normal vagina. It has been suggested that the diagnosis can be made when three of the four features of characteristic discharge, pH > 4.5, clue cells, and positive sniff test are noted.[66] It must be stressed that the diagnosis is based upon multiple parameters in a patient who has symptoms, as all of these indicators of bacterial vaginosis are insensitive in asymptomatic patients and in fact will persist in only the small minority of such patients without therapy.[61]

While some noted authorities feel that *G. vaginalis* is solely a sexually transmitted infectious agent and recommend that the male sexual partner always receive the same medication as the woman,[50] this is not the general view. *G. vaginalis* has been isolated commonly from patients with stable, monogomous sexual relationships who only rarely had isolation of more traditional sexually transmitted diseases,[58,61] as well as from children without prior sexual contact.[60] Furthermore, the prevalence of vaginal isolation of *G. vaginalis* in sexually active adolescents is not significantly different from the prevalence in virginal adolescents.[67] Finally concurrent male therapy has not been shown to consistently improve cure rates for bacterial vaginosis.[16,68] Still there is little question that the male sexual partner can carry *G. vaginalis* in the urethra and serve as a potential source of persistent infection. Thus, although routine male therapy cannot be recommended, contact therapy in recurrent cases of bacterial vaginosis seems prudent.

While triple sulfa vaginal cream was proposed as effective therapy for bacterial vaginosis in the original study of Gardner and Dukes,[48] subsequent evidence as to poor long term cures with this agent have led them to declare that "sulfa drugs are ineffective in treating this infection."[50] Still, sulfa is widely used by many clinicians. Sulfa has been shown effective in controlling symptoms *during therapy,* likely due to the fact that it masks odor through its effect on vaginal pH and through a dilutional effect.[62] Once therapy is discontinued, virtually all women have a recurrence of signs and symptoms of bacterial vaginosis as well as isolation of *G. vaginalis* from the vagina.[62] This is not surprising in view of the fact that *G. vaginalis* is almost totally resistant to sulfa and that sulfa drugs have a very limited anaerobic spectrum.[65] Other agents that have been proposed as effective in treating bacterial vaginosis in the past but which are now felt to be ineffective include oral tetracycline (including doxycycline), ampicillin, and erythromycin.

Metronidazole in a dosage of 500 mg twice daily for 7 days has proven highly effective[62,68] and should be considered the regimen of choice for bacterial vaginosis. Metronidazole's success is likely due to the agent's well-recognized efficacy against anaerobic bacteria and due to the activity of the hydroxymetronidazole metabolite against *G. vaginalis.*[16] While single dose therapy with 2 g of metronidazole has been advocated,[69] this has been found less effective than the 7-day regimen, particularly if patients were assessed for recurrence several weeks after therapy.[68,70]

Other alternative regimens that have proven successful include vaginal tetracycline, 100 to 200 mg in a cream base one or two times daily for 7 days[48] or cephalexin, 500 mg orally four times daily also for a week.[16] The vaginal tetracycline regimen usually induces vaginal candidiasis and appropriate prophylactic therapy for this is recommended. Therapy of asymptomatic bacterial vaginosis is usually unwarranted since the abnormal discharge will persist for 6 months in only 22 percent of such cases without therapy.[61] Whether the anaerobic bacterial overgrowth that typifies the condition may increase the risk of postpartum or postoperative infectious morbidity is undetermined. These concerns warrant well-designed prospective investigations and may also warrant therapy of selected asymptomatic patients. Table 23–2 summarizes the drugs that are currently felt to be useful in the treatment of bacterial vaginosis.

ENDOCERVICITIS SYNDROMES

Endocervical infections may be responsible for an increase in purulent but usually nonirritating vaginal discharge. The three recognized causes of endocervicitis, *Neisseria gonorrhoeae, Chlamydia trachomatis,* and *Herpesvirus hominis,*[3,16] will be considered. They should be suspected when none of the three previously discussed infectious vaginitis syndromes are diagnosed, especially when microscopic evaluation of vaginal discharge reveals many inflammatory cells. When this is the case, an aspirate of endocervical mucus should be examined microscopically and if a purulent discharge is evident, appropriate Gram stains and cultures obtained.

Gonorrhea

Gonorrhea continues to be an epidemic disease of worldwide proportions. Penicillin has long been the treatment for gonorrhea and is discussed in detail in Chapter 14. The discovery of β-lactamase-producing strains of Neisseria gonorrhoeae by Ashford et al. (1976) and Phillips (1976) has explained treatment failures.[71,72]

The symptomatic patient usually shows a vaginal discharge or dysuria. Barlow et al. showed that microscopic examination of cultures from infected sites produces the diagnosis in only 60 percent of females conpared to 95 percent of males.[73] Cultures should be

TABLE 23–2. DRUGS USEFUL IN THE TREATMENT OF BACTERIAL VAGINOSIS

Drug Name	Dosage	Comments
Systemic		
Metronidazole	500 mg PO every 6 hr for 7 days	Most effective therapy
	2 g PO single dose	Less effective, higher recurrence
Cephalexin	500 mg PO every 6 hr for 7 days	
Local		
Tetracycline in cream base	100–200 mg once or twice daily for 7 days	High incidence of candidiasis

taken from the urethral orifice, vagina, endocervical, and anal canals. Omission of the anal culture will cause a missed diagnosis in almost 5 percent of infected patients. Repeated cultures may support initial negative results. Chipperfield and Catterall, using urethral and endocervical cultures, showed in 209 female patients that 91 percent were positive on first culture.[74] They were able to substantiate the diagnosis in another 7.1 percent by repeating the culture. Barlow and Phillips also showed that despite 85.6 percent positive cultures, only 60 percent of the women were symptomatic.[75]

Treatment for uncomplicated genitourinary gonorrhea as outlined by the Centers for Disease Control appears in Table 23–3.[76] All patients should be tested for syphilis and follow-up cultures obtained in 3 to 7 days after treatment. Spectinomycin should only be used in cases of β-lactamase-producing *N. gonorrhoeae* or in those who fail to respond to other antimicrobial treatment.[77] Tetracycline is contraindicated during pregnancy (Chap. 2).

Treatment of *N. gonorrhoeae* infections is mandatory if the complications of infertility, pelvic inflammatory disease, and possible disseminated infection are to be prevented. The sexual partner(s) should also be treated.

Chlamydia trachomatis

C. trachomatis, a bacterialike organism that is an obligatory intracellular parasite sensitive to the action of some antibiotics, is the most prevalent significant sexually transmitted organism. It has surpassed *N. gonorrhoeae* in frequency by a factor of three to five times, particularly in adolescents and young women.[67] While the organism displays a strict tissue tropism for columnar epithelium in the adult female reproductive tract and thus does not cause a true vaginitis, it is a common cause of mucopurulent cervicitis.[3] It should be suspected in any patient who shows a yellow mucopus from the endocervix and who has significant numbers of polymorphonuclear leukocytes in a properly collected specimen of cervical mucus.[3] With the increased availability and reliability of chlamydial culture techniques as well as antigen detection

TABLE 23–3. TREATMENT OF UNCOMPLICATED GENITOURINARY *NEISSERIA GONORRHOEAE* AND PENICILLINASE-PRODUCING *NEISSERIA GONORRHOEAE*

Uncomplicated genitourinary *Neisseria gonorrhoeae*
1. Either amoxicillin 3 g or ampicillin 3.5 g PO single dose, with probenecid 1 g PO single dose
or
2. Tetracycline 500 mg PO qid for 7 days, or doxycycline 100 mg PO bid for 7 days
or
3. Penicillin G procaine 4.8 million units IM at two sites, plus probenecid 1 g PO single dose
or
4. 1 followed by 2.
Penicillinase-producing *Neisseria gonorrhoeae*
1. Spectinomycin 2 g IM single dose
or
2. Cefoxitin 2 g IM single dose, plus probenecid 1 g PO single dose
or
3. Cefotaxime 1 g IM single dose

Adapted from Centers for Disease Control: Sexually transmitted diseases guidelines. Morbid Mortal Week Rep 31 (Suppl):338, 1982.

and immunofluorescent cytologic techniques, the diagnosis should be actively and definitively confirmed in most areas. Recognition and prompt therapy of chlamydial endocervicitis is essential to prevent upper tract infection with the organism. This will hopefully allow prevention of the significant sequelae of chlamydial pelvic inflammatory disease: tubal infertility, ectopic pregnancy, and chronic pelvic pain.[78]

Therapy of choice for chlamydial endocervicitis is tetracycline HCl 500 mg four times daily for 7 to 10 days or doxyclycline hyclate 100 mg twice daily for 7 to 10 days. Alternative are erythromycin base 500 mg four times daily for at least 7 days, or sulfamethoxazole 1 g twice daily for 10 days.[79] Erythromycin is the drug of choice in pregnancy. Sexual contacts of women with chlamydial infections should always receive treatment.

Herpesvirus hominis

The cervicitis caused by Herpesvirus is virtually always in association with a primary infection and associated with vulvar herpes.[2] Management of this condition is considered in the next section.

HERPES VULVOVAGINITIS

The herpes simplex virus is a DNA-containing virus specific to humans. There are two antigenic groups (type I and type II). Type I herpes virus, initially found only in the oral cavity, has been seen in as many as 30 percent of genital herpes infections.

Primary genital infection with herpes virus (usually type II) may present without clinical manifestations or with both localized and systemic reactions. The patient may experience fever, malaise, inguinal adenopathy, erosions, labial edema, and painful ulcerations. Small vesicles usually present on the labia minora, inner labia majora, or cervix. The vesicles often enlarge, rupture, and ulcerate before spontaneous healing. The ulcers last from 1 to 3 weeks in primary infection and last for a shorter period without systemic manifestations in recurrent infection. The virus then goes into a latent phase within the nerve ganglia and may recur with any form of stress. Recurrent lesions tend to be more localized and less painful. The diagnosis may be accomplished by observing intranuclear inclusion bodies on Pap smear or a positive culture.

Until recently, treatment success has been limited, as reflected by the wide number of treatment regimens that have been proposed. Some of these are listed in Table 23–4. The spontaneous healing of the ulcers makes it difficult to assess the efficacy of treatment regimens. Symptomatic treatment includes the local use of sitz baths and analgesics as necessary.

Acyclovir has become the mainstay of treatment for vulvar herpes. Topical acyclovir in initial genital mucocutaneous disease reduced the duration of viral shedding, hastened the resolution of lesions, and decreased symptoms.[89] With severe vulvar infections intravenous therapy was found to be even more effective.[90] This probably was related to better drug delivery to the site of virus replication. A study addressing itself to oral acyclovir treatment of primary genital herpes infections showed the drug to be effective in reducing viral shedding, new lesion formation, and duration of new lesions in both men and women.[91]

The treatment of recurrent genital herpes has been more difficult. Topical acyclovir, although shortening the duration of virus shedding in men, did not result in shortened duration of lesions or symptom relief in men or women.[89] Topical acyclovir was also found to have no clinical benefit in the treatment of recurrent herpes labialis in the noncompromised patient.[92] It would appear that topical acyclovir is not effective in the treatment of recurrent genital or labial herpes in the noncompromised host.

Oral acyclovir has shown efficacy in reducing the duration of viral shedding and the

TABLE 23–4. TOPICAL THERAPY OF HERPETIC VULVOVAGINITIS

Agent	Comments	References
2 Deoxy-D-glucose	Inhibits synthesis or elongation of macromolecules required for envelope biogenesis and recognition phenomenon Effective in this study	80
3% Adenine arabinoside	Inhibits DNA synthesis Ineffective	81
5% Idoxuridine	Inhibits DNA synthesis Not effective in herpetic vulvovaginitis	82 83
Neutral-red photodynamic inactivation	Oncogenic potential Not effective	84
Proflavine photodynamic inactivation	Oncogenic potential Not effective	85
Burrow's solution	Soothing for local relief only	86
Ether	Painful Ineffective	
Nonoxynol-9	Nonionic surfactant Not effective	87
Povidone iodine douche (Betadine)	Antiseptic Antiviral 2 tsp betadine per quart warm water	88
Povidone iodine sitz bath	4 oz betadine solution to warm tub two to three times daily	

time necessary to complete healing in recurrent herpes. In addition, new lesion formation was decreased.[93]

Acyclovir is an acyclic analogue of deoxyquanosine. Acylovir acts as a selective substrate for viral thymidine kinase. The herpesvirus-specified thymidine kinase acts to concentrate acyclovir in the herpes-infected cell. This is done by phosphorylating it to the monophosphate derivative. Cellular kinase then converts the monophosphate derivated to acyclovir triphosphate, which is the active form of the drug.[94] The triphosphate derivative is both a competitive inhibitor of the viral DNA polymerase and DNA chain terminator, thus acting to inhibit viral DNA synthesis.[95]

Recent studies have shown acyclovir to be effective in the oral form in treating initial and recurrent episodes as well as in suppressing recurrent episodes of genital herpes.[96–98]

Dosages of acylovir are listed in Table 23–5. Side effects are rare with the ointment. The intravenous form may lead to inflammation, phlebitis, rash or hives, and transient elevations of the serum creatinine. The oral form may cause nausea, vomiting, headache, diarrhea, vertigo, and arthralgias. Dosages should be reduced in patients with acute or chronic renal impairment.

ATROPHIC VAGINITIS (MENOPAUSAL AND PREPUBERTAL)

Atrophic vaginitis is most often found in postmenopausal women and in those who have been rendered anestrogenic through removal of their ovaries. The vaginal mucosa and vulva are usually thin and quite pale, and rugal folds are usually missing. The discharge

TABLE 23–5. USE OF ACYCLOVIR IN PATIENTS WITH HERPES GENITALIS NONIMMUNOCOMPROMISED HOST—NORMAL RENAL FUNCTION

Agent	Indication	Dosage
Acyclovir 5% ointment	Initial herpetic episode	Six times a day for 7 days
Acyclovir powder for intravenous use	Severe initial herpetic episode	5 mg/kg infused over 1 hr, every 8 hr for 7 days
Acyclovir capsules	Initial episode	200 mg every 4 hr 5 times a day for 10 days
	Recurrent episode	200 mg every 4 hr 5 times a day for 5 days
	Chronic suppressive therapy	200 mg tid for 6 months or longer

is not usually diagnostic, but examination under the microscope is necessary to rule out candidiasis, trichomoniasis, or other forms of vaginitis.

Treatment consists of hormonal replacement by the judicious use of estrogen locally or systemically (Chap. 17). Dosage in each patient must be individualized regardless of the form of estrogen used. The minimal dosage that achieves the desired therapeutic effect is the correct dosage. Since estrogens are absorbed from the vaginal mucosa, they should be avoided in estrogen-sensitive tumors of the breast or uterus.[99] In addition, they are ineffective in vulvar dystrophies where 2 percent testosterone propionate in petrolatum is the drug of choice.

At the other end of the age spectrum, prepubertal vulvovaginal irritations are also in part related to the anestrogenic status of the child. This results in a thin glycogen-depleted vaginal epithelium which lacks lactobacilli and acidic pH protection from low virulence organism infection. Additionally, a lack of external physical protection of the vaginal opening by labial fat pads and pubic hair and typically poor perineal hygiene can make contamination, principally from rectal sources, more frequent and significant. These susceptibility factors make infections and inflammations of the vulva the only common gynecologic disorders in premenarchal girls. Unlike in the adult, vulvovaginitis in the child most often starts as a primary nonspecific hygenic vulvitis, with relatively infrequent secondary vaginal involvement. The foundation of therapy is improved local hygiene. Rarely short courses of topical estrogen are necessary. Local or systemic antimicrobial agents are rarely necessary or effective.

The primary adult vaginitis syndromes, (trichomoniasis, candidiasis, and bacterial vaginosis) are rarely if ever a cause of clinical vaginitis in the child.[60] Two specific etiologic agents of true premenarchal vaginitis deserve emphasis: *N. gonorrhoeae* and *C. trachomatis.* It has long been recognized that *N. gonorrhoeae* is capable of infecting the thinned, anestrogenic prepubertal vagina. There is now good evidence that chlamydia can infect the atrophic vagina as well.[100] Any prepubertal child with a profuse, purulent or white, homogeneous vaginal discharge should be tested for both of these organisms. Their isolation is an indication for a full sexual abuse investigation, using all available medical, microbiologic, social, and legal resources.[100] Sexual abuse should also be considered in the child with vulvar irritation unresponsive to therapy.

Childhood gonorrhea is treated with procaine penicillin, 100,000 U/kg intramuscularly plus 25 mg/kg of probenecid orally. Tetracycline is the drug of choice for chlamydia in children over the age of 8, with erythromycin or sulfonamides the drugs of choice

TABLE 23–6. RECOMMENDED TREATMENT FOR OTHER VULVOVAGINAL INFECTIONS

Disease	Drug/Therapy	Dose	References
Syphilis			
Primary, secondary, and early latent (less than 1 year duration)	Benzathine penicillin	2.4 million units in divided doses each buttock	101
	Penicillin allergy: tetracycline or erythromycin	500 mg orally four times a day for 15 days	
During pregnancy	Benzathine penicillin	2.4 million units in divided doses each buttock (Charles prefers 2.4 million units in divided doses each buttock each week for 3 consecutive weeks)	101–104
	Penicillin allergy: erythromycin	500 mg orally four times a day for 15 days (Charles prefers 750 mg orally four times a day for 20 days)	101–104
Late latent (more than 1 year duration)	Benzathine penicillin	2.4 million units in divided doses each buttock every week for 3 consecutive weeks	101
	Penicillin allergy: tetracycline or erythromycin	500 mg orally four times a day for 30 days	101
Granuloma inguinale (agent: Calymmatobacterium granulomates)	Tetracycline or erythromycin	500 mg four times a day for 14 days	102
Chancroid (agent: Hemophilus ducreyl)	Sulfonamides (sulfisoxazole)	1 g four times a day for 2 weeks	103
Condylomata acuminata	25% podophyllin in tincture of benzoin	1. Wash lesions with soap and water within 4 hr of application	104
		2. Do not apply to vagina or cervix	104
		3. Systemic toxic effects have been reported	105, 106
		4. Contraindicated in the gravid patient	107, 108
	Eliminate other infections		109
	Trichloracetic acid	1. Dilute 30–50% 2. Protect surrounding tissues 3. Neutralize with sodium bicarbonate after a few minutes 4. Bathe thoroughly within 30 min	109, 110
	Topical 5-fluorouracil		110
	Cryosurgery, electrocoagulation, laser vaporization		110
Molluscum contagiosum	Superficial incision and extrusion of contents Dermal curettage Cryotherapy	Benign, self-limited infection, therapy rarely necessary	112

(continued)

TABLE 23–6. (*Continued*)

Disease	Drug/Therapy	Dose	References
Lymphogranuloma venereum (agent: *Chlamydia trachomatis,* subgroup A)	Sulfonamides (sulfisoxazole, sulfadiazine	1 g four times a day for 3 weeks	111
	Tetracycline	500 mg four times a day for 1 week followed by 250 mg four times a day for 2 weeks	111
	Doxycycline hyclate	100 mg two times a day for 2 weeks	111

under that age due to the well-known risk of dental staining with tetracycline.

OTHER VULVOVAGINAL INFECTIONS

It is beyond the scope of this text to include each drug for every vulvovaginal infection; however, Table 23–6 lists and comments upon current drugs recommended for treating other predominantly vulvar infections.

REFERENCES

1. Friedrich EG: Vaginitis. In Vulvar Disease. Philadelphia, Saunders, 1976, pp 1–25
2. Eschenbach DA: Vaginal infection. Clin Obstet Gynecol 26:186, 1983
3. Brunham RC, Paavonen JR, Stevens CE, et al.: Mucopurulent cervicitis—The ignored counterpart in women of urethritis in men. N Engl J Med 311:1, 1984
4. Drake TE, Mallbach HE: Candida and candidiasis, parts 1,2. Postgrad Med 53:83, 120, 1973
5. Oriel JD, Partridge BM, Denny MJ, et al.: Genital yeast infections. Br Med J 4:761, 1971
6. Eddie DAS: The laboratory diagnosis of vaginal infection caused by trichomonas and candida (monilial) species. J Med Micro Biol 1:153, 1968
7. McHennon MT, Smith TM, McLennon CE: Diagnosis of vaginal mycosis and trichomoniasis: Reliability of cytologic smear, wet smear and culture. Obstet Gynecol 40:231, 1972
8. Sobel JD: Epidemiology and pathogenesis of recurrent vulvovaginal candidiasis. Am J Obstet Gynecol 152:924, 1985
9. Haller I: Mode of action of clotrimazole: Implications for therapy. Am J Obstet Gynecol 152:939, 1985
10. Syverson RE, Buckley H, Gibian J, et al.: Cellular and humoral immune status in women with chronic vaginitis. Am J Obstet Gynecol 134:624, 1979
11. Miles MR, Olsen L, Rogers A: Recurrent vaginal candidiasis: Importance of an intestinal reservoir. JAMA 230:1836, 1977
12. Van Slyke KK, Michel VP, Rein MF: Treatment of vulvovaginal candidiasis with boric acid powder. Am J Obstet Gynecol 141:145, 1981
13. Horowitz BJ, Edelstein SW, Lippman L: *Candida tropicalis* vulvovaginitis. Obstet Gynecol 66:229, 1985
14. Witkin SS, Yu IR, Ledger WJ: Inhibition of *Candida albicans*-induced lymphocyte proliferation by lymphocytes and sera from women with recurrent vaginitis. Am J Obstet Gynecol 147:809, 1983
15. Witkin SS: Defective immune responses in patients with recurrent candidiasis. Infect Surgery September 1985, pp 677–680
16. Eschenbach DA: Vaginal syndromes. In Spagna VA, Prior RB (eds): Sexually Transmitted Diseases. A Clinical Syndrome Approach. New York, Marcel Dekker, 1985, pp 127–159
17. Sargent EC Jr, Pasquale SA: Evaluation of monistat cream (miconazole nitrate 2%) in reduced regimen for treatment of vulvovaginal candidiasis. J Reprod Med 19:67, 1977
18. Oates JK, Davidson F: Treatment of vaginal candidiasis with clotrimazole. Postgrad Med J 50(Suppl):99, 1974
19. Masterton G, Napier I, Henderson J: Three-day clotrimazole treatment in candidal vaginitis, Br J Vener Dis 53:126, 1977

20. Fleury F, Hughes D, Floyd R: Therapeutic results obtained in vaginal mycoses after single-dose treatment with 500 mg clotrimazole vaginal tablets. Am J Obstet Gynecol 152:968, 1985
21. Lebherz T, Guess E, Wolfson N: Efficacy of single-versus multiple-dose clotrimazole therapy in the management of vulvovaginal candidiasis. Am J Obstet Gynecol 152:965, 1985
22. Loendersloot EW, Goormans E, Wiesenhaan PE, et al.: Efficacy and tolerability of single-dose versus six-day treatment of candidal vulvovaginitis with vaginal tablets of clotrimazole. Am J Obstet Gynecol 152:953, 1985
23. Forssman L, Milsom I: Treatment of recurrent vaginal candidiasis. Am J Obstet Gynecol 152:959, 1985
24. Swate TE, Weed JC: Boric acid treatment of vulvovaginal candidiasis. Obstet Gynecol 43:893, 1974
25. Mead PB: Fungi. In Monif GRG (ed): Infectious Diseases in Obstetrics and Gynecology (2nd ed.). Philadelphia, Harper & Row, 1982, pp 323–350
26. Eschenbach DA, Hummel D, Gravett MG: Recurrent and persistent vulvovaginal candidiasis: Treatment with ketoconazole. Obstet Gynecol 66:248, 1985
27. Sobel JD. Management of recurrent vulvovaginal candidiasis with intermittent ketoconazole prophylaxis. Obstet Gynecol 65:435, 1985
28. Tucker WS, Snell BB, Island DP, et al.: Reversible adrenal insufficiency induced by ketoconazole. JAMA 253:2413, 1985
29. Catteral RD, Nicol CS: Is trichomonal infestation a venereal disease? Br Med J 1:1177, 1960
30. Rein JF, Chapel TA: Trichomoniasis, candidiasis and the minor venereal diseases. Clin Obstet Gynecol 18:73, 1975
31. Fleury FJ: Adult vaginitis. Clin Obstet Gynecol 24:407, 1981
32. Perl G: Errors in diagnosis of trichomonas vaginales infection: As observed among 1199 patients. Obstet Gynecol 39:70, 1972
33. Durel P, Roiron V, Seboulet A, Borel LJ: Systemic treatment of human trichomoniasis with a derivative of nitroimidazole, 8823 R.R. Br J Vener Dis 36:21, 1960
34. Morton RS: Metronidazole in the single dose treatment of trichomonal vaginitis in men and women. Br J Vener Dis 48:525, 1972
35. Dykers JR: Single-dose metronidazole for trichomonal vaginitis: Patient and consort. N Engl J Med 293:23, 1975
36. Fleury FJ, VanBergen WS, Prentice RL, et al.: Single dose of two grams of metronidazole for trichomonas vaginalis infection. Am J Obstet Gynecol 128:320, 1977
37. Lossick JG: Single dose metronidazole treatment for vaginal trichomoniasis. Obstet Gynecol 56:508, 1980
38. Thurner J, Meingassner JG: Isolation of trichomonas vaginalis resistant to metronidazole (letter). Lancet 2(8092 pt 1):738, 1978
39. Meingassner JG: Strain of trichomonas vaginales resistant to metronidazole and other 5-nitroimidazoles. Antimicrob Agents Chemother 15(2):254, 1979
40. Kane PO, McFadzeam JA, Squires S: Absorption and excretion of metronidazole. Br J Vener Dis 37:276, 1961
41. Stambaugh JE, Feo LG, Manther RW: The isolation and identification of the urinary oxidative metabolites of metronidazole in man. J Pharmacol Exp Ther 161:373, 1968
42. Mead PB, Gibson M, Schentag JJ, Ziemniak JA: Possible alteration of metronidazole metabolism by phenobarbital. N Engl J Med 306:1490, 1982
43. Mead PB, Hager WD, Spence MR: Trichomoniasis: Reinfection or resistance? Contemp Ob/Gyn June 1985, pp 141–148
44. Voogd CE, vaan der Stel JJ, Jacobs JA: The mutagenic action of nitroimidazoles: I. Metronidazole, nimorazole, dimetridazole and ronidazole. Mutat Res 26:483, 1974
45. Legator MS, Connor TH, Stocker M: Detection of mutagenic activity of metronidazole and niridazole in body fluids of humans and mice. Science 188:1118, 1975
46. Rosenkranz HS, Speck WT: Mutogenicity of metronidazole activation by mammalian liver microsomes. Biochem Biophys Res Commun 66:520, 1975
47. Rustia M, Shubik P: Induction of lung tumours and malignant lymphomas in mice by metronidazole. J Natl Cancer Inst 48:721, 1972
48. Gardner HL, Dukes CD: *Haemophilis vaginalis* vaginitis: A newly defined specific infection previously classified "nonspecific" vaginitis. Am J Obstet Gynecol 69:962, 1955
49. Gardner HL, Dampeer TK, Dukes CD: The

prevalence of vaginitis: A study in incidence. Am J Obstet Gynecol 73:1080, 1957

50. Brown D, Kaufman RH, Gardner HL: *Gardnerella vaginalis* vaginitis: The current opinion. J Reprod Med 29:300, 1984
51. Lapage SP: *Haemophilus vaginalis* and its role in vaginitis. Acta Pathol Microbiol Scand 52:34, 1961
52. Dunkelberg W, Hefner JD, Patow WE, et al.: *Haemophilus vaginalis* among asymptomatic women. Obstet Gynecol 21:629, 1962
53. Frampton J, Lee Y: Is *Haemophilus vaginalis* a pathogen in the female genital tract. Br J Obstet Gynaecol 71:436, 1964
54. Davidson AJL, Layton KB: Vaginitis and *Haemophilus vaginalis.* Med J Aust 1(Suppl 10):757, 1968
55. Tashjian JH, Coulam EB, Washington JA: Vaginal flora in asymptomatic women. Mayo Clin Proc 51:557, 1976
56. Levison ME, Corman LC, Carrington ER, Kaye D: Quantitative microflora of the vagina. Am J Obstet Gynecol 127:80, 1977
57. Corishley CM: Mirobial flora of the vagina and cervix. J Clin Pathol 30:745, 1977
58. McCormack WM, Hayes CH, Rosner B, et al.: Vaginal colonization with *Corynebacterium vaginal (Haemophilus vaginalis).* J Infect Dis 136:740, 1977
59. Levison ME, Trestman I, Quach R, et al.: Quantitative bacteriology of the vaginal flora in vaginitis. Am J Obstet Gynecol 133:139, 1979
60. Hammerschlag MR, Alpert S, Rosner I, et al.: Microbiology of the vagina in children: Normal and potentially pathogenic organisms. Pediatrics 62:57, 1978
61. Bump RC, Zuspan FP, Buesching WJ, et al.: The prevalence, six-month persistence, and predictive values of laboratory indicators of bacterial vaginosis (nonspecific vaginitis) in asymptomatic women. Am J Obstet Gynecol 150:917, 1984
62. Pheifer TA, Forsyth PS, Durfee MA, et al.: Nonspecific vaginitis: Role of *Haemophilus vaginalis* and treatment with metronidazole. N Engl J Med 63:1429, 1978
63. Chen KCS, Forsyth PS, Durfee MA, et al.: Amine content of vaginal fluid from untreated and treated patients with nonspecific vaginitis. J Clin Invest 63:828, 1979
64. Spiegel CA, Amsel R, Eschenback D, et al.: Anaerobic bacteria in nonspecific vaginitis. N Engl J Med 303:601, 1980
65. Vontver LA, Eschenbach DA: The role of *Gardnerella vaginalis* in nonspecific vaginitis. Clin Obstet Gynecol 24:439, 1981
66. Amsel R, Totten PA, Spiegel CA, et al.: Nonspecific vaginitis: Diagnostic criteria and microbial and epidemiologic associations. Am J Med 74:14, 1983
67. Bump RC, Sachs LA, Buesching WJ: Sexually transmissible infectious agents in sexually active and virginal asymptomatic adolescent girls. Pediatrics (in press)
68. Swedberg J, Steiner JF, Deiss F, et al.: Comparison of single-dose vs one-week course of metronidazole for symptomatic bacterial vaginosis. JAMA 254:1046, 1985
69. Minkowski WL, Baker CJ, Alleyne D, et al.: Single dose oral metronidazole therapy for *Garnerella vaginalis* vaginitis in adolescent females. J Adolesc Health Care 4:113, 1983
70. Eschenbach DA, Critchlow CW, Watkins H, et al.: A dose duration study of metronidazole for the treatment of nonspecific vaginitis. Scand J Infect Dis 40(Suppl):73, 1983
71. Ashford WA, Golash RG, Hemming VG: Penicillinase-producing neisseria gonorrhoeae. Lancet 2:657, 1976
72. Phillips I: Beta-lactamase producing penicillin-resistant gonococcus. Lancet 2:656, 1976
73. Barlow D, Nayyar K, Phillips I, et al.: Diagnosis of gonorrhoea in women. Br J Vener Dis 52:326, 1976
74. Chipperfield EJ, Catterall RD: Reappraisal of gram-staining and culture techniques for diagnosis of gonorrhea in women. Br J Vener Dis 52:36, 1976
75. Barlow D, Phillips I: Gonorrhoea in women: Diagnostic, clinical, and laboratory aspects. Lancet 1:761, 1978
76. Centers for Disease Control: Sexually transmitted diseases guidelines. Morbid Mortal Week Rep 31(Suppl):33S, 1982
77. Thornsberry C, Jaffer H, Brown ST, et al.: Spectinomycin resistant neisseria gonorrhoea. JAMA 237:2405, 1977
78. Bump RC, Fass RJ: Pelvic Inflammatory Disease. In Spagna VA, Prior RB, (eds): Sexually Transmitted Diseases. A Clinical Syndrome Approach. New York, Marcel Dekker, 1985, pp 187–220
79. Centers for Disease Control: *Chlamydia trachomatis* infections: Policy guidelines for prevention and control. Morbid Mortal Week Rep 34(Suppl):53S, 1985
80. Blough HA, Giuntoli RL: Successful treat-

ment of human genital herpes infection with 2-deoxy-D-glucose. JAMA 241:2798, 1979
81. Adams GH, Benson EA, Alexander ER, et al.: Genital herpetic infection in men and women: Clinical course and effect of topical application of adenine arabenoside. J Infect Dis 133(Suppl):A151, 1976
82. Taylor PK, Doherty NR: Comparison of the treatment of herpes genitales in men with proflavine photoinactivation, idoxuridine ointment and normal saline. BR J Vener Dis 51:125, 1975
83. Kibrick S, Katz AS: Topical idoxuridine in recurrent herpes simplex. Ann NY Acad Sci 173:83, 1970
84. Myers MG, Oxman MN, Clark JE, et al.: Failure of neutral-red photodynamic inactivation in recurrent herpes simplex virus infection. N Engl J Med 293:945, 1975
85. Kaufman RH, Adam E, Mirkovic RR: Treatment of genital herpes simplex virus infection with photodynamic inactivation. Am J Obstet Gynecol 132:861, 1968
86. Corey L, Reeves WC, Chiang WT, et al.: Ineffectiveness of topical ether for the treatment of genital herpes simplex virus infection. N Engl J Med 299:237, 1978
87. Vontver LA, Reeves WC, Rattray M: Clinical course and diagnosis of genital herpes simplex virus infection and evaluation of topical surfactant therapy. Am J Obstet Gynecol 133:548, 1979
88. Wilbanks GD, Chez RA: How to diagnose and treat genital herpes. Contemp Obstet Gynecol 16:81, 1980
89. Corey L, Nahmias AJ, Guinan M, et al.: A trial of topical acyclovir in genital herpes simplex infections. N Engl J Med 306:1313, 1982
90. Mindel A, Adler MW, Sutherland S: Intravenous acyclovir treatment for primary genital herpes. Lancet 1:697, 1982
91. Bryson Y, Dillon M, Lovett M, et al.: Treatment of first episodes of genital herpes simplex virus infections with oral acyclovir. N Engl J Med 308:916, 1983
92. Spruance SI, Schnipper LE, Averall JC, Jr: Treatment of herpes simplex labialis with topical acyclovir in polyethylene glycol. J Infect Dis 146(1):85, 1982
93. Nilsen AE, Aasen T, Halos AM: Efficacy of oral acyclovir in the treatment of initial and recurrent genital herpes. Lancet 2:571, 1982
94. Elion GB, Furnam PA, Fyfe JA, et al.: Selectivity of action of an antiherpetic agent, 9-(2-hydroxyethoxymethyl) quanine. Proc Natl Acad Sci USA 74(12):2716, 1977
95. Furnam PA, St. Clair MH, et al.: Inhibition of herpes simplex virus-induced DNA polymerase activity and viral DNA replication by 9-(2-hydroxyethoxymethyl) quanine and its triphosphate. J Virol 32(1):72, 1979
96. Mertz GJ, Critchlow CW, et al.: Double-blind placebo-controlled trial of oral acyclovir in first-episode genital herpes simplex virus infection. JAMA 252:1147, 1984
97. Reichman RC, Badger GJ, Mertz GJ, et al.: Treatment of recurrent genital herpes simplex infections with oral acyclovir. A controlled trial. JAMA 251:2103, 1984
98. Douglas JM, Critchlow C, Benedetti J, et al.: A double blind study of oral acyclovir for suppression of recurrences of genital herpes simplex virus infection. N Engl J Med 310:1151, 1984
99. Rigg LA, Herman HW, Yen SCC: Absorption of estrogen from vaginal cream. N Engl J Med 298:195, 1978
100. Bump RC: *Chlamydia trachomatis* as a cause of prepubertal vaginitis. Obstet Gynecol 65:384, 1985
101. Centers for Disease Control: Syphilis: CDC recommended treatment schedules. J Infect Dis 134:97, 1976
102. Charles D: Infections in Obstetrics and Gynecology. Philadelphia, Saunders, 1980, p 38
103. Charles D: Infections in Obstetrics and Gynecology. Philadelphia, Saunders, 1980, p 39
104. Charles D: Infections in Obstetrics and Gynecology. Philadelphia, Saunders, 1980, p 49
105. Montalde DH, Grombrone JP, Courney NG, et al.: Podophyllin poisoning associated with the treatment of condyloma accumulation. Am J Obstet Gynecol 119:1130, 1974
106. Slater GE, Rumack BH, Peterson RG: Podophyllin poisoning. Systemic toxicity following cutaneous application. Obstet Gynecol 52:94, 1978
107. Graber EA, Barber HRK, O'Rourke JJ: Simple surgical treatment for condyloma accumulation of the vulva. Obstet Gynecol 29:247, 1967
108. Chamberlain MJ, Reynolds AL, Yeoman WB: Toxic effects of podophyllin application in pregnancy. Br Med J 3:391, 1972
109. Woodruff JD: Identifying and treating the acuminate wart. Contemp Ob/Gyn 7:125, 1976

110. Camisa C: *Condyloma acuminatum* and other human papillomavirus-induced diseases. In Spagna VA, Prior RB (eds): Sexually Transmitted Diseases. A Clinical Syndrome Approach. New York, Marcel Dekker, 1985, pp 309–332
111. Fiumara NJ: The Sexually Transmissible Diseases, Vol. 25, No 3. Chicago, Year Book Medical Publishers, 1978
112. Lambert DR, Yoder FW: Ectoparasites and molluscum contagiosum. In Spagna VA, Prior RB (eds): Sexually Transmitted Diseases. A Clinical Syndrome Approach. New York: Marcel Dekker, 1985, pp 333–355

24

Antibiotic Therapy

Nancy K. Eberhard, James A. Visconti, and William E. Copeland, Jr.

It is useful to regard bacterial infections of the female genital tract as alterations in the relationship between the host and her normal bacterial flora. When normal vaginal flora gain access to the upper tracts and multiply, pelvic infection may result. Surgical or obstetrical procedures, foreign bodies, and exogenous pathogenic bacteria may produce a change in the location and number of endogenous organisms sufficient for infection to be manifested (Fig. 24–1). Principal among aerobic organisms are the gram-positive aerobic streptococci and the gram-negative rods, including *Escherichia coli*. The anaerobic spectrum of organisms, including *Bacteroides fragilis,* peptostreptococci, streptococci, and *Clostridia* organisms has provided a significant contribution to the etiology of pelvic infections. Other than *Neisseria gonorrhoeae, Chlamydia trachomatis, Listeria monocytogenes,* and aerobic β-hemolytic streptococci (groups A and B), exogenous pathogens are rarely implicated in pelvic infections.

When clinical symptoms suggest an infection of the lower genital tract, cultures may be useful to identify the presence of exogenous bacteria that might be responsible for clinical infection. Cultures obtained transvaginally or transcervically are unlikely to be clinically useful unless one of these organisms is isolated. The specific diagnosis of salpingitis and pelvic inflammatory disease is more difficult because of the inaccessibility of the upper genital tracts. Clinical diagnosis is accurate in only 65 percent of patients with visually documented pelvic inflammatory disease.[1] Culture data are helpful but not possible to obtain without the use of invasive techniques (culdocentesis or laparoscopy), which increase patient discomfort and risk. Any cultures taken directly from infected tissues at surgery are accurate if processed correctly and are helpful in choosing an appropriate treatment plan.

Monif has described the "progressive anaerobic syndrome," a useful concept to explain many of the clinical features of pelvic infection.[2] The initial insult occurs as a disruption of the integrity of the upper genital tract through surgery, delivery, or presence of a foreign body (e.g., an intrauterine device, IUD). Aerobic bacteria produce the initial in-

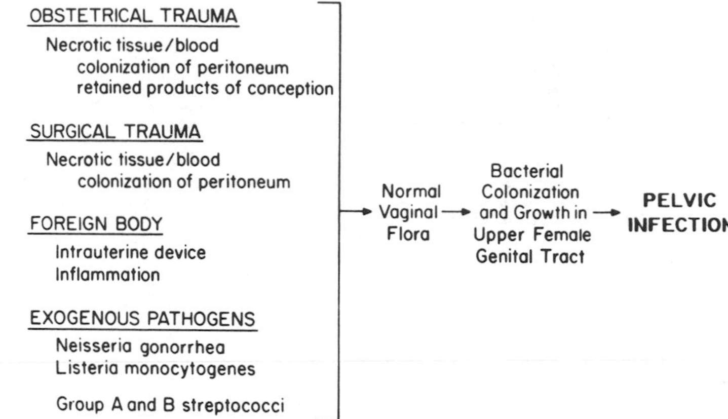

Figure 24-1. Surgical or obstetrical procedures, foreign bodies, and exogenous pathogenic bacteria may produce a change in the location and number of endogenous organisms sufficient for infection to manifest.

fection and, as these organisms multiply and destroy tissue, available oxygen is consumed and a progressively anaerobic and acidotic environment is produced. This is followed by the secondary invasion of facultative aerobes and subsequently the obligate anaerobes. This progression can often be arrested in the early stages by antimicrobials without anaerobic activity, if the diagnosis is made early. Infections of longer duration or greater severity, including tubovarian abscesses, require the addition of antibiotics with an anaerobic spectrum. Whether the early utilization of antimicrobials effective against anaerobes will improve long-term results is still unknown. However, this concept accounts for the reported excess of antimicrobial agents of limited spectrum as prophylactic drugs in gynecologic surgery.

The rationale for clinical use of antibiotics in pelvic infections is based on numerous factors. The single most important concept is that of the polymicrobial nature of these mixed aerobic-anaerobic infections. Penicillin remains an excellent choice for the majority of anaerobic organisms, with the significant exception of *B. fragilis*. Most gram-positive cocci, specifically aerobic streptococci, are also sensitive to penicillin therapy. Antibiotics effective against *B. fragilis* include clindamycin, chloramphenicol, β-lactamase-resistant cephalosporins, extended-spectrum penicillins, and metronidazole. The aerobic gram-negative rods significant in pelvic infections are usually sensitive to the various aminoglycosides.

Multiple regimens of various antibiotics have been investigated in pelvic infections without one specific combination demonstrating a definite superiority based on acute response or long-term sequelae. This has been documented in both acute salpingitis[3] and postpartum[4-6] endometritis. In recent studies, the most significant feature in altering both short- and long-term outcome was early diagnosis and treatment.[7]

Chlamydia trachomatis has emerged as a pathogen in acute pelvic inflammatory disease.[8-10] This protozoan is responsible for a variety of infections, including lymphogranuloma venereum, neonatal conjunctivitis, nonspecific urethritis in the male, and perhaps preterm delivery. *C. trachomatis* is now implicated as an etiologic agent in acute salpingitis as well as being identified in an asymptomatic carrier state in approximately 5 percent of the population. The treatment of choice for *C. trachomatis* is tetracycline 500 mg four times daily for 7 days or doxycycline 100 mg twice daily for 7 days. Erythromycin 500 mg four times daily for 7 days is an effective substitute in patients allergic to the tetracyclines.

On occasion, antibiotic therapy, regardless of bacterial spectrum, is ineffective. These conditions should strongly suggest abscess formation, retained products of conception, or presence of a foreign body such as an IUD. These conditions should be corrected to maximize the effect of the administered medication.

Antimicrobial drugs can prevent infection in some surgical patients, but are not without risk. Potential adverse effects include toxic or allergic drug reactions and superinfection. It should be noted that an effective prophylactic antibiotic regimen need not be active against all potential pathogens.

Physicians have a bewildering array of antimicrobial agents at their disposal. The number of agents and their doses, side effects, and actions make it nearly impossible to think of them in an organized manner. Accordingly, they are discussed in the following sections as chemically related groups of drugs. The material on each group of drugs is subdivided into similar areas (mechanism, pharmacology, indications, dosing, adverse effects) for ease of retrieval.

PENICILLINS

Pharmacology and Preparations

The penicillins remain among the most effective and least toxic of available antimicrobials. The various preparations (Table 24–1) of the penicillins are obtained by chemical or biologic modifications of the 6-aminopenicillanic acid nucleus of this compound. Penicillins act by inhibiting bacterial cell wall synthesis, but many different mechanisms are involved in this process.

The potassium salt of penicillin V is better absorbed than the sodium salt. Penicillin G, methicillin, carbenicillin, and nafcillin are all highly acid labile, which accounts for their poor bioavailability. Patients should be advised to ingest penicillins 1 hour before meals, or 2 hours after meals, because the presence of food delays and impairs their absorption.

Once in the bloodstream penicillins bind to serum proteins to varying degrees. Despite

TABLE 24–1. PENICILLIN AND CEPHALOSPORIN PREPARATIONS AVAILABLE IN THE UNITED STATES

Penicillins	Cephalosporins
Natural penicillins Benzylpenicillin G Phenoxymethylpenicillin (V)	First-generation Cephalothin, cephapirin, cephaloridine, cephalexin, cephradine, cefaclor, cefodroxil, cefonacid, ceforanide
Penicillinase-resistant penicillins Methicillin Nafcillin Isoxazolyl penicillins Cloxacillin Dicloxacillin Oxacillin	Second-generation Cefoxitin, cefamandole, cefuroxime, cefotetan
Aminopenicillins Ampicillin Amoxicillin Cyclacillin	Third-generation Cefotaxime, ceftizoxime, ceftriaxone, ceftazidime, cefoperazone, moxalactam
Antipseudomonas penicillins Carbenicillin Indanyl carbenicillin Ticarcillin Ureidopenicillins Mezlocillin Piperacillin Azlocillin	

many studies, the precise influence of protein-binding on therapy is a clouded issue. Only unbound drug exerts antibacterial activity, and bound drug cannot enter a microorganism or diffuse into tissue. Penicillins are distributed to the lungs, liver, kidney, muscle, and bone in sufficient quantities to treat infections.

The major pathway of penicillin elimination is renal, resulting in high urine concentrations. A portion of all of these agents is metabolized, but much is eliminated without degradation. Most penicillins are actively secreted into the bile, producing concentrations that exceed those in serum. Penetration, however, is poor in the presence of common duct obstruction. Because most penicillins are rapidly secreted into the urine, their half-lives in serum are short. Therefore, renal impairment is important when considering their elimination, since it prolongs the half-life of several agents. Even in the presence

TABLE 24–2. RECOMMENDED PENICILLIN MAINTENANCE DOSAGES FOR ADULT PATIENTS WITH NORMAL AND REDUCED RENAL FUNCTION*

Drug	PO Dose	Normal Renal Function IM Dose	IV Dose
Penicillin G (1.7 mEq K^+/mil. units)	1.0 g every 6 hr before meals	600,000–1.2 million units	10–12 mu up to 40 mil. u/day
Procaine		300,000 units	1.2 mil. u every 24–72 hr
Benzathine		600,000 units	1.2 mil. u every 15–30 days
Penicillin V	0.250–0.5 g every 6 hr before meals		
Methicillin		1–2 g every 4–6 hr	8–12 g/day (2 g every 4 hr)
Nafcillin	0.250 g every 6 hr ac	0.5–1.0 g every 4–6 hr	4–12 g/day (1–2 g every 4–6 hr)
Oxacillin	0.5–1.0 g every 6 hr		8–12 g/day (2 g every 4 hr)
Cloxacillin	0.25–0.5 g every 6 hr before meals		
Dicloxacillin	0.25–0.5 g every 6 hr ac	0.25–0.5 g every 6 hr	
Ampicillin	0.250–0.5 g every 6 hr ac	0.25–0.5 g every 6 hr	4–12 g/day (1 g every 6 hr)
Amoxicillin	0.25 g every 8 hr		
Carbenicillin disodium (4.7 mEq Na^+/g)			24–36 g/day (2–3 g every 2 hr)
Indanyl carbenicillin	0.382–0.764 g every 6 hr		
Ticarcillin (5.2–6.5 mEq Na^+/g)		1 g every 6 hr	6–18 g/day (2 g every 4–6 hr)
Piperacillin (~2 mEq Na^+/g)			6–18 g/day (2–4 g every 6 hr)
Mezlocillin (~2 mEq Na^+/g)			6–18 g/day (2–4 g every 6 hr)

*(*Adapted from Bennett WM et al.*[11])

of marked renal impairment (creatinine clearance <20 ml/min), urinary levels of ampicillin, carbenicillin, and ticarcillin are adequate for effective therapy. Urinary levels of indanyl carbenicillin may not be adequate when renal function is significantly reduced.

Recommended penicillin dosages for adults with renal insufficiency are also given in Table 24–2. The renal excretion of all penicillins can be impaired by probenecid, increasing serum levels and prolonging drug half-life. The major use of probenecid is to increase serum levels of penicillin G, ampicillin, and amoxicillin in the treatment of gonorrhea by single-dose administration.

Penicillin G is available as two repository salts for IM use only, procaine penicillin G and benzathine penicillin G. Procaine penicillin G produces detectable blood levels for 12 hours. Doubling the dose does not double the blood level, unless the drug is administered in different body sites. This is the pri-

Mild Renal Failure (>50 ml/min)	Moderate Renal Failure (50 ml/min to 10 ml/min)	Severe Renal Failure (<10 ml/min)
600,000–20 mu/day (every 4–6 hr)	5–20 ml/units/day (every 8–12 hr)	5 mu/day (every 12–18 hr)
1–2 g every 4 hr	1–2 g every 4 hr	1–2 g every 8–12 hr
2 g every 4 hr	2 g every 4 hr	2 g every 4 hr
0.25–0.5 g every 6 hr	0.25–0.5 g every 6 hr	0.25–0.5 g every 6 hr
0.25–0.5 g every 6 hr	0.25–0.5 g every 6 hr	0.25–0.5 g every 6 hr
0.25–0.5 g every 6 hr	0.25–0.5 g every 6–12 hr	0.25 g every 12–16 hr
0.25–0.5 g every 8 hr	0.250 g every 6–12 hr	0.250 g every 12–16 hr
2–3 g every 8–12 hr	2–3 g every 12–24 hr	2–3 g every 24–48 hr
3 g every 8–12 hr	3 g every 12–24 hr	3 g every 24–48 hr
6–24 g/day (4 g every 6 hr)	12 g/day (1–4 g every 8 hr)	8 g/day (1–4 g every 12 hr)
12–18 g/day (1.5–4 g every 6 hr)	9 g/day (1.5–3 g every 8 hr)	6 g/day (1.5–2 g every 8 hr)

mary rationale for splitting the 4.8 million units of procaine penicillin G into two sites to treat gonorrhea. Benzathine penicillin G provides detectable blood levels for 4 weeks. Mixtures of procaine penicillin and benzathine penicillin are available, but their use is irrational since this preparation actually dilutes the level of benzathine penicillin.

Antibacterial Activity

Streptococci

Streptococci of the *Streptococcus pyogenes* (group A), *St. agalactiae* (Group B), *St. viridans, St. pneumoniae* (pneumococcus), peptostreptococci, and the anaerobes have remained extremely sensitive to penicillin G.[12-14] Group D streptococci include *St. bovis,* which is penicillin-sensitive, and the true enterococci (*Enterococcus faecalis, St. fecium, St. durans,* and *St. liquifaciens*), which have always been relatively resistant to penicillin. The levels of penicillin V and the aminopenicillins needed to inhibit these organisms are about the same. Ampicillin, amoxicillin, and the ureidopenicillins, however, may be more active against enterococci. The semisynthetic antistaphylococcal penicillins have the advantage over methicillin in their effectiveness against not only penicillinase-resistant staphylococci but against other gram-positive organisms as well.

The population at risk of developing bacterial endocarditis includes patients with rheumatic heart disease, congenital heart disease, idiopathic hypertrophic subaortic stenosis (IHSS), and prosthetic valves. The most recent recommendations[15] from the American Heart Association for the prevention of bacterial endocarditis are given in Table 24–3.

Staphylococci

Both *Staphylococcus aureus* and *S. epidermis* have become increasingly resistant to penicillin G. Greater than 80 percent of hospital-acquired staphylococci are resistant to penicillin G because of β-lactamase production. Staphylococci resistant to penicillin G are also resistant to the aminopenicillins, ampicillin, amoxicillin, cyclacillin, carbenicillin, the ureidopenicillins and ticarcillin. *S. aureus* or *S. epidermis* resistant to methicillin are also resistant to oxacillin, nafcillin, and cloxacillin.

Neisseria

Neisseria are more sensitive to penicillin G than to penicillin V. They are almost as sensitive to ampicillin as to penicillin G but carbenicillin is much less active. For practical purposes, the antistaphylococcal agents have only minimal activity against *N. meningitidis* or *N. gonorrhoeae*. Antibiotics and the doses used to treat gonorrhea are shown in Table 24–4.

Clostridium

Penicillin G is effective against most of the gram-positive bacilli that are clinically important including *Cl. tetani, Cl. perfringens, Corynebacterium diphtheriae, Bacillus anthracis,* and *Listeria monocytogenes*. While the antistaphylococcus agents are less active than penicillin G, they do adequately inhibit all these organisms except Listeria. Other species of *Clostridium* may resist penicillin, ampicillin, and cephalosporins while showing susceptibility to chloramphenicol and metronidazole.[16]

Bacteroides

There are a number of gram-negative rods of clinical importance that are sensitive to penicillin G. *Fusobacterium nudeatum, B. melanenogenicus,* and *B. oralis* are inhibited by penicillin G and, to a lesser extent, to penicillin V. Intravenous administration provides adequate levels. The antistaphylococcal agents do not show good activity against these organisms.

There is still considerable disagreement about the agents of choice in the treatment of intra-abdominal anaerobic infections, in which *B. fragilis* is an important pathogen. At present, clindamycin, cefoxitin, metronidazole, and chloramphenicol seem to be agents of choice followed by secondary agents including penicillin G and extended spectrum penicillins. In spite of this, penicillin G succeeds in eradicating most pelvic in-

TABLE 24–3. BACTERIAL ENDOCARDITIS PROPHYLAXIS

1. For *genitourinary tract and gastrointestinal tract surgery* and instrumentation

The Committee on Rheumatic Fever and Infective Endocarditis of the Council on Cardiovascular Disease in the Young recommends prophylaxis for the following: cystoscopy, prostatic surgery, urethral catheterization (especially in the presence of infection), urinary tract surgery, vaginal hysterectomy, gallbladder surgery, colonic surgery, esophageal dilation, esophageal varices, colonoscopy, upper GI endoscopy with biopsy or proctosigmoidoscopic biopsy. Patients at risk for bacterial endocarditis undergoing such procedures should receive prophylactic antibiotics. Bacteremia less often accompanies other genitourinary and gastrointestinal tract procedures, and endocarditis has developed subsequent to those procedures rarely, if ever. These include percutaneous liver biopsy, upper GI endoscopy or proctosigmoidoscopy without biopsy, barium enema, uncomplicated vaginal delivery, and brief ("in and out") bladder catheterization with sterile urine. If infection is not suspected, the following gynecologic procedures do not routinely require prophylaxis: uterine dilatation and curettage, cesarian section, therapeutic abortion, sterilization procedures, or intrauterine device insertion or removal. However, because patients with prosthetic heart valves and those with surgically constructed systemic-pulmonary shunts appear to be at especially high risk for infective endocarditis, it may be prudent to administer prophylactic antibiotics for these low-risk procedures to such patients

Standard regimen

A. Ampicillin 2.0 g IM or, IV plus gentamicin 1.5 mg/kg IM or IV, given 1/2 to 1 hour before procedure. One follow-up dose may be given 8 hours later

Oral regimen for minor or repetitive procedures in low-risk patients

B. Amoxicillin 3.0 g orally 1 hour before procedure and 1.5 g 6 hours later

For penicillin-allergic patients

C. Vancomycin 1.0 g IV slowly over 1 hour, plus gentamicin 1.5 mg/kg IM or IV given 1 hour before procedure. May be repeated once 8–12 hours later after initial dose

2. For *dental procedures* that cause gingival bleeding and oral/respiratory tract surgery

Standard regimen

A. Penicillin V 2.0 g orally 1 hour before procedure then 1.0 g 6 hours after initial dose. For patients unable to take oral medications give 2 million units of aqueous penicillin G IV or IM 30–60 minutes before procedure; 1 million units 6 hours later may be substituted for the oral form

For patients with prosthetic valves and others with highest risk of endocarditis

B. Ampicillin 1.0–2.0 g IM or IV plus gentamicin 1.5 mg/kg IM or IV, 1/2 hour before procedure, followed by 1.0 g oral penicillin V 6 hours after initial dose. Alternatively, the parenteral regimen may be repeated once 8 hours later

For penicillin-allergic patients

C. Oral: Erythromycin 1.0 g orally 1 hour before procedure, then 500 mg 6 hours after initial dose

D. Parenteral: vancomycin 1.0 g IV slowly over 1 hour, starting 1 hour before procedure. No repeat dose is necessary

3. For patients undergoing *cardiac surgery*

Patients undergoing open-heart surgery are at risk for bacterial endocarditis. The choice of antibiotic prophylaxis (usually a penicillinase-resistant penicillin or a first-generation cephalosporin) should be influenced by the hospital's antibiotic susceptibility data. The Divisions of Infectious Diseases or Clinical Microbiology could be contacted for specific information

Adapted from Shulman ST et al.: 1984. By permission of the American Heart Association, Inc.[15]

fections. Carbenicillin may be effective, but a substantial percentage of *B. fragilis* strains are resistant. Ticarcillin is active against most anaerobes, including *B. fragilis,* but the role of this agent in pelvic infections needs further investigation.

Other Gram-Negative Organisms

The activity of penicillins against gram-negative enteric bacilli depend on the susceptibility patterns of the local organisms. In general, penicillin G will inhibit some *E. coli* and *Proteus mirabilis* found in urinary tract in-

TABLE 24–4. ANTIBIOTICS AND TREATMENT SCHEDULES FOR VENEREAL DISEASES

Gonorrhea

Urethritis or cervicitis. Amoxicillin, 3 g orally at once plus 1 g of probenecid once followed by tetracycline, 500 mg given orally four times daily for 7 days. This regimen is effective for chlamydia trachomatis as well as gonorrhea. Doxycycline, 100 mg twice daily, may be used in place of tetracycline. Tetracycline should be avoided in pregnant patients. Patients who cannot tolerate oral tetracycline or are unlikely to complete a seven day oral regimen can be given Penicillin G procaine 4.8 million units (administered in two injections) plus 1 g of probenecid by mouth

Anal and pharyngeal. Anal gonorrhea in women can be treated like urethritis or cervicitis. The penicillin G procaine and tetracycline regimens used for urethral gonorrhea are probably adequate to treat pharyngeal gonorrhea. Trimethoprim-sulfamethoxazole, nine tablets daily for 5 days, is an alternate for treatment of pharyngeal gonorrhea

Gonorrhea in pregnancy. Pregnant women can be treated with the same regimens of penicillin G procaine or amoxicillin as other patients. Tetracyclines are not recommended during pregnancy. Spectinomycin, 2 g IM once, is effective and probably safe for pregnant women allergic to penicillin

Pelvic inflammatory disease

Hospitalized patients may be administered cefoxitin, 2 g IV four times daily plus doxycycline 100 mg IV twice daily until improvement followed by doxycycline 100 mg orally twice daily to complete 10 days of therapy. Alternative therapy is doxycycline 100 mg IV twice daily plus metronidazole 1 g twice daily IV until improvement followed by doxycycline 100 mg orally twice daily plus metronidazole 1 g orally twice daily to complete 10 days of therapy

Outpatients may be given cefoxitin 2 g IM once plus probenicid 1 g once orally followed by doxycycline 100 mg orally twice daily for 10 days. Alternate therapy is tetracycline HCL 500 mg orally four times daily for 10 days

Syphilis

Primary, secondary or latent syphilis known to be of less than 1 year's duration can be treated effectively with penicillin G benzathine, 2.4 million units IM in a single injection. Alternative therapy is tetracycline 500 mg orally four times daily for 15 days or erythromycin 500 mg orally four times daily for 15 days

Late syphilis (more than 1 year's duration) may be treated with penicillin G benzathine, 2.4 million units IM weekly for 3 weeks. Alternative therapy is tetracycline or erythromycin 500 mg orally four times daily for 30 days

Syphilis in pregnancy. Pregnant women with syphilis should be treated with penicillin in doses appropriate to the stage of the disease and follow-up quantitative serologic tests should be performed monthly until delivery. Retreatment in succeeding pregnancies is unnecessary in the absence of clinical or serologic evidence of new infection. Pregnant women allergic to penicillin should be given erythromycin, but the effectiveness of erythromycin for treatment of syphilis is uncertain, and careful follow-up of mother and child is recommended. In a newborn with a positive serologic test for syphilis where there is no definite history of adequate treatment of the mother, prompt therapy of the infant is recommended

fections, but penicillin G shows a more limited antibacterial spectrum than ampicillin. Penicillin V has poor activity against gram-negative bacilli and the antistaphylococcal agents possess no activity against these organisms.

The aminopenicillins inhibit about 85 percent of *E. coli* and *P. mirabilis* isolated in the community.[17] Most *Klebsiella, Enterobacter, Serratia,* indole-positive *Proteus (P. morganii* and *P. vulgaris),* and *Providencia* are resistant. Although most *Salmonella typhii* are sensitive, some isolates from Central America are resistant. Many *Sa. typhimurium* are resistant and at present most *Shigella sonnei* are resistant, except for *Sh. flexneri,* which is inhibited by ampicillin.

Carbenicillin and ticarcillin are active against *E. coli* and *P. mirabilis.* Ticarcillin has less activity than ampicillin against streptococci and *Haemophilus influenzae* but is more active against many gram-negative bacilli. Both contain a significant amount of sodium and in high doses may cause edema and hypokalemia. These drugs have a significant effect on platelet function and may be a risk factor for bleeding. In addition to their activity against *Pseudomonas aeruginosa,* they are active against many *Enterobacter,* most indole-positive *Proteus,* some *Serratia,* most *Providencia,* and *Acinetobacter* organisms.[18] Table 24–4 summarizes the antibiotics and their doses used in the treatment of syphilis.

The most recent semisynthetic ureidopenicillins (piperacillin, mezlocillin, and azlocillin) offer a broader spectrum that includes increased activity against *P. aeruginosa*. Piperacillin has greatest activity against *Pseudomonas*. All three are readily hydrolyzed by β-lactamase; therefore, resistant strains may be encountered. Piperacillin is also very active against *H. influenzae* and *N. gonorrhoeae*. All three penicillins are active against *E. coli, Proteus sp.,* and *S. marcescens*. Piperacillin and mezlocillin are active against *B. fragilis*. Although these drugs are safe and effective in gynecologic infections, they offer no advantage over other proven agents such as cefoxitin. The addition of clavulanic acid, a β-lactamase inhibitor, to amoxicillin and ticarcillin has resulted in combination products useful against *H. influenzae, B. fragilis,* and other β-lactamase producers. These agents may prove useful in the treatment of mixed infections.

Adverse Effects

All of the penicillins can produce untoward reactions. Hypersensitivity reactions are the major adverse effect. Allergic reactions to penicillin are estimated to occur in 2 to 5 percent of the general population; approximately 10 percent of patients who have previously been exposed to penicillin will experience an allergic reaction.[19] Penicillin preparations administered by the parenteral route are associated with a higher incidence of sensitivity reactions (procaine penicillin IM ~ 5 percent; penicillin G IV ~ 2.5 percent; penicillin G, PO ~ 0.3 percent) than are oral products.[20] Ampicillin produces about twice as many rashes (7 percent) as do other penicillins and is particularly likely to develop in patients with infectious mononucleosis, cytomegalovirus infection, or leukemics receiving allopurinol. Other reactions that have been noted with the various penicillins include:

1. Coombs' positivity, hemolytic anemia being rare.
2. Nephritis, interstitial with fever and eosinophilia, appears to be most common with methicillin.
3. Hepatitis and elevations of serum glutamic oxaloacetic transaminase (SGOT).
4. Bleeding tendency because of platelet dysfunction seen with carbenicillin, ticarcillin and other extended-spectrum penicillins.
5. Diarrhea, commonly with ampicillin- and pencillinase-resistant products.
6. Pain and tenderness at injection site, especially with benzathine products.
7. Stomatitis, glossitis.
8. Convulsions, usually associated with high-dose parenteral therapy in patients with renal insufficiency.
9. Central nervous system reactions (not seizures) in some patients receiving procaine penicillin G, probably due to the procaine.
10. Hyperkalemia and potassium penicillin G (contains 1.7 mEq potassium ion/1 million units).
11. Hypernatremia and excess sodium load with carbenicillin (contains 4.7 mEq sodium ion/g) and ticarcillin (contains 5.2 mEq sodium ion/g).

CEPHALOSPORINS

Pharmacology

Cephalosporins are compounds containing 7-amino cephalosporanic acid and are derived by a number of modifications of cephalosporin C. These agents are similar to penicillin in respect to structure, mechanism of action, and general antimicrobial activity. Like penicillins, cephalosporins inhibit peptoglycan transpeptidase and D-alanine carboxypeptidase in bacterial cells; thus, they prevent cross-linking of muramic acid-containing peptidoglycan strands. This results in a defective bacterial cell wall which is osmotically unstable.[21] The β-lactam moiety, unlike that in the 5-member penicillin ring, is attached to a 6-member ring in the cephalosporins. It is this structural characteristic which makes cephalosporins more resistant to penicillinase. The currently available cephalosporins can be divided into three general classes based on their spectra of activity. The classes are referred to as the first-, second-, and third-generation cephalosporins. (See Table 24–1.)

The pharmacokinetic characteristics of the cephalosporins have been studied extensively. The primary route of excretion of the cephalosporins is renal, mainly by glomerular filtration and tubular secretion. Cephalothin and cephapirin are also metabolized (20 to 30 percent) to the less active desacetyl metabolite. From 60 to 80 percent of both cephalothin and cephapirin are eliminated in the unchanged form by renal tubular secretion. Cefazolin is primarily cleared by glomerular filtration. Table 24–5 summarizes dosing adjustments of selected cephalosporins needed in patients with renal impairment.

Cefoxitin is not strictly considered a cephalosporin, because it is derived from cephamycin C and contains a 7-α methoxy moiety which is responsible for resistance to β-lactamase.[22]

Antibacterial Activity

The cephalosporins are drugs of choice only for infections caused by *Klebsiella*. Urinary tract infection with *Klebsiella* is not uncommon in reproductive-age women, and may be particularly difficult to eradicate during pregnancy. Combination therapy with two agents

TABLE 24–5. RECOMMENDED CEPHALOSPORIN DOSES FOR ADULT PATIENTS WITH NORMAL AND REDUCED RENAL FUNCTION[11,35,36,38]

Drug	Normal Renal Function	Moderate Renal Function	Severe Renal Failure (<10 ml/min)
Cephalothin	1–2 g every 4 hr IV	1–2 g every 4–6 hr	1 g every 8 hr
Cefazolin	250–500 mg IV every 6–8 hr	250 mg every 6 hr	0.25–1.0 g every 24 hr
Cephapirin	1–2 g every 4 hr IV	1–2 g every 4–6 hr	1 g every 8 hr
Cefamandole	1–2 g every 4–6 hr	0.5–2.0 g every 8 hr	1 g every 12 hr
Cefoxitin	1–2 g every 6–8 hr	1–2 g every 8–12 hr	1.0–2.0 g every 24–48 hr
Cephalexin	250–500 mg every 6 hr PO	250 mg every 6 hr	250 mg every 24 hr
Cefaclor	250–500 mg every 8 hr	0.125–0.5 every 8 hr	0.125 g every 8 hr
Cefotaxime	2 g every 6–8 hr	2 g every 6–8 hr	1 g every 6–8 hr
Moxalactam	4 g every 8 hr	1–2 g every 8 hr	Further adjustment only necessary for patient with hepatic and renal insufficiency
Ceftizoxime	1–2 g every 8–12 hr	0.5–1 g every 12 hr	0.5–1.0 g every 48 hr
Cefoperazone	1–2 g every 12 hr	1–2 g every 12 hr	1–2 g every 12 hr

showing bactericidal urinary concentrations in vitro is often required.

Gram-Positive Organisms

The cephalosporins are active against most gram-positive organisms including penicillinase-producing staphylococci. Methicillin-resistant staphylococci are generally resistant to cephalosporins regardless of in vitro sensitivity testing results.

Gram-Negative Organisms

Cephalothin, cefazolin, cephapirin, and cephradine are considered effective against three common gram-negative bacilli, that is, *E. coli, P. mirabilis,* and *Klebsiella*.[23-25] Though these agents have some activity against *Haemophilus influenzae,* ampicillin and chloramphenicol are considered the agents of choice.[26] The first-generation cephalosporins have marginal effects on the enterobacteriaceae (*Serratia; Enterobacter; Enterococci; Salmonella; Shigella;* and indole-positive *Proteus* including *P. morganii, P. vulgaris, P. rettgeri; Citrobacter;* and *Providencia*), *Pseudomonas,* and *Bacteroides* organisms.

Cefoxitin has an extended spectrum of activity over the first generation cephalosporins and has more in vitro activity against β-lactamase-producing bacteria. It is effective against indole-positive *Proteus* (*P. morganii, P. rettgeri,* and *P. vulgaris*), *Serratia, Providencia,* and *Bacteroides fragilis*.[27-29] Cefoxitin is, however, not as active as penicillin against other anaerobes: peptostreptococci, *Fusobacteria,* and *Clostridia*.[28] It is also less effective than penicillin or ampicillin against *St. pneumoniae, St. pyogenes, H. influenzae,* and has poor activity against *Enterobacter, Citrobacter, Acinetobacter,* and *Pseudomonas*.[28] Though gentamicin remains the drug of choice in *Serratia* infections, resistant strains may respond to cefoxitin.[30] For treating anerobes, the increased activity of cefoxitin against bacteroides has proved useful, particularly when treating mixed infections caused by both aerobic and anaerobic pathogens where *B. fragilis* is suspected to be the primary pathogen.

Prophylaxis

The cephalosporins are useful agents for gynecologic surgical antimicrobial prophylaxis.[31] The first generation agents are especially suited for this purpose, as they provide adequate coverage for common pathogens and are lower in cost than second- and third-generation agents. Newer cephalosporins with longer half-lives may prove cost effective in this area, as administration costs of less expensive agents may override the higher drug cost of these agents. Prophylatic antibiotics of any type should be administered immediately prior to surgery and for no more than 24 hours thereafter. The issue of how long prophylatic antibiotics need to be given postoperatively remains controversial; however, 24 hours is considered the maximum length of time.

The benefit of prophylactic antibiotics for patients undergoing vaginal hysterectomy has been clearly established.[31,32] Cefazolin 1 to 2 g is given IM or IV preoperatively and may be repeated in 8 hours.[32] Although the benefit of antibiotic prophylaxis has not been clearly established in patients undergoing abdominal hysterectomy, the same regimen may be used.

Prophylactic antibiotics are generally not necessary for patients undergoing elective repeat cesarean section. Risk factors warranting prophylaxis include primary cesarean section, premature rupture of membranes, onset of labor prior to procedure, obesity, and hematocrit less than 30 percent.[31] If antimicrobial prophylaxis is desired, cefazolin 1 g is given IV after cord clamping then every 8 hours for two doses.[32] Alternatively, ampicillin 1 g IV may be administered after cord clamping, then 2 and 8 hours postoperatively.[32]

Many studies have been undertaken to determine the value of prophylactic antibiotic therapy to decrease febrile morbidity after cesarean section.[33] These investigations have compared the effectiveness of a specific antibiotic(s) to a placebo in a prospective manner. Findings have shown consistently that prophylactic antibiotics compared with a placebo are effective in decreasing the incidence of febrile morbidity related to endometritis, wound infection, and urinary tract infection. Advantages to such therapy include less prolonged hospitalization, postpartum fever, and patient discomfort. Limitations have included expense and an inability to avoid serious postoperative infections.

The ideal choice of antibiotic therapy has not been established, and each physician is recommended to determine a profile of those persons at moderate or high risk for developing pelvic infection. Conditions known to predispose to postpartum wound infection or endometritis would include prior labor, ruptured amniotic membranes for 6 hours or more, multiple vaginal examinations, and lower socioeconomic patients.

A single antibiotic with broad-spectrum coverage against most pelvic pathogens seems to be as effective as two or more antibiotics. No cephalosporin or penicillin preparation has clearly been found to be more effective than the other. Administering the drug shortly after cord clamping is considered to be as effective as administering the drug preoperatively. An antibiotic needs to be prescribed for 12 hours or less postoperatively, thereby eliminating potential drug complications. Hypersensitivity and anaphylactic shock at the time of surgery are quite uncommon and negligible if screening is done beforehand.

Persons with postoperative complications usually have febrile morbidity attributed to endometritis. Serious pelvic pathogens must be considered, and appropriate cultures obtained before changing antibiotic therapy. Irrigation of the uterus, bladder flap, pelvic cavity, and wound with a diluted antibiotic solution (e.g., cefoxitin or cefamandole 2 g in 1 L normal saline) may be an alternative to parenteral therapy during surgery. The incidence of endometritis following cesarean section has been reported to decrease dramatically despite surgical sites being potentially devascularized and contaminated. More prospective investigations are necessary at several institutions although early reports are promising.[23] The patients should be chosen in a randomized manner with the drug being given in a double-blind manner.

Preparations and Doses

Cephalothin, cefazolin, and cephapirin have very similar therapeutic effectiveness and antimicrobiologic activity.[23,24,34,35] Cefazolin may have some advantages since it causes the least pain on IM injection, can be administered either IM or IV, and attains higher serum and tissue levels. It therefore can be administered less frequently, and in smaller doses. Recommended doses of cephalothin and cephapirin and their microbiologic spectra are similar. The authors are unaware of reports in the literature indicating cephapirin to be any more or less effective than cephalothin, and therefore these two drugs should be considered interchangeable. However, since cephalothin has been shown to be the most stable cephalosporin against inactivation by the cephalosporinases produced by some strains of *S. aureus,* it should be considered the cephalosporin of choice for treating difficult staphylococcal infections. Cephradine and cephalexin are also similar and can be considered therapeutically equivalent[25] when oral therapy is necessary. At equivalent doses, cefazolin achieves serum levels that are between two and four times those of cephalothin.[35,36]

Cefoxitin is more active than first-generation cephalosporins against gram-negative bacilli. It has an extended spectrum which includes enterobacteriaceae, *H. influenzae,* and *Neisseria*. It is less active against *S. aureus* but is therapeutically effective. It is active against many strains of *B. fragilis* and related anaerobes and this makes it useful for treating certain mixed aerobic-anaerobic infections.

Cephalexin is the prototype oral cephalosporin. Its antibacterial spectrum is very similar to cephalothin, although it is less active against penicillinase-producing staphylococci.

Cefaclor is a second-generation oral cephalosporin. It has extended activity against gram-negative organisms including *E. coli, K. pneumoniae, P. mirabilis,* and *H. influenzae*. The bioavailability of oral cephalosporins is not affected by the presence of food in the stomach, although lower and delayed peak serum concentrations are obtained.

The third-generation cephalosporins have only fair activity against gram-positive organisms, but they have an expanded spectrum against gram-negative organisms and anaerobes. When antimicrobial spectra are compared, this group of agents is somewhat heterogenous. Most strains of *E. coli, Klebsiella, Haemophilus, Neisseria, Citrobacter diversus, Proteus,* and *Morganella* are susceptible to the third-generation agents.[37-40] As a class, approximately 50 percent of *pseudomonas aeruginosa* isolates show resistance to these agents.[37] Cefoperazone and ceftazidime are more active against *P. aeruginosa,* although this increase in antipseudomonal activity is coupled with a decrease in activity versus other pathogens. Of the group, moxalactam has predictable activity against most strains of *Bacteroides fragilis*.[37,39,40]

The elimination half-lives of these drugs vary within the group. Ceftriaxone can be dosed every 24 hours, ceftizoxime and cefoperazone every 8 to 12 hours, whereas cefotaxime requires dosing every 6 to 8 hours.[37,40] The usual doses of selected cephalosporins are shown in Table 24–5.

Cost-Effectiveness

The purchase of cephalosporins often represents the largest single drug expenditure in most United States hospitals. Where the cephalosporins are comparative and are marketed by more than one company, significant cost savings can be achieved by competitive bidding. The use of third-generation cephalosporins, especially those with longer elimination half-lives, can be cost effective, as their broad spectra may eliminate the need for additional antibiotic use. Although these drugs are more expensive on a gram-per-gram basis, their high potency and longer dosage intervals may result in lower daily cost of therapy to the patient when administration fees are considered.

Adverse Effects

The cephalosporins may be associated with the production of serious untoward effects including hypersensitivity reactions, hematologic reactions, nephrotoxicity, and local reactions such as thrombophlebitis. Allergic reactions may occur. The precise incidence of cross-reactivity between penicillins and cephalosporins is not well defined. Cephalosporins probably should not be administered to individuals who have immediate-type reactions such as urticaria or anaphylaxis to the administration of penicillins. Cephalosporins may elicit allergic reactions in patients who are not allergic to penicillin. Such reactions include anaphylaxis, serum sickness, eosinophilia, fever, and skin eruptions. Therapy with cephalothin and cephaloridine have been associated with a positive Coombs' test, but hemolytic anemia is uncommon. Prolongation of the prothrombin time (PT) has been reported after 5 to 7 days of therapy, especially in malnourished patients and vitamin K may be administered if necessary to improve clotting function. Ten milligrams of vitamin K once per week is now recommended in any patient receiving moxalactam. Colonization and superinfection have been reported in 2 to 5 percent of patients receiving cephalosporins and is more common in patients receiving second- and third-generation agents. Leukopenia has been rarely reported with high doses (> 12 g/day) and is reversible in 2 to 7 days after therapy is discontinued.

Central nervous system toxicity with mental confusion has been reported after high doses in patients with renal failure. Reversible renal tubular necrosis may result from cephaloridine administration. Pain and sterile abscesses at injection sites and phlebitis have been reported. Cefamandole, moxalactam, and cefoperazone has been associated with a disulfiram-like reaction with nausea and vomiting, flushing, and hypotension happening about 30 minutes after administration. The oral cephalosporins have been associated with abdominal distress, diarrhea, hypersensitivity reactions, and rarely, antibiotic-induced pseudomembranous colitis.

TETRACYCLINES

Tetracyclines have a broad spectrum of antimicrobial activity, are relatively well absorbed after oral administration, and are generally well tolerated with few serious adverse effects. Tetracyclines, however, are regarded as the drugs of choice for relatively few microbial pathogens because of their often unpredictable and incomplete coverage of most pathogenic species.

Pharmacology

Tetracyclines block the binding of transfer RNA-amino acid complexes to the ribosome, thus making amino acids unavailable to messenger RNA for protein synthesis.

The major differences in the various tetracycline products relate to their pharmacokinetic characteristics (Table 24–6). The completeness of oral absorption when taken on an empty stomach ranges from 60 to nearly 100 percent with various preparations. Food interferes with absorption. Divalent ions, calcium, aluminum, magnesium, as well as iron preparations, and sodium bicarbonate impair absorption significantly.

Peak serum levels with a 250-mg oral dose of tetracycline are 1 to 3 mcg/ml at 1 to 2 hours and up to 5 mcg/ml with a 500-mg dose.[41] Intravenous therapy with tetracycline, doxycycline, or minocycline gives levels of 15 to 30 mcg/ml depending on the rate of infusion and dose. Intramuscular administration is not recommended due to severe pain and poor absorption. Tetracyclines penetrate tissue and body fluids well. Liver and bile levels are five to ten times higher than simultaneous serum levels. Protein-binding ranges from 55 to 80 percent for all tetracyclines except oxytetracycline, which is 30 percent bound.

Elimination of tetracyclines is primarily by the gastrointestinal tract and urinary tract. Tetracycline and oxytetracycline give the highest urinary levels and are sometimes preferred for urinary tract infections. In patients with impaired renal function, doxycycline may be administered without reduction in dosage and is the drug of choice for extrarenal infections. In these patients, the half-life of tetracycline and oxytetracycline increases to about 100 hours. The half-lives of chlortetracycline, doxycycline, and minocycline are about doubled by impaired renal function.

Tetracyclines cross the placental barrier and relatively high concentrations are found in human milk and therefore should not be prescribed to nursing mothers. Tetracyclines should not be used for the treatment of urinary tract infections in pregnant women (Chap. 2). Doxycycline and minocycline are more convenient for patients due to twice-daily dosing and are least affected by concomitant food.

Clinical Uses—Spectrum of Activity

The tetracyclines are active against many gram-positive and gram-negative bacteria as well as rickettsia, mycoplasma, and chlamydia. The antibacterial spectrum, although broad, is often unpredictable. Most gonococci, *H. influenza,* and *St. pneumoniae* are sensitive, but there is increasing resistance among each of the species. Resistance among gram-positive bacteria include about 50 percent of *S. aureus,* 30 percent of β-hemolytic streptococci, and virtually all enterococci. Susceptibility of *E. coli, P. mirabilis, Klebsiella, Shigella,* and *Salmonella* organisms is quite variable. Most strains of indole-positive *Proteus, Serratia, P. aeruginosa, Providencia,* and *Enterobacter* are resistant. Activity against anaerobes is erratic—as many as 40 percent of peptostreptococci, 40 percent of

TABLE 24–6. PHARMACOKINETICS OF TETRACYCLINES[42,43]

Product	Adult Dose		% Oral Absorption	Half-Life (hr)	Peak Serum Concentration (mcg/ml)	Excretion
	Oral	*IV*				
Demeclocycline (Declomycin)	250–300 mg four times a day		70	15	2–4	40% renal
Doxycycline (Vibramycin)	100 mg every 12 hr first day, then 100–200 mg/day in one or two doses	200 mg initially, then 100 mg every 12 hr	90	15 (15–36) ESRD*	2–6 PO 15–30 IV	10% renal
Minocycline (Minocin, Vectrin)	200 mg initially, then 100 mg every 12 hr	200 mg initially, then 100 mg every 12 hr	100	17 (17–30) ESRD	2–4 PO 15–30 IV	Metabolized
Tetracycline	250–500 mg four times a day	250–500 mg every 12 hr should not exceed 2 g/day	80	10	2–4 PO 15–30 IV	60% renal

* ESRD = End-stage renal disease.

B. melanerogenicus, and 30 to 60 percent of *B. fragilis* are resistant.

The analogues of tetracyclines show similar spectra of activity. An exception would be minocycline, which is more active against *S. aureus* and *Nocardia asteroides*. In all instances, other antimicrobials are considered the agents of choice for infection involving these pathogens. Minocycline and doxycycline are somewhat more active against anaerobes and facultative gram-negative bacilli. While doxycycline is the best tetracycline against anaerobes, one-third of *B. fragilis* strains remains resistant at readily achievable blood concentrations.

Adverse Effects

Common Effects

Gastrointestinal side effects are common and include nausea, vomiting, anorexia, unpleasant taste, pruritis, and diarrhea. Superinfections are common and include oral candidiasis and vulvovaginitis. Hypersensitivity reactions are also common and include rashes, fever, and eosinophilia. Photosensitivity may occur with any tetracycline, especially with demeclocycline. Photosensitivity may be avoided with a sunscreen preparation. Vestibular toxicity is unique to minocycline and has been reported in up to 90 percent of patients receiving this drug. This effect is dose-related and reversible.

Tetracyclines are deposited in developing teeth during early stages of calcification and may cause a dose-related yellow-brown mottling effect. There may also be disturbances in fetal bone growth. These potential complications contraindicate the use of tetracycline in children under 8 years old and in any pregnant woman.

Intravenous administration frequently causes thrombophlebitis. Increases in blood urea nitrogen (BUN) may occur because of the inhibition of hepatic protein synthesis while catabolism continues. In the presence of impaired renal function there may be increasing acidosis, hyperphosphatemia, anorexia, nausea, vomiting, weight loss, and severe electrolyte disturbances. These effects may be noted with any tetracycline other than doxycycline.

Uncommon Effects

Hepatotoxicity ranges from mildly abnormal liver function tests to severe hepatic failure with jaundice followed by azotemia, acidosis, shock, and death. Hepatotoxicity is usually related to excessive dose (>2 g/day), pregnancy, renal disease, or previous hepatic disease. Pregnant women also appear to have a greater than normal chance of developing pancreatitis following tetracycline administration. Because many alternative drugs are available, tetracyclines should be avoided entirely in the pregnant patient.

Rare Effects

The ingestion of outdated tetracycline has been associated with the Fanconi syndrome. Pseudomembranous enterocolitis has also been rarely reported. A number of recent cases of injury to the esophagus have been reported with tetracyclines, especially doxycycline capsules. The pH of a solution of doxycycline in water is about 1.0 and when passage of such capsules down the esophagus is delayed, injury is likely to result. Patients should be counseled to swallow tetracycline products with a glass of water with the patient in an upright position. These drugs should not be taken immediately before bedtime or when lying down.

CHLORAMPHENICOL

Pharmacology

Chloramphenicol has bacteriostatic activity through an inhibition of microbial protein production by suppressing peptidyl transferase activity on the 50 S-subunit of the ribosome.

It is well absorbed after oral administration with peak blood levels of 3 to 6 mcg/ml following a 500-mg dose and 8 to 15 mcg/ml following a 1-g dose. Absorption from IM injection is poor. Peak serum concentrations with intravenous administration in the usual doses are 10 to 20 mcg/ml, depending on the infusion rate. Chloramphenicol penetrates well into tissues and body fluids because of its high lipid solubility. Most of the drug is inactivated by conjugation with glucuronide in the liver. The half-life of 2 to 3 hours in patients with normal liver function increases in the presence of severe hepatic disease with jaundice. Chloramphenicol may inhibit the metabolism of tolbutamide, phenytoin, and warfarin, and increases in half-lives of these drugs have been reported.[44] Most of the drug is excreted in the urine with about 5 percent excreted unchanged. Renal failure results in the accumulation of nontoxic metabolites with minimal influence on the half-life of the active form. Severe liver disease increases the potential for high levels of free chloramphenicol due to decreased glucuronide conjugation. Serum concentrations greater than 25 mcg/ml should be avoided due to potential for hematologic toxicity.[42]

Chloramphenicol is available for oral and intravenous use. The usual dose is 50 to 100 mg/kg/day in four divided doses. Maximum doses for adults with severe renal disease are 2 to 3 g/day. Ascites or jaundice due to liver disease is a relative contraindication to chloramphenicol.

Antibacterial Activity

Chloramphenicol is highly active in vitro against all anaerobic microorganisms. This drug is indicated for a variety of bacterial, rickettsial, and chlamydial infections. Because of hematologic toxicity, its use is usually limited to typhoid fever, ampicillin-resistant *H. influenzae,* and certain central nervous system suppurative infections. Chloramphenicol has failed in a small number of *B. fragilis* sepsis patients even though the organism was sensitive in vitro. Chloramphenicol is the drug of choice for treatment of typhoid fever and other systemic *Salmonella* infections. Chloramphenicol should *not* be used to treat infections caused by staphylococci, *St. pneumoniae,* or β-hemolytic streptococci. These microorganisms are susceptible in vitro to chloramphenicol, but safer, more effective therapy is available. Penicillin G is the drug of choice for all anaerobic infections except those caused by *B. fragilis*. Activity against aerobic gram-negative bacilli is erratic, but *E. coli, Shigella,* and *P. mirabilis* are generally sensitive. About 30 to 60 percent of *Klebsiella, Citrobacter,* indole-positive *Proteus, Providencia,* and *Serratia* are susceptible, but *P. aeruginosa* is almost always resistant.

Adverse Effects

The most important toxic effect of chloramphenicol is bone marrow suppression, which occurs in a dose-related form and as an idiosyncratic reaction. Dose-related bone marrow suppression occurs particularly when plasma concentrations exceed 25 mcg/ml with daily doses of 4 g or more and with prolonged therapy. The clinical picture is characterized by anemia, pancytopenia, and increased serum iron concentration. Serious granulocytopenia is rare if treatment with chloramphenicol is discontinued when white blood cell counts decrease to less than 4000/mm^3 and the neutrophil percentage decreases to less than 40 percent.[42] Recovery from dose-related bone marrow suppression usually occurs within 3 weeks after use of the drug has been stopped.

Idiosyncratic aplastic anemia is rare. It has only been documented in cases where the drug is administered orally, usually in persons who have received prolonged therapy and especially in those who have received the drug on multiple occasions.[45] Idiosyncratic aplastic anemia is unrelated to dose. Other side effects include nausea, vomiting, glossitis, stomatitis, diarrhea, and pseudomembranous colitis.

ERYTHROMYCIN

Erythromycin is a macrolide antimicrobial with activity against most gram-positive bacteria, many anaerobes, *Mycoplasma pneu-*

monia and Legionella pneumophilia (Legionnaire's disease).

Pharmacology

Erythromycin inhibits protein synthesis by binding with the 50 S-ribosomal subunit, thereby interfering with the site where amino acids are transferred to protein. The drug is bacteriostatic but may be bactericidal at high concentrations. It is available as estolate, ethylsuccinate, gluceptate, lactobionate, and stearate salts.

Absorption of all erythromycin preparations is mainly in the duodenum. The bioavailability of oral preparations depends on formulation, the gastric acidity and emptying time, and the effect of multiple dosing.[46] Erythromycin base is acid labile and therefore commercially available as an enteric-coated tablet (resistant to gastric acid). The stearate is less water soluble and therefore protected to some extent against gastric acid. The ethylsuccinate is partially dissociated in the intestine, and once absorbed, it is hydrolyzed to free erythromycin. Erythromycin estolate is acid stable and dissociates in the intestine and becomes hydrolyzed in the blood to the free base.

Peak blood levels of active drug after a 500-mg oral dose usually range from 3 to 10 mcg/ml. Serum levels obtained with a 500-mg IV infusion of the lactobionate are 8 to 12 mcg/ml. Peak blood levels are seen 30 to 90 minutes after oral administration, and the half-life is 1.5 to 2.5 hours.

Erythromycin is excreted primarily in the bile while only 2 to 5 percent is excreted in the urine. Erythromycin is present in maternal milk and crosses the placental barrier (although fetal levels are <25 percent of maternal blood levels).[47]

Antibacterial Activity

Erythromycin is active against most gram-positive bacteria, including streptococci such as *St. pneumoniae,* group A and B β-hemolytic streptococci, and most enterococci. Most strains are sensitive to concentrations of 0.5 mcg/ml or less at neutral pH. The activity of erythromycin increases at a pH of 8. Susceptibility of *S. aureus* is variable: Most community-acquired strains are susceptible, but up to 50 percent of hospital-acquired strains are resistant in institutions where the drug is extensively used.

H. influenzae, Neisseria, C. diphtheriae, Pasteurella mutlocida, Listeria, brucella, rickettsia, mycoplasma, chlamydia, and treponemes strains are usually sensitive. Activity versus anaerobic bacteria is erratic.[48] Less than half of *F. nucleatum* and *B. fragilis* are susceptible to 4 mcg/ml. Most anaerobic gram-positive cocci are susceptible. Aerobic and facultative gram-negative bacteria are resistant but may be susceptible to urinary levels in alkaline media.

Indications

The parenteral use of erythromycin is limited because of the frequency of thrombophlebitis. In most instances the drug is given orally where the primary uses are for respiratory tract infections. Penicillins are preferred for most of these infections but erythromycin is a suitable alternative for patients who are penicillin-sensitive. Erythromycin is the agent of choice for *M. pneumoniae* and Legionnaires' disease.[42] The American Heart Association recommends erythromycin as an alternative to penicillin for both treatment and prevention of pharyngeal infections caused by group A β-hemolytic streptococci. For venereal disease, erythromycin is an alternative agent for penicillin-allergic patients with syphilis or pregnant patients with uncomplicated gonorrhea. (See Table 24–4). It may also be used as an alternative to tetracyclines for genital infections due to *C. trachomatis*. Cystitis and pyelonephritis caused by gram-negative bacilli may be treated with erythromycin and urine alkalinization with 12 to 15 g of sodium bicarbonate daily.

Dosage

Adult oral doses range from 250 to 1000 mg (30 to 60 mg/kg/day) every 6 hours. The usual dose is 500 mg every 6 hours. No dosage adjustment is necessary in renal failure.

Intravenous preparations are usually administered in 1 to 4 g/day in two to four divided doses.

Adverse Reactions

The major adverse reactions with oral preparations are epigastric distress, nausea, and diarrhea. These are dose-related and rarely ecessitate discontinuing the drug.

The most serious toxicity is cholestatic hepatitis, which occurs only with the estolate salt. Symptoms include fever, abdominal pain, nausea, vomiting, jaundice, and dark urine. The onset usually occurs 10 to 20 days after initial exposure or immediately after reexposure. Laboratory abnormalities include leukocytosis, eosinophilia with increased bilirubin, alkaline phosphatase, and serum alanine aminotransferase. Most patients improve promptly when the drug is discontinued. Hypersensitivity reactions such as rash and drug fever are rare. Intramuscular administration is extremely painful and is therefore not recommended. Intravenous administration may cause pain during infusion with a high incidence of phlebitis.[42]

CLINDAMYCIN

Clindamycin inhibits the initiation of peptide chain synthesis, and is similar to chloramphenicol and erythromycin. Clindamycin is bactericidal against some, but not all, susceptible bacteria.

Pharmacokinetics

Oral preparations are nearly completely absorbed. Peak serum levels of 3 to 5 mcg/ml are achieved at 30 to 45 minutes after oral administration of 300 mg of clindamycin hydrochloride or palmitate. Concurrent food administration has little effect on serum levels. There is only a modest increase in peak levels with repeated dosing at 6- to 8-hour intervals. Intramuscular injections of 300 mg produce levels of 3 to 5 mcg/ml, while 600-mg doses give peak levels of about 8 mcg/ml. Intravenous administration of 600 mg yields peak levels of 10 to 45 mcg/ml.[42] Clindamycin is extensively distributed throughout body tissues with the exception of the eye and central nervous system. The half-life is 2 to 3 hours and only slightly increased in renal failure. Half-life increases dramatically (~ five times) in hepatic failure. Clindamycin readily (10 to 20 percent) crosses the placental barriers.[47]

Spectrum of Activity

Clindamycin is active against most gram-positive bacteria, streptococci (not enterococci), and *S. aureus*. Most anaerobic bacteria are susceptible to clindamycin at 0.5 mcg/ml or less. This includes *B. fragilis,* which accounts for 75 percent of anaerobic bacteremias and is a major isolate in female genital tract infections.

Indications

One indication for clindamycin is serious infection in which *B. fragilis* is an established or suspected pathogen. This includes intraabdominal sepsis, infections of the female upper genital tract, and selected soft tissue infection. In most instances the drug is combined with another agent that is active against aerobic gram-negative bacilli, since these conditions are usually mixed aerobic-anaerobic infections.

Dosage

Clindamycin preparations are the hydrochloride, the 2-palmitic acid ester and the 2-phosphoric acid ester. The two esters are not biologically active and must be hydrolyzed in the blood. Clindamycin hydrochloride is recommended for oral use with adult doses of 150 to 450 mg every 6 to 8 hours, usually 300 mg every 6 hours. Concurrent food administration has little effect on serum levels. IM or IV doses are usually 300 to 600 mg every 6 to 8 hours or 900 mg every 8 hours for severe infections. No dose modification is necessary in renal failure. The usual parenteral dose in patients with severe liver disease is 300 mg every 8 hours.

Adverse Reactions

Major adverse reactions are gastrointestinal complications ranging from common, uncomplicated diarrhea to serious pseudomembranous colitis. This colitis is believed to be caused by an enterotoxin produced by *C. difficile,* and probably occurs in about 0.01 percent of cases. While both the oral and parenteral forms of clindamycin may cause pseudomembranous colitis, there appears to be a modest increase in the incidence of this complication with oral administration.[49] Treatment consists of discontinuing clindamycin, avoiding antiperistaltic medications such as diphenoxylate, and oral treatment with metronidazole or vancomycin to decrease overgrowth of *C. difficile*.

Other side effects include a morbilliform rash in 3 to 5 percent of patients. Transient abnormalities of liver function are relatively common. These are not dose-related and they return to baseline values when the drug is discontinued or treatment continued.

METRONIDAZOLE

At physiologic pH, metronidazole[50–53] is taken up by aerobic and anaerobic bacteria. Sensitive anaerobic organisms contain low-redox-potential electron transport proteins. Metronidazole is reduced by these proteins and unstable intermediate compounds in this reaction apparently inhibit DNA synthesis, causing cell death.

Pharmacokinetics

Oral preparations of metronidazole are nearly completely absorbed. One hour after a single 500-mg dose, a peak serum concentration of approximately 10 mcg/ml is achieved. Peak levels are not decreased with concommitant food administration, however, the time to achieve peak concentrations may be delayed. Serum concentrations rise with repeated dosing until a steady state is obtained. Intravenous dosing of 500 mg every 8 hours yields minimum serum concentrations between 5.6 and 21 mcg/ml and maximum concentrations of 14 to 60 mcg/ml. Metronidazole is not significantly bound to serum proteins and is well distributed throughout body fluids and tissues including pelvic organs.[51]

The serum half-life of metronidazole is approximately 8 hours in patients with normal renal function. The drug is metabolized extensively by hepatic oxidative enzymes, and no dosage adjustment is necessary for patients in renal failure.[52] Although dosing regimens have not been developed for patients with impaired hepatic function, the plasma clearance of the drug is reduced in this population.

Spectrum of Activity

Metronidazole possesses activity solely against facultative or obligate anaerobic bacteria. Metronidazole is active against most gram-negative anaerobic bacilli, including *B. fragilis*. It also possesses activity against *Clostridia* species including *C. perfringens*. Anaerobic, non-spore-forming gram-positive bacilli, including *Propionibacterium spp.,* are relatively resistant to metronidazole. Both anaerobic gram-positive and gram-negative cocci are susceptible to metronidazole. Metronidazole is active against anaerobic protozoa including *Trichomonas vaginalis*.[50]

Indications

Metronidazole is indicated in the treatment of certain vaginal infections (Chap. 23) and infections in which *B. fragilis* is implicated, and can be combined with agents possessing aerobic activity in empiric therapy until culture results have been obtained. Due to its broad anaerobic spectrum and considerably lower cost, metronidazole is often preferred over clindamycin.

Metronidazole is also an alternative to oral vancomycin in the treatment of *C. difficile* enterocolitis, a recognized side effect of many antimicrobial agents, at a great cost savings compared to vancomycin treatment.[53]

Dosing

In the treatment of anaerobic bacterial infections, an IV loading dose of 15 mg/kg followed by 7.5 mg/kg every 6 hours is recommended, although the pharmacokinetic parameters of the drug indicate less frequent dosing could be equally effective. In the treatment of trichomonal infections, metronidazole may be administered either as a single 2-g dose or a regimen of 250 mg orally three times daily for 7 days. The latter regiment is preferred for patients with recurrent infection. The sexual contacts of infected individuals should receive treatment.

The single dose regimen may be used in this instance.

Adverse Reactions

The incidence of adverse side effects associated with metronidazole is low. A metallic taste in the mouth, and gastrointestinal side effects including anorexia, nausea, vomiting, and some diarrhea have occurred. Metronidazole may produce a disulfiramlike reaction in some patients who ingest alcohol during therapy; patients should therefore be counseled to avoid alcohol intake during treatment. Neurologic side effects such as ataxia, dizziness, and confusion have been reported, as well as reversible neutropenia and discoloration of the urine to a reddish-brown color.

Prolonged high-dose metronidazole has been linked with mutagenicity in laboratory animals. The use of metronidazole in the low-dosage range used in humans has not been linked with carcinogenesis in humans, although extensive long-term studies have not been undertaken. Avoidance of the medication during the first trimester of pregnancy is recommended.

AMINOGLYCOSIDES

Pharmacology

Aminoglycoside antibiotics in clinical use include streptomycin, kanamycin, gentamicin, tobramycin, netilmicin, and amikacin. They bind irreversibly to bacterial ribosomes, blocking the recognition step in protein synthesis and causing misreading of the genetic code.

The aminoglycosides are (1) bactericidal for a wide range of gram-positive and gram-negative species and mycobacteria, (2) minimally absorbed from the gut, (3) their dosage is more accurately calculated on the basis of lean rather than total body weight, and (4) elimination occurs almost entirely by the kidney.

These antibiotics are well absorbed by IM injection producing peak serum levels after about 1 hour. Less than 1 percent of an oral dose is absorbed and the resultant serum levels are usually insignificant in patients with normal renal function. Repeated oral dosing may result in accumulation in patients with impaired renal function. These drugs have similar volumes of distribution and are minimally protein bound. Aminoglycosides are distributed in extracellular fluid volume which constitutes about 30 percent of lean body weight (about 20 L in the average adult). Intrathecal administration is necessary to ensure adequate concentration in the cerebrospinal fluid (CSF). Placental tissue levels are approximately 25 to 50 percent of those in the serum. These drugs have a marked affinity for renal cortical tissue, accumulating in concentrations that are 10 to 50 times those in serum. Aminoglycosides are eliminated from the body by renal glomerular filtration. The half-life of 2 to 3 hours in patients with normal renal function is markedly increased in the renally impaired patient.

Antimicrobial Activity

All aminoglycosides are negligibly bound to plasma proteins and excreted primarily unchanged by the kidneys. Although the average half-life in patients with normal renal function is 2 to 3 hours, it may range from 0.5 to 10 hours. Patients with impaired renal function excrete the drug more slowly and the half-life in an anuric patient may range from 50 to 80 hours.

Indications for monitoring serum levels of aminoglycosides include: (1) assuring that peak concentrations are in the therapeutic range, (2) patients not responding to therapy, (3) patients with conditions associated with lower peak levels (e.g., obesity and expanded extracellular fluid volume), (4) patients who develop signs or symptoms of ototoxicity or nephrotoxicity, (5) patients undergoing dialysis, and (6) patients who have received more than 5 days of therapy—even those without obvious impaired renal function.

Gentamicin, Tobramycin, Netilmicin, and Amikacin

All these agents are indicated for serious aerobic gram-negative infections including those in which *P. aeruginosa* is suspected of being an etiologic agent. Where possible, culture and sensitivity results as well as resistance patterns should guide the physician in the selection of one of these agents.

Tobramycin is similar to gentamicin, and bacteria highly resistant to gentamicin are usually also resistant to tobramycin. While most strains of *Pseudomonas* are sensitive to tobramycin and gentamicin, tobramycin may be inhibitory at one-third the concentration of gentamicin. *Serratia* may be less sensitive to tobramycin than to gentamicin. Amikacin is similar to gentamicin but active against many isolates of *Proteus* and *Serratia* that are resistant to gentamicin and tobramycin.

Seriously ill patients should receive a loading dose in order to initially achieve therapeutic plasma concentrations (Table 24–7). For tobramycin or gentamicin this should be 2 mg/kg, for amikacin this should be 7.5 mg/kg, and for netilmicin 1.3 to 2.2 mg/kg. Although these drugs do not completely distribute to adipose tissue, it is recommended to administer the loading dose based upon total body weight in a critically ill patient to avoid subtherapeutic levels. Amikacin should be considered only where organisms are resistant to gentamicin, tobramycin, and netilmicin. The initial maintenance dose should be based on the nomogram in Table 24–8.[56] This nomogram is based upon average data and should be employed for initial therapy only. The recommended dosing interval for gentamicin and tobramycin for patients with creatinine clearance <50 ml/min is 12 hours, and 24 hours for those with a creatinine clearance <10 ml/min. An IV dose should be administered over 30 minutes. In patients with relatively stable renal function, peak plasma concentration can be obtained by sampling 60 minutes after the loading dose infusion is completed and again immediately before the maintenance dose. These values may be used to calculate steady state peak and trough levels. In patients with unstable renal function or those who did not have drug levels drawn after the loading dose, serum levels may be drawn 60 minutes after the infusion is complete and immediately before the next dose. These values represent peak and trough levels. Where gentamicin, tobramycin, netilmicin, or amikacin are administered intramuscularly, peak serum levels should be drawn at 1 to 1½ hours for gentamicin, amikacin, and tobramycin and again immediately before the next dose. Peak and trough levels should be checked every 3 to 4 days to avoid toxicity and assure therapeutic levels.

Peritonitis and suppurative pelvic disease (including pelvic inflammatory disease,

TABLE 24–7. AMINOGLYCOSIDE DOSES IN ADULTS WITH NORMAL AND IMPAIRED RENAL FUNCTION

	Desirable Serum Level (mg/ml)				Impaired Renal Functions	
Antibiotic	***Peak***	***Trough***	**Toxic Range (mg/ml)**	**Dosage, Normal Renal Function IM or IV (mg/kg/bw)***	***Initial Loading Dose (mg/kg/bw)***	***Maintenance Dose***
Gentamicin	5–8	<2	>10–12	IM/IV 1.5–2.0 every 8 hr	1.5–2.0	Adjusted based on creatinine clearance
Netilmicin	6–10	<2	>16	IM/IV 1.3–2.2 every 8 hr	1.3–2.2	
Tobramycin	5–8	<2	>10–12	IM/IV 1.5–2.0 every 8 hr	1.5–2.0	Same as above
Amikacin	15–25	<8–10	>30–35	IM/IV 5.0–7.5 every 8 hr	5.0–7.5	Same as above

* In obese patients, doses should be calculated based on "ideal" or "lean" body weight: Male = 160 lb + 5 lb/in. over 5 ft, female = 100 lb + 5 lb/in. over 5 ft.
Adapted from Guisti DL, 1973;[54] Jackson EA, McLeod DC, 1974,[55] with permission.

TABLE 24–8. MAINTENANCE DOSE SELECTION (AS PERCENTAGE OF CHOSEN LOADING DOSE) OF AMINOGLYCOSIDE TO CONTINUE PEAK SERUM LEVELS INDICATED*

		Percentage of Loading Dose Required for Dosage Interval Selected		
Creat. Clear. (ml/min)	Half-Life (hr)	8 hr	12 hr	24 hr
90	3.1	84	—	—
80	3.4	80	91	—
70	3.9	76	88	—
60	4.5	71	84	—
50	5.3	65	79	—
40	6.5	57	72	92
30	8.4	48	63	86
25	9.9	43	57	81
20	11.9	37	50	73
17	13.6	33	46	70
15	15.1	31	42	67
12	17.9	27	37	61
10	20.4	24	34	56
7	25.9	19	28	47
5	31.5	16	23	41
2	46.8	11	16	30
0	69.3	8	11	21

* According to desired dosing interval and the patient's correct creatinine clearance.
Adapted from Sarubbi FA, Hull HJ, 1978.[56]

chorioamnionitis, postpartum endomyometritis, and postsurgical infections) are generally caused by a mixture of anaerobic and facultatively aerobic organisms. These infections usually respond well to a combination of antibiotics designed to cover this spectrum. If there is any likelihood of the presence of the gonococcus, penicillin G or ampicillin should be added. Although aminoglycosides are not drugs of choice, they cover unsuspected *S. aureus* and *S. epidermidis, Salmonella,* and *H. influenzae* until more effective and safer therapy can be selected.

The aminoglycosides are not effective against anaerobic bacteria, anaerobic cocci, most strains of streptococci (including β-hemolytic streptococci and *St. viridans*), enterococci, and pneumococci. Staphylococci are readily inhibited by aminoglycosides, but penicillins and cephalosporins provide much safer therapy for infections due to these organisms.

Adverse Effects

Allergic reactions such as eosinophilia and rash occur in approximately 1 percent of patients receiving aminoglycosides. The most important adverse effects of this group of drugs are toxic rather than allergic in nature, affecting the auditory-vestibular apparatus and the kidneys. These reactions can be roughly correlated to the length of treatment, preexisting renal impairment, and other factors. It is not clear whether the toxicity is primarily related to an excessively high peak serum concentration or to an excessively high trough concentration.

Two types of ototoxicity have been observed. Cochlear damage manifested by varying degrees of high-tone hearing loss and vestibular impairment with nystagmus, nausea, and vertigo. There is considerable disagreement as to the evidence of ototoxicity (and its reversibility) caused by aminoglycosides.

The ototoxic effects of aminoglycosides are potentiated by coadministration of ethacrynic acid, furosemide, and mannitol.

Aminoglycosides may damage the proximal tubular cells of the kidney. The resultant clinical picture is that of acute tubular necrosis of greater or lesser degree. The mechanism of this phenomenon is not established; however, it is known that these antibiotics accumulate in renal cortical tissue in concentrations that greatly exceed those in serum and persist there for days following a single dose of drug. Renal damage is usually reversible if the aminoglycoside is discontinued at the first signs of renal dysfunction such as a rising BUN, serum creatinine, or the presence of protein and tubular cells in the urine.

Other potentially important adverse reactions include neuromuscular blockade. This effect is similar to that produced by *d*-tubocurarine. Patients with myasthenia gravis or severe hypoglycemia as well as patients who have recently received other neuromuscular-blocking drugs appear to be particularly sensitive to this effect. The propensity of the various congeners to block neuromuscular transmission is neomycin > streptomycin > kanamycin and amikacin > gentamicin and tobramycin. Blockade can be partially or completely reversed by the intravenous administration of calcium salts.

VANCOMYCIN

Vancomycin is a glycopeptide antibiotic not structurally related to any other available antibiotic. Its primary mode of bactericidal action is by inhibition of bacterial cell wall synthesis by blocking peptidoglycan formation.[57,58]

Pharmacokinetics

Vancomycin is minimally absorbable by the GI tract. Intravenous administration of 1 g of vancomycin yielded 2-hour postdose levels of approximately 25 mcg/ml.[59] Vancomycin distribution is best described by a two- or three-compartment open model, with a terminal half-life of approximately 6 hours in patients with normal renal function.[59,60] The bulk of the scientific literature indicates that vancomycin is excreted solely by a renal mechanism, although vancomycin clearance shows a poor linear correlation with measured creatinine clearance, and two studies suggest the existence of a nonrenal route of elimination.[60,61] The half-life of the drug appears to increase in both renal and hepatic insufficiency.[60,61] Vancomycin is moderately distributed to body tissues but has poor central nervous system penetration.

Spectrum of Activity

Vancomycin exhibits excellent activity against gram-positive cocci and bacilli and is the drug of choice in the treatment of methicillin-resistant *S. aureus*. The great majority of *Clostridia* are susceptible to vancomycin, leading to its use in antibiotic-associated colitis. Gram-negative bacilli are not sensitive to the drug, although it is effective against gram-negative cocci.

Indications

Vancomycin is the drug of choice in the treatment of methicillin-resistant *S. aureus* infections and is the classic therapy for *C. difficile* colitis.

Dosage

Vancomycin 500 mg can be administered every 6 to 12 hours in the treatment of systemic infections. Serum concentrations should be monitored in patients with serious infections and/or renal (hepatic) impairment. Predose levels of 5 to 10 mg/ml and postdose concentrations of 30 to 40 mg/ml have been recommended.

Oral doses of 125 mg every 6 hours have been shown effective in the treatment of *C. difficile* colitis.[62]

Adverse Reactions

Rapid infusion rates of vancomycin can result in a histaminelike reaction, commonly including erythema and flushing of the neck (red neck syndrome). These symptoms are sometimes accompanied by hypotension and tachycardia and can generally be avoided by administering a 500-mg dose in 250 ml of fluid and infusing the dose over at least 1 hour.

Ototoxicity in the form of tinnitus or hearing loss has been associated with excessive serum concentrations (>80 mcg/ml). Nephrotoxicity has not been clearly related to serum concentrations, and it is thought that newer purer preparations of vancomycin have less nephrotoxic potential. Other adverse reactions reported with vancomycin therapy include thrombophlebitis, allergic reactions (especially rash), drug fever, and leukopenia.

REFERENCES

1. Jacobson L, Westrom L: Objectivized diagnosis of acute pelvic inflammatory disease. Am J Obstet Gynecol 105:1088, 1969
2. Monif GRG, Welkos SL: Infectious morbidity due to *Bacteroides fragilis* in obstetric patients. Clin Obstet Gynecol 19:131, 1976
3. Ledger WJ: Laparoscopy in the diagnosis and management of patients with suspected salpingo-oophoritis. Am J Obstet Gynecol 138: 1012, 1980
4. di Zerega G, Yonekura L, Roy S, et al.: A comparison of clindamycin-gentamicin and penicillin-gentamicin in the treatment of post-cesarean section endomyometritis. Am J Obstet Gynecol 134:238, 1979
5. Sweet RL, Ledger WJ: Cefoxitin: Single-agent treatment of mixed aerobic-anaerobic pelvic infections. Obstet Gynecol 54:193, 1979
6. Platt LD, Yonekura ML, Ledger WJ: The role of anaerobic bacteria in postpartum endomyometritis. Am J Obstet Gynecol 135:814, 1979
7. Westrom L: Effect of acute pelvic inflammatory disease on fertility. Am J Obstet Gynecol 121:707, 1975
8. Mardh PA, Ripa T, Svensson L, et al.: *Chlamydia trachomatis* infection in patients with acute salpingitis. N Engl J Med 296:1377, 1977
9. Paavonen J: *Chalmydia trachomatis* in acute salpingitis. Am J Obstet Gynecol 138:957, 1980
10. Ripa KT, Svensson L, Treharne JD, et al.: *Chlamydia trachomatis* infection in patients with laparoscopically verified acute salpingitis. Am J Obstet Gynecol 138:960, 1980
11. Bennett WM, Muther RS, Parker RA, et al.: Drug prescribing in renal failure: Dosing guidelines for adults. Am J Kidney Dis 3:155, 1983
12. Finland M, Garner C, Wilcox C, et al.: Susceptibility of pneumococci and *Haemophilus influenzae* to antibacterial agents. Antimicrob Agents Chemother 9:274, 1976
13. Finland M, Garner C, Wilcox C, et al.: Susceptibility of beta-hemolytic streptococci to 65 antibacterial agents. Antimicrob Agents Chemother 9:11, 1976
14. Sutter VL: Susceptibility of anaerobic bacteria to 23 antimicrobial agents. Antimicrob Agents Chemother 10:736, 1976
15. Shulman ST, Amren DP, Bisno AL, et al.: Prevention of bacterial endocarditis: A statement for health professionals by the Committee on Rheumatic Fever and Infective Endocarditis of the Council on Cardiovascular Disease in the Young. Circulation 70:1123A, 1984
16. Finefold SM: Anaerobic infections. Arch Intern Med 139:144, 1979
17. Neu HC: Antimicrobial activity and human pharmacology of amoxicillin. J Infect Dis 129:123, 1974
18. Neu HC, Garvey GJ: Comparative *in vitro* activity and clinical pharmacology of ticarcillin and carbenicillin. Antimicrob Agents Chemother 8:462, 1972
19. Pitts JC: Allergic penicillin reactions. J Kansas Med Soc 72:322, 1971
20. Maheras MG: Penicillin hypersensitivity. Minn Med 52:1811, 1969
21. Sanders WF Jr, Sanders CC: Toxicity of antibacterial agents: Mechanism of action on mammalian cells. Annu Rev Pharmacol Toxicol 19:53, 1979
22. Miller AK, Celozzi E, Pelak BA, et al.: Cephamycins: A new family of β-lactam. Antibiot Antimicrob Agents Chemother 5:25, 1974
23. Elliott J, Flaherty J: Comparison of lavage or intravenous antibodies at cesarean section. Obstet Gynecol 67:29, 1986

24. Thrupp LD: Newer cephalosporins and "extended spectrum" penicillins. Annu Rev Pharmacol 14:435, 1974
25. Klastersky J, Daneau D, Weerts D: Cephradine: Antibacterial activity and clinical effectiveness. Chemotherapy 18:191, 1973
26. Medical Letter on Drugs & Therapeutics 26:19, 1984 Revised Edition. New Rochelle, NY, The Medical Letter, Inc., 1984
27. Kirby ER, William MM, Fang IW, et al.: Clinical pharmacology of cefamadole compared with cephalothin. Antimicrob Agents Chemother 9:653, 1976
28. Tally FP, Miao PV, O'Keefe JP, et al.: Cefoxitin therapy of anaerobic and aerobic infections. J Antimicrob Chemother 5:101, 1979
29. Wise R: Use of antibiotics: Cephalosporins. Br Med J 2:40, 1978
30. Yu, VL: *Serratia marcescens:* Historical perspective and clinical review. N Engl J Med 300:887, 1979
31. Cartwright PS, et al.: The use of prophylactic antibiotics in obstetrics and gynecology. A review. Obstet Gynecol Surv 39:537, 1984
32. Duff P, Park RC: Antimicrobial prophylaxis in vaginal hysterectomy: A review. Obstet Gynecol 55:1935, 1980
33. Rayburn WF: Prophylactic antibiotics during cesarean section: An overview of prior clinical investigations. Clin Perinatol 10:461, 1983
34. Kirby ER, William MM, Fang IW, et al.: Clinical pharmacology of cefamadole compared with cephalothin. Antimicrob Agents Chemother 9:653, 1976
35. Nightingale CH, Grlene DS, Quintiliani R: Pharmacokinetics and clinical use of cephalosporins. J Pharmacol Sci 64:1899, 1975
36. Barza M, Miao VW: Antimicrobial spectrum pharmacology and therapeutic use of antibiotics: Part 3. Cephalosporins. Am J Hosp Pharmacol 34:521, 1977
37. Barriere SL, Flaherty JF: Third generation cephalosporins: A critical evaluation. Clin Pharmacol 3:351, 1984
38. Quintiliani R, Nightingale C: Drugs five years later: Cefazolin. Ann Intern Med 89:650, 1978
39. Fass RJ: Comparative in vitro activities of third-generation cephalosporins. Arch Intern Med 143:1743, 1983
40. Neu HC: The new beta-lactamase-stable cephalosporins. Ann Intern Med 97:408, 1982
41. Barr WH, Gerbracht LM, Letcher K, et al.: Assessment of the biologic availability of tetracycline products in man. Clin Pharm Ther 13:97, 1972
42. Wilson WR, Cockerill FR: Tetracyclines, chloramphenicol, erythromycin and clindamycin. Mayo Clin Proc 58:92, 1983
43. Barza M, Scheife RT: Tetracyclines. J Maine Med Assoc 67:368, 1976
44. Christensen LK, Skousted L: Inhibition of drug metabolism by chloramphenicol. Lancet 2:1397, 1969
45. Holt R: Bacterial degradation of chloramphenicol. Lancet 1:1259, 1967
46. Nicholas P: Erythromycin: Clinical review. NY State J Med 77:2088, 1977
47. Philipson A, Sabath LD, Charles D: Transplacental passage of erythromycin and clindamycin. N Engl J Med 288:1219, 1973
48. Sutter LV, Finegold SM: Susceptibility of anaerobic bacteria to 23 antimicrobial agents. Antimicrob Agents Chemother 10:736, 1976
49. Bartlett JG: Antibiotic-associated diarrhea. In Remington JS, Swartz MN (eds): Current Clinical Topics in Infectious Diseases. New York, McGraw-Hill, 1980, pp 240–264
50. Molavi A, Lefrock JL, Prince RA: Metronidazole. Med Clin N Am 66:121, 1982
51. Ralph ED: Clinical pharmacokinetics of metronidazole. Clin Pharmacokinet 8:43, 1983
52. Jensen JC, Gugler R: Single and multiple dose metronidazole kinetics. Clin Pharmacol Ther 34:481, 1983
53. Teasley DG, Gerding DN, Olson MM, et al.: Prospective randomized trial of metronidazole versus vancomycin for clostridium-difficile-associated diarrhea and colitis. Lancet 2:1043, 1983
54. Giusti DL: The clinical use of antimicrobial agents in patients with renal and hepatic insufficiency: The aminoglycosides. Drug Intell Clin Pharmacol 7:540, 1973
55. Jackson EA, McLeod DC: Pharmacokinetics and dosing of antimicrobial agents in renal impairment. Am J Hosp Pharmacol 31:36, 1974
56. Sarubbi FA, Hull HJ: Amikacin serum concentrations: Predictions of levels and dosage guidelines. Ann Intern Med 89:612, 1978
57. Geraci JE, Hermans PE: Vancomycin. Mayo Clin Proc 58:88, 1983
58. Watanakunakorn C: Mode of action and in vitro activity of vancomycin. J Antimicrob Chemother 14(Suppl D):7, 1984

59. Moellering RC: Pharmacokinetics of vancomycin. J Antimicrob Chemother 14(Suppl D):43, 1984
60. Rotschafer JC, Crossley K, Zaske DE, et al.: Pharmacokinetics of vancomycin: observations in 28 patients and dosage recommendations. Antimicrob Agents Chemother 22: 391, 1982
61. Brown N, Ho DW, Fong KL, et al.: Effects of hepatic function on vancomycin clinical pharmacology. Antimicrob Agents Chemother 23:603, 1983
62. Keighley MRB, Burdon DW, Arabic Y, et al.: Randomized controlled trial of vancomycin for pseudomembranous colitis and postoperative diarrhea. Br Med J 2:1667, 1978

25

Urologic Disorders

James K. Crane and Richard C. Bump

Increasingly sophisticated investigative techniques have advanced our knowledge of the dynamics of lower urinary tract function and have allowed a more precise diagnosis of voiding disorders. These advances have led to more rational pharmacologic approaches to alleviate symptoms associated with these disorders. This chapter discusses drugs used in the treatment of certain urologic disorders in women. Their use should be based upon a thorough history, physical examination, and urodynamic evaluation. Only through proper evaluation and knowledge of lower urinary tract function can the proper pharmacologic agent be chosen.

CLINICAL NEUROLOGY OF THE LOWER URINARY TRACT

A complete description of the neurophysiology of the lower urinary tract is beyond the intended scope of this chapter. The interested reader is referred to excellent chapters in several basic textbooks[1-5] for reviews of the complexities and controversies surrounding neuro-urology. We will, however, present a short overview of this subject since it forms the basis for pharmacologic therapy of lower urinary tract disorders.

The lower urinary tract, consisting of the bladder, the urethra, and their supporting structures, has two basic functions. These are the storage of urine and, under appropriate circumstances, the active expulsion of urine. These are basically functions of the peripheral autonomic nervous system that is, in turn, subject to facilitation, inhibition, and coordination by higher neurologic levels. It is useful to conceptualize central nervous system modulation of the lower urinary tract by describing four loops identified by Bradley.[3,4] These interdependent loops connect the cerebral cortex, the brain stem micturition center, the sacral micturition center, and the lower urinary tract. They provide for volitional control of detrusor muscle contraction (loop I, cerebral–brain stem loop), for sustained duration of detrusor muscle contraction to allow complete bladder emptying (loop II, brain stem–sacral loop), for coordination of urethral sphincter relaxation and

TABLE 25-1. THERAPEUTICALLY ORIENTED CLINICAL CLASSIFICATION OF NEURO-UROLOGIC DYSFUNCTION

Detrusor instability (hyperreflexia)
Coordinated sphincters
Striated sphincter dyssynergia
Smooth muscle sphincter dyssynergia
Detrusor hypotonia (areflexia)
Coordinated sphincters
Nonrelaxing striated sphincter
Nonrelaxing smooth muscle sphincter
Denervated striated sphincter
Normally functioning detrusor
Unstable striated sphincter
Unstable smooth muscle sphincter
Striated sphincter dyssynergia
Smooth muscle sphincter dyssynergia

Adapted from Krane and Siroky.[2]

detrusor muscle contraction during micturition (loop III, brain stem–vesical–sacral sphincter loop), and for volitional control of the striated component of the urethral sphincter mechanism (loop IV, cerebral–sacral loop).

Dysfunction of a central loop can be idiopathic, a result of an irritative process in or around the lower urinary tract, or can be due to lesions of the brain, spinal cord, or peripheral nerves. Most frequently, the underlying central cause of a voiding dysfunction is unknown and/or not specifically treatable. Thus, therapy is aimed at relief of symptoms based upon a knowledge of the functional status of both the bladder and the urethra as determined by appropriate testing. A useful, therapeutically-oriented clinical classification of neuro-urologic dysfunction, modified from Krane and Siroky[2] and based on the functional status of both the bladder and the urethra, is presented in Table 25–1. The aim of therapy is to modify the dysfunctional status of the bladder and urethra pharmacologically to achieve symptom relief. This pharmacologic manipulation is almost always with agents that have autonomic affects. Thus a knowledge of autonomic control of the lower urinary tract is essential to select appropriate pharmacologic agents.

The autonomic nervous system's effects on the bladder and urethra are summarized in Table 25–2 and illustrated in Figures 25–1 and 25–2. The parasympathetic (cholinergic) division is micturition promoting and is facilitated by central loops II and III and controlled volitionally by loops I and IV. Cholinergic stimulation of the lower urinary tract results in detrusor muscle contraction and inhibition of the smooth muscle component of the urethral sphincter mechanism.

Sympathetic (adrenergic) discharge, along with central inhibition of parasym-

TABLE 25-2. AUTONOMIC NERVOUS SYSTEM

	Parasympathetic	Sympathetic	
Origin	S2–S4	T10–L2	
Preganglionic fiber	Long	Short	
(neurotransmitter)	Acetylcholine	Acetylcholine	
Postganglionic fiber	Short	Long	
(neurotransmitter)	Acetylcholine	Norepinephrine	
		Alpha	***Beta***
Urethra (smooth muscle)	Relax	Contract→	Relax
Detrusor	Contract	Relax* ←	Relax

* Alpha: direct detrusor effect → contract; depression of parasympathetic ganglion → relax; net effect → relax.

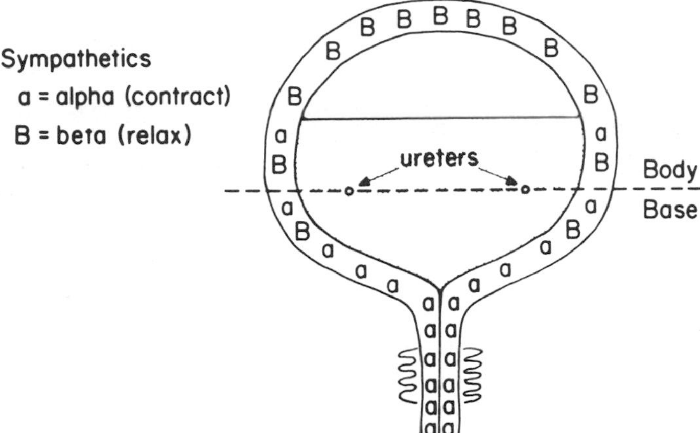

Figure 25–1. Filling phase. The filling phase is mostly a sympathetic process with α-contraction of the bladder base and urethra, β-relaxation of the dome, and α-inhibition of the increasing stimulus of the parasympathetics to discharge as the bladder fills.

pathetic activity, promotes urine storage. Sympathetic β-adrenergic fibers terminate predominantly in the detrusor and their stimulation effects detrusor muscle relaxation. α-adrenergic fibers terminate primarily in the urethra and their stimulation effects contraction of urethral smooth muscle. While some α fibers terminate directly in the detrusor muscle and stimulate detrusor contraction, the main α effect is via inhibition of peripheral parasympathetic ganglion activity, resulting in a net α-adrenergic affect on the detrusor of relaxation. The few β-adrenergic fibers that terminate in the urethra promote smooth muscle relaxation, but this local effect is small compared with the α-adrenergic effect.

THE URETHRAL SPHINCTER MECHANISM

Intraluminal urethral pressure is determined by approximately equal contributions from (1) the smooth muscle and connective tissues of the urethra and periurethra, (2) the striated muscle of the urethra and pelvic floor, and (3) the urethral mucosa and submucosal vascular plexus.[6] Autonomic control of the smooth muscle component has already been

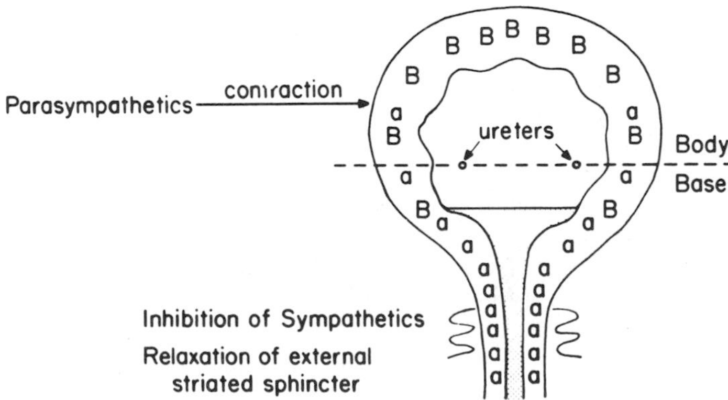

Figure 25–2. Expulsion phase. Expulsion of urine occurs when there is parasympathetic stimulation of the body with inhibition of the sympathetic system of the base. The external sphincter responds to somatic control.

discussed. The striated external sphincter is somatically innervated via the internal pudendal nerves. The mucosal and submucosal vascular plexus component is maintained by the trophic effects of estrogen. Each of these three determinants can be manipulated pharmacologically to influence intraurethral pressure and alleviate symptoms under certain clinical circumstances.

STRESS URINARY INCONTINENCE

Stress urinary incontinence is a condition defined as the involuntary loss of urine when the intravesical pressure exceeds the maximum intraluminal urethral pressure in the absence of a detrusor contraction.[7] It is not generally felt to be a neurologic disorder but rather represents a neurologically intact lower urinary tract in an anatomic dislocation. Stress incontinence results from inadequate transmission of increases in intra-abdominal pressure to the proximal urethra due to its displacement outside the abdominal cavity. When the pressure transmission differential from the bladder to the urethra exceeds the maximum urethral closure pressure, stress incontinence results. The presence of stress urinary incontinence thus depends upon three interrelated factors: (1) the intensity of the increase in intra-abdominal pressure; (2) the percentage of the increase in intra-abdominal pressure transmitted to the urethra, which is dependent upon the position of the urethra with respect to the urogenital diaphragm; and (3) the resting urethral closure pressure. Anything that will increase urethral closure pressure, increase the pressure transmission ratio, or decrease the force of the valsalva stress can help alleviate the symptom. In certain instances pharmacologic agents can be used to improve urethral closure pressure (and perhaps improve pressure transmission) to control the symptom of stress urinary incontinence. This may be particularly applicable for patients with mild to moderate stress urinary incontinence who would like to avoid surgery.

EVALUATION OF LOWER URINARY TRACT DYSFUNCTION

When evaluating urologic dysfunction, questionnaires have been found to be useful because they allow a more uniform and complete approach to the patient. There are several questionnaires that are available for this purpose.[8–10] In addition to a careful history, a thorough physical examination with a neurologic assessment is mandatory. An appropriate urodynamic evaluation based on both the patient's symptoms and her physical findings is critical for accurate diagnosis and successful therapy. Baseline studies may include the measurement of immediate postvoiding residual urine volumes, cystometry, stress testing, and endoscopy. For complex voiding dysfunction, accurate assessment of both the urethra and detrusor is essential to allow specific therapy. This will often require the services of specialized facilities capable of performing simultaneous urethrocystometry, resting and stressed urethral pressure profilometry, urethral sphincter electromyography, and complex uroflowmetry.

After an assessment of this sort, proper choice of drug therapy becomes more rational and has a greater chance of success. It is useful to classify drugs as to their action in promoting urine storage or urine expulsion, and then to subclassify them as to their primary site of action in the lower urinary tract. Figure 25–3 does this graphically for agents that have been useful in the therapy of urinary tract dysfunction. These drugs are further discussed in Tables 25–3 and 25–4 and in the next section.

DRUGS THAT PROMOTE URINE EVACUATION

Bethanechol (Duvoid, Myotonachol, Urecholine)

Bethanechol is a synthetic choline ester that acts principally by stimulation of muscarinic cholinergic receptors to increase detrusor tone and decrease bladder capacity.

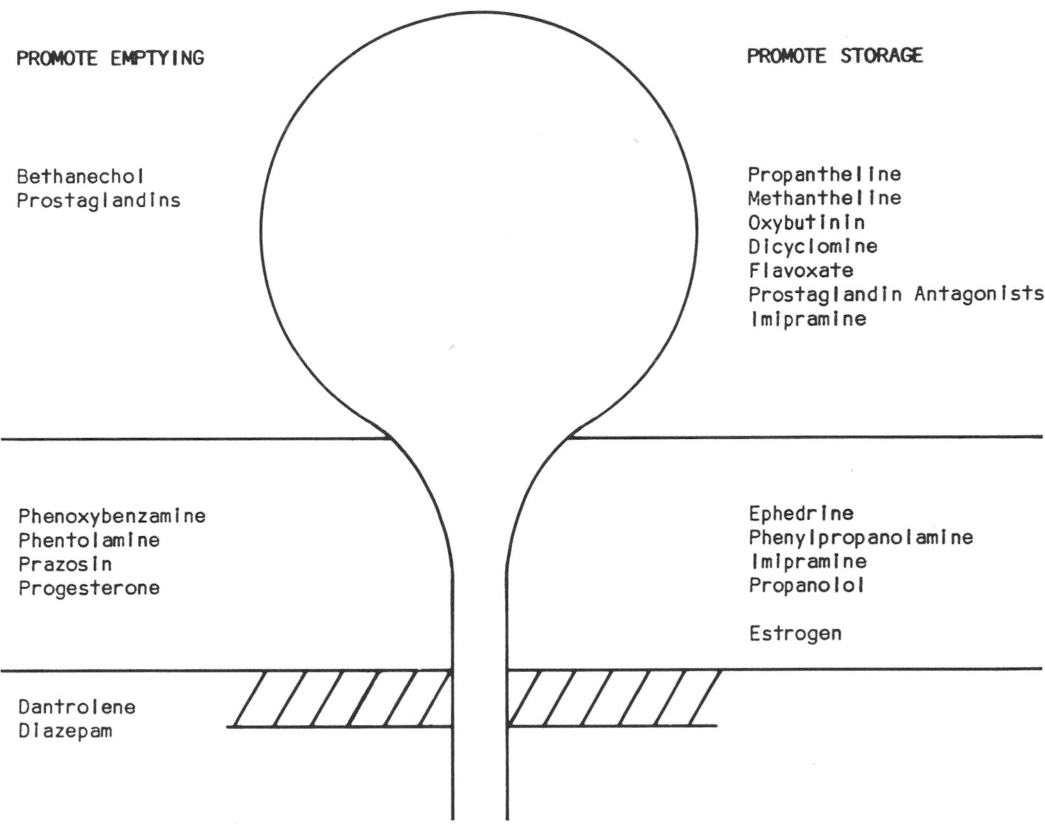

Figure 25–3. Pharmacology of the lower urinary tract.

Despite its widespread use, the literature is not firm on the efficacy of bethanecol in stimulating physiologic detrusor contractions in the majority of patients with hypotonic or atonic bladders. Wei..ı and associates found that in the normal male, doses as high as 100 mg orally did not significantly affect the carbon dioxide cystometrogram.[11]

In voiding, there is a synchronous contraction of the detrusor with opening of the bladder neck and urethra. Bethanechol-induced contractions are not always synchronous, and the outlet may not relax because of the weak nicotinic properties of bethanechol that stimulate the sympathetic ganglia, increasing outlet resistance.[12] Combination therapy with bethanechol and an α-adrenergic antagonist is one approach to decreasing outflow resistance in this situation.

Bethanechol is available for oral or subcutaneous administration. The subcutaneous dosage is usually 2.5 to 10.0 mg every 4 to 6 hours, and the oral dosage is 10 to 100 mg four times a day. By the subcutaneous route, a significant rise in intravesical pressure is noted within 10 minutes, and most activity disappears in 2 hours.[13] When taken orally, the onset of action is slower (30 to 60 minutes) but is maintained for 2 to 6 hours.[13]

Side effects of bethanechol therapy can include lacrimation, flushing, sweating, gastrointestinal disturbances (abdominal

TABLE 25–3. DRUGS THAT MAY AID IN URINE EVACUATION

Agent	Mode of Action	Dosage	Adverse Reactions
Bethanechol (Duvoid, Myotonachol, Urecholine)	Stimulates parasympathetic nervous system	10–100 mg PO three to four times a day	Lacrimation, flushing, sweating, gastrointestinal disturbances, headaches, visual disturbance
		2.5–10.0 mg SC three to four times a day	
Phenoxybenzamine (Dibezyline)	α-Adrenergic blocker	10–20 mg PO one to three times a day	Postural hypotension, miosis, nasal stuffiness, sweating, dryness of mouth, tachycardia. Animal study carcinogenesis.
Prazosin (Minipress)	Postsynaptic α-adrenergic blocker	1–5 mg PO three to four times a day	Postural hypotension (may be severe with first dose), tachycardia, headaches, drowsiness, nausea, dry mouth
Diazepam (Valium)	Centrally acting skeletal muscle relaxant; antianxiety agent	2–10 mg PO three to four times a day	Sedation, ataxia, fatigue
Dantrolene (Dantrium)	Skeletal muscle relaxant	25–150 mg PO two to four times a day	Generalized weakness, severe hepatotoxicity

cramps, nausea, vomiting) difficulty with visual accommodation, headaches, and bronchospasm.

The most common gynecologic use for bethanechol is in the atonic, postoperative bladder. Lapides suggests the following guidelines for the use of bethanechol in patients with an atonic bladder.[14] If the patient is using a urethral catheter, this should be removed, or if a suprapubic catheter is in place, it should be clamped. Bethanechol is then given as a dose of 10 mg subcutaneously every 4 hours; this dose may be decreased to 7.5 mg if the patient is debilitated. The patient's urinary function is evaluated by noting the volume voided at each micturition and the time of micturition as related to time of drug administration. The patient is catheerized approximately 24 hours after initiation of drug therapy, and this is timed to follow the last voiding induced by the injection of bethanechol. When the residual is less than 30 ml, the subcutaneous dose is decreased to 2.5 mg. If the patient continues to respond, the regimen is converted to 50 to 100 mg orally four times a day. This is then progressively tapered.

One needs to be aware of the anatomic and functional status of the bladder outlet before initiating therapy. Often postoperative urinary retention is the result of the patient's inability to relax the urethral sphincter. If the patient is able to increase bladder pressure via either detrusor contraction or Valsalva or Credé maneuvers, it is unlikely that effecting a further increase in bladder tone via cholinergic stimulation will allow her to void. Bethanechol is contraindicated in bladder outlet obstruction and also in patients with asthma, peptic ulcer disease, enteritis, bowel obstruction, hyperthyroidism, and cardiac disease.

Phenoxybenzamine (Dibezyline)

Phenoxybenzamine hydrochloride is a long acting α-adrenergic receptor blocking agent that effectively lowers urethral pressure for

TABLE 25-4. DRUGS THAT MAY AID IN URINE STORAGE

Generic Name	Mode of Action	Dosage	Adverse Reactions
Propantheline (Probanthine)	Inhibits parasympathetic nervous system	15–30 mg PO two to four times a day	Dryness of mouth, blurred vision, constipation, tachycardia, mydriasis, drowsiness
Methantheline (Banthine)	Inhibits parasympathetic nervous system	50–100 mg PO three to four times a day	Anticholinergic effects as above
Oxybutynin (Ditropan)	Inhibits parasympathetic nervous system, local anesthetic, smooth muscle relaxant	5 mg PO two to four times a day	Anticholinergic effects as above (less severe and less frequent)
Dicyclomine (Bentyl)	Inhibits parasympathetic nervous system, smooth muscle relaxant	10–30 mg PO three to four times a day	Anticholinergic effects as above but less frequently
Flavoxate (Urispas)	Very weak parasympathetic inhibitor, local anesthetic, smooth muscle relaxant	100–200 mg PO three to four times a day	Anticholinergic effects as above are rare. Not a potent drug
Imipramine (Tofranil)	Anticholinergic, α- and β-adrenergic agonist, smooth muscle relaxant	25–50 mg PO three to four times a day	Sweating, weakness, fatigue, headache, and anticholinergic effects as above (but all are rare), withdrawal
Ephedrine	Adrenergic stimulation	15–50 mg PO three to four times a day	Central nervous system stimulation, palpitations, gastrointestinal disturbance, hyperexcitability, nervousness, hypertension, insomnia
Phenylpropanolamine (Propadrine)	α-Adrenergic stimulator	25–50 mg PO three to four times a day	As above
(Ornade)	α-Adrenergic stimulator (antihistamine)	One capsule (75 mg) two times a day	As above plus drowsiness
(Entex LA)	α-Adrenergic stimulator (expectorant)	One capsule (75 mg) two times a day	As above
Propranolol (Inderal)	β-Adrenergic blocker	10–40 mg PO three to four times a day	Bradycardia, hypotension, depression, gastrointestinal disturbances, bronchospasm. Not potent
Estrogen	Trophic hormone for urethral mucosa and submucosal vascular plexus; enhances α-adrenergic effects	Oral or vaginal replacement dosage	Those associated with estrogen replacement therapy

several hours. There is no firm evidence that the drug has a significant effect on the bladder or the striated urethral sphincter.

Phenoxybenzamine can be used in patients with neurogenic bladder of a short-term nature and is useful in rehabilitating decompensated or atonic bladders when used in combination with bethanechol.[15-19] Since bethanechol has a weak nicotinic effect leading to increased resistance in the urethra, the combination of bethanechol and phenoxybenzamine will increase bladder contractability and decrease urethral resistance. Another use for the drug is in patients with detrusor instability combined with spasm of the smooth muscle component of the urethral sphincter mechanism. Therapy of this form of vesicosphincter dyssynergia can be with α-adrenergic blockade alone or in combination with anticholinergic agents.

Kleeman states that the therapeutic dose of phenoxybenzamine should rarely exceed 10 mg/day, and doses over 30 mg/day commonly produce adverse side effects such as sweating, dryness of the mouth, and tachycardia.[20] The maximum effect of the drug is not usually realized until 4 to 14 days after initiation of therapy or a change in dose. Daily doses exceeding 10 mg should be given in divided schedules every 8 to 12 hours. The drug may cause postural hypotension, tachycardia, miosis, and nasal stuffiness; however, side effects are rare using 10 mg/day. Another α-adrenergic antagonist, prazosin, has become the preferred agent of this class because of its lower overall side effect incidence and because animal studies have recently implicated phenoxybenzamine as a carcinogen.

The short acting α-adrenergic blocker, phentolamine (Regitine) has been used diagnostically to identify patients who may be candidates for prolonged therapeutic trials with phenoxybenzamine or prazosin.[21,22]

Prazosin (Minipress)

Prazosin is an antihypertensive agent that is felt to relax smooth muscle via blockade of postsynaptic α-adrenergic receptors. Due to this more selective site of blockade, prazosin effects equivalent relaxation of urethral smooth muscle with a lower incidence of side effects, particularly tachycardia, than phenoxybenzamine. It has been shown to effectively lower urethral pressure in dogs[23] in vivo and relax noradrenaline stimulated human urethral preparations in vitro.[24] Recent studies have also suggested that the agent may relax the striated sphincter through central mechanisms.[25] The drug has been used successfully to treat obstructive symptoms in patients with smooth muscle vesicosphincter dyssynergia.[24]

The indications for prazosin use in urinary tract dysfunction are identical to those described for phenoxybenzamine. Side effects are similar although less frequent and severe. A peculiar sensitivity to the drug's postural hypotensive effect is sometimes seen when therapy is initiated. Manifested by dizziness, palpitations, and sudden syncope, this first dose phenomenon is felt to be due to an exaggerated acute postural hypotension. For this reason therapy is usually started with a 1 mg dose at bedtime, and gradually increased up to a maximum daily dose of 15 to 20 mg in divided doses, titrated against the patient's response.[26]

Diazepam (Valium)

As noted earlier, a significant portion of urethral resistance is the result of skeletal muscle activity. Pharmacologic modulation of the striated sphincter has been directed toward the use of skeletal muscle relaxants. These have been used for the treatment of lower tract dysfunctions that have been the result of a nonrelaxing striated sphincter with or without associated detrusor instability, skeletal muscle vesicosphincter dyssynergia. This dysfunction can occur acutely postoperatively, idiopathically, or as the result of suprasacral cord lesions, neuropathies, advanced multiple sclerosis, or local irritative diseases. It is best diagnosed with complex uroflowmetric studies using striated sphincter electromyography.

Oral diazepam is effective in reducing anxiety through its depressant action on the brain stem reticular system. In addition, it also has some relaxant effect on striated muscle through its polysynaptic inhibitory action. Stanton et al., in their work with women who had undergone colposuspension surgery, found that 10 mg given as a nightly dose was more effective than phenoxybenzamine, bethanechol chloride, and intravesical prostaglandin E_2 (PGE_2) in shortening the time to spontaneous voiding postoperatively.[27] The patient population, however, was quite small. While evidence of the efficacy of oral diazepam as a significant skeletal muscle relaxant is not overwhelming, it is the most widely used agent for the control of the nonrelaxing external sphincter and has been unquestionably successful in some patients. What portion of such success is due to the drug's antianxiety effects, independent of its muscle relaxing effects, is unknown.

Dantrolene (Dantrium) and Baclofen (Lioresal)

Investigators have reported some success with dantrolene (Dantrium) and baclofen (Lioresal) in urologic patients with neurogenic and nonneurogenic bladders.[28-30] Baclofen inhibits both monosynaptic and polysynaptic reflexes in the central nervous system and does not have the sedating effects of diazepam. Kiesswelter and Schober showed baclofen to be effective in treating patients with inhibited neurogenic bladders in multiple sclerosis and in those patients with detrusor-sphincter dyssynergia.[29] The drug was ineffective in bladder spasms due to cerebral lesion. Side effects are significant and include weakness, insomnia, drowsiness, rash, dizziness, and hallucinations with abrupt withdrawal.

Dantrolene is a potent muscle relaxant that acts on excitation–contraction coupling. It does not appear to have any effect on peripheral nerves or neuromuscular junctions. Murdock et al. had success using this drug in treating external sphincter spasm.[30] They chose patients who otherwise might have undergone surgery consisting of pudendal neurectomy or external sphincterotomy and obtained favorable results. The most consistent side effect at the high doses frequently needed to achieve sphincter relaxation is distressing generalized weakness. These doses also increase the risk of severe hepatotoxicity during prolonged use.[26] These side effects limit the usefulness of dantrolene as an option for treatment of vesicosphincter dyssynergia.

DRUGS THAT AID IN THE STORAGE OF URINE

Propantheline (Probanthine)

The predominant action of propantheline is interference with transmission at parasympathetic endings by competition with acetylcholine or similar agents. When used in clinically effective doses, propantheline has no effect on the tone of the empty bladder, urethral outlet pressures, or sensation. It will, however, abolish uncontrolled bladder contractions without significantly increasing residual urine, unless very high doses are used. When given orally, its onset of action occurs at 30 minutes and its duration of action is approximately 4 hours.[36] Finkbeiner and Bissada recommend the following adult dosage regimen.[32] The initial oral dosage is 15 mg four times daily. This dose will usually decrease or abolish the amplitude and frequency of uncontrolled contractions and increase bladder capacity without a significant increase in residual urine. If the desired effect is not achieved, the dosage may be increased until either the desired effect is achieved, undesired side effects occur, or significant residual urine volumes ensue. An oral dose of 30 mg four times a day is the maximum a patient can usually tolerate.

Side effects of propantheline include dryness of mouth, blurred vision, constipation, tachycardia, and mydriasis. These drugs should therefore be used with caution in patients with heart disease and avoided in those with glaucoma, myasthenia gravis, and bowel or urinary obstruction.

In gynecology, the principal use of propantheline is for idiopathic detrusor instability defined as a bladder that on filling shows uninhibited contractions above 15 cm H_2O, either spontaneously or provoked with physical activity, without a detectable neurologic or local lesion. Propantheline in these cases in an effective drug with a relatively low cost. Another antimuscarinic agent, methantheline, has similar, though less potent, effects on detrusor activity dose for dose.

Oxybutynin Chloride (Ditropan)

Oxybutynin chloride is a moderately strong cholinergic blocker and a strong direct smooth muscle relaxant with local anesthetic activity.[33] It has less anticholinergic effect but greater antispasmodic effect on the detrusor muscle than atropine.[34] Using a 5-mg oral dose, the onset of action is 1 hour, with peak effectiveness within 3 to 6 hours. In patients with uncontrolled detrusor contractions, cystometrograms have demonstrated a decrease in amplitude and/or a decrease in frequency of uncontrolled contractions. Some patients have shown an increase in bladder volume.[33] Fredericks et al. found oxybutynin exposure in rabbits to be a potent inhibitor of barium chloride-induced contractions.[35] Thompson and Lavretz, in study of patients with neurovesical reflex activity (uninhibited bladders, eneuresis, and primary muscle spasm), found oxybutynin to have antispasmodic and anticholinergic effects.[36]

Oxybutynin has also been shown to be useful in those patients with urethralgia and vesicalgia due to infection, postoperation inflammation, irradiation, or following removal of catheters.

Side effects are similar to, although generally less severe than, those seen with propantheline. It is an excellent drug for use in those patients with uninhibited contractions secondary to infection, operation, or radiation and in patients with idiopathic detrusor instability, as an adjuct to retraining drills. The usual dosage is 5 mg two to four times daily.

Dicyclomine (Bentyl, Pasmin)

Dicyclomine has been used widely in a number of gastrointestinal disorders for some time. Like oxybutynin it has a direct smooth muscle relaxant effect along with antimuscarinic activity. Awad et al. evaluated this drug in patients with uninhibited bladder contractions and found that the symptoms of urge and urge incontinence were cured in all of the female patients using 20 mg three times a day for 4 to 8 weeks.[37] Side effects included difficulty in visual accommodation and mild dryness of the mouth. None of the patients in their study had a detectable neurologic disorder, so treatment was purely symptomatic. A noticeable improvement in symptoms was not usually observed for 7 to 10 days after beginning therapy, so an 8-week course was necessary to achieve a maximum effect in most cases. Dicyclomine is a less potent agent than oxybutinin but has a lower incidence and severity of adverse anticholinergic side effects.

Flavoxate Hydrochloride (Urispas)

Flavoxate hydrochloride is a flavone derivative that has a direct smooth muscle relaxant and anesthetic effects as well as minimal anticholinergic activity.[38] There is controversy as to the relative efficacy of flavoxate with respect to its ability to inhibit the unstable detrusor. Both Wein[26] and Khanna[34] conclude that it is not a potent drug and is unlikely to improve symptoms associated with detrusor instability when other, less expensive agents have failed. However, due to its very low incidence and severity of side effects, it is a reasonable agent to consider when other agents prove unacceptable due to intolerable side effects.

Flavoxate appears to be an effective drug for relief of the symptoms of dysuria, urgency, nocturia, suprapubic pain, frequency, and incontinence that may occur in cystitis, prostatitis, urethritis, urethrocystitis, and urethrotrigonitis. In cases of urinary tract infection, it can be used in conjunction with the appropriate antibiotic.

Side effects have been very infrequent at a dose of one to two 100-mg tablets three to four times a day. The drug is contraindicated in obstructive conditions, achalasia, or gastrointestinal hemorrhage, and should be used with caution in patients with glaucoma.

Imipramine (Tofranil)

The tricyclic antidepressent imipramine is a dibenzazepine derivative whose urologic mechanism of action is predominantly via its combined α- and β-adrenergic stimulating and anticholinergic properties. These effect an increase in urethral smooth muscle tone and a decrease in detrusor tone. Maclean first reported the benefits from imipramine use in children with enuresis using an effective dose of 25 mg at bedtime.[40] Labay and Boyarsky, using an in vitro canine model, found imipramine capable of relaxing the bladder musculature and blocking the cholinergic effect of acetycholine.[41] Mahoney et al., in examining the sphincter-augmenting effect of imipramine in children, felt that the drug exerted its beneficial effect by augmenting the tone of the involuntary urethral sphincter.[42] Work by Benson et al. indicated that imipramine significantly decreased both bethanechol (cholinergic blockade) and barium-induced (antispasmodic or musculotropic) bladder contractions.[43] Thus it seems to have some direct inhibitory effect on the detrusor independent of its adrenergic and anticholinergic actions.

The dose of imipramine in adults is 25 mg four times daily. Children and elderly patients require a lower dosage of 5 to 20 mg four times daily. Beneficial effects on urinary continence are usually not seen for several days to weeks. Before therapy is begun, organic disease should be ruled out before a functional basis is assumed. Side effects include sweating, weakness, fatigue, headache, anticholinergic effects, and obstructive urinary symptoms. Some children have undergone personality changes. The drug should be used with caution in those patients with hypertension and cardiovascular disease. Imipramine is contraindicated in patients using monoamine oxidase inhibitors because of the possible potentiation of sympathomimetic substances in these patients resulting in hypertensive crisis. Common monoamine oxidase inhibitors are toanylcypromine (Parnate), phenelzine (Nardil), and parqylene (Eutonyl) (Chap. 26). Abrupt withdrawl of imipramine after prolonged therapy has resulted in nausea, abdominal distress, headache, and malaise.[44] Gradual tapered dose discontinuation, especially in children and in patients on high doses, is recommended.

Ephedrine

Ephedrine sulfate stimulates both the α- and β-adrenergic receptors to release norepinephrine, which then acts directly on the effector cells.[45] Diako and Taub used ephedrine in doses of 40 to 200 mg daily in four divided doses to improve urinary incontinence of mild to moderate nature.[46] It was of little benefit in cases with an uninhibited neurogenic bladder or with severe stress incontinence. In addition, tachyphylaxis is occasionally seen with the agent.[32] Side effects include hypertension, palpitations, insomnia, and anxiety. It should be used with caution in patients with hypertension, glaucoma, heart disease, and hyperthyroidism and avoided in patients on digitalis.

Phenylpropanolamine (Propadrine, Ornade [combination], and Entex LA [combination])

Phenylpropanolamine seems to have the same peripheral effects as ephedrine with less central stimulation and without the tendency for tachyphylaxis. Awad et al.[47] found it to be effective in 11 of 13 women with stress urinary incontinence. Side effects were uncommon, and any beneficial response depended on the therapy being continuous. The agent has also proven effective in the therapy of the unstable female urethra,[48] a condition diagnosed with simultaneous urethrocystometry. Unstable urethra is increasingly recognized as a common cause of sensory urgency, sensory urgency incontinence and chronic urethral syndrome.[49,50]

Ornade is a combination drug containing 75 mg phenylpropanolamine and 12 mg of chlorpheniramine maleate. Since it contains the antihistamine, drowsiness may be an undesirable side effect. This is avoided with Entex LA, another combination agent that also contains 75 mg of phenylpropanolamine with the expectorant guaifenesin. Phenylpropanolamine preparations have the same potential side effects, though less severe, and same contraindications as ephedrine.

Propranolol

Propranolol, through its β-blocking effect, may potentiate α-receptors and increase outlet resistance. Gleason et al. found propranolol to be useful in treating stress incontinence in five women scheduled for incontinence surgery when a 10-mg dose was given four times a day.[51] A trial of propranolol may have merit for patients with cardiovascular or hypertensive disease in whom α-stimulators are contraindicated[16] and who want to avoid surgery for stress urinary incontinence.

Estrogen and Progesterone

Several investigators have reported subjective improvement in the symptom of stress urinary incontinence when estrogen replacement was used in hypoestrogenic incontinent women.[52–55] Estrogen may influence urethral function via its trophic effect on the urethral mucosa, the submucosal vascular plexus, and the connective tissue of the pubovesical and pubourethral ligaments[56] and by enhancing the effects of α-adrenergic stimulation of urethral smooth muscle.[57] Estrogen has been shown to increase maximum urethral pressure,[54] urethral length,[54,58] and mean urethral pressures.[59] It also has been shown to enhance bladder to urethra pressure transmission in stress incontinent postmenopausal women.[54,55] While there have been reports that fail to support the benefits of estrogen therapy,[60] a trial of estrogen replacement seems appropriate, particularly for women who develop mild to moderate stress incontinence for the first time postmenopausally. Administration can be either orally or intravaginally. Contraindications and the need for periodic progestin administration with an intact uterus are well known (Chap. 20).

There is some controversy as to progesterone's effects on urethral pressure.[54,61] There is evidence that it may decrease smooth muscle tone via enhancement of the β-adrenergic response in the urethra. The therapeutic implications of this observation have not been reported.

PROSTAGLANDINS AND PROSTAGLANDIN INHIBITORS

Prostaglandins E_2 and prostaglandin $F_{2\alpha}$ ($PGF_{2\alpha}$) are released during the nervous stimulation of the bladder, and studies have shown this to cause an increased detrusor muscle activity.[62,63] It has been hypothesized that a reduction in circulating prostaglandin levels may help to reduce detrusor hypercontractility. Indomethacin is a prostaglandin synthetase inhibitor which has been shown by Ghoneim et al. to reduce urethral resistance observed during vesical distention.[64]

Cardozo and Stanton undertook a study to compare bromocriptine and indomethacin in the treatment of detrusor instability.[65] Primary detrusor instability was diagnosed in 66 percent, multiple sclerosis in 19 percent, cerebrovascular accident in 9 percent, and other upper motor neuron lesions in 6 percent. Indomethacin was found to be useful in treating the symptom of freqency with detrusor instability, but bromocriptine was not helpful. Neither drug was effective against urgency or urge incontinence and side effects with indomethacin and bromocriptine were numerous (nausea, vomiting, dizziness).

There have also been reports showing beneficial effects on urinary retention from intravesical instillation of prostaglandins. Prostaglanam E_2 was able to increase tone in patients with hypotonic bladders[66] and $PGF_{2\alpha}$ was able to decrease significantly the frequency of urinary retention following vaginal hysterectomy.[67]

Investigation of the effects of prostaglandins and prostaglandin synthetase inhibitors on the lower urinary tract continues and should help clarify their role in the clinical management of urologic dysfunction.

REFERENCES

1. Wein AJ, Raezer DM: Physiology of micturition. In Krane RJ, Siroky MB, (eds): Clinical Neuro-Urology. Boston, Little, Brown, 1979, pp 1–34.
2. Krane RJ, Siroky MB: Classification of neurourologic disorders. In Krane RJ, Siroky MB, (eds): Clinical Neuro-Urology. Boston, Little, Brown, 1979, p 143–58
3. Bradley WE: The neurology of micturition. In Ostergard DR (ed): Gynecologic Urology and Urodynamics. Baltimore, Williams & Wilkins, 1980, pp 11–27
4. Ostergard DR: The neurological control of micturition and integrated voiding reflexes. In Ostergard DR (ed): Gynecologic Urology and Urodynamics. Baltimore, Williams & Wilkins, 1980, pp 29–42
5. Torrens MJ: Neurophysiology. In Stanton SL (ed): Clinical Gynecologic Urology. St. Louis, Mosby, 1984, pp 13–21
6. Rud T, Andersson KE, Asmussen M, et al.: Factors maintaining the intraurethral pressure in women. Invest Urol 17:343, 1980
7. International Continence Society Committee on Standardisation of Terminology, Hald T (chairman). The standardisation of terminology of lower urinary tract function. Glasgow, International Continence Society, 1984
8. Hodgkinson CP: Stress urinary incontinence—1970. Am J Obstet Gynecol 108:1149, 1970
9. Corlett RC, Jr: Gynecologic urology, part 1. Curr Probl Obstet Gynecol 12(1):32, 1978
10. Robertson JR: Genitourinary Problems in Women. Springfield, Ill., Thomas, 1978, p 32
11. Wein AJ, Hanno PM, Dixon DO, et al.: The effect of oral bethanechol chloride on the cystometrogram of the normal male adult. J Urol 120:330, 1978
12. Yalla SV, Rossier AB, Fam B: Synchronous cystosphincterometry in patients with spinal cord injury. Urology 6:777, 1975
13. Diokno AC, Lapides J: Action of oral and parenteral bethanecol on decompressed bladder. Urology 10:23, 1977
14. Lapides J: Urecholine regimen for rehabilitating the atonic bladder. J Urol 91:658, 1964
15. Krane RJ, Olsson CA: Phenoxybenzaminde in neurogenic bladder dysfunction: II. Clinical considerations. J Urol 110:653, 1973
16. Khanna OP: Disorders of micturition: Neuropharmacologic basis and results of drug therapy. Urology 8:316, 1976
17. Stockamp K: Treatment with phenoxybenzamine of upper urinary tract complications caused by intravesical obstruction. J Urol 113:128, 1975
18. Krane RJ, Olsson CA: Phenoxybenzamine in neurogenic bladder dysfunction—clinical considerations. J. Urol 110:653, 1973
19. Khanna OP: Disorders of micturition: Neuropharmacologic basis and results of drug therapy. Urology 8:316, 1976
20. Kleeman FJ: Phenoxybenzamine: Letter to the editor. J Urol 117:814, 1977
21. McCarthy TA: Propantheline and phentolamine testing. In Ostergard DR (ed). Gynecologic Urology and Urodynamics. Baltimore, Williams & Wilkins, 1980, pp 175–179
22. Diokno AC: Evaluation of the neurologically obstructed patient. In Krane RJ, Siroky MB, (eds): Clinical Neuro-Urology. Boston, Little, Brown, 1979, pp 111–121
23. MacGregor RJ, Diokno AC: The α-adrenergic blocking action of prazosin hydrochloride on the canine urethra. Invest Urol 18:426, 1981
24. Andersson KE, Ek A, Hedlund H, et al.: Effects of prazosin on isolated human urethra and in patients with lower motor neuron lesions. Invest Urol 19:39, 1981
25. Gajewski J, Downie JW, Awad SA: Experimental evidence for a central nervous system site of action in the effect of α-adrenergic blockers on the external urinary sphincter. J Urol 132:403, 1984
26. Wein AJ: Applied pharmacology. In Stanton

SL (ed): Clinical Gynecologic Urology. St. Louis, Mosby, 1984, pp 441–461
27. Stanton SL, Cardozo LD, Kerr-Wilson R: Treatment of delayed onset of spontaneous voiding after surgery for incontinence. Urology 13:494, 1979
28. From A, Heltberg A: A double-blind trial of baclofen (Lioresal) and diazepam in spasticity due to multiple sclerosis. Acta Neurol Scand 51:158, 1975
29. Kiesswelter H, Schober W: Lioresal in the treatment of neurogenic bladder dysfunction. Urol Int 30:63, 1975
30. Murdock M, Sax D, Krane RJ: Use of dantrolene sodium in external sphincter spasm. Urology 8:133, 1976
31. Kiesswelter H, Popper L: A cystometrographic study to assess the influence of atropine, propantheline and mebeverine on the smooth muscle of the bladder. Br J Urol 44:31, 1972
32. Finkbeiner AE, Bissada NK: Drug therapy for lower urinary tract dysfunction. Urol Clin North Am 7:3 1980
33. Diokno AC, Lapides J: Oxybutynin: A new drug with analgesic and anticholinergic properties. J Urol 108:307, 1972
34. Khanna OP: Non surgical therapeutic modalities. In Krane RJ, Siroky MB (eds): Clinical Neuro-Urology. Boston, Little, Brown, 1979, pp 159–196
35. Fredericks CM, Anderson GF, Kreulen DC: A study on the anticholinergic and antispasmodic activity of oxybutynin (Ditropan) on rabbit detrusor. Invest Urol 12:317, 1975
36. Thompson IM, Lavretz R: Oxybutynin in bladder spasm, neurogenic bladder and enuresis. Urology 8:452, 1976
37. Awad SA, Bryreak S, Downie JW, et al.: The treatment of the uninhibited bladder with dicyclomine. J Urol 117:161, 1977
38. Setrikar I, Ravaer MT, Dare P: Pharmacological properties of peperideno ethyl-3-methylflavone 8-carboxylate hydrochloride, a smooth-muscle relaxant. J Pharmacol Exp Ther 130:356, 1960
39. Kohler RP, Morales PA: Cystometric evaluation of flavoxate hydrochloride in normal and neurogenic bladder. J Urol 100:729, 1968
40. Maclean REG: Imipramine hydrochloride (Tofranil) and enuresis. Am J Psychiatry 117:551, 1960
41. Labay P, Boyarsky S: The action of imipramine on the bladder musculacture. J Urol 109:385, 1973
42. Mahoney DT, Laferte RD, Mahoney JE: Observations on sphineteric augmenting effect of imipramine in children with urinary incontinence. Urology 1:317, 1973
43. Benson GS, Sarshek SA, Raezer D, et al.: Bladder muscle contractility: Comparative effects and mechanisms of action of atropine, propantheline, flavoxate and imipramine. Urology 9:31, 1977
44. Petti TA, Law W III: Abrupt cessation of high-dose imipramine treatment in children. JAMA 246:768, 1981
45. Irnes IR, Nickerson M: Drugs acting on post-ganglionic adrenergic nerve endings and structures innervated by them. In Goodman LS, Gilman A (eds): The Pharmacologic Basis of Therapeutics, ed. 3. New York, Macmillian, 1965, pp 505–526
46. Diokno AC, Taub M: Ephedrine in treatment of urinary incontinence. Urology 5:624, 1975
47. Awad SA, Downie JW, Kiruluta HG: Alpha-adrenergic agents in urinary disorders of the proximal urethra: Part 1. Sphincter incontinence. Br J Urol 50:332, 1978
48. Fossberg E. Beisland HO, Sander S: Sensory urgency in females: Treatment with phenylpropanolamine. Eur Urol 7:157, 1981
49. Ulmsten U, Henriksson L, Iosif S: The unstable female urethra. Am J Obstet Gynecol 144:93, 1982
50. Kulseng-Hanssen S: Prevalence and pattern of unstable urethral pressure in one hundred seventy-four gynecologic patients referred for urodynamic evaluation. Am J Obstet Gynecol 146:895, 1983
51. Gleason DM, Reilly RJ, Bottacini MR, et al.: The urethral continence zone and its relation to stress incontinence. J Urol 112:81, 1974
52. Raz S, Ziegler M, Caine M: The role of female hormones in stress incontinence. Paper read before the Congress of the International Society of Urology, Amsterdam, 1973
53. Musiani U: A partially successful attempt at medical treatment of urinary-stress incontinence in women. Urol Int 27:405, 1972
54. Rud T: The effects of estrogens and gestagens on the urethral pressure profile in urinary continent and stress incontinent women. Act Obstet Gynecol Scand 59:265, 1980
55. Hilton P, Stanton SL: The use of intravaginal oestrogen cream in genuine stress incontinence. Br J Obstet Gynecol 90:940, 1983
56. Hilton P, Varma TR: The menopause. In Stan-

ton SL (ed): Clinical Gynecologic Urology. St. Louis, Mosby, 1984 pp 343–353

57. Caine M, Raz S: Some clinical implications of adrenergic receptors in the urinary tract. Arch Surg 110:247, 1975
58. Van Geelen JM, Doesburg WH, Thomas CMG, Martin CB: Urodynamic studies in the normal menstrual cycle; the relationship between hormonal changes during the menstrual cycle and the urethral pressure profile. Am J Obstet Gynecol 141:384, 1981
59. Bump RC, Friedman CL: Intraluminal urethral pressure measurements in the female baboon: Effects of hormonal manipulation. Presented at the Annual Meeting of the Gynecologic Urology Society, San Diego, 1985
60. Walter S, Worl H, Barlebo H, Jensen HK: Urinary incontinence in postmenopausal women treated with estrogens: A double-blind clinical trial. Urol Int 33:135, 1978
61. Raz S, Seigler M, Caine M: The effect of progesterone on the adrenergic receptors of the urethra. Br J Urol 45:131, 1973
62. Abrams PH, Feneley RCL: The actions of prostaglandins on the smooth muscle of the human urinary tract in vitro. Br J Urol 47:909, 1976
63. Bultitude MI, Huls NH, Shuttleworth KED: Clinical experimental studies on the action of prostaglandins and their synthesis inhibitors on detrusor muscle in vitro and in vivo. Br J Urol 48:631, 1976
64. Ghoneim MA, Fretin JA, Gagno DJ, et al.: The influence of vesical distention on the urethral resistance to flow: A possible role for prostaglandins? J Urol 116:739, 1976
65. Cardozo LD, Stanton SL: A comparison between bromocriptine and indomethacin in the treatment of detrusor instability. J Urol 123:399, 1980
66. Desmond AD, Bultitude MI, Hills NH, Shuttleworth KE: Clinical experience with intravesical prostaglandin E2. A prospective study of 36 patients. Br J Urol 52:357, 1980
67. Jaschevatzky OE, Anderman S, Shalit A, et al.: Prostaglandin F2alpha for prevention of urinary retention after vaginal hysterectomy. Obstet Gynecol 66:244, 1985

26

Endometriosis, Dysmenorrhea, and Pelvic Pain

Jeffrey M. Dicke

The treatment of endometriosis, dysmenorrhea, and chronic pelvic pain often represents a therapeutic challenge to the family physician and gynecologist. These are common conditions with significant implications regarding the patient's physical and emotional well-being. Medical management has formerly been limited to the use of agents that were relatively ineffective or undesirable because of potential side effects. Recent advances in the pathophysiology of these disorders have resulted in the development of many new agents that are more specific and effective in their ability to provide relief from these conditions, while causing fewer adverse effects. The following is a brief discussion of these disease entities including their etiology, pathophysiology, and therapy.

ENDOMETRIOSIS

Endometriosis is a pathologic entity resulting from the proliferation and function of endometrial glands and stroma in various extrauterine locations. The ovary is the most common site of occurrence with bilateral involvement in approximately 50 percent of patients. Other frequently affected structures include the uterosacral, round and broad ligaments, rectovaginal septum, and pelvic peritoneum covering the uterus, fallopian tubes, rectum, sigmoid, and bladder. Less frequently endometriosis involves the cervix, vagina, vulva, appendix, small bowel, and laparotomy scars, with occasional occurrence in extraabdominal locations such as the pleura, lung, skeletal muscle, and bone.

The proliferation of such aberrant endometrial tissue is dependent upon ovarian hormones. Cyclic ovarian function typically stimulates proliferation and characteristic menstrual changes of ectopic endometrial implants resulting in peritoneal irritation, sequestration, and scarring. In the absence of viable ovaries such implants regress.

The etiology of endometriosis is uncertain although a variety of mechanisms have been proposed. The most credible theories may be grouped as follows:

1. Transplantation theories, which imply

dissemination of endometrial glands and stroma via transtubal regurgitation, as advanced by Sampson in 1921,[1] or spread through lymphatic or vascular channels.

2. Metaplasia theories, which suggest ectopic-functioning endometrium results from atypical development of germinal epithelium and various parts of pelvic peritoneum that are embryologically derived from totipotential coelomic epithelial cell elements.
3. Induction theories, which propose that chemical mediators from the uterine cavity are transported to extrauterine locations where they stimulate metaplasia of local cells.

The incidence of endometriosis in the general population is not known with certainty, although the frequency of the disease is estimated to be 1 to 2 percent. A potential polygenic/multifactorial mode of transmission is suggested by the fact that endometriosis is seven times more prevalent and is generally more severe in women whose first-degree relatives are also affected. In women with infertility, endometriosis has been demonstrated laparoscopically in 15 to 25 percent of cases. In women with known endometriosis, the frequency of infertility is estimated to be 30 to 40 percent.[2] Such women often present as nulliparas in their 20s or early 30s with a history of delayed childbearing or involuntary infertility. The progress of the disease is related to the number of uninterrupted progestational cycles, and improvement is noted during periods of anovulation and amenorrhea. Thus, it is not a disease of premenarchal, pregnant, or postmenopausal females.

Endometriosis may have either an acute or chronic presentation, and the site of involvement determines the symptomatology. The four most common manifestations of the disease include infertility, dysmenorrhea and pelvic pain, dyspareunia, and menstrual irregularities. Symptomatology is not proportional to the extent of disease. Patients with extensive palpable disease may be relatively asymptomatic, while those with relatively small peritoneal implants may experience significant pain resulting from fibrosis and stretching of the involved peritoneum.

Although there are no pathognomonic signs or symptoms of endometriosis, the combination of acquired progressive dysmenorrhea, dyspareunia, and pelvic pain in conjunction with tender cul-de-sac nodularities and adnexal enlargement are highly suggestive of this disorder. Such a clinical diagnosis should always be confirmed laparoscopically to avoid prolonged hormonal therapy of unconfirmed disease. Endometriotic implants appear as brown or black nodules frequently surrounded by hemorrhagic areas, fibrosis, and adhesions. Larger lesions, known as endometriomas, often involve ovaries and intestines. Thus, as Kistner notes, the diagnosis is "suggested by history, corroborated by the pelvic exam, and verified by endoscopy and/or biopsy."[3]

Therapy for endometriosis is surgical and/or hormonal. Surgical treatment is considered to be either conservative or radical, depending upon intent. Conservative surgery is that done to preserve and improve reproductive potential, while radical surgery attempts to alleviate the disease completely. Ectopic endometrial implants typically soften and regress with cessation of cyclic ovarian function. Thus, hormonal therapy is aimed at inhibiting both the proliferation and subsequent bleeding of aberrant endometrium by pharmacologically providing a pseudopregnancy or pseudomenopause. The following is a discussion of agents used for such purposes.

Danazol (Danocrine)

First available for clinical and animal studies in 1967, danazol is a synthetic (2,3-isoxyl) derivative of 17 α-ethinyl testosterone. An orally active pituitary gonadotropin inhibitory agent, danazol has no estrogenic or progestational activity and only mild androgenic activity. It is well absorbed orally with maximum serum concentrations achieved within

2 to 4 hours. Gonadotropin secretion or release is inhibited even though overt sex hormone activity is not manifested. Although there are conflicting data regarding the effect of danazol on gonadotropin release, it is thought to act as an impeded androgen, interrupting the midcycle gonadotropin surge, and suppressing endometrial growth and enzyme pathways controlling ovarian steroidogenesis.

Evidence also suggests that danazol has direct actions at the gonadal and endometrial levels with probable competitive blocking of estrogen and progesterone receptors. Over several weeks, plasma levels of estradiol and estrone are markedly suppressed, resulting in peripheral changes similar to castration or menopause. Atrophy of the vaginal mucosa, uterine endometrium, and the aberrant endometrium of endometriosis may occur. Studies evaluating the effect of danazol therapy on pituitary, thyroid, and adrenal function in relatively small numbers of women reveal a decrease in thyroid-binding globulin, thyroid-stimulating hormone (TSH), T_3, and T_4 with slight increases in free T_4 and free T_3 index.[4] Metyrapone challenge tests to evaluate pituitary-adrenal response reveal a normal ability of the pituitary to secrete adrenocorticotropic hormone (ACTH) and of the adrenal gland to respond.[5] Glucose tolerance and serum concentrations of prolactin, cortisol, and testosterone are unaffected by danazol therapy.[5] Likewise, no changes in fibrinolysis, coagulation, or platelet function have been demonstrated.[6]

Clinical Uses

Several large studies utilizing danazol 200 mg four times daily for periods of 3 to 18 months have demonstrated good clinical success.[7–9] The average course of therapy was 6 months, with the goal of treatment being to achieve suppression and atrophy of endometrial deposits. Effective treatment therefore was usually accompanied by complete amenorrhea. (Amenorrhea, vaginal cytology, and endometrial biopsies provide evidence of the pseudomenopausal state and are measures of the effectiveness of danazol therapy.) Subjective symptomatology showed improvement after only a few weeks of therapy, with eventual amelioration of dysmenorrhea and pelvic pain in 90 to 100 percent of all patients.[6,10] Clinical findings on pelvic exam revealed a slower response and provided a measure of the adequacy of therapy duration. Gradual improvement in pelvic induration and tenderness occurred in 80 to 90 percent of patients after 3 to 7 months of treatment.[5,6]

The optimum regimen for danazol administration remains controversial. The usual dosage of danazol in North America is 800 mg/day, although recent evidence suggests that lower doses may also be efficacious. Low et al.[11] conducted a randomized trial to investigate the efficacy of different doses of danazol in the treatment of endometriosis. Their results indicated that for mild endometriosis 200 mg/day of danazol is effective therapy with fewer side effects than higher doses. These results corroborate the findings of Moore[12] and Chalmers[13] who reported that mild–moderate pelvic endometriosis could be managed successfully with lower doses of danazol. However, these studies as well as others also indicate that more severe disease requires 600 to 800 mg daily for approximately 6 months, at which time the need for further therapy is reassessed. Regular ovulatory menses usually returns within 1 to 3 months following discontinuation of therapy, thus relieving the pseudomenopausal state and its beneficial effect on endometriosis. The interval between cessation of therapy, rate of recurrence, and subsequent progression of the disease is variable. Approximately one-third of study populations experienced exacerbation of symptoms within the first year.[8,10]

Pregnancy rates subsequent to danazol therapy vary markedly. Chances are dependent on the severity of disease, the dosage and duration of danazol treatment, and the presence or absence of other factors impairing fertility. Initial studies of patients with mild endometriosis treated with danazol for infertility reported pregnancy rates of 38 to

83 percent.[14] However, a recent collaborative effort involving 75 patients (the largest series to date) with mild endometriosis treated with danazol for infertility reported an overall pregnancy rate of only 28 percent with a viable pregnancy rate of 20 percent.[14] This led the authors to suggest that the pregnancy rate in patients with infertility and mild endometriosis treated with danazol is less than previously reported and possibly no greater than the spontaneous pregnancy rate. Uncorrected pregnancy rates of 46 to 56 percent have been reported following danazol therapy of moderate endometriosis, while somewhat lower rates can be expected when danazol is utilized postoperatively in patients with severe endometriosis.[15]

Danazol has also been approved for the treatment of severe fibrocystic disease of the breast, a disorder characterized by pain, tenderness, and nodularity exacerbated premenstrually. In clinical studies using 50 to 800 mg (usually 100 to 400 mg) of danazol daily for 3 to 6 months, relief of pain and nodularity was achieved in 54 to almost 90 percent of patients. These signs and symptoms recurred in approximately one-third of patients 11 to 32 months following cessation of therapy. The manufacturer claims the disease may recur in one-half of patients within 1 year after discontinuation of the drug. The long-term safety and cost-effectiveness are not well established for such use.[16]

Side Effects and Precautions

The side effects of danazol are generally the result of its primary pharmacologic actions. Those attributable to inhibition of the pituitary-gonadal axis include symptoms referable to depressed ovarian function, such as vasomotor instability, breast changes, and vaginitis, and have been reported to occur in 1.5 to 4.5 percent of 704 treated women.[3] Side effects attributable to danazol's androgenic activity and their incidence include acne (13.4 percent), hirsutism (5.8 percent), edema (5.8 percent), weight gain (2.8 percent), voice change (2.8 percent), and oiliness of skin (1.8 percent).[4] General side effects reported in a small percentage of patients include emotional (depression, anxiety, fatigue), gastrointestinal (nausea, vomiting, diarrhea, constipation), and musculoskeletal complaints. These effects were those recorded by patients treated with 800 mg/day. Studies in progress indicate that the incidence of side effects is decreased in women maintained on lesser dosages.[17,18]

A disadvantage of danazol therapy and a potentially limiting factor in its use is cost. Current retail cost often exceeds $1 per 200-mg capsule. This may render danazol unavailable to patients with limited budgets and should be considered when evaluating the advantages and disadvantages of therapy.

Other Steroids

Since signs and symptoms of endometriosis regress during pregnancy and for a varying length of time thereafter, gestation has long been suggested as a prophylactic and therapeutic modality. Such regression is thought to be the result of anovulation and amenorrhea induced by pituitary-gonadal suppression. If pregnancy is not a desirable or obtainable means of therapy, anovulation may be achieved using estrogens, progestins, androgens, or a combination thereof.

Estrogens

Based on the observation that endometriosis is associated with ovulatory cycles, constant estrogen administration has been used to inhibit ovulation and suppress further growth of the aberrant endometrium. The daily administration of large doses of estrogen results in symptomatic improvement but little change in the size and location of ectopic endometrial implants.[19] Despite subjective improvement, prolonged estrogen administration is associated with a variety of serious side effects including cystic and adenomatous hyperplasia of the endometrium, thrombophlebitis, breakthrough bleeding, peripheral edema, nausea, and vomiting (Chap. 20). Furthermore, estrogen-stimulated proliferative growth of endometrium will not cause regression of the disease. Because of potential side effects and alternate methods of therapy, the routine use of estrogens is currently considered unacceptable in treating endometriosis.

Progestins

The use of progestational agents to inhibit ovulation has been advocated. Progestational agents are generally better tolerated with fewer complications than estrogen administration (Chap. 20). With progestational therapy, gonadotropin release is inhibited and ovarian steroid production is reduced. Progesterone also exerts a direct effect on the endometrium, resulting in endometrial atrophy. With excessive suppression of estrogen, breakthrough bleeding may occur and necessitate low dose estrogen to stabilize the endometrium. Other side effects are minor and include weight gain, depression, breast tenderness, and vaginitis. Depomedroxyprogesterone acetate 100 mg every 2 weeks for 2 months, followed by 200 mg each month for 4 to 6 months has been used to achieve subjective remission. A disadvantage of progestin therapy in the patient desiring pregnancy is delayed ovulation for possibly 6 to 12 months following the cessation of treatment.

Androgens

Androgens are thought to be effective in treating endometriosis by acting directly on areas of endometriosis. Androgen therapy is unique among hormonal treatments for endometriosis, because neither gonadotropin release, ovarian steroid production, nor ovulation is inhibited. The use of androgens has centered around their effectiveness in relieving both dysmenorrhea and dyspareunia. Methyltestosterone 5 to 10 mg daily for 6 to 12 weeks has been shown to provide symptomatic improvement in approximately 80 percent of patients, although most patients experienced a recurrence of symptoms within several months after discontinuation.[3] Pregnancy rates following therapy have been reported to be 10 to 60 percent.[20] A comparison with untreated patients is difficult because of the lack of standardization. Androgens may cause virilization of female fetuses, so early pregnancy must be excluded if menses are delayed (Chap. 2). Side effects of androgen treatment include acne, menstrual irregularities, hirsutism, clitoromegaly, hoarseness, and hepatocellular jaundice.

Estrogen/Progestin Combination Therapy

The observation that pregnancy induces both subjective and objective improvement in patients with endometriosis is the basis for administration of estrogen and progestin in a manner simulating the hormonal profile in pregnancy. Similar to true pregnancy, the pseudopregnant state results in the decidualization, necrosis, and resorption of aberrant endometrium.

A common regimen involves the continuous use of oral contraceptives with an initial dose of one tablet daily. After several weeks, this is increased to two or three tablets daily, with additional increases as necessary to prevent breakthrough bleeding. An exacerbation of symptoms may occur during the initial 2 to 3 months of therapy, which resolves following decidual necrosis and absorption. Subjective improvement has been reported in various studies in approximately 85 to 90 percent of patients.[21,22] Objective improvement as manifested by the regression of endometrial nodules has also been noted to occur within 4 months of treatment.[22] Recurrence of symptoms has been shown to occur in approximately one-third of patients, commonly within 1 year.[21] Treatment is usually continued for 6 to 9 months, with spontaneous ovulation often occurring within 6 to 8 weeks following therapy. Corrected pregnancy rates after pseudopregnancy treatment vary from 26 to 72 percent. Interpretation is difficult because of the variety of drugs used, patient preselection, and lack of standards for therapy and effectiveness. Spontaneous rupture of endometriomas has been reported in patients with severe disease treated with induction of pseudopregnancy.[20] Other complications of oral contraceptive therapy include reproductive system and systemic side effects (Chap. 16).

DYSMENORRHEA AND CHRONIC PELVIC PAIN

Historical Perspective

Dysmenorrhea has presented a therapeutic challenge to physicians throughout the ages with popular remedies of the past rooted in traditions having little scientific basis. Ancient Greek medicine described the analgesic effect of sweet wine, fennel root, and rose oil when applied to the external genitalia of menstruating women. Chinese women were treated with moxibustion, wherein a cone of wormwood on a slice of ginger was placed on a specific point on the abdomen, ignited, and allowed to burn down to the skin. In the mid-1800s bilateral oophorectomy became popular for the treatment of dysmenorrhea and other functional disorders.

At the turn of the century, a number of plant extracts and synthetic chemicals were used, with opium being the most popular. Nitroglycerine was recommended for symptoms of vasomotor lability and pallor. The association between dysmenorrhea and ovulation was first noted in the 1930s, with Sturgis and Albright, in 1940, the first investigators to demonstrate that estrogens suppress ovulation by inhibiting pituitary gonadotropins.[23] Pending the development of oral contraceptives, estrogens remained the treatment of choice for dysmenorrhea. Following their introduction, oral contraceptives became the preferred hormonal therapy for dysmenorrhea, although with further elucidation of side effects the risks of such treatment became arguably greater than the benefits.

In 1965, Dickles postulated the role prostaglandins (PGs) play in the etiology of dysmenorrhea, and in 1971 Vane speculated that aspirinlike compounds act by inhibiting PG synthesis. Dickles subsequently suggested that antiinflammatory agents might be used to treat dysmenorrhea, and since then the efficacy of PG synthesis inhibitors has been demonstrated in multiple clinical studies.[24] Future development of drugs that act more specifically on uterine PGs may allow the physician an even more effective means of treating the symptoms of dysmenorrhea and chronic pelvic pain.

The exact incidence of dysmenorrhea is difficult to quantitate with certainty although it is estimated that 52 percent of post pubescent females are affected and that 10 percent are disabled for 1 to 3 days each month. Dysmenorrhea represents the single most common cause of work and school absenteeism among young women.[25] Primary dysmenorrhea, or menstrual discomfort in the absence of pelvic pathology, generally begins with the initiation of ovulatory cycles and thus first occurs 6 to 12 months following menarche and becomes progressively worse with time. The characteristic history is that of colicky lower quadrant pain radiating to the thighs and lower back. In greater than 50 percent of patients this pain is accompanied by one or more systemic symptoms including diarrhea (60 percent) and headache (45 percent). The pain usually occurs immediately prior to menstruation and symptoms may continue for several hours up to 3 days. The diagnosis of primary dysmenorrhea is suggested by the above historical features in conjunction with a normal pelvic examination.

Menstrual pain initially occurring later in reproductive life is known as secondary dysmenorrhea and is related to pelvic pathology or anatomic abnormalities. These may include endometriosis, myomas, pelvic inflammatory disease, polyps, or Müllerian anomalies resulting in outflow obstruction. The pain of secondary dysmenorrhea contrasts with primary dysmenorrhea in that it often begins several days before menstruation and may occur at various times during the menstrual cycle. Furthermore, treatment of secondary dysmenorrhea is less amenable to drug manipulation and more curable by operative intervention.

Etiology

The pathophysiology of primary dysmenorrhea is thought to involve a variety of factors including uterine blood flow, myometrial activity, ovarian–pituitary hormones, cervical factors, and, most recently, prostaglandins.

Uterine blood flow has been advanced as a possible factor in the etiology of dysmenorrhea based on studies recording local endometrial blood flow in dysmenorrheic women during pain.[26] Decreases in local endometrial blood flow were noted during uterine contractions and correlated with maximal colicky pain. The relation between blood flow and pain demonstrated by these recordings has led to the hypothesis that primary dysmenorrhea may result from uterine ischemia occurring secondary to uterine hyperactivity or to other factors acting on the uterine vasculature.

Using microtransducer catheters, myometrial hyperactivity during painful menstruation was demonstrated in almost all dysmenorrheic women.[26] In women with primary dysmenorrhea the following aberrations of uterine activity have been demonstrated: elevated basal tone (> 10 mm Hg), elevated intrauterine active pressure, increased frequency of contractions (> five per 10 minutes), and dysrhythmic uterine activity. Concomitant with such abnormal uterine activity is a reduction in uterine blood flow resulting in uterine ischemia and pain characteristic of primary dysmenorrhea. Although previous investigators sought to ascribe the pain of dysmenorrhea to specific contractile patterns, such as regular or dysrhythmic activity, no single activity pattern has been shown to be responsible.[26]

Estrogen and progesterone may have a role in the pathology of dysmenorrhea since anovulatory women seldom experience such discomfort, and therapy with oral contraceptives is effective in relieving dysmenorrhea. The mechanism wherein ovarian steroids are involved in the pathophysiology of dysmenorrhea is unknown, although it has been suggested that these steroids may affect uterine production of and response to prostaglandins.

Vasopressin stimulates myometrial activity and exerts a direct effect on the vasculature to decrease uterine blood flow.[27] Although its precise role in the etiology of primary dysmenorrhea is not clearly defined, recent evidence suggests a link between arginine vasopressin (AVP) and painful menstruation. Increased plasma levels of AVP have been demonstrated in dysmenorrheic women, and AVP and prostaglandins have been shown to act synergistically upon the uterus.[28] The above suggest a potentially important role for AVP in the genesis of primary dysmenorrhea.

Cervical obstruction and subsequent retention of menstrual secretion as a cause of painful menstruation is a theory of dysmenorrhea ascribed to Hippocrates.[28] Early reports indicating improvement of dysmenorrhea following cervical dilatation gave credence to this concept. More recent evaluation of such therapy has demonstrated an occasionally favorable but usually temporary response. Further observations arguing against this theory include the lack of dysmenorrhea in cases of known cervical stenosis, its occurrence in patients with unobstructed and profuse menstrual flow, and the pain secondary to mechanical obstruction (as in hematometra) being dissimilar in character to typical dysmenorrhea. Although cervical obstruction alone may not be a direct cause of dysmenorrhea, it may delay the discharge of menstrual fluid. Uterine distension may result, and myometrial hyperactivity can occur from the increased absorption of prostaglandins from the menstrual fluid.

Role of Prostaglandins

Prostaglandins are oxygenated metabolites of certain 20-carbon polyunsaturated, essential fatty acids and are composed of a central five-membered ring with two side chains. Precursor fatty acids are membrane bound in cells and require release by phospholipase enzymes before PG synthesis can be initiated (Fig. 26-1). A variety of stimuli are known to activate phospholipase for PG biosynthesis. These include chemical, neural, mechanical, and hormonal stimuli including estrogen and progesterone. Prostaglandin synthesis occurs throughout the body with all cell types demonstrating the capacity for converting fatty acids into PGs. The ratio of different PGs varies in different tissues and within the same tissue depending on the circumstances.

Uterine PG synthesis is apparently initiated by lysosomal enzymes released late in the menstrual cycle. The action of these enzymes, induced by the alteration in the hormonal environment, may be responsible for the release of phospholipids from the cell membrane. These phospholipids provide the common denominator, arachidonic acid, along with other fatty acids necessary for prostaglandin synthesis. The initial step in the conversion of arachidonic acid to PGs is the formation of prostaglandin G_2, a cyclic endoperoxide. This reaction is inhibited by nonsteroidal anti-inflammatory agents.[29] Prostaglandins E_2 and F_2 are subsequently formed from prostaglandin G_2. Progesterone induces PG production. Since primary dysmenorrhea is observed only during ovulatory cycles, progesterone may function to regulate endometrial PG production.

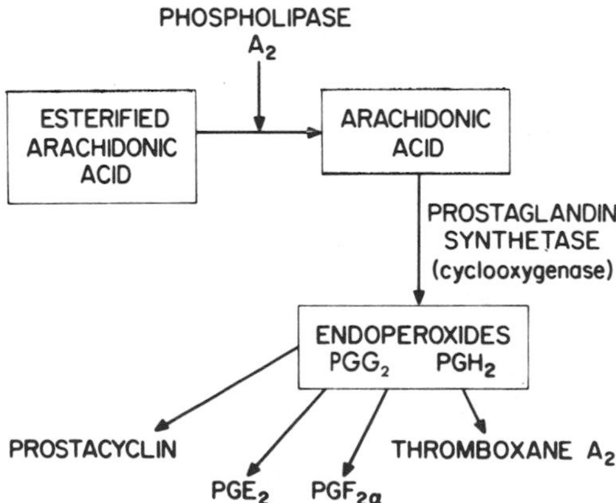

Figure 26–1. PGSI inhibition of prostaglandin biosynthesis.

A role for PGs in primary dysmenorrhea is suggested by the observation that the concentrations of prostaglandins E_2 and F_2, present in the endometrium throughout the cycle, are maximal at the time of menstruation.[30] Increased PG levels have been demonstrated in endometrial jet-wash specimens, menstrual blood, and endometrial tissue from patients with primary dysmenorrhea. Additional evidence suggesting a direct relation between PG synthesis and primary dysmenorrhea includes the following:

1. Plasma concentrations of the metabolite of prostaglandins $F_{2\alpha}$ ($PGF_{2\alpha}$) (15-keto, 13, 14-dihydro-$PGF_{2\alpha}$) are higher in women with primary dysmenorrhea.
2. Side effects of $PGF_{2\alpha}$ administration, either as an abortifacient or for the induction of term labor, include nausea, vomiting, headache, diarrhea, and cramps that are similar to the symptoms of primary dysmenorrhea.
3. Certain PG synthesis inhibitors have been shown to be effective in the therapy of primary dysmenorrhea.

A recent theory advanced by Henzel and Izu to explain the mechanism of action of PGs in producing dysmenorrhea is as follows: Lysosomal enzymes released as a result of the changing balance of ovarian hormones at menstruation activate phospholipases. These stimulate the release of phospholipids, which are rearranged into arachidonic acid and other PG precursors, which are then converted to PGs by the enzyme complex PG synthetase.[30] Prostaglandins so formed subsequently cause myometrial hyperactivity, vascular constriction, decreased uterine blood flow, and tissue ischemia, resulting in the typical symptoms of dysmenorrhea.

An approach to the diagnoses and treatment of the women with the premenstrual syndrome has been described recently.[31] Pharmacologic options in the management of primary dysmenorrhea include oral contraceptives (OCs) and prostaglandin synthetase inhibitors (PGSI). Oral contraceptives are well suited to the treatment of primary dysmenorrhea in young, sexually active women desiring contraception. Combination-type OCs have been utilized effectively for this purpose since their introduction and provide symptomatic relief in 90 percent or more of women so treated for primary dysmenorrhea (Chap. 19). Following initiation of OC therapy, endometrial tissue is suppressed, resulting in decreased menstrual fluid volume, and ovulation is inhibited. This mimics the hormonal environment of the early proliferative phase when PG levels are at their nadir. These changes are thought to account for a general reduction in menstrual fluid PG levels and subsequent symptomatic relief of women treated with OCs.

If contraception is not required, or oral contraceptives are contraindicated, the most appropriate alternative for the treatment of primary dysmenorrhea is a PGSI. These compounds do not inhibit the pituitary ovarian axis or induce the pejorative metabolic effects of the OC. As a group PGSI can be divided into two classes: (1) the aryl carboxylic acids, which include the salicyclic acids (aspirin) and fenemates (mefenamic acid, flufenamic acid); and (2) the aryl alkanoic acids, consisting of the aryl propionic acids (indomethacin). The mechanism of action of these agents is thought to involve their suppression of PG synthesis via inhibition of the prostaglandin synthetase (cyclooxygenase) enzyme. The resulting decreased levels of PGs correlate with reduced intrauterine pressure and significant relief of pain. The following is a review of the cumulative experience with currently available PGSIs. Table 26-1 lists dosages for the various brands of these drugs.

Aspirin

Aspirin is still the most commonly used PGSI. Low cost and wide availability make it well suited for treatment of mild dysmenorrhea. Unfortunately, one tablet (0.5 g) given four times daily for 3 days is not significantly more effective than placebo or acetaminophen (0.5 g four times daily for 3 days).[32] The recommended dose of aspirin for analgesia is 0.3 to 1.0 g every 3 to 4 hours.[33] Higher doses of either aspirin or acetaminophen may prove to be more effective. One trial has demonstrated this potential, as 62 percent of patients on 1.0-g doses of acetaminophen achieved relief.[34]

Indolacetic Acid Derivatives

In 1953, before prostaglandins were recognized as a factor in dysmenorrhea, women taking phenylbutazone for treatment of rheumatic disease experienced a decrease in menstrual pain.[35] Despite this finding, phenylbutazone has not been widely used to treat dysmenorrhea, because it is poorly tolerated by many patients. Nausea, vomiting, epigastric discomfort, and skin rashes are the most frequently reported side effects, while more serious effects include edema, peptic ulcer, and hematologic toxicity (aplastic anemia,

TABLE 26-1. DRUGS TO TREAT DYSMENORRHEA AND CHRONIC PELVIC PAIN

Drug	Dosages for Treatment of Dysmenorrhea
Indolacetic acids	
Indomethacin	25-mg capsules three times a day
(Indocin)	50-mg capsules three times a day
Indeneacotic acid	
Sulindac (Clinoril)	N/A
Propionic acids	
Naproxen	250 mg × 2 stat, then
(Naprosyn)	250 mg every 4–6 hr
Naproxen sodium	275 mg × 2 stat, then
(Anaprox)	275 mg every 6–8 hr
Ibuprofen (Motrin)	400 mg three times a day
Fenoprofen	
(Nalfon)	200 mg every 4–6 hr
Fenemate	
Mefenamic acid	250 mg × 2 stat, then
(Ponstel)	250 mg every 6 hr

Abbreviation: N/A = not applicable.

leukopenia, agranulocytosis, and thrombocytopenia). Another member of this pharmacologic class, indomethacin (Indocin), has been evaluated in 12 clinical trials involving a total of 350 women.[36] An average of 68 percent (range 58 to 100 percent) of women reported excellent to complete relief, while 19 percent of patients (range 0 to 29 percent) experienced minimal or no pain relief. The average placebo response was 16 percent. Of the 134 side effects reported from these trials, the majority involved the central nervous system (72 patients reporting headaches and dizziness) and gastrointestinal system (49 patients). The usual dose of indomethacin for primary dysmenorrhea is 25 to 50 mg three times daily which is begun either prior to the onset of menses or when symptoms occur.

Propionic Acid Derivatives

Propionic acid derivatives provide good pain relief in dysmenorrhea without the bothersome central nervous system effects of indomethacin. Drugs included in this classification are ibuprofen (Motrin), fenoprofen (Nalfon), naproxen (Naprosyn), and naproxen sodium (Anaprox).

Naproxen and its sodium salt have been evaluated in 19 trials totaling 712 women.[36] In 17 of these trials pain relief percentages were reported with an average of 62 percent of patients (range 13 to 100 percent) indicating complete or excellent relief of symptoms, while 21 percent (range 7 to 38 percent) achieved only minimal or no relief of symptoms. The placebo response averaged 16 percent. The significant pain relief using either agent compared to placebo is associated with a marked reduction in uterine tonicity. The sodium content of each 275-mg tablet of naproxen sodium is 25 mg (1 mEq). A total of 62 side effects were reported, with the majority referrable to the central nervous system (headache and fatigue). Lower back discomfort and minor gastrointestinal symptoms were the next most common. Only three women reported side effects as their reason for discontinuing therapy in the ten trials providing this information. Most data support a dose of 550 mg (two tablets of naproxen sodium) started with the onset of symptoms, then 275 mg every 4 to 6 hours until symptoms abate.

Ibuprofen has been investigated in 11 trials including 308 women.[36] Measurable decreases in menstrual fluid PG levels, uterine pressures, and good to excellent pain relief have been reported in patients receiving this agent. Of the seven trials reporting percentages of patients with pain relief, an average of 66 percent (range 42 to 87 percent) achieved excellent or complete pain relief, while 22 percent (range 13 to 39 percent) reported minimal or no pain relief. A placebo response averaged 17 percent, ranging from 2 to 30 percent. In the usual dosages of 400 mg every 4 to 8 hours, reported side effects are minimal, consisting primarily of occasional nausea.

Fenemates

Flufenamic and mefanamic acid have been investigated in 9 trials totaling 279 women.[39] An average of 90 percent of patients (range 88 to 100 percent) reported excellent or complete pain relief in the five studies specifying pain relief percentages. Minimal or no relief of symptoms was reported in 4 percent and 14 percent of subjects in two mefanamic acid trials. The placebo response ranged from 0 to 16 percent. A total of 22 side effects were reported with the majority being minor gastrointestinal complaints. If diarrhea occurs, mefenamic acid should be discontinued because of its association with ulceration or inflammation of either the upper or lower gastrointestinal tract. The use of mefanamic acid to treat moderate pain should not exceed 1 week, since serious gastrointestinal effects or nephrotoxicity have been associated with prolonged use.

Mefanamic acid may have two advantages over the other PSGIs. First, it not only inhibits PG synthesis, but also reduces the activity of already synthesized PGs.[37] Second, in patients with menorrhagia, a significant reduction in menstrual blood loss has been described.[38] Treatment is begun with the onset of symptoms, using 250 to 500 mg initially followed by 250 mg every 6 hours.

In summary, PGSIs are effective therapy for primary dysmenorrhea. The fenemates appear to be the most efficacious as indicated by the percentage of patients achieving complete relief of menstrual signs and symptoms. Side effects referrable to the fenemates ibuprofen and naproxen are infrequent, mild, and primarily gastrointestinal in nature for the fenemates and ibuprofen and central nervous system related for naproxen. Indomethacin has the highest incidence of side effects, most involving the central nervous system.

Based on the data from studies to date, it can be anticipated that anywhere from 9 to 22 percent of dysmenorrheic women will not respond to treatment with PGSIs. Other pelvic pathology to be ruled out should include endometriosis, pelvic inflammatory disease, and uterine myomas. As indicated in multiple trials, with the exception of indomethacin, side effects of PGSI therapy are an uncommon cause of patient discontinuation of therapy.

The following dosages of PGSIs are those employed most frequently in trials to date: fenemates, 250 to 500 mg, 3 to 4 times daily; ibuprofen, 400 mg, 3 to 4 times daily; naproxen, 250 mg, 4 times daily; naproxen sodium, 275 mg, 3 to 4 times daily; indomethacin, 25 to 50 mg, 3 times daily. Pretreatment with PGSIs is not considered necessary. Therapy is usually initiated with the onset of symptoms (usually corresponding to the onset of menstruation) and continued for 2 or 3 days. Such a schedule minimizes prolonged treatment, decreases the likelihood of side effects, and guards against potential teratogenic effects with early pregnancy usage.

Other Drugs

Many other medications have been utilized in the management of primary dysmenorrhea. Anticholinergic agents, such as methoscopolamine bromide (Pamine) and methantheline bromide (Banthine), are atropine-like medications. Their inhibition of the parasympathetic nervous system produces some degree of uterine relaxation, but may be accompanied by unwanted effects such as tachycardia, dry mouth, blurred vision, and urinary retention. β-adrenergic receptor stimulants, such as isoxsuprine (Vasodilan) and terbutaline (Bricanyl, Brethine), have the potential to produce relaxation in the nonpregnant uterus.[39] The response to these agents is variable, and side effects such as tachycardia and nervousness may limit their use. Isoxsuprine is significantly less effective than placebo in relieving pain of dysmenorrhea and may even increase uterine vascular congestion.[40] Terbutaline is significantly more effective than placebo in relieving symptoms of dysmenorrhea, but has not been used extensively to treat this disorder.[41]

Guidelines for Managing Chronic Pelvic Pain

Careful evaluation of the patient's history and a thorough physical examination is important for the diagnosis and proper treatment of dysmenorrhea and chronic pelvic pain. The absence of obvious pelvic pathology indicates the patient may be a suitable candidate for medical management.

Of the currently available classes of drugs, the prostaglandin synthetase inhibitors have been shown to be highly effective with minimal side effects. The fenemates, such as Ponstel, have some advantage over the propionic derivatives, such as Naprosyn and Motrin, since they inhibit the activity of PGs already formed. Indoleacetic acid derivatives have proven efficacy but with a high incidence of side effects. Despite its relative low cost, aspirin may be significantly less effective in the recommended doses in comparison to other medications. Anticholinergic agents and β-adrenergic receptor stimulants may have some future use in the treatment of dysmenorrhea and pelvic pain, but are currently not popular because of their variable response and side effects.

Exploratory surgery, usually by laporoscopy, is indicated in the presence of pelvic pathology or if medical management fails after at least a 3-month trial.

REFERENCES

1. Sampson JA: The life history of ovarian hematomas (hemorrhagic cysts) of endometrial müllerian type. Am J Obstet Gynecol iv:451, 1922
2. Dmowski WP, Radwanska E: Endometriosis and infertility. Acta Obstet Gynecol Scand (Suppl)123:73, 1984
3. Kistner RW: Management of endometriosis in the infertile patient. Fertil Steril 26:1151, 1975
4. Thorell JI, Rannevik G, Dymling JF: Effect of danazol on thyroid function in women. Postgrad Med J 55(Suppl 5):33, 1979
5. Young MD, Blackmore WP: The use of danazol in the management of endometriosis. J Int Med Res 5(Suppl 3):86, 1977
6. Fraser IS: Danazol—A steroid with a unique combination of actions. Scot Med J 24:147, 1979
7. Mettler L, Semm K: Clinical and biochemical experiences with danazol in the treatment of endometriosis in cases with female infertility. Postgrad Med J 55(Suppl 5):27, 1979
8. Dmowski WT, Cohen MR: Antigonadotropin (danazol) in the treatment of endometriosis. Am J Obstet Gynecol 130:41, 1978
9. Audebert AJM, Emperaire JC, Larrve CS: Endometriosis and infertility: A review of sixty-two patients treated with danazol. Postgrad Med J 55(Suppl 5):10, 1979
10. Greenblatt RB, Tzigounis V: Danazol treatment of endometriosis: Long-term follow up. Fertil Steril 32:518, 1979
11. Low RAL, Roberts ADG, Lees DAR: A comparative study of various dosages of danazol in the treatment of endometriosis. Br J Obstet Gynaecol 91:167, 1984
12. Moore EE, Harger JH, Rock JA, Archer DF: Management of pelvic endometriosis with low dose danazol. Fertil Steril 36:15, 1981
13. Chalmers JA: Treatment of endometriosis with reduced dosage schedules of danazol. Scot Med 27:143, 1982
14. Butler L, Wilson E, Belisle S, et al.: Collaborative study of pregnancy rates following danazol therapy of stage I endometriosis. Fertil Steril 41:373, 1984
15. Ronnberg L, Jarvinen PA: Pregnancy rates following various therapy modes for endometriosis in infertile patients. Acta Obstet Gynecol Scand Suppl 123:69, 1984
16. Danazol for fibrocystic disease of the breast. Med Lett 23:5, 1981
17. Chalmers JA, Shervington PC: Follow-up of patients with endometriosis treated with danazol. Postgrad Med J 55(Suppl 5):44, 1979
18. Ward GD: Dosage aspects of danazol therapy in endometriosis. J Int Med Res 5(Suppl 3):75, 1977
19. Hoskins AL, Woolf RB: Stilbestrol-induced hyperhormonal amenorrhea for the treatment of pelvic endometriosis. Obstet Gynecol 5:113, 1955
20. Hammond CB, Haney AF: Conservative treatment of endometriosis. Fertil Steril 30:497, 1978
21. Kistner RW: The treatment of endometriosis by inducing pseudopregnancy with ovarian hormones. Fertil Steril 10:539, 1959
22. Hammond CB, Rock JA, Parker RT: Conservative treatment of endometriosis: The effects of limited surgery and hormonal pseudopregnancy. Fertil Steril 7:756, 1976
23. Sturgis SH, Albright F: The mechanism of estrin therapy in the relief of dysmenorrhea. Endocrinology 26:68–72, 1940
24. Henzel MR, Massey S, Hanson FW et al.: Primary dysmenorrhea: The therapeutic challenge. J Reprod Med 25(Suppl 4):226, 1980
25. Dawood MY: Dysmenorrhea. Clin Obstet Gynecol 26:719, 1983
26. Akerlund M: Pathophysiology of dysmenorrhea. Acta Obstet Gynecol 87(Suppl):27, 1979
27. Akerlund M, Anderson KE: Vasopressin response and terbutaline inhibition of the uterus. Obstet Gynecol 48:528, 1976
28. Voto SJ, Essig GF: Primary dysmenorrhea: Current concepts. Ohio St Med J 80:606, 1984
29. Samuelsson B, Granstrom E, Green K, et al.: Prostaglandin and thromboxanes. Annu Rev Biochem 47:997, 1978
30. Henzel MR, Izu A: Naproxen and naproxen sodium in dysmenorrhea: Development from in vitro inhibition of prostaglandin synthesis to suppression of uterine contractions in women and demonstration of clinical efficacy. Acta Obstet Gynecol Scand 87(Suppl):105, 1979
31. Pariser S, Stern S, Shank S, et al.: Premenstrual syndrome: Concerns, controversies, and treatment. Am J Obstet Gynecol 153:599, 1985
32. Janbu T, Lokken P, Nesheim BI: Effect of acetylsalicylic acid, paracetamol and placebo on pain and blood loss in dysmenorrheic women. Acta Obstet Gynecol Scand 87(Suppl):81, 1979
33. Flower RJ, Moncada S, Vane JR: Analgesic-antipyretics and anti-inflammatory agents. In

Gilman AG, Goodman LS, Gilman A (eds): The Pharmacological Basis of Therapeutics, ed. 6. New York, Macmillan, 1980, pp 682–728

34. Layes Molla A, Donald JF: A comparative study of ibuprofen and paracetamol in primary dysmenorrhea. J Int Med Res 2:395, 1974
35. Fox WW: Butazolidine: Letter to the editor. Lancet 1:195, 1953
36. Owen PR: Prostaglandin synthetase inhibitors in the treatment of primary dysmenorrhea. Am J Obstet Gynecol 148:96, 1984
37. Simon LS, Mills JA: Nonsteroidal anti-inflammatory drugs. N Engl J Med 302(22):1238, 1980
38. Anderson AB, et al.: Reduction of menstrual blood loss by prostaglandin synthetase inhibitors. Lancet 1:774, 1976
39. Koelle, GB: Neurohumoral transmission and the autonomic nervous system. In Goodman LS, Gilman A (eds): The Pharmacological Basis of Therapeutics, ed. 5. New York, Macmillan, 1975, pp 404–444
40. Rubin A: Isoxsuprine for the treatment of dysmenorrhea: A double-blind study of 143 subjects. Obstet Gynecol 19:9, 1962
41. Akerlund M, Andersson KE, Ingemarsson I: Effect of terbutaline on myometrial activity, uterine blood flow, and lower abdominal pain in women. Br J Obstet Gynecol 83(9):673–678, 1976

27

Chemotherapy in Gynecologic Oncology

John G. Boutselis and James A. Roberts

A remarkable advancement in the management of cancer has been the demonstration that certain disseminated malignancies may be controlled or cured using chemotherapy.[1] Although surgery and radiation remain the primary regional modes for treating gynecologic malignancies, adjuvant chemotherapy provides the only means of systemic therapy for disseminated disease.[1] Promising results have been shown using adjuvant drugs in treating trophoblastic and ovarian neoplasms. Investigations are also continuing in determining the efficacy of adjuvant chemotherapy in widespread squamous cell carcinoma of the vulva or cervix and endometrial adenocarcinoma.

This chapter reviews general principles of cancer chemotherapy, particularly as they relate to cellular biology and kinetics. The proposed mechanisms of action, usual dose ranges, and adverse effects are described for each of the commonly used agents, classified in Table 27–1. The role of these drugs in the management of gynecologic malignancies is then briefly discussed; however, the treatment of each specific malignancy is beyond the scope of this chapter.

PRINCIPLES OF CANCER CHEMOTHERAPY

Principles of chemotherapy are derived from their original successful application to the treatment of choriocarcinoma, Burkitt's lymphoma, acute lymphocytic leukemia, Hodgkin's disease, Wilms' tumor, Ewing's sarcoma, and testicular carcinoma.[2] The one common denominator in these tumors is a rapid proliferation of cells. Conversely, tumors with a slower growth rate are usually less responsive to antineoplastic agents. Utilizing the L-1210 mouse leukemia model, it has been established that a given dose of an effective chemotherapeutic drug kills a constant fraction of cells regardless of the number of cells present in a tumor (fractional kill hypothesis).[3] A single course of drug therapy may result in a 90 percent decrease of a 10^{10} (10 billion) cell population/cm^3 of tumor. With each succeeding dose, the number of surviving cells is proportionately decreased. Li et al. have demonstrated this hypothesis of fractional kill through the use of the human chorionic gonadotropin (HCG) tumor marker in choriocarcinoma.[4]

TABLE 27-1. CLASSIFICATION OF CURRENTLY USED CHEMOTHERAPEUTIC AGENTS

I	Alkylating agents
	Cyclophosphamide (Cytoxan)
	Melphelan (Alkeran)
	Chlorambucil (Leukeran)
	Triethylenethiophosphoramide (Thiotepa)
	Mechlorethamine (Mustargen)
II	Antimetabolites
	Methotrexate (Amethopterin)
	5-Fluorouracil (5-FU, Fluorouracil)
	6-Mercaptopurine (6MP) (Purinethol)
III	Antibiotics
	Dactinomycin (Cosmegen)
	Doxorubicin (Adriamycin)
	Bleomycin (Blenoxane)
	Mitomycin-C (Mutamycin)
	Mithramycin (Mithracin)
IV	Plant alkaloids—Vinca alkaloids (periwinkle drugs)
	Vinblastine (Velban)
	Vincristine (Oncovin)
V	Hormones (progestins)
	Medroxyprogesterone acetate (Depo-Provera)
	Hydroxyprogesterone caproate (Delalutin)
	Megestrol acetate (Megace)
VI	Other drugs (miscellaneous)
	Hydroxyurea (Hydrea)
	Cis-Diamininodichloroplatinum II (Platinol)
	Tamoxifen (Nolvadex)
	Hexamethylmelamine
	Dacarbazine (DTIC)
	Nitrosourea (Carmustine)

Variables to be considered in administering chemotherapy include the immunocompetence of the host, the volume of the tumor, the growth rate, the number and sensitivity of cells entering the resting phase of the cell cycle (G-0), the specific agents, and the dose schedules utilized.

Cell Growth Kinetics

To understand growth kinetics of cancer cells with uncontrolled proliferative characteristics, one must understand the kinetics of *normal* cell growth. Cell growth kinetics may be divided into three tissue groups (expanding, static, and renewing) that relate to parenchymal cell production and loss. The *expanding* tissues (kidney, liver, endocrine glands) are composed of differentiated cells that do not require replacement and will survive the lifetime of the organism. They maintain their ability to replicate and replace accidental cell loss. *Static* tissues (nerve and striated muscle) are highly differentiated, and these cells have lost their capacity to divide. *Renewing* tissues (bone marrow, gastrointestinal mucosa, epidermis, and hair follicles) are composed of differentiated cells with a short life span; these are constantly renewed from a stem cell or clonogenic subpopulation. Cancer cells possess the attribute of uncontrolled cell growth and most closely resemble the renewing cell tissues since they depend on the stem cell or a subpopulation of cells.[3]

The Cell Cycle

Cell growth kinetics are best illustrated in Figure 27-1, which depicts the cell cycle. The S, G-1, and M phases are relatively constant for any cell type. As the G-1 phase becomes more prolonged, the cell enters a resting or nondividing phase (G-0). The resting cell can either enter into the dividing cell cycle or remain as a permanently nondividing cell and eventually die. Hence, the G-0 phase can act as a reservoir from which cell proliferation can occur.[5]

The metabolic characteristics of the various phases of the cell cycle are important to the clinician, since various chemotherapeutic agents have damaging effects at one or more phases of the life cycle of the cell (Table 27-2). In general, some agents are characterized as being cell cycle-specific or phase-specific, while other agents are cell cycle-nonspecific or phase nonspecific. The distinction between specific and nonspecific agents is relative rather than absolute.

High doses of phase-specific agents have been used intermittently when a tumor has a rapid growth potential. The continuous ex-

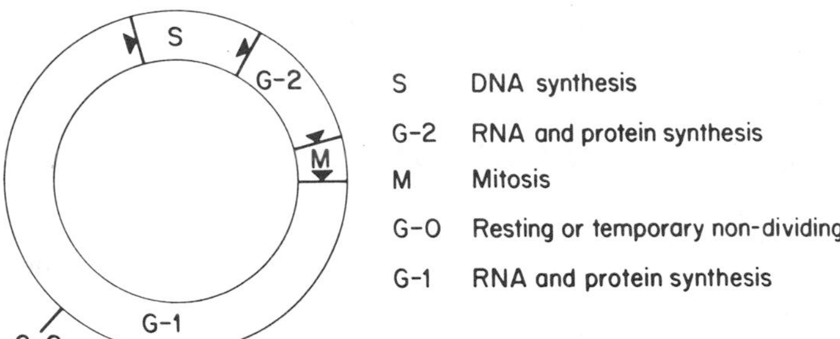

Figure 27–1. The cell life cycle.

posure of a tumor to cycle- and phase-specific drugs should destroy any resistant, resting tumor cells which eventually enter the more drug-sensitive proliferating cycle.[5]

MECHANISMS OF ACTION

The mechanisms of action of chemotherapeutic agents relate to the different phase of the cancer cell cycle and whether or not the agents are cycle-nonspecific or cycle-specific.[6] Although antineoplastic agents vary in their mechanisms of action, they all destroy rapidly proliferating cells by interfering with one or more of the sequences in cell replication.

TABLE 27–2. RELATION BETWEEN THE CELL CYCLE AND DAMAGING EFFECTS FROM CHEMOTHERAPEUTIC AGENTS

Cycle-nonspecific agents
- Alkylating agents
- Antibiotics

Cycle-specific agents
- Antimetabolites
- Plant alkaloids
- Miscellaneous group

Phases of the cell cycle and effective agents
- S (DNA synthesis) = alk. agents, methotrexate (MTX), 5-FU, H. urea, 6-MP, cytosine arabinoside, (ARC-C), actinomycin D, adriamycin
- G-2 (RNA + protein synthesis) = alk. agents, 5-FU, actinomycin D
- M (mitosis) = alk. agents, vincristine, vinblastine, bleomycin, nitrogen mustard
- G-O (resting) = alk. agents, adriamycin, actinomycin D, mitomycin D, bleomycin
- G-1 (RNA + protein synthesis) = alk. agents, MTX, 5-FU, actinomycin D

Alkylating Agents

This is the single most commonly used group of antineoplastic agents. These agents produce carbonium ions which alkylate or cross-link with amino, carboxyl, phosphate, or sulfhydryl groups present in cells. The highly nucleophilic number 7 nitrogen in quanine, a DNA purine base, is a likely site for this covalent bond. This bonding results in an altered structional configuration of quanine and abnormal base pairs. Cross-linking with guanine pairs stops DNA function and may cause DNA strand breaks. This results in the inhibition of nearly all cellular function and leads to cell death. The alkylating agents act during the G-0 to M cell phases of the cell cycle. These drugs are cycle-nonspecific agents, since they do not depend on DNA synthesis for their effect and are best suited for slow-growing bulky tumors. The cells, which remain unaltered after alkylating therapy, are more susceptible to attack by cycle-specific agents.

Antimetabolites

Antimetabolites are a large heterogenous group of cycle-specific or phase-specific agents which act by inhibiting essential metabolic processes that are necessary for DNA or RNA synthesis. The most common folic acid antagonist, methotrexate, acts to prevent the reduction of folic acid to folinic acid. It combines with the enzyme, dihydrofolinic acid reductase, to interfere with the formation of tetrahydrofolinic acid, a substance needed for thymidine and purine synthesis. Hence, it behaves as an enzyme-blocking agent, inhibiting DNA and RNA synthesis.

5-Fluorouracil (5-FU) is the most effective and widely prescribed pyrimidine analogue. It binds with thymidylate synthetase after being incorporated into the nucleic acid complex. Thymidine deficiency results from this enzyme inhibition, and cell replication is prevented.

Antibiotics

Antibiotics are phase- or cycle-nonspecific agents which form a complex with DNA. This is caused by a selective binding at the guanine-cytosine segment to block the enzyme, DNA-dependent RNA synthetase, and inhibit the formation of messenger RNA and subsequent cell protein synthesis. These agents may also cause single and double DNA chain breaks resulting in DNA malfunction. It is this mechanism of action that results in the synergism between these agents and radiation therapy.

Plant Alkaloids

The plant alkaloids vinblastine sulfate and vincristine, from the periwinkle plant, *Vinca rosea,* are cycle-specific agents which arrest mitosis during metaphase by binding to the protein necessary for mitotic spindle formation.

Hormones

Although the mechanisms of action are poorly understood, hormones seem to induce their therapeutic effect by binding with specific receptor proteins. This complex then interacts with the chromatin to alter RNA-directed protein synthesis. The major advantage of this group is the relative lack of toxicity.

Other Drugs

cis-*Platinum*

The biochemical properties of *cis*-platinum are similar to that of the alkylating agents which cause interstrand and intrastrand cross-links in DNA. Its action is cell cycle-nonspecific by inhibiting translation of DNA precursors for DNA and protein synthesis. Analogues of this drug, which are less toxic, are presently under study.

Hexamethylamine

Hexamethylamine acts in an unknown manner. It was originally thought to be a member of the alkylating agent group but its action is more similar to the antimetabolites.

Hydroxyurea

Hydroxyurea enhances radiosensitivity, perhaps by freezing cells into the relatively radiosensitive, late phase of G-1 rather than permitting them to proceed to the radioresistant S-phase of the cycle. This mode of action may make this a most useful drug for cell cycling and combination with a cycle-specific drug.

Tamoxifen

Tamoxifen is an antiestrogen-like compound, similar to clomiphene in chemical structure, which competes with circulating estrogen at intracellular receptor sites in the cytoplasm and nucleus complex. It may also induce a therapeutic effect by altering prostaglandin production.

DOSES AND ROUTES OF ADMINISTRATION

The doses and routes of administration of the various agents are listed in Tables 27–3 and 27–4. The goal of adjunctive chemotherapy is maximal tumor cell kill with minimal toxic

TABLE 27-3. DOSAGE REGIMENS AND SIDE EFFECTS OF THE VARIOUS CHEMOTHERAPY AGENTS

Drug	Dose and Route of Administration	Acute Side Effects	Toxicity
Alkylating agents			
Cyclophosphamide (Cytoxan)	750–1,000 mg/m² IV as single dose every 3 weeks	Nausea and vomiting	Bone marrow (BM) depression (thrombocytopenia), hemorrhagic cystitis, alopecia
Melphalan (Alkeran)	0.2 mg/kg/day PO × 5 days, 4–6 weeks	Nausea and vomiting	BM depression (thrombocytopenia)
Chlorambucil (Leukeran)	0.1–0.2 mg/kg/day PO Decrease dose with BM depression	Nausea and vomiting with high dose	BM depression
Thiotepa (triethylenethiophosphoramide)	0.2 mg/kg/day IV × 5 days	Nausea and vomiting	BM depression
DTIC (carbazine)	150–250 mg/m²/day × 5	Nausea and vomiting	BM depression and hepatotoxicity
Antimetabolites			
Methotrexate (amethopterin)	15–25 mg OD/IV or IM × 5 days for choriocarcinoma. Dose variable with type malignancy.	Usually none; stomatitis	BM toxicity, liver or renal failure; GI disturbance as acute stomatitis, nausea, vomiting and diarrhea; alopecia; pulmonary toxicity
5-Fluorouracil (5-FU, fluorouracil)	12–15 mg/kg IV weekly 12–15 mg/kg IV/OD × 5 days per month 5 mg/kg OD/IV × 5 days as part of act fu cy	Nausea and vomiting	Liver fibrosis rare. BM depression, stomatitis, ileitis, alopecia, diarrhea, cerebellar ataxia
6-Mercaptopurine (6MP, Purinethol)	2.5–5.0 mg/kg PO daily	Nausea and vomiting	BM depression, hepatotoxicity, dermatitis, mucosal ulceration
Antibiotics			
Dactinomycin (actinomycin D, Cosmegen)	12-15 mcg/kg IV daily × 5 days (0.5 mg/day × 5 days)	Pain with extravasation and local skin necrosis; nausea, vomiting, diarrhea, cramps	BM depression, GI symptoms, skin rash; pigmentation and desquamation if had previous irradiation
Doxorubicin (adriamycin)	40–100 mg/m² IV every 3 weeks (maximum dose 550 mg/m²)	Nausea and vomiting; local phlebitis, fever, extravasation necrosis, red urine	BM depression, stomatitis; cardiotoxicity related to cumulative dose
Bleomycin (Blenoxane)	10–20 mg/m² IV or IM one to two times per week (maximum dose total of 400 mg)	Nausea, vomiting, fever, chills, localized pain, stomatitis, skin blisters	Pulmonary fibrosis, BM depression, GI symptoms, skin changes, alopecia, kidney toxicity

(continued)

TABLE 27-3. (*Continued*)

Drug	Dose and Route of Administration	Acute Side Effects	Toxicity
Mitomycin C (mutamycin)	0.05 mg/kg OD/IV × 6 days, then alternate days until total dose of 50 mg	Nausea and vomiting, extravasation necrosis	BM depression, nausea, vomiting, oral ulceration, diarrhea, irreversible thrombocytopenia
Mithramycin (Mithracin)	0.02–0.05 mg/kg	Nausea and vomiting, hypocalcemia	BM depression, hepatotoxicity
Plant Alkaloids (periwinkle drugs)			
Vinblastine (Velban)	0.1–0.2 mg/kg IV per week	Localized severe and prolonged extravasation, skin reaction, headache, nausea and vomiting, parasthesia, stomatitis	BM suppression (especially neutropenia), alopecia, muscle weakness, peripheral neuropathy, depression
Vincristine (Oncovin)	1.5 mg/m^2 IV per week in vincristine, actinomycin D, cyclophosphamide (VAC); 0.4–1.4 mg/m^2 IV weekly in adults, 2 mg/m^2 weekly in children	Extravasation, local inflammation	Neuropathy, constipation, paralytic ileus, weakness and loss of reflexes, foot cramp, hoarseness, depression, BM toxicity (mild), alopecia
Antineoplastic hormones			
Medroxyprogesterone acetate (Depo-Provera)	400–800 mg IM or PO per week	None	Occasional liver function abnormality, alopecia and hypersensitivity with any of the progestational agents, fluid retention
Hydroxyprogesterone caproate (Delalutin)	1,000 mg IM two times per week	None	Same as above
Megestral acetate (Megace)	120–320 mg daily	None	Same as above with caution in cardiac patients
Miscellaneous drugs			
Hydroxyurea (Hydrea)	80 mg/kg PO every 3 days during radiation therapy or 20–30 mg/kg PO daily	Anorexia and nausea	BM depression, alopecia, stomatitis, diarrhea, megaloblastic anemia
Cis-Diammine di-chloroplatinum (*cis*-platinum)	50–100 mg/m^2 IV every 3 weeks	Severe nausea and vomiting	Renal toxicity, neurotoxicity, ototoxicity, moderate BM depression, decreased mg

TABLE 27-3. (*Continued*)

Drug	Dose and Route of Administration	Acute Side Effects	Toxicity
Hexamethylmelamine	4–8 mg/kg PO daily 2 weeks per month, or 3 weeks every 6 weeks	Nausea and vomiting	BM depression, CNS depression, peripheral neuropathy
Tamoxifen citrate (Nolvadex)	10–20 mg PO daily	Nausea	Minimal, if any

TABLE 27-4. MULTIPLE-AGENT CHEMOTHERAPY REGIMENS

Drug	Dose and Route of Administration		Acute Side Effects	Toxicity
MAC				
Methotrexate Actinomycin D Chlorambucil	0.3 mg/kg IM or IV 0.01 mg/kg IV 0.2 mg/kg PO Cytoxan 3–5 mg/kg/day IV in place of chlorambucil	Five times daily every 2–3 weeks	Refer to individual drug for acute side effects	Potential severe BM depression, gut toxicity, alopecia, dermatitis, nausea, stomatitis
VAC				
Vincristine	1.5 mg/m² weekly × 4–6 weeks, then every 2 weeks		Refer to individual drug for acute side effects	BM toxicity; neurologic toxicity; alopecia, constipation, stomatitis, dermatitis, ileus
Actinomycin D Cyclophosphamide	0.5 mg 8 mg/kg When used with x-ray therapy (XRT), give vincristine only until XRT completed.	Five times daily every 4–6 weeks		
PAC				
Cis-platinum Adriamycin Cyclophosphamide	50 mg/m² 50 mg/m² 500 mg	IV every 3 weeks	Refer to individual drug for acute side effects	Potential severe BM toxicity; stomatitis; renal toxicity; cardiotoxicity

effects. The highest tolerable dose of each agent is to be used until either (1) tumor cells are successfully eradicated, or (2) tolerable signs of reversible toxicity are maximized. For chemotherapy to be most effective, the tumor must be decreased to a subclinical or occult size following surgery or radiation. Otherwise, presumed tumoricidal doses during continuous or intermittent therapy may achieve inadequate concentrations in these less accessible tissues. The tumor size is also important to follow during therapy, since tumor growth would indicate a drug failure and the development of a resistant clone of cells. A drug regimen is considered ineffective only after a trial of two or more courses of chemotherapy.

SINGLE VERSUS COMBINATION THERAPY

Although single-agent chemotherapy may be used in certain circumstances, most disseminated gynecologic malignancies are more effectively treated with multiple agents. This varies with the type of malignancy and stages of disease.

Single-agent chemotherapy is more commonly used for slow-growing solid tumors, while rapidly proliferating solid tumors may be more amenable to combination chemotherapy. Combination chemotherapy ideally acts synergistically by increasing the fractional kill of tumor through their different mechanisms of action. Table 27–3 describes the various single agents presently used in treating a number of highly malignant neoplasms, while Table 27–4 describes some of the most common agents used in combination chemotherapy.[5]

ADVERSE EFFECTS

The physician must be familiar with any potential immediate or delayed toxic effects before any agent is administered (Table 27–3). Immunosuppression is the most common side effect, especially with continuous drug therapy. No myelosuppressing agent should be given without initial and periodic blood counts. Recommended dosages and regimens are very schedule-dependent, but should be decreased in the presence of myelosuppression or if drug elimination processes are impaired. The best indicators of hematopoetic reserve are the neutrophil and platelet counts. Therapy should be delayed if the white blood count is less than 3000 mm^3, neutrophil count is less than 1500 mm^3, or platelet count is less than 100,000 mm^3. Furthermore, any drug should be discontinued if signs of severe toxicity develop. This usually occurs in 1 to 3 weeks after beginning the administration of most agents.

Mild signs of toxicity are frequent and include nausea, vomiting, diarrhea, hair loss, and slight temperature elevations. The patient should be aware of these effects and report them to the physician when treated on an out-patient basis.

Supportive care of adverse effects is necessary. Treatment frequently consists of pain relief or management of infectious or myelosuppression complications. Pain is dependent on tumor aggressiveness, tumor location, and patient sensitivity. Drugs used to relieve pain include narcotics, mild analgesics, and Brompton's cocktail (morphine 5 mg, cocaine 10 mg, and 95 percent ethanol/20 ml).[7] Brompton's cocktail may be given with a phenothiazine every 4 hours to prevent rather than to treat the pain. Transfusion is recommended to replace specific blood cell lines. A blood transfusion is usually necessary if the patient is remarkably symptomatic or if the hematocrit is 24 percent or less. Platelet transfusion is necessary if the count is less than 20,000/mm^3 and if spontaneous bleeding occurs. Multiple vitamins are routinely prescribed to anyone taking a chemotherapy agent. Infectious morbidity and mortality are increased with myelosuppression and impaired host defenses. Fever evaluations with surveillance cultures, removal of indwelling catheters, and isolation precautions are indicated.

TABLE 27–5. ROLE OF CHEMOTHERAPY IN THE MANAGEMENT OF VARIOUS GYNECOLOGIC NEOPLASMS*

Neoplasm	Role of Surgery and XRT	Role of Chemotherapy
Squamous cancer of cervix		
Stage IB, IIA	1. Radical hysterectomy with pelvic lymphadenectomy *or* T & C plus ext. radiation	Chemotherapy is less promising for squamous carcinoma than other gynecologic malignancies. Drug regimens have included:
Stage II-B, III, IV	2. Complete radiation therapy (plus hydroxyurea)	1. Bleomycin + mitomycin + vincristine
Radiation failures	3. Total pelvic exenteration when lesion resectable and deemed operable	2. As above + *C.* platinum 3. Bleomycin + methotrexate 4. Adriamycin + methotrexate 5. Hydroxyurea + radiation 6. *C.* platinum + methotrexate 7. Adriamycin + 5-fluorouracil 8. Cytoxan, adriamycin, bleomycin, vincristine, actinomycin D (Barker) 9. *Cis*-platinum and dichloromethotrexate
Squamous cancer of vagina	1. Complete radiation is procedure of choice 2. Radical pelvic surgery for recurrent cancer	5-Flurouracil cream if intraepithelial neoplasia See squamous cancer of cervix
Squamous cancer of vulva	1. Radical vulvectomy, groin lymphadenectomy. Pelvic node dissection when indicated 2. Radical vulvectomy and pelvic radiation in selected cases	See squamous cancer of cervix
Adenocarcinoma cervix	T & C[1] plus external radiation	Adriamycin fluorouracil, cytoxan (See squamous cancer of cervix)
Special gonadal-stromal ovarian tumors		
Granulosa cell tumor	1. TAHBSO 2. Debulk if needed 3. Irradiation	VAC or Act Fu Cy
Thecoma	TAHBSO	Unnecessary
Sertoli-Leydig tumors	USO or TAHBSO	VAC or Act Fu Cy
Gynandroblastoma	TAHBSO	VAC or Act Fu Cy
Lipin cell tumor	USO or TAHBSO + irradiation	VAC or Act Fu Cy in advanced stages
Secondary (metastatic) ovarian tumors Metastatic from breast, GI tract, and lymphatic system to ovary	1. Locate primary tumor. 2. Treatment of metastatic tumor is secondary to that of the primary tumor site therapy	Varies with primary tumor
Endometrial carcinoma		
Stage I, G-1	1. TAHBSO	No chemotherapy indicated in Stage IA, G-1
All other stage I	2. T & C + TAHBSO; ext. rad. with myometrial invasion; T & C + ext. rad. plus TAHBSO	Extrapelvic metastases requires chemotherapy:

(*continued*)

TABLE 27–5. (*Continued*)

Neoplasm	Role of Surgery and XRT	Role of Chemotherapy
Stage II Stage II and IV	3. T & C + radical hysterectomy and pelvic lymphadenectomy; T & C + ext. rad. with TAHBSO 4. TAHBSO	1. Estrogen and progesterone receptors may be guide. Provera 500 mg three times per week × five doses. Then Megace: Megace 240 mg/PO daily × 1 year 2. ADR and cytoxan nine times per 3 weeks × 12 courses 3. Platinum may be added to CTX and ADR 4. Tamoxifen
Endometrial sarcoma	1. Ext rad. and TAHBSO in 6 weeks 2. Radical surgery may be used in ca/sa or sarcoma botryoides	Progestational chemotherapy in stromal sarcoma. Advanced sarcoma may be treated with: 1. VAC 2. VAC-DTIC 3. ADR 4. Platinum
Leiomyosarcoma	TAHBSO	Low mitotic count—no chemotherapy
Fallopian tube carcinoma	1. TAHBSO 2. Radiation therapy is controversial	ADR + CTX ± *C.* platinum Melphelan may be used with minimal disease
Epithelial cancer of ovary (mesotheliomas) Serous carcinoma Mucinous carcinoma Endometrial carcinoma Clear cell carcinoma	TAHBSO + omentectomy (maximum primary surgical effort to reduce tumor to less than 2 cm in diameter); diaphragm and periaortic biopsies, appendectomy, peritoneal washings	*Single-drug therapy (stage IA)* 1. Melphalan 0.2 mg/kg/day IV 5 days/month 2. Cytoxan 1000 mg/m² IV every 3 weeks 3. Thiotepa 0.2 mg/kg/day IV for 5 days/month 4. Leukoran 0.1–0.2 mg/kg/day PO 5. *C.* platinum 50 mg/m² IV every 3 weeks 6. Adriamycin 60–90 mg/m² IV every 3 weeks 7. Hexamethylmelamine 280 mg/m² × 14 days every 4 weeks *Multiple drugs (advanced disease)* 1. ADR + CTX as above, plus *C.* platinum 50 mg/m² IV every 3 weeks 2. Adriamycin 60 mg/m² IV every 3 weeks; cytoxan 100 mg IV every 3 weeks 3. Intraperitoneal ADR, 5-FU, *cis*-platinum
Germ-cell ovarian tumors		
Pure dysgerminomas	USO or TAHBSO + total abdominal radiation therapy	Chemotherapy optional (VAC) for pure dysgerminomas. Otherwise, VAC, MAC, *cis*-platinum-vinblastine-bleomycin, or Act Fu Cy for all other germ-cell tumors

TABLE 27–5. (*Continued*)

Neoplasm	Role of Surgery and XRT	Role of Chemotherapy
Endodermal sinus	USO or TAHBSO	*VAC*:
Embryonal carcinoma	USO or TAHBSO	Vinc. 1.5/m² IV weekly × 12 weeks
Choriocarcinoma	USO or TAHBSO	ADR 60 mg/m² IV every 3 weeks
Malignant immature teratoma	USO or TAHBSO	CTX 1000 mg/IV every 3 weeks *MAC*:
Mixed germ-cell tumors	TAHBSO	MTX 0.3 mg/kg IM or IV } daily × 5 days
Polyembryoma	TAHBSO	Act. D 0.01 mg/kg IV } every 4 weeks CTX 4 mg/kg IV } (trophoblast element) *Act Fu Cy*: Act. D. 0.01 mg/kg IV } daily × 5 days 5-FU 5 mg/kg IV } every 4 weeks CTX 5 mg/kg IV
Hydatidiform mole	1. Suction and sharp currettage uterus 2. Hysterectomy for sterilization	If persistent β-subunit hCG after 2 months or plateau or rising titer, treat with methotrexate (20 mg/day IM × 5 days every 10–14 days until weekly negative hCG × 3 weeks) or actinomycin D (0.5 mg IV × 5 days, every 10–14 days). Then interval hCG for 1 year.
Invasive mole	Need examination of removed uterus for positive diagnosis	If diagnosis can be made, treat as above with 25 mg methotrexate (or actinomycin D) daily × days.
Choriocarcinoma (low risk)	1. Hysterectomy with localized uterine lesions, while on methotrexate only if sterilization desired 2. Chemotherapy otherwise	Methotrexate 25 mg IM or IV or actinomycin D 0.5 mg IV daily × 5 days every 10–14 days until negative β-subunit hCG for 3 weeks
Choriocarcinoma (high risk) (100,000 IU/24-hr urine or 40,000 mIU/ml serum) Initial high hCG Delayed therapy (4 + months) Brain or liver metastasis Resistant to single agent Following term pregnancy	1. Surgery may be used to remove localized lesion resistant to chemotherapy (uterus, liver, lung, etc.) 2. External radiation—2,000–3,000 rads for brain or liver metastasis 3. Radiation until patient is stabilized for use of chemotherapy	1. MTX 15 mg IM, actinomycin D 0.5 mg IV and chlorambucil 10 mg PO = all given daily × 5 days every 12–14 days until negative β-subunit hCG weekly for 3 weeks, as with mole. 2. Modified Bagshawe regimen[†]

Day	*Hour*	*Treatment*
	0600	Hydroxyurea 500 mg PO
1	1200	Hydroxyurea 500 mg PO
	1800	Hydroxyurea 500 mg PO
	1900	Actinomycin D 200 mcg IV

(*continued*)

TABLE 27-5. (*Continued*)

Neoplasm	Role of Surgery and XRT	Role of Chemotherapy		
			2400	Hydroxyurea 500 mg PO
		2	0700	Vincristine 1 mg/m² IV
			1900	MTX 100 mg/m² IV
				MTX 200 mg/m² IV infusion in 12 hr
				Actinomycin D 200 mcg IV
		3	1900	Actinomycin D 200 mcg IV
				Cytoxan 500 mg/m² IV
				Folic acid 14 mg IM
		4	0100	Folic acid 14 mg IM
			0700	Folic acid 14 mg IM
			1300	Folic acid 14 mg IM
			1900	Actinomycin 500 mcg IV
		5	0100	Folic acid 14 mg IM
			1900	Actinomycin 500 mcg IV
		6	No Rx	
		7	No Rx	
		8	1900	Cytoxan 500 mg/m² IV
				Adriamycin 30 mg/m² IV

* Abbreviations: T & C— tandem and culpostat internal radiation (radium and cesium): TAHBSO—total abdominal hysterectomy, bilateral salpingo-oophorectomy; USO—unilateral salpingo-oophorectomy.

† Currently used at Southeast Regional Center for Trophoblastic Disease.

GUIDELINES FOR THE USE OF CHEMOTHERAPY IN TREATING GYNECOLOGIC MALIGNANCIES

Chemotherapy is used in gynecology to eliminate microscopic metastatic tumors or for palliation of advanced, disseminated, or recurrent disease. Table 27–5 illustrates the relation between chemotherapy and other therapeutic modalities in the management of specific neoplasms. Surgery for treating choriocarcinoma has been replaced by methotrexate or actinomycin D therapy. Similarly, in germ-cell tumors of the ovary, multiagent chemotherapy has resulted in cure rates otherwise unattainable by surgery alone. For ovarian epithelial tumors, a combination of therapeutic modalities includes an initial maximal surgical debulking effort, followed by the utilization of appropriate chemotherapeutic agents. There is still a need for continued research in the management of metastatic squamous cell carcinomas of the cervix using surgery and/or radiation along with adjunctive chemotherapy.

Although chemotherapeutic agents are considered valuable adjuncts to standard therapeutic modalities, their effectiveness is often difficult to assess and requires continued clinical trials. The effectiveness of chemotherapy has been enhanced by new protocols and revisions in drug scheduling. The additional use of immunotherapy may also be promising, but it too requires years of refinement to assess its clinical value.[8] Undoubtedly, newer drugs and new forms of drug delivery will be developed through research efforts and will place chemotherapy at greater heights of successful treatment of gynecologic malignancies.

REFERENCES

1. Smith JP, Rutledge F: Advances in chemotherapy for gynecologic cancer. Cancer 36:669, 1975
2. Barber H: Chemotherapy. In Van Nagell JR, Barber HR (eds): Modern Concepts of Gynecologic Oncology. Boston, Wright, 1982, pp 539–564
3. Morrow CP, Townsend DE (eds): Chemotherapy. In Synopsis of Gynecologic Oncology. New York, Wiley, 1981, pp 415–448
4. Li MD, Hertz R, Spencer DB: Effects of methotrexate upon choriocarcinoma and chorioadenoma. Proc Exp Biol Med 93:361, 1956
5. Disaia P, Creasman W: Clinical Gynecologic Oncology. St. Louis, Mosby, 1981, Chap 11, pp 285–298
6. McGowan D: Gynecologic Oncology. New York, Appleton-Century-Crofts, 1978, Chap 5, pp 92–145
7. Mount BM, Ayemian I, Scott JF: The use of Brompton mixture in treating chronic pain of malignant disease. CMA J 115:122, 1976
8. Barber H: Immunotherapy and immunopotentiation. In Barber H (ed): Manual of Gynecologic Oncology. Philadelphia, Lippincott, 1980, p 130

28

Parenteral Nutrition

Robert A. Wolk and William F. Rayburn

Parenteral nutrition (PN) was first applied in 1968 by Dudrick et al.[1] and has been used widely in patients unable to eat or tolerate enteral feedings. Parenteral nutrition has been used in pre- and postoperative surgical patients, neonates, persons with a short bowel syndrome, and in patients requiring bowel rest, such as severe inflammatory bowel disease, as well as burn, cancer, and trauma patients.[2] However, reports of PN use in gynecological and obstetric patients are limited. As more complex situations have developed, PN has become a useful therapy in those women who are unable to meet their nutritional needs orally or enterally.

Parenteral nutrition has changed significantly from Dudrick's first report,[1] progressing from a protein, dextrose and salt solution to a more complex and complete solution containing individual amino acids, dextrose, fat emulsion, vitamins, trace elements, and electrolytes.[2] The availability of more complete products, protocols for use, and standardized solutions, along with proper clinical and laboratory monitoring, has reduced the potential for toxic, metabolic and infectious complications. Parenteral nutrition is now accepted as potentially life saving but requires prudent use to minimize cost and wastage and complications.[2]

This chapter will provide an overview of the experience for administering PN solutions to women with gynecologic and obstetric complications. The methods for monitoring and special considerations for the care of these women will also be reviewed.

INDICATIONS

Gynecology

Parenteral nutrition had been used rarely in gynecology patients.[3-10] Complex situations, especially for those with oncologic conditions have suggested PN to be a valuable therapy, however. Undesired effects from radiation,

This chapter is adapted from Rayburn W, Wolk R, Mercer N, Roberts J: Parenteral nutrition in obstetrics and gynecology. Obstet Gynecol Surv 41:200, 1986. Adapted with kind permission from Williams & Wilkins Co., Baltimore, MD.

chemotherapy, and surgery may reduce oral or enteral intake at a time of increased nutritional demand. Women with weight losses of 10 percent or more of body mass or who are unable to have adequate oral or enteral intake for several days should be started on PN support.[3] These women have usually suffered from major illnesses and even minor therapeutic procedures may be life-threatening.

Parenteral nutrition improves nitrogen balance, weight gain, wound healing, and enhances fistula closure.[2,11,12] Improvements in the tolerance to radiation and chemotherapy, immunologic status, and survival rates are also benefits from PN.[3]

Obstetrics

Most reports on the use of PN during pregnancy have been relatively recent.[3,7,13–19] Most information is anectodal but suggests that PN is safe and effective.[3,7,13–18] These reports usually involve one or two cases involving women with either prolonged severe hyperemesis gravidarum or inadequate absorption or assimilation of nutrients as in inflammatory bowel disease or recurrent pancreatitis.[3] The duration of therapy has ranged from 2 to 365 days (average 23 days) and included a few cases with prolonged home PN.[3] This therapy has been used primarily within the second half of pregnancy, while the cases reported in early gestation were for women with hyperemesis gravidarum.[3]

Deliveries at or beyond 38 weeks have occurred in 39 percent (15 of 38) of cases reported recently in the obstetric literature.[3] Preterm deliveries were related less to maternal nutritional problems and more to a worsening of the primary medical or obstetric complication. In most cases PN was usually discontinued several weeks before delivery. Cesarean sections were performed in many but not most of the cases. An appropriately sized rather than growth-retarded infant was delivered in 61 percent (23 of 38) of these reported pregnancies.[3] Many infants found to be small were thought to be growth retarded before PN was initiated. While PN appears to be safe and effective, several questions need to be answered about fetal metabolism and PN utilization.

NUTRITIONAL ASSESSMENT AND REQUIREMENTS

A patient's nutritional condition and energy requirements must be known before selecting the proper PN formula. The patient's general condition must include a history of any weight loss or gain, dietary habits, disease state(s), and gestational age. The physical examination should include the recording of her height, weight, skin appearance, vital signs, fluid status, and specific organ review, especially gastrointestinal tract function.[2] Risk factors contributing to malnutrition include malabsorption syndromes, medications (steroids, immunosuppressants, chemotherapy), surgery, anorexia, protracted emesis, and sepsis.[3,11,12] A normal or above ideal body weight is not a guarantee of adequate nutrition.[3,11,12]

Visceral protein mass, measuring synthetic capacity, and muscle mass reflecting nitrogen "stores" and balance should also be evaluated. Visceral protein mass is reflected by serum albumin, transferrin, and retinol-binding protein levels.[2,11] The immune status may be affected by malnutrition as seen by low total lymphocyte counts and anergic skin tests.[2,11] Skin induration greater than 10 mm at 48 hours indicates a positive reaction to such antigens as mumps, PPD, and Candida. Nitrogen balance and muscle mass may be evaluated by periodic urine urea nitrogen or creatinine height index determinations.[2,11,19] A 24-hour urine collection for urea nitrogen and creatinine is necessary to make these assessments. The creatinine clearance is particularly useful to monitor in pregnant patients.[5,20] Periodic anthropometric measurements (triceps skinfold thickness, mid-arm circumference) may be helpful for assessing body fat and muscle mass. Some major assessment parameters are described in Table 28-1.

Once nutritional status is assessed, PN requirements may be determined. Little if anything is known about specific PN requirements for obstetric and gynecology patients. The National Research Council–American Academy of Science has established recommended daily allowances (RDA) for oral intake (Table 28-2).[21] These standards are based on the oral intake of healthy nonpregnant women and may not be adequate for gynecology and obstetric patients with inadequate nutrition, chronic disease(s), severe infection, metabolic disorders, or other conditions. These values must be extrapolated and adjusted for any variable oral absorption or aberrant liver metabolism. Nutrients must be supplied to meet the woman's calorie needs and maintain a positive nitrogen balance. Once assessment has been completed, the next step is to select an appropriate PN solution.

TABLE 28-1. NUTRITIONAL ASSESSMENT PARAMETERS

	Degree of Impairment				
	Normal	***Mild***	***Moderate***	***Severe***	**Calculations/Limitations**
Weight	<10%	10–20%	20–30%	30%	Percent weight loss = $\frac{\text{Usual weight-current weight}}{\text{Usual weight}}$ Weight change may reflect increased or decreased hydration and not change in lean body mass
Albumin (g%)	3.5	3.5–3.0	3.5–2.5	2.5	Due to long half-life of about 20 days, visceral depletion and repletion will not be detected rapidly. Serum levels may be affected by hepatic and renal disease, congestive heart failure, chronically draining wounds, and hemodilution especially during pregnancy
Transferrin (mg)	200–350	200–180	180–160	160	Modified in the presence of hepatic and renal disease, congestive heart failure, and chronically draining wounds
Total lymphocyte count (cells/mm³)	1800	1800–1500	1500–900	900	Total lymphocyte count = $\frac{\text{\% lymphocytes} \times \text{WBC}}{100}$ Many factors to cause a decrease in TLC include chemotherapy, sepsis, and trauma
Skin test antigens (mm)	15	15–10	10–5	5–0 (anergy)	Factors other than malnutrition may affect duration such as chemotherapy, medications, and sepsis
Nitrogen balance	2–4 g	Zero	Small neg	Large neg	IV INTAKE = (gN/L × L/d) – (UUN + 3) Not accurate in patients with fistulas, burns, or draining wounds

Adapted from Parenteral and Enteral Nutrition Manual, ed 3, 1984.[2]

TABLE 28–2. ESTIMATES OF DAILY ORAL DIETARY NEEDS FOR WOMEN ACCORDING TO AGE

Nutrient	Age 11–14	Age 15–18	Age 19–50	Pregnancy	Lactation	Age 51 +
Energy (kcal)	2200	2100	2000	+300	+500	1800
Protein (g)	46	46	44	+30	+20	44
Vitamin A (mcg)	800	800	800	+200	+400	800
Vitamin D (mcg)	10	10	7.5–5	+5	+5	5
Vitamin E (mg)	8	8	8	+2	+3	8
Vitamin C (mg)	50	60	60	+20	+40	60
Folic acid (mcg)	400	400	400	+400	+100	400
Niacin (mg)	15	14	13	+2	+5	13
Riboflavin (mg)	1.3	1.3	1.2	+0.3	+0.5	1.2
Thiamine (mg)	1.1	1.1	1	+0.4	+0.5	1
Vitamin B_6 (mg)	1.8	2	2	+0.6	+0.5	2
Vitamin B_{12} (mcg)	3	3	3	+1	+1	3
Calcium (mEq)	60	60	40	+20	+20	40
Iron (mg)	18	18	18	+3	+3	10
Zinc (mg)	15	15	15	+5	+10	15
Phosphorus (mM)	26–39	26–39	26–39	+13	+13	26
Magnesium (mEq)	25	25	25	+12.5	+12.5	25
Iodine (mcg)	150	150	150	+25	+50	150

Adapted from National Research Council, 1980.[21]

SELECTING A PARENTERAL NUTRITION SOLUTION

Providing nutrients in the proper quantities may be a major challenge. It is important to evaluate the route of administration, recommended daily requirements, and disease and malnourished state. Standardized PN solutions at many hospital pharmacies make ordering easier, more efficient, cost effective, and safer. Advice and assistance from a hospital-based PN team is strongly encouraged.

Calories

Total calories in PN solutions come primarily from dextrose (3.4 kcal/g) and fat (9 kcal/g) and to a lesser degree from protein (4 kcal/g). Maintenance energy needs described as resting metabolic expenditure (RME) may be calculated using Wilmore's normogram[12] or the Harris–Benedict equation for women:[22]

$$\text{RME (kcal)} = 655 + 9.563\,(W) + 1.85\,(H) - 4.676\,(A)$$

where W = weight in kg, H = height in cm, and A = age in years.

Increased energy requirement increments for various stress conditions have been identified (Table 28–3). Early reports by Oldham and Sheft have documented that at least 36 kcal/kg body weight is required to maintain a positive nitrogen balance during pregnancy,[23] and this figure is typical for other types of patients as well. Most case reports of pregnant women receiving PN support reported 2000 to 3000 kcal being given per day for adequate maternal weight gain and fetal growth.

Dextrose

Dextrose is the most common energy source available because it is usually well tolerated and readily mixed with PN additives. It is available commercially and can be prepared by pharmacies in 5 to 35 percent final concentrations. The concentration of dextrose to

TABLE 28–3. INCREMENTS FOR INCREASED ENERGY REQUIREMENTS*

Select appropriate factors from A and B and multiply by RME to determine total energy requirement

A. Physical Activity	
	Factor†
Confined to bed	1.2
Out of bed	1.3
B. Clinical Condition	
	Factor†
Starvation	0.7
Fever	1 + .13 per degree C
Elective surgery	1–1.2
Peritonitis	1.2–1.5
Soft tissue trauma	1.14–1.37
Multiple fractures	1.2–1.35
Severe infection	1.4–1.8
Burn (based on size)	1.0–2.05

* Total energy requirement is predicted by product of activity factor × RME.
† Figures represent maximum increases and must be adjusted as recovery and convalessence proceeds.
Adapted from Silberman H, Eisenberg D (eds), 1982.[11]

be used is based on patient's need, tolerance, and infusion site. Because of the high osmotic load, only PN solutions with less than 600 mOsm should be infused peripherally. As the osmolarity increases, a greater chance of phlebitis and venospasm occurs requiring the use of a central line. A 5 to 10 percent dextrose-containing solution can be used peripherally, while 20 to 35 percent dextrose is used centrally.[2] Examples of calorie and protein combinations are listed in Table 28–4. Dextrose is well tolerated by gynecology and obstetric patients although special concerns for stricter glucose control is required in pregnancy for fetal growth interests.[3] When determining the amount of dextrose to provide it is important to remember that the liver dextrose utilization rate is estimated at 0.4–1.2 g/kg/hr.[2] Exceeding this may lead to hyperosmolar and dehydration hyperglycemia.

Fat

Fat emulsion (FE) is usually provided to prevent essential fatty acid deficiency (EFAD) and to provide concentrated calories. Fat emulsion is available as concentrations of 10 (1.1 kcal/ml) or 20 percent (2 kcal/ml) soybean oil in 250- and 500-ml bottles. The composition is displayed in Table 28–5.

Symptoms of fatty acid deficiency appear in 4 to 6 weeks while biochemical changes become evident as early as 1 to 2 weeks. This may be avoided with the administration of 10 percent fat emulsion 2 to 3 times weekly.

A fat emulsion may be administered concomitantly with parenteral nutrition solutions in a piggyback manner, but distal to any filter used. This is advantageous with peripheral parenteral nutrition because the fat emulsion's isotonicity (10 percent 300 mOsm/L, 20 percent 330 mOsm/L) will reduce the final osmolarity of the PN solution delivered to the vein. Proper monitoring of maternal serum triglycerides and cholesterol levels makes FE a safe therapy. For rates greater than 30 ml/hr, the manufacturer recommends a test dose because of rare allergic reactions.

Gynecology patients and patients in general should tolerate fat emulsions well unless underlying problems like hyperlipidemia, diabetes mellitus, or chronic renal failure exist. These patients can usually tolerate up to 60

TABLE 28-4. EXAMPLES OF POSSIBLE PARENTERAL NUTRITION REGIMENS

	Central Formulation		Peripheral Formulation	
	Regimen 1	*Regimen 2*	*Regimen 1*	*Regimen 2*
Final dextrose concentration (%)	25	35	10	10
Final protein concentration (%)	4.25	4.25	2.5	2.5
Calories per liter	1020	1360	440	440
Typical number liters given per day	2	1	2	3
Calories provided/day	2040	1360	880	1320
Plus				
Fat emulsion 10% 500 ml/day				
Total calories*	2590	1910	1430	1870
Or				
Fat emulsion 20% 500 ml/day				
Total calories*/day	3040	2360	1880	2320

* Calories determined based on glucose and protein, and fat emulsion provided.

percent of the total calories as FE, however, fat emulsion should never exceed 3.5 g/kg in adults.[2]

Fat therapy for pregnant women is not as clear. Theoretic concerns exist about fat deposition within the placenta possibly leading to placental insufficiency, spontaneous uterine contractions, and effects of lipids on fetal metabolism.[3,16,20,24] Several case reports have shown that infants do not have any apparent ill effects or deliver prematurely despite preliminary assertions that FE may be unsafe in pregnancy.[14,16,19,25]

While Luukkainen et al.[26] used rapid infusion of FE to induce labor in pregnancies at 40 to 46 weeks gestation, no significant uterine activity was induced when a standard dose of FE was used in preterm pregnancies. Infarctions of the placenta may be possible from FE emboli, but this has never been observed. We recommend FE be limited to 40 percent of total calories in pregnancy. Table 28-4 illustrates examples of PN regimens with acceptable FE combinations.

TABLE 28-5. REPRESENTATIVE COMPOSITION OF SOYBEAN OIL, FAT EMULSION

	Soybean Oil	
	10%	*20%*
Calories (kcal)	550	1000
Fat (g)	50	100
Fatty acid components (%)		
Linoleic acid	50	50
Oleic acid	26	26
Palmitic acid	10	10
Linolenic	9	9
Egg phosphatides	1.2	1.2
Glycerin	2.25	2.25
Volume (ml)	500	500
Osmolarity (mOsm/L)	300	330

Adapted from Parenteral and Enteral Nutrition Manual, ed 3, 1984.[2]

Amino Acids

Recommended dietary allowances for protein for the average adult is 0.8 g/kg/day.[21] In general, most patients on PN typically receive and do well on 1 to 1.5 g/kg. An additional 30 g/day is required for pregnant women to meet fetal development needs.[21] Moderate stress such as trauma and major surgery may rarely increase daily protein needs up to 2 g/kg and for burn patients up to 3.5 g/kg to maintain a positive nitrogen balance.[2,12,27]

Synthetic amino acids are used because of the low level of complications and compatibility in the PN solution. Amino acids are typically available as 2.5, 3.5, 4.25, and 5 percent final concentrations of the compounded PN solution. Table 28–4 provides examples on calorie and protein PN regimens.

ELECTROLYTES

Recommended daily allowances are only established for calcium, phosphorous, and magnesium.[21] Electrolyte ranges that are well tolerated in PN therapy are listed in Table 28–6.[2] Wide ranges of sodium, chloride, and potassium and narrower ranges of calcium, phosphorous, and magnesium are well tolerated if renal function is adequate.[2] Pregnant women have slightly higher needs than gynecologic patients for calcium, potassium, phosphorous, and magnesium because of fetal bone development and lean tissue synthesis.[21] Examples of standard electrolytes, per liter, for obstetric and gynecologic patients are listed in Table 28–6.

Monitoring serum electrolyte levels should prevent an overdose or deficiency and allow fine tuning if needed. Albumin levels should be determined because calcium levels vary proportionally with serum albumin (decrease of albumin by 1 g/dl will produce a drop of 0.8 mEg/L of calcium).[11]

FLUID REQUIREMENTS

Fluid requirements are important because they define the amount of PN that can be provided. Typical maintenance fluid requirements may be calculated by using the data in Table 28–7.[2] Losses from nasogastric tubes, vomiting, diarrhea, ostomy, and fistulae need to be replaced. Ideally, they should be replaced in equal volumes using a fluid to match those specific losses of fluids and electrolytes (see Table 28–7).[28] Use of the PN solution for fluid replacement is not advised, since specific solutions to replace fluid losses will allow greater control and avoid complications from changes in the PN rate.

VITAMINS

Dietary allowances for ten vitamins have been established by the National Research Council. American Medical Association guidelines have established requirements for an additional three vitamins.[29] Twelve of these vitamins are found in the three currently available multivitamin products for PN. Daily requirements are met using the preparations after converting from oral to intravenous doses by assuming oral absorption rates to be 25 to 50 percent of the dose given.[21] Concentrations of vitamins listed in Table 28–8 are those found in a single dose used daily in 1 L of the parenteral solutions.

TABLE 28–6. ELECTROLYTES FOR GYNECOLOGY AND OBSTETRIC PATIENTS

Electrolyte	Daily Range*	Typical Standard/Liter†
Calcium	10–15 mEq	4.5 mEq (gynecology) 9 mEq (obstetric)
Magnesium	8–24 mEq	5 mEq
Potassium	90–240 mEq	40 mEq
Sodium	60–150 mEq	35 mEq
Acetate	80–120 mEq	30 mEq
Chloride	60–150 mEq	35 mEq
Phosphorus	30–50 mmol	12 mmol

* Electrolyte supplementations may need to be adjusted based on patient's liver, renal, and cardiac status.
† Typical patient receives 2 to 3 L/day.
Adapted from Parenteral and Enteral Nutrition Manual, ed 3, 1984.[2]

TABLE 28–7. MAINTENANCE FLUID AND FLUID REQUIREMENTS

Maintenance Fluids	
Weight	*Fluid required*
0–10 kg	100 ml/kg plus
10–20 kg	50 ml/kg plus
>20 kg	20 ml/kg
Replacement Fluids	
Fluid Lost	*Replacement*
Urine output	0.45% saline
Insensible	Water or 5% dextrose
Gastric	0.45% saline
Stool	0.45% saline with $NaHCO_3$ or 5% dextrose Lactated Ringers
Drains	0.9% saline

Most patients require the addition of 10–40 mEq of potassium chloride per liter to their saline solutions.

Adapted from Parenteral and Enteral Nutrition Manual, ed 3, 1984.[2] Wolk R, Swartz R, 1985.[28]

TABLE 28–8. FAT AND WATER SOLUBLE VITAMINS, TRACE ELEMENTS, AND DRUGS TO BE ADDED TO PARENTERAL NUTRITION SOLUTIONS FOR GYNECOLOGIC AND OBSTETRIC PATIENTS*

	Daily Recommendation	
1. Multivitamins Package (Per Day)		
Ascorbic acid	100.0	mg
Vitamin A	1,000.0	mcg
Vitamin D	5.0	mcg
Thiamine HCl	3.0	mg
Riboflavin	3.6	mg
Pyridoxine HCl	4.0	mg
Niacinamide	40.0	mg
Pantothenic acid	15.0	mg
Vitamin E	10	mg
Biotin	60	mcg
Folic acid	400	mcg
Cyanocobalamn (Vitamin B_{12})	5.0	mcg
2. Phytoniadione (Vitamin K_1)	5–10	mg (per week)
3. Trace Elements Per Day		
Zinc	4.0	mg (gynecology)
	6.0	mg (obstetric)
Copper	1.0	mg
Manganese	0.8	mg
Chromium	0.010	mg
4. Drugs		
Heparin	500–1000	units/L
Insulin, regular (if necessary)	0.5	units/10 g infused glucose (initially)

* Further additives during pregnancy and lactation include additional iron dextran (20 mg weekly for long-term therapy), and iodine (2–3 mcg/kg daily if long term).

Adapted from Parenteral and Enteral Nutrition Manual, ed 3, 1984.[2] *Rayburn W, et al. 1985.*[3]

Once-a-day dosing of the vitamin package should meet the needs for gynecology and obstetric patients. Vitamin K is not included in the multivitamin package because of compatibility problems. A separate weekly dose of 5 to 10 mg should be sufficient for clotting factor synthesis (see Table 28–8).[29]

TRACE ELEMENTS

Several trace elements are supplied in standard formula to meet daily nutritional needs. The National Research Council has established daily allowances for zinc, iron, and iodine,[21] while the AMA Department of Foods and Nutrition has recognized copper, chromium, manganese, cobalt (as vitamin B_{12}), and zinc as being essential trace elements to be supplemented in PN solutions.[30] Only a small fraction of oral doses are considered to be absorbed.[21] Several trace element preparations are available to provide sufficient amounts of zinc, copper, chromium, and manganese for gynecologic patients. A representative formulation of trace elements that meets the AMA guidelines for intravenous nutritional requirements is shown in Table 28–8.

Zinc is needed in higher doses for women who are pregnant or have excess diarrhea or an ostomy.[2,21] Pregnancy requires an additional 2 mg/d, while persons with an ostomy and excess diarrhea may require 12 mg/L of small bowel fluid loss and 17 mg/kg of stool or ileostomy loss.[2,21]

It is necessary to supply iodine to women, especially during pregnancy.[21] Gynecologic PN patients usually receive adequate amounts of iodine if providone-iodine solutions are used during central venous catheter dressing changes. Additional iodine is unnecessary for short-term alimentation during pregnancy but might be recommended and provided parenterally as 2 to 3 mcg/kg body weight if therapy is long-term.[21] Gynecologic patients should receive iodine only if a deficiency occurs.

Iron should be supplemented for the additional erythrocyte production during pregnancy.[21] Unlike pregnant patients, gynecologic patients do not need supplemental iron dextran unless an iron deficiency anemia is diagnosed.[2] The recommended amount of elemental iron is 3 mg per day or 750 mg during the entire pregnancy.[21] While intravenous iron dextran is contraindicated by the manufacturer, several authors have used infusions to correct anemias in the second or third trimesters.[31–35] A small intravenous test dose of 0.5 ml (25 mg) in 50 to 100 ml of normal saline is required over 1 to 2 hours to test for any allergic reaction. The test dose is required before supplementation begins. Because total dose infusion is rarely associated with side effects, smaller doses of 20 mg every week may be appropriate to prevent anemia during long term parenteral nutrition.[31,32]

DRUGS

The two most common drug additives are heparin and regular insulin. Heparin is provided as 0.5 to 1 unit/ml of PN, to reduce the formation of a fibrin sheath and phlebitis (see Table 28–8).[2] Heparin has also been reported to potentially lessen the seeding of catheters with microorganisms that might become responsible for bringing infection to the catheter.[36] Regular insulin may be added to PN if glucose intolerance develops (see Table 28–8). Suspensions of insulin (mostly intermediate or long acting preparations) are not compatible with PN, so only regular insulin should be added. Insulin should be provided initially by the subcutaneous route or with an intravenous drip.[2] These routes of administration provide tighter glucose control without disruption of the PN provided. Two-thirds to three-quarters of the subcutaneous dose may then be added to the PN solution.

Serum glucose levels and urine fractionals should be followed closely for 1 to 2 days when starting PN in gynecologic patients and less frequently, but routinely, thereafter. These levels should not usually exceed 200 mg% for nonpregnant women, with stricter control being desired during pregnancy for fetal interests. Measuring glycosuria is inadequate in pregnant women because of the increased glomerular filtration, so serum or capillary blood glucose levels should be measured four times daily. Strict control consists of glucose values ranging between 60 and 120 mg%. Glucose levels exceeding 140 mg% should be avoided.

Because of an increased risk of catheter sepsis and possible incompatibility with PN, medications such as antibiotics, pressor agents, and steroids should be infused through a separate intravenous line. Exceptions to this rule would be in emergencies, when this is the only intravenous access, and after checking the compatibility literature. This is important to prevent medication deactivation or precipitation formation. The nutritional support service or pharmacy should be consulted if questions occur.

ADMINISTRATION AND DISCONTINUATION

Examples of PN formulations for use in gynecology and obstetric patients are given in Table 28–4. A daily combination of 2 L of a standard central formulation (using 25 percent dextrose) or 3 L of a standard peripheral formulation (using 10 percent dextrose) with 500 ml of a 10 or 20 percent fat emulsion and 75 to 85 g of protein should provide 1800 to 3000 kcal. This will meet the needs of obstetric and gynecologic patients, as well as most other patients. Additional fluids for hydration or replacement of fluids should be given through another intravenous line and without interruption of the PN.

Infusion of a hyperosmolar solution may be undertaken after the catheter placement has been confirmed and once a satisfactory intravenous solution has been chosen. An example of an infusion setup with a parenteral nutrition solution and fat emulsion is shown in Figure 28–1. Volumetric pumps are used to infuse both types of solutions.

Parenteral nutrition solutions should be ordered daily and sent to the pharmacy the evening beforehand. This will permit an adequate time for compounding the solutions

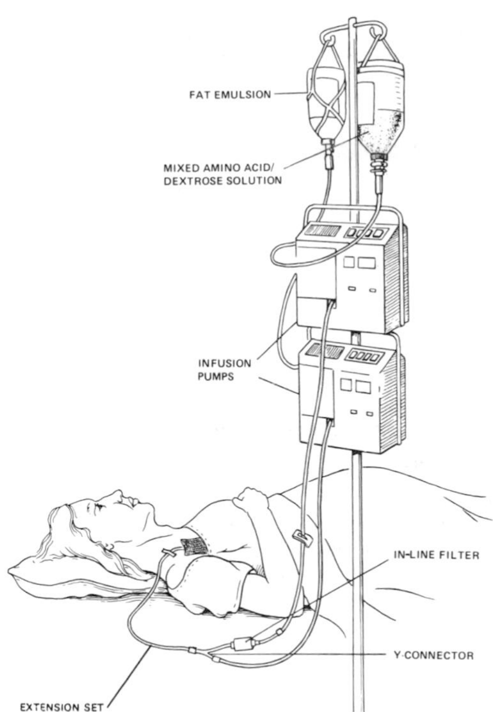

Figure 28–1. Example of parenteral nutrition administrative system.

and a greater awareness of cost considerations. Blood and urine metabolic studies listed in Table 28–9 should be assessed periodically. Metabolic complications are infrequent with close monitoring. Proper monitoring will prevent complications and deficiencies. Recommended monitoring intervals of specific urine or serum values as well as general parameters and catheter care are shown in Table 28–9.

Infusions of hypertonic dextrose solutions should be slow initially (40 ml/hr or 1 L/d), then increased as the woman's pancreas adjusts to tolerate the concentrated glucose challenges. Rates for persons receiving solutions containing 25 percent dextrose or more should begin more slowly at 30–45 ml/hr and increase at 20 ml/hr/day increments until achieving the desired rate. The maintenance rate of infusion is dependent on daily caloric needs but does not usually exceed 120 ml/

TABLE 28–9. RECOMMENDED MONITORING DURING PARENTERAL NUTRITION

	Suggested Frequency	
	First Week or Until Patient Is Stable	***Later Period***
General		
Volume of infusage	Daily	Daily
Oral intake (if any)	Daily	Daily
Urine output, ostomy output, fistula, NG	Daily	Daily
Weight	Daily	Daily
Height	Initially	—
Temperature	Daily	Daily
Anthropometric measurements	Initially	Every 3 weeks
Metabolic		
Blood		
Complete blood count, platelets	Weekly	Weekly
Total lymphocytes	Initially	Monthly
Electrolytes (Na, K, Cl, CO_2)	Daily	Twice weekly
BUN	Twice weekly	Twice weekly
Ca, PO_4	Twice weekly	Weekly
Total protein/albumin	Weekly	Weekly
Glucose	Daily	Twice weekly
Liver function tests (SGOT, SGPT, LDH, Alkaline phosphatase, bilirubin D/T)	Twice weekly	Weekly
Mg	Weekly	Weekly
Cholesterol, triglycerides	Weekly	Weekly
PT, PTT	Weekly	Weekly
Fe, TIBC	Weekly	Optional
Transferrin (estimated from TIBC)	Weekly (optional)	Weekly (optional)
Aminogram	Optional	Optional
Urine		
Glucose	Four times daily	Twice daily
Specific gravity	Four times daily	Daily
Creatinine	Initially	prn
Urea nitrogen	Weekly (optional)	Weekly (optional)
Catheter		
Route and date placed, chest film confirmation of position	Initally	prn
Tubing change	Daily or every other day	Daily or every other day
Dressing change	Daily or every other day	Daily or every other day
Date removed, and reason for removal	As indicated	
Catheter tip cultures	As indicated	
Blood cultures	As indicated	

Abbreviations: BUN, blood urea nitrogen; D/T, direct/total; Fe, iron; LDH, lactic acid dehydrogenase; NG, nasogastric; PT, prothrombin time; PTT, partial thromboplastin time, SGOT, serum glutamic oxaloacetic transaminase; SGPT, serum glutamic pyruvic transaminase; TIBC, total iron-binding capacity.

Adapted from Parenteral and Enteral Nutrition Manual, ed 3, 1984.[2]

hr.[2,11] Serum or capillary blood glucose determinations need to be performed regularly if the woman is pregnant or if glucosuria (3 to 4+) is present in the gynecologic patient.

The solution may be safely discontinued by reversing the infusion rate in a manner opposite that in which it was started. The transition to enteral or oral support should be initiated before parenteral therapy is discontinued regardless of the manner for discontinuing PN. As tolerance to enteral feedings increases, intravenous support may be decreased appropriately. Otherwise, sudden discontinuation of a hypertonic dextrose infusion may lead to symptomatic hypoglycemia.

COMPLICATIONS

Technical

The insertion of an intravenous line is a surgical procedure which requires strict aseptic technique. Central rather than peripheral infusions are used in most obstetrics and gynecology patients, since therapy is intended to be long term (14 days or more) and catheter placement is not too difficult. Central infusions are also preferred if renal or cardiac impairment exists. A subclavian rather than jugular venipuncture is preferred when a central line is used. A chest x-ray film should be obtained immediately after catheter insertion to verify proper catheter tip placement above the right atrium.[2,11]

Catheter insertion may cause complications, even by the most experienced physcians.[2] A pneumothorax is the most common complication of subclavian venipuncture, occurring in 1 to 6 percent of attempted catheterizations.[11] The next most frequent complication is the puncture of a nearby artery, usually the subclavian artery. Air embolism, a rare but potentially fatal complication, may occur during either percutaneous catheterization, routine intravenous tubing changes, or inadvertent disconnecting of the tubing. This complication requires immediate attention and treatment. A routine chest film to localize the catheter tip, near the right atrium, should alert the physician to other technical complications listed in Table 28–10.

Use of the intravenous line for central venous pressure readings and removing or infusing blood should be avoided except in emergencies or when this is the only access. Changes of the dressing, intravenous tubing, and filter should be daily according to strict protocol.

Sepsis

If sepsis is suspected, PN should be started only after blood cultures have been drawn and antimicrobial therapy has been started. Cultures of the blood drawn through the catheter tip and a peripheral site should be tested for aerobes, anaerobes, and fungi.[2] Sepsis during therapy may be manifested by fevers, sudden glucose intolerance, hypotension, oliguria, or general deterioration in the clinical condition. The catheter should be removed in the presence of septic shock, culture-proven bacteremia or fungemia, focal infection at the insertion site, persistent unexplained fever, and embolic phenomenon.

Infection of the catheter is suspected in approximately 5 percent of patients.[11] Once removed, the solution and infusion line should be cultured. Reinsertion with a new intravenous tubing and solution at a different site should not be attempted for at least six hours after beginning a broad spectrum antibiotic therapy.

Respiratory Compromise

The infusion of a high glucose-containing parenteral nutrition solution may lead to an overproduction of carbon dioxide and resultant increased respiratory work.[2,11] Women who are being weaned from the ventilator may benefit by the substitution of a dextrose solution with more FE (up to 50 percent) to reduce carbon dioxide production and respiratory work. Once the weaning is complete, the previous PN regimen should be reinstituted.

TABLE 28–10. COMPLICATIONS ASSOCIATED WITH PARENTERAL NUTRITION

	Complications	
	Common	***Uncommon***
Technical	Pneumothorax Subclavian artery puncture Subclavian hematoma Thromboembolism Catheter malposition	Hemothorax Hydromediastinum Innominate or subclavian vein laceration Carotid artery injury Air embolism Catheter embolism Thoracic duct laceration Cardiac perforation and tamponade Brachial plexus injury Horner's syndrome Phrenic nerve paralysis
Sepsis	Catheter sepsis	Septic shock Infusion site infection Unexplained fever
Respiratory	Pneumothorax	Respiratory failure
Metabolic	Hyperglycemia Hypoglycemia Hyperkalemia Hypokalemia Hyperphosphatemia Hypophosphatemia Hypertriglyceridemia Elevated hepatic enzymes	Hypermagnesemia Deficiencies in trace elements (zinc, chromium, copper) Hypercalcemia

Adapted from Parenteral and Enteral Nutrition Manual, ed 3, 1984.[2]

Metabolic

Metabolic complications include acid-base, fluid, and electrolyte imbalances, and those from the PN itself such as cholestasis and increased liver function tests. These abnormalities may be detected early or avoided with regular monitoring (see Table 28–10).

The most common metabolic imbalance is hyperglycemia which is most likely present during the initial 3 days of parenteral nutrition.[2,11] Endogenous insulin secretion increases gradually as the infusion rate or concentration is increased, and insulin therapy is often avoided. If glucose intolerance becomes apparent, insulin may be administered subcutaneously or intravenously until serum glucose is controlled. Once control is achieved, insulin may be added to the PN solution. The initial dose of regular insulin is usually 10 to 15 units/L of hypertonic dextrose but may be increased if necessary.

Hypoglycemia from a sudden decrease or cessation in infusion may explain any diaphoresis, confusion, or agitation in the patient. Reinstitution of the nutritional solution or starting 10 percent dextrose in water is preferred over administering an ampule of 50 percent dextrose.

Hyperkalemia may occur if the woman is not sufficiently anabolic or able to fully utilize the administered potassium. Other causes of hyperkalemia include tissue necrosis, decreased renal function, systemic sepsis, and low cardiac output. The amount of infused potassium should be reduced, or rarely, withheld until serum levels return to normal. Intravenous bicarbonate, glucose, and insulin may be necessary if cardiac toxicity is found. Once she becomes anabolic, hypokalemia may develop and an obligatory requirement for intracellular potassium becomes present. Doses of 40 mEq/L of potassium are usually sufficient but patient needs may reach 200 mEq day.[2]

Elevations in serum calcium, phosphate, or magnesium may result from the initial infusion if she is in a severe catabolic state. Increased serum concentrations of these electrolytes may result in muscle weakness or central nervous system depression. In contrast, low serum concentrations of calcium, phosphate, and magnesium are uncommon with proper supplementation. Lethargy, mental confusion, hyperreflexia, and anemia are associated findings. These complications are usually found initially during increasing anabolism and protein synthesis.

Fat emulsion in dosages exceeding 3.5 g/kg/day or more than 60 percent of the total calories may precipitate a fat overload syndrome.[2,11] This finding is characterized by fever, liver damage, coagulation disorders, lethargy, and hyperlipidemia. Reduction in fat emulsion is usually sufficient to resolve this problem. Serum triglyceride needs to be monitored regularly to insure safe utilization of FE.

Unique to PN are transient changes in a patient's liver function tests. These elevations usually peak about 10 to 14 days and may rise three- to sevenfold above baseline. Alkaline phosphatase and transaminases are the most common enzymes to rise, although bilirubin will occasionally become elevated. The histologic examination may show fatty infiltration, bile stasis with periportal inflammation and parenchymal changes, and fibrosis. After another 2 or 3 weeks, elevated liver function tests usually return to normal while liver changes resolve once the PN is stopped. While a number of causes have been proposed, it appears that overfeeding the patient is an important factor. A review of the patient's caloric requirements and a reduction if necessary should be considered.

Deficiencies of the trace elements zinc, chromium, and copper are usually with long-term PN though large or prolonged ostomy output or diarrhea may result in copper or zinc deficiency.[2] Manifestations of these deficiencies include glucose intolerance (chromium), anemia and neutropenia (copper), and hair loss or seborrheic dermatitis (zinc). Therefore, a trace element solution should be administered daily in the parenteral solution. Little is known about effects from an excess of these infused elements.

SPECIAL CONSIDERATIONS

Preexisting Cardiac, Liver, or Renal Failure

The liver, renal, and cardiac status must be considered and may require modifications in nutritional therapy. Renal and liver disease may require less fluid and more protein restrictions. Potassium, phosphorus, and magnesium supplementation may also require reduction because of the reduced glomerular filtration of renal failure. An increase in dextrose concentration is appropriate for central formulations to compensate for fluid restrictions.

Sodium restriction may be necessary to control fluid status in the presence of any cardiac or liver failure. Certain trace elements may need to be restricted in either severe renal failure (zinc, chromium) or liver failure (copper, manganese).

Close monitoring of the patient's fluid intake and output, weight, and changes in mental status is necessary. Serum electrolytes and renal and liver function testing require more frequent determinations.

Preoperative and Postoperative Therapy

Because a woman undergoing surgery may develop glucose intolerance from increased catecholamine release, it is recommended that the PN rate be reduced by half or switched to a 10 percent dextrose solution while in the operating room. The prior infusion rate may be resumed within 24 to 48 hours postoperatively if the patient remains normoglycemic.

Sufficient replacement of potassium and amino acids is necessary if a cesarean section is to be performed. A decrease in insulin requirements is to be expected after removal of the placenta. The need for continued glucose monitoring and a decreased requirement for insulin are to be anticipated.

Lactation

No known reports exist about breastfeeding during parenteral nutrition, but we see no reason to discourage lactation if the mother is so inclined. Formula supplementation for the infant may be necessary depending on the adequacy of the mother's milk supply. The infant's growth should be monitored closely as a means of determining adequate nutrition. Daily oral dietary needs for the lactating woman are essentially the same as those for pregnancy (see Table 28–3).

Cost Considerations

This therapy is expensive ($200 to $500 per day) with costs ranging from 25 to 100 times greater than enteral feedings. Even for short-term therapy, expenses of several thousand dollars are not unusual to defray costs for preparing and administering solutions, equipment, and monitoring of nutritional status and complications. Enteral nutrition by oral supplements or tube feeding should therefore be considered before PN is started. If sufficient calories and protein are not consumed or if bowel rest is indicated, then PN should be initiated. The patient's needs, anticipated length of therapy, and hospital stay must be considered. The cost of PN is not directly covered by diagnostic related group (DRG) reimbursement although malnutrition cofactors may offset part of the cost and therefore may represent an additional cost to the hospital. Home PN therapy is less expensive than hospitalization, and Medicare, Medicaid, and insurance carriers will pay for home PN, however, qualifications are always changing and regulations should be reviewed beforehand.

Minimizing expenses during PN is also important. Careful planning, ordering solutions the day before, and use of standardized solutions when possible may save pharmacy and nursing time and costs, and reduce product waste.

Home Therapy

While used rarely in obstetric or gynecologic patients, home PN may be necessary for those persons requiring long-term support. Candidates include patients with Crohn's disease, radiation enteritis, cancer requiring chemotherapy, bowel fistuli or obstructions, a severe malabsorption syndrome, and short-gut syndrome.[2,18] Persons requiring bowel rest or preoperative nutrition may also be candidates. In pregnant women, the limited experience has been favorable, and appropriately grown infants have been delivered.[14,16,17,25]

Up to 2 weeks may be required for education and mastery of the technique. Both the woman and a family member or close friend must have proficiency in aseptic technique, handling of a permanent right atrial catheter, care of the intravenous line, dressing changes, and solution compounding.

SUMMARY

Despite 18 years of PN availability, published reports of its use for gynecology and obstetric patients are limited. Most information is anecodotal but suggests that this form of therapy is safe and effective. Parenteral nutrition should be instituted when nutritional requirements are not met by oral or enteral routes of consumption. It is safe and effective as long as monitoring of the patient's clinical condition and biochemical status is routine. Because of its high cost, PN should be used in very select cases and should be short term when possible.

REFERENCES

1. Dudrick SJ, Wilmore DW, Vars HM, et al.: Long-term total parenteral nutrition with growth, development, and positive nitrogen balance. Surgery 64:134, 1968
2. Parenteral and Enteral Nutrition Team: Parenteral and Enteral Nutrition Manual, ed 3. Ann Arbor, Michigan, University of Michigan Medical Center, 1984
3. Rayburn W, Wolk R, Mercer N, et al.: Parenteral nutrition in obstetrics and gynecology. Obstet Gynecol Surv 41:200, 1986
4. Berman ML, Hamrell CE, LaGasse LD, et al.: Parenteral nutrition by peripheral vein in the management of gynecologic oncology patients. Gynecol Oncol 7:318, 1979
5. Ford JH, Dudan RC, Bennett JS, et al.: Parenteral hyperalimentation in gynecologic oncology patients. Gynecol Oncol 1:70, 1972
6. Fuller AF, Griffiths CT: Ovarian cancer cachexia—surgical interactions. Gynecol Oncol 8:301, 1979
7. Hew LR, Deitel M: Total parenteral nutrition in gynecology and obstetrics. Obstet Gynecol 55:464, 1980
8. Joyeux H, Dubois, JB, Solassol C, et al.: Cycise intermittent parenteral (CPN). The first adjuvant therapy for radio-chemotherapeutic combination in advanced ovarian tumors (AOT). 13th International Cancer Congress, part D, Research and Treatment, 1986 pp 171–178
9. Lavery IC, Steiger E, Fazio VW: Home parenteral nutrition in management of patients with severe radiation enteritis. Dis Colon Rectum 23:91, 1980
10. Tunca JC: Impact of cisplatin multiagent chemotherapy and total parenteral hyperalimentation on bowel obstruction caused by ovarian cancer. Gynecol Oncol 12:219, 1981
11. Silberman H, Eisenberg D (eds): Parenteral and enteral nutrition for the hospitalized patient. E. Norwalk, Connecticut, Appleton-Century-Crofts, 1982
12. Wilmore DW: The metabolic management of the critically ill. New York, Plenum, 1980
13. Benny PS, Legge M, Aickin DR: The biochemical effects of maternal hyperalimentation during pregnancy. NZ Med J 88:283, 1978
14. Cox KL, Byrne WJ, Ament ME: Home total parenteral nutrition during pregnancy: A case report. JPEN 5:246, 1981
15. Gineston JL, Capron JP, Delcenserie R, et al.: Prolonged total parenteral nutrition in a pregnant woman with acute pancreatitis. J Clin Gastroenterol 6:249, 1984
16. Seifer D, Silberman H, Catanzarite V, et al.: Total parenteral nutrition in obstetrics. JAMA 253:2073, 1985
17. Rivera-Alsina ME, Saldana LR, Stringer CA: Fetal growth sustained by parenteral nutrition in pregnancy. Obstet Gynecol 64:138, 1984
18. Weinberg RB, Sitrin MD, Adkins GM, et al.: Treatment of hyperlipidemic pancreatitis in pregnancy with total parenteral nutrition. Gastroenterology 83:1300, 1982
19. DiConstanzo JD, Martin J, Cano N., et al.: Total parenteral nutrition with fat emulsions during pregnancy—nutritional requirements: A case report. JPEN 6:534, 1982
20. Heller L: Parenteral nutrition in obstetrics and gynecology. Current concepts in parenteral nutrition. The Hague, Nijhoff, 1977, pp 179–186
21. National Research Council, National Academy of Science. Recommended Dietary Allowances, ed 3. Washington, D.C. 1980
22. Harris JA, Benedict FG: Biometric studies of basal metabolism in man. Carnegie Institute, Washington, D.C. Publication No. 279, 1919
23. Oldham H, Sheft BB: Effect of caloric intake on nitrogen utilization during pregnancy. J Am Diet Assoc 27:847, 1951
24. Elphick MC, Filshie GM, Hull D: The passage of fat emulsion across the human placenta. Br J Obstet Gynaecol 85:610, 1978
25. Tresadern JC, Falconer GF, Turnberg LA, et al.: Maintenance of pregnancy in a home parenteral nutrition patient. JPEN 8:199, 1984
26. Luukkainen T, Jarvinen PA, Pyrola T: Induction of labour with intravenous fat emulsion at term. J Obstet Gynecol Br Common 71:45, 1964
27. Cerra F: Profiles in nutritional management: The trauma patient, Northbrook, Illinois Abbott Laboratories, 1982
28. Wolk R, Swartz R: Nutritional support for patients with renal failure. Nutritional Support Services 6:2, 38, 1985
29. AMA Nutritional Advisory Group, Shils ME (Chairperson): Multivitamin preparations for parenteral use. JPEN 3:258, 1979
30. AMA Guidelines for essential trace element preparations for parenteral use. JPEN 3:263, 1979
31. Evans L: Parenteral iron in pregnancy. In Wallerstein, R, Mettiel S (eds): Iron in Clinical

Medicine. Berkeley, California, University of California Press, 1958, pp 161–171
32. Fahmy K: Systemic reactions with total dose infusion of iron dextran complex in obstetric patients. Int J Gynecol Obstet 16:170, 1978
33. Mays T: Intravenous iron dextrane therapy in the treatment of anemia occurring in surgical, gynecologic and obstetric patients. Surg Gynecol Obstet 143:381, 1976
34. Oluboyede O, Ogunbode O, Ayeall O: Iron deficiency anemia during pregnancy: A comparative trial of treatment by iron-poly complex Ferastral[R] given intramuscularly and iron dextran by total dose infusion. E Afr Med J 57:626, 1980
35. Sood SK, Ramachandran K, Rani K: W.H.O. sponsored collaborative study: The effect of parenteral iron administration in the control of anemia of pregnancy. Br J Nutr 42:399, 1979
36. Bailey MJ: Reduction of catheter-associated sepsis in parenteral nutrition using low-dose intravenous heparin. Br Med J 1:1671, 1979
37. Lavin JP, Gimmon Z, Miodovnik M, et al.: Total parenteral nutrition in a pregnant insulin-requiring diabetic. Obstet Gynecol 59:660, 1982
38. Stowell JC, Bottsford JE, Rubel HR: Pancreatitis with pseudocyst and cholelithiasis in third trimester of pregnancy: Management with total parenteral nutrition. South Med J 77:502, 1984
39. Webb GA: The use of hyperalimentation and chemotherapy in pregnancy: A case report. Am J Obstet Gynecol 137:263, 1980

Appendix I

Chemical Properties of Drugs

Brian D. Andresen

Name	Structure (page number)*	Molecular Weight	pKa	$T_{1/2}$ (hr)	% Protein Binding
Anesthetics, local					
Bupivacaine	600	288	8.1	2.7	96
Lidocaine	200	234	7.9	1.6	64
Mepivacaine	600	246	7.6	1.9	77
Analgesics, nonnarcotic					
Aspirin	606	180	3.5	2–5 (<3 gm) 16–19 (>3 mg)	50–90
Acetaminophen	608	151	9.5	2–2.4	25
Ibuprofen	616	206	4.4	2	99
Indomethacin	614	357	5.5	4–12	92–99
Phenylbutazone	610	308	4.5	29–175	98
Naproxen	616	230	5	10–17	98–99
Analgesics, narcotic					
Meperidine	—	247	8.7	2.4–4	65–75
Morphine	624	285	8	1.9–3.1	35
Pentazocine	627	285	9	2	60–70
Methadone	632	309	8.6	18–97	71–87
Naloxone	630	327	8	1–1.7	—
Codeine	622	299	8.2	3–4	7
Antianxiety Agents					
Chlordiazepoxide	693	299	4.8	5–30	94–97
Diazepam	657	284	3.3	24–48	94–98
Oxazepam	657	286	1.7, 11.6	6–25	90
Lorazepam	657	321	1.3, 11.5	9–16	90

(*continued*)

Name	Structure (page number)*	Molecular Weight	pKa	$T_{1/2}$ (hr)	% Protein Binding
Antiarrhythmics					
Procainamide	200	235	9.2	2.2–4	15
Propranolol	202	259	9.4	2–6	90–96
Anticoagulants					
Heparin	319	6,000–20,000	—	1.5–2	95
Warfarin	114	308	4.8	35–45	>99
Anticonvulsants					
Carbamazepine	672	236	—	18–65	70–80
Phenobarbital	655	232	7.2	48–144	50–60
Phenytoin	201	252	8.3	8–60	87–93
Primidone	664	218	—	3.3–12.5	0
Trimethadione	668	143	—	12–24	0
Valproic acid	669	144	4.8	13–21	80–90
Antidepressants					
Amitryptyline	712	277	9.4	32–40	82–96
Imipramine	713	280	—	3.5	85–92
Antihistamines					
Chlorpheneramine	378	275	9.2	30	172
Diphenhydramine	377	255	8.3	4–10	98
Pseudoephedrine	506	165	9.9, 5.8	9–16	—
Antihypertensives					
Diazoxide	267	230	8.7	21–36	90–93
Hydralazine	255	160	7.1	2–4	88–90
Methyldopa	265	211	2.2, 9.2, 10.6, 12	8	<20
Antimicrobial Agents					
Gentamicin	39	477	8.2	2–3	<10
Kanamycin	39	484	7.2	2.5	0–3
Cefoxitin	—	427	—	1	65–80
Cephalothin	20	396	5.5	0.5–1	70
Cefazolin	—	454	2.3	2	84
Chloramphenicol	36	323	5.5	1.6–3.3	60–80
Clindamycin	29	424	7.5	2–4	94
Erythromycin	28	733	8.8	1.4	73
Metronidazole	80	171	2.5	6–12	<20
Nitrofurantoin	54	238	7.2	0.3–0.6	25–60
Ampicillin	16	349	2.5, 7.2	1–1.5	15–29
Benzyl penicillin	12	334	2.8	0.5	65
Sulfamethoxazole	7	253	5.7	7–12	62
Sulfisoxazole	—	267	4.9	3–7	84
Doxycycline	34	444	3.4, 7.7	15–24	25–31
Tetracycline	34	444	3.3, 7.7	1.3–1.6	20–40
Antipsychotic Drugs					
Chlorpromazine	—	318	9.3	16–30	98–99
Lithium	—	6.9	6.8	8–35	0
Prochlorperazine	679	373	8.1	23	—
Thioridazine	680	370	9.5	26–36	96–99

Name	Structure (page number)*	Molecular Weight	pKa	$T_{1/2}$ (hr)	% Protein Binding
Antituberculosis Drugs					
Ethambutol	46	204	6.9, 9.5	6–8	8–40
Isoniazid	45	137	2.0, 3.9	0.7–4	low
PAS (para-amino salicylic acid)	43	153	1.7, 3.2	0.5–1.5	50–70
Rifampin	46	822	1.7, 7.9	1.5–5	70–90
Streptomycin	40	581	—	2–3	20–30
Antiulcer Drugs					
Cimetidine	383	252	7	2	18–26
Bronchodilators					
Terbutaline	285	225	8.8, 10.1, 11.2	3.4	25
Theophylline	283	180	0.7, 8.8	3–13	53–65
Cardiac Glycosides					
Digoxin	195	780	—	30–40	20–40
Corticosteroids					
Betamethasone	409	393	—	≥5	—
Cortisone	406	360	—	0.5–2	90
Dexamethasone	410	392	—	3–4.5	77
Hydrocortisone	406	362	—	1.5–2	90–95
Prednisone	414	358	—	3.4–3.8	70
Diuretics					
Chlorothiazide	216	295	6.7, 9.5	13	20–80
Furosemide	219	330	3.8	0.3–1.6	91–99
Hydrochlorothiazide	216	297	7.9, 9.2	2–15	—
Hypoglycemic Agents					
Insulin (regular)	—	6,000	—	1.5–2	1–10
Tolazamide	463	311	3.5, 5.7	7	—
Tolbutamide	463	270	5.3	3–27	95–97
Sedatives					
Flurazepam	657	387	1.9, 8	47–100	—
Secobarbital	654	238	7.4	20–28	46–70
Thyroid/Antithyroid Drugs					
Methimazole	422	114	—	6–7	—
Propylthiouracil	422	170	7.8	1.2–1.5	75
Thyroxine	420	776	2.2, 6.7, 10.1	144–168	>99
Triiodothyroxine	—	690	—	35–60	>99
Tocolytic Agents					
Ritodrine	—	287	—	2–10	—
Terbutaline	516	225	8.8, 10.1, 11.2	3.4	25
Isoxsuprine	516	301	8.0, 9.8	1.25	—
Uterine Stimulants					
Oxytocin	303	1,007	—	0.08–0.1	30
Methylergonovine	302	339	—	—	—

(*continued*)

Name	Structure (page number)*	Molecular Weight	pKa	$T_{1/2}$ (hr)	% Protein Binding
Miscellaneous					
Caffeine	210	194	3.5	3.5	1–5
Ethanol	732	46	14	4.33	1–5
Tetrahydrocannabinol	—	314	—	—	>99
Amphetamine	510	135	9.9	10–30	—
Lysergic acid (LSD-25)	728	323	—	1.7–3.0	—
Cocaine	596	303	8.4	1	—
Methaqualone	660	250	2.5	16–42	80

*The structure of each drug may be found on the page number shown in Csáky TZ, Barnes, BA: Cutting's Handbook of Pharmacology: The Actions and Uses of Drugs, ed. 7., Norwalk, Conn., Appleton-Century-Crofts, 1984.

Appendix II

Cost Comparisons Between Commonly Prescribed Drugs

Paul E. Hafner

Prices listed in this appendix are wholesale prices based on 100 doses, unless otherwise noted. The data were gathered from the 1984–1985 *American Druggist Blue Book* or January 1985 *Medi-Span Pricing Guide*. These prices are for relative cost comparison only; the actual cost to the patient will vary from one pharmacy to another. This table does not consider the frequency of administration or the duration of therapy.

Product	Pharmaceutical Company	Wholesale Cost per 100 ($)
Decongestants/Antihistamines		
Sudafed 60 mg tab	Burroughs-Wellcome	7.91
Pseudoephedrine HCl 60 mg tab	Various	1.25 (VRL)
Actifed tab	Burroughs-Wellcome	9.02
Dimetapp tab	A. H. Robins	20.35
Ornade cap	Smith Kline	28.80
Drixoral tab	Schering	21.05
Hista tapp	Upster Smith	4.90
Trinalin	Schering	27.27
Entex-LA	Norwich Eaton	21.48
Antibiotics		
Polycillin 500 mg cap	Bristol	31.54
Ampicillin 500 mg cap	Various	11.29–13.31
Keflex 500 mg cap	UpJohn	113.61
Vibramycin 100 mg cap	Pfizer	151.00
Doxycyline Hyclate 100 mg cap	Various	53.38–92.10

(*continued*)

Product	Pharmaceutical Company	Wholesale Cost per 100 ($)
Achromycin-V 500 mg cap	Lederle	10.94
Tetracycline HCl 500 mg cap	Various	4.57–5.10
Erythrocin 250 mg tab	Abbott	11.78
Erythromycin Stearate 250 mg tab	Various	7.22–8.73
Erythromycin base 250 mg	UpJohn	6.86
Septra tabs	Burroughs-Wellcome	27.47
Septra DS tabs	Burroughs-Wellcome	45.08
Cotrim DS	Lemmon	25.00
Bactrim tabs	Roche	27.46
Macrodantin 50 mg cap	Eaton	25.26
Nitrofurantoin 50 mg cap	Various	8.63–9.68
Gantrisin 500 mg tab	Roche	8.97
Sulfisoxazole 500 mg tab	Various	2.30–3.31
Ceclor 500 mg cap	Lilly	174.17
Duricef 500 mg cap	Mead-Johnson	116.78
Metronidazole 250 mg	Various	17.45–43.80
Flagyl 250 mg tab	Searle	74.46
Protostat	Ortho	54.60
Metryl	Lemmon	23.90
Velosef 500 mg	Squibb	118.70
Anspor 500 mg	Smith Kline	95.60
Antidepressants		
Elavil 50 mg tab	MSD	25.90
Amitriptyline 50 mg tab	Various	2.82–8.79
Tofranil 50 mg tab	Geigy	33.79
Imipramine HCl 50 mg tab	Various	4.01–7.88
Vivactil 10 mg tabs	MSD	25.51
Sinequan 50 mg cap	Pfizer	24.33
Desyrel 50 mg	Mead-Johnson	23.57
Parnate 10 mg	Smith Kline	15.50
Nardil 15 mg	Parke-Davis	11.60
Antianxiety Drugs		
Valium 5 mg tab	Roche	22.36
Librium 25 mg cap	Roche	31.24
Chlordiazepoxide HCl 25 mg cap	Various	2.19–2.44
Tranxene 7.5 mg cap	Abbott	27.57
Ativan 2 mg tab	Wyeth	36.49
Serax 15 mg cap	Wyeth	22.88
Miltown 400 mg tab	Wallace	26.14
Meprobamate 400 mg tab	Various	1.64–2.07
Vistaril 25 mg cap	Pfizer	32.31
Atarax 25 mg tab	Roerig	32.31
Hydroxyzine HCl 25 mg tab	Various	8.85–9.44
Xanax 1 mg	UpJohn	40.79
Halcion 0.25 mg	UpJohn	25.35
Klonopin 1 mg	Roche	18.77
Antihypertensives		
Aldomet 250 mg tab	MSD	17.95
Apresoline 25 mg tab	CIBA	11.27

Product	Pharmaceutical Company	Wholesale Cost per 100 ($)
Hydralazine 25 mg tab	Various	1.50–2.79
Inderal 40 mg tab	Ayerst	17.04
HydroDiuril 50 mg tab	MSD	9.29
Hydrochlorothiazide 50 mg tab	Various	1.11–2.19
Diuril 500 mg tab	MSD	9.29
Chlorothiazide 500 mg tab	Various	5.70–6.94
Lasix 40 mg tab	Hoechst-Roussel	12.45
Dyazide cap	Smith Kline	18.15
Minipress 2 mg	Pfizer	22.44
Lopressor 50 mg	Geigy	19.20
Tenormin 50 mg	Stuart	39.86
Insulins		
Regular U-100	Squibb	8.28/vial
Regular U-100	Lilly	8.14
NPH U-100	Squibb	8.28
NPH U-100	Lilly	8.14
Lente U-100	Squibb	8.28
Lente U-100	Lilly	8.14
Humulin-R 10 ml	Lilly	12.42
Humulin-N 10 ml	Lilly	12.42
Semilente U-100	Lilly	8.14
Anticonvulsants		
Dilantin 100 mg cap	Parke-Davis	8.28
Sodium phenytoin 100 mg cap	Various	0.90–2.29
Phenobarbital sodium 32 mg tab	Various	0.33–1.90
Mysoline 250 mg tab	Ayerst	12.89
Primidone 250 mg tab	Various	5.25
Tegretol 200 mg tab	Geigy	20.64
Tridione 300 mg cap	Abbott	12.66
Zarontin 250 mg cap	Parke-Davis	22.33
Depakene 250 mg cap	Abbott	25.26
Vulvovaginal Candidiasis Preparations		
Mycostatin Vag tabs 100,000 U	Squibb	8.91/15
Nilstat Vag tabs 100,000 U	Lederle	6.90
Nystatin Vag tabs 100,000 U	Various	2.64–2.68/15
Monistat 7 tabs	Ortho	10.05
Monistat 3 tabs	Ortho	9.31
Monistat 7 Vag cream	Ortho	9.31/47 g
Gyne-Lotrimin 100 mg tabs	Schering	9.08/7
Gyne-Lotrimin Vag Cr 7 day	Schering	8.62/45 g
Mycelex-G 100 mg tabs	Miles	8.87/7
Mycelex-G 500 mg	Miles	7.92
Mycelex Vag Cr 7 day	Miles	8.44/45 g
Nonspecific Vaginitis Preparations		
Tetracycline cap—see Antibiotics		
Ampicillin cap—see Antibiotics		
Metronidazole tab—see Antibiotics		
Sultrin Vag Cr	Ortho	12.39/78 g
Triple Sulfa Vag Cr	Various	2.65–3.50/78 g

(continued)

Product	Pharmaceutical Company	Wholesale Cost per 100 ($)
Estrogens		
Estrace 1 mg tab	Mead-Johnson	9.31
Diethylstilbestrol 0.5 mg tab	Various	2.52
Premarin 0.625 mg tab	Ayerst	11.59
Conjugated estrogens 0.625 mg tab	Various	5.64–6.95
Estrovis 100 mcg tab	Parke-Davis	40.99
Menest 0.625 mg tab	Beecham	8.11
Evex 0.625 mg tab	Syntex	8.62
Ogen 0.625 mg tab	Abbott	11.59
Estinyl 0.05 mg tab	Schering	19.03
β-Adrenergic Tocolytic Agents		
Vasodilan 10 mg tab	Mead-Johnson	23.76
Isoxsuprine HCl 10 mg tab	Various	2.44–2.50
Brethine 2.5 mg tab	Geigy	11.86
Bricanyl 2.5 mg tab	Astra	10.96
Yutopar 10 mg tab	Merrell-National	42.64
Antiemetics		
Phenergan 25 mg supp	Wyeth	9.25/12
Compazine 25 mg supp	Smith Kline	11.80/12
Oral Contraceptives		
Ortho Novum 1/50 21 or 28	Ortho	10.93/cycle
Norinyl 1/50 21 or 28	Syntex	10.53/cycle
Ovral 21 or 28	Wyeth	12.50/cycle
Ovcon-50 21 or 28	Mead-Johnson	9.24/cycle
Norlestrin 1/50 21 or 28	Parke-Davis	10.27/cycle
Demulen 21 or 28	Searle	12.00/cycle
Ortho Novum 1/35 21 or 28	Ortho	10.93/cycle
Norinyl 1/35 21 or 28	Syntex	10.53/cycle
LoOvral 1/35 21 or 28	Wyeth	12.10/cycle
Brevicon 21 or 28	Syntex	10.45/cycle
Modicon 21 or 28	Ortho	10.98/cycle
Ovcon 35 21 or 28	Mead-Johnson	9.24/cycle
Loestrin 1/20 21	Parke-Davis	10.27/cycle
Loestrin 1.5/30	Parke-Davis	10.27/cycle
Ortho Novum 10/11 28's	Ortho	10.98/cycle
Ortho Novum 7/7/7	Ortho	10.98/cycle
Triphasil	Searle	12.10/cycle
Norlestrin 2.5/50	Parke-Davis	10.63/cycle
Demulen 1/35 28's	Searle	11.00/cycle
Drugs for Pelvic Pain		
Danocrine 200 mg cap	Winthrop	124.87
Indocin 25 mg cap	MSD	27.14
Clinoril 150 mg tab	MSD	46.80
Naprosyn 250 mg tab	Syntex	44.76
Anaprox 275 mg tab	Syntex	43.34
Motrin 400 mg tab	UpJohn	17.31
Rufen 400 mg	Boots	10.80
Advil 200 mg	Whitehall	6.68
Nuprin 200 mg	Bristol-Myers	7.34

Product	Pharmaceutical Company	Wholesale Cost per 100 ($)
Ponstel 250 mg cap	Parke-Davis	32.09
Bayer 325 mg tab	Glenbrook	2.64
Aspirin 325 mg tab	Various	0.66–1.17
Tylenol 325 mg tab	McNeil	4.01
Acetaminophen 325 mg tab	Various	1.20–1.62
Urologic Disorders		
Urecholine 10 mg tab	MSD	28.95
Bethanechol HCl 10 mg tab	Various	2.79
Dibenzyline 10 mg cap	Smith Kline	17.70
Anticholinergics/Antispasmodics		
Ditropan 5 mg tab	Marion	21.88
Bentyl 10 mg cap	Merrell-National	8.50
Dicyclomine HCl 10 mg cap	Various	1.38–1.73
Probanthine 15 mg tab	Searle	21.62
Propantheline HBr 15 mg tab	Various	2.15–2.91
Urispas 100 mg tab	Smith Kline	22.85

Appendix III

Adverse Interactions Between Drugs

R. Michael Gendreau

Drugs	Interaction	Proposed Mechanism
Aminoglycosides		
Cephaloridine	Increased nephrotoxicity	Not established
Cephalothin	Increased nephrotoxicity	Not established
Curaiform drugs	Neuromuscular blockade	Additive
Digoxin	Possible decreased digoxin effect	Inhibition of gastrointestinal absorption
Ethacrynic acid	Increased ototoxicity	Additive
Polymyxins	Increased nephrotoxicity	Additive
Ampicillin		
Contraceptives, oral	Decreased contraceptive effect	Not established
Anesthetics, general		
Antihypertensive drugs	Hypotension	Usually additive
Antacids		
Digoxin	Decreased drug levels	Decreased digoxin absorption
Indomethacin	Decreased drug levels	Decreased indomethacin absorption
Isoniazid	Decreased isoniazid effect with aluminum antacids	Decreased absorption of isoniazid
Salicylates	Decreased salicylate levels	Increased renal clearance
Tetracyclines, oral	Decreased tetracycline levels	Decreased tetracycline absorption
Anticoagulants, oral		
Anabolic and androgenic steroids	Increased anticoagulant effect	Not established
Barbiturates	Decreased anticoagulant effect	Induction of microsomal enzymes
Carbamazepine	Decreased anticoagulant effect	Induction of microsomal enzymes
Cimetidine	Increased anticoagulant effect	Inhibition of microsomal enzymes

Drugs	Interaction	Proposed Mechanism
Contraceptives, oral	Decreased anticoagulant effect	Increased factor VII and X (prothrombin may decrease)
Dextrothyroxine	Increased anticoagulant effect	Not established
Hypoglycemics	Increased sulfonylurea hypoglycemia	Inhibition of microsomal enzymes
Indomethacin	Increased bleeding risk	Inhibition of platelet function
Metronidazole	Increased anticoagulant effect	Inhibition of microsomal enzymes
Miconazole	Increased anticoagulant effect	Not established
Phenylbutazone or oxyphenbutazone	Increased anticoagulant effect	Displacement from binding sites; inhibition of microsomal enzymes
Phenytoin	Increased phenytoin toxicity with dicumarol	Inhibition of microsomal enzymes
Rifampin	Decreased anticoagulant effect	Induction of microsomal enzymes
Salicylates	Increased bleeding time	Inhibition of platelet function
(more than 2 g/day)	Increased hypoprothrombinemic effect	Reduction in plasma prothrombin
Sulfinpyrazone	Increased anticoagulant effect	Not established
Sulfonamides	Increased anticoagulant effect	Inhibition of microsomal enzymes; displacement from binding sites
Thyroid hormones	Increased anticoagulant effect	Increased clotting factor catabolism
Barbiturates		
β-Adrenergic blockers	Decreased β-blocker effect	Induction of microsomal enzymes
Anticoagulants, oral	Decreased anticoagulant effect	Induction of microsomal enzymes
Antidepressants, tricyclic	Decreased antidepressant effect	Induction of microsomal enzymes
Chloramphenicol	Increased barbiturate effect	Inhibition of microsomal enzymes
Contraceptives, oral	Decreased contraceptive effect	Induction of microsomal enzymes
Corticosteroids	Decreased steroid effect	Induction of microsomal enzymes
Digitoxin	Decreased digitoxin effect	Induction of microsomal enzymes
Doxycycline	Decreased doxycycline effect	Induction of microsomal enzymes
Meperidine	Increased CNS depression	Increased meperidine metabolites
Phenothiazines	Decreased phenothiazine effect	Induction of microsomal enzymes
Rifampin	Decreased barbiturate effect	Induction of microsomal enzymes
Valproic acid	Increased phenobarbital effect	Decreased phenobarbital metabolism
Benzodiazepines		
Cimetidine	Increased effect of chlordiazepoxide and diazepam	Inhibition of microsomal enzymes
β-adrenergic (see Sympathomimetic Amines)		
Cephaloridine		
Aminoglycoside antibiotics	Increased nephrotoxicity	Not established
Ethacrynic acid	Increased nephrotoxicity	Additive
Furosemide	Increased nephrotoxicity	Additive
Cephalothin		
Aminoglycoside antibiotics	Increased nephrotoxicity	Not established
Chloramphenicol		
Barbiturates	Increased barbiturate effect	Inhibition of microsomal enzymes
Phenytoin	Increased phenytoin toxicity	Inhibition of microsomal enzymes

(*continued*)

Drugs	Interaction	Proposed Mechanism
Cimetidine		
Anticoagulants, oral	Increased anticoagulant effect	Inhibition of microsomal enzymes
Benzodiazepines	Increased effect of chlordiazepoxide	Inhibition of microsomal enzymes
Theophylline	Increased theophylline toxicity	Inhibition of microsomal enzymes
Contraceptives, oral		
Ampicillin	Decreased contraceptive effect	Induction of microsomal enzymes
Anticoagulants, oral	Decreased anticoagulant effect	Increased factor VII and X (prothrombin may decrease)
Barbiturates	Decreased contraceptive effect	Induction of microsomal enzymes
Carbamazepine	Decreased contraceptive effect	Induction of microsomal enzymes
Guanethidine	Decreased guanethidine effect	Not established
Hypoglycemics, oral	Increased glucose levels	Increased glucose tolerance
Phenytoin	Decreased contraceptive effect	Induction of microsomal enzymes
Primidone	Decreased contraceptive effect	Induction of microsomal enzymes
Tetracyclines	Decreased contraceptive effect	Not established
Diazepam	Slower diazepam elimination	Impaired metabolism
Corticosteroids		
Barbiturates	Decreased corticosteroid effect	Induction of microsomal enzymes
Diuretics (except spironolactone and triamterene)	Increased potassium loss	Additive
Ephedrine	Decreased dexamethasone effect	Not established
Estrogens	Usually increased corticosteroid effect	Increased protein-binding
Phenytoin	Decreased corticosteroid effect	Induction of microsomal enzymes
Rifampin	Decreased corticosteroid effect	Induction of microsomal enzymes
Danazol		
Estrogens	Decreased estrogen effects	Inhibition of gonadotropins
Diazoxide		
Anesthetics, general	Hypotension	Usually additive
Phenytoin	Decreased anticonvulsant effect	Not established
Sympathomimetic amines	Decreased antihypertensive effect	Pharmacologic antagonism
Digoxin		
Antacids, oral	Decreased digoxin effect	Decreased digoxin absorption
Diuretics (except K^+ sparing)	Increased digoxin toxicity	Hypokalemia
Sympathomimetic amines	Increased tendency to cardiac arrhythmia	Additive
Ergot Alkaloids (ergotamine, ergotrate, cafergot and similar agents)		
Ephedrine	Postpartum hypertension	Additive
Methoxamine	Postpartum hypertension, headaches	Additive
Propranolol	Headaches, vasoconstriction	Additive
Sympathomimetics	Hypertension, headaches	Additive
Estrogens		
Anticoagulants	Usually decreased anticoagulant effect	Increased coagulation factors

Drugs	Interaction	Proposed Mechanism
Corticosteroids	Potentiation of corticosteroid (esp. anti-inflammatory) effects, esp. with hydrocortisone	Possibly due to increased steroid being protein bound
Hypoglycemics	Increased blood glucose levels	Decreased glucose tolerance
Oxytocin	Increased uterine contractility	Not established
Phenobarbital	Decreased drug levels	Induction of microsomal enzymes
Vitamins	Decreased folate levels	Not established
Furosemide		
Cephaloridine	Increased nephrotoxicity	Additive
Corticosteroids	Increased potassium loss	Additive
Digitalis drugs	Increased digitalis toxicity	Hypokalemia
Indomethacin	Decreased antihypertensive and natriuretic effect	Prostaglandin inhibition
Lithium	Increased lithium toxicity	Decreased renal lithium clearance
Phenytoin	Reduced diuresis	Not established
Propranolol	Increased β-blockade	Not established
Heparin		
Aspirin	Increased bleeding risk	Inhibition of platelet function
Hydralazine		
Anesthetics, general	Hypotension	Usually additive
Sympathomimetic amines	Decreased antihypertensive effect	Pharmacologic antagonism
Hypoglycemics, oral		
Contraceptives, oral	Increased blood glucose levels	Decreased glucose tolerance
Dicumarol	Increased hypoglycemia	Inhibition of microsomal enzymes
Propranolol	Prolonged hypoglycemia	Reduced glycogenolysis
	Masks tachycardia and tremor	β-receptor blockade
	Hypertension during hypoglycemia	Blocked β effects of epinephrine
Rifampin	Decreased hypoglycemic effect	Induction of microsomal enzymes
Salicylates	Increased hypoglycemia, especially with chlorpropamide	Displacement from binding sites; additive
Indomethacin		
Antacids, oral	Decreased indomethacin effect	Decreased indomethacin absorption
Anticoagulants, oral	Increased bleeding risk	Inhibition of platelet function
β-adrenergic blockers	Decreased antihypertensive effect	Possibly by prostaglandin inhibition
Diuretics	Decreased antihypertensive and natriuretic effect of thiazides and furosemide	Possibly by prostaglandin inhibition
Lithium	Increased lithium toxicity	Decreased renal lithium clearance
Sympathomimetic amines	Severe hypertension	Not established
Influenza Vaccine		
Theophylline	Increased theophylline effect	Decreased theophylline metabolism
Insulin		
Anticoagulants, oral	Decreased glucose levels	Decreased protein-binding
Corticosteroids	Increased glucose levels	Antagonism
Diuretics (thiazide)	Increased glucose levels	Antagonism

(*continued*)

Drugs	Interaction	Proposed Mechanism
Oral contraceptives	Increased glucose levels	Decreased glucose tolerance
Phentolamine	Increased insulin secretion	Blockade of adrenergic suppression of insulin secretion
Propranolol	Increased insulin activity, hypoglycemia	Pharmacologic action
Salicylates	Decreased glucose levels	Decreased protein-binding
Sulfonamides	Decreased glucose levels	Decreased protein-binding
Iron, oral		
Tetracyclines	Decreased tetracycline effect	Decreased tetracycline absorption
Isoniazid		
Aluminum antacids	Decreased isoniazid effect	Inhibition of isoniazid absorption
Phenytoin	Increased phenytoin toxicity	Inhibition of microsomal enzymes
Lithium		
Diuretics (except spironolactone and triamterene)	Increased lithium toxicity	Decreased renal lithium clearance
Indomethacin	Increased lithium toxicity	Decreased renal lithium clearance
Methyldopa	Increased lithium toxicity	Not established
Phenothiazines	Decreased phenothiazine levels	Not established
Meperidine		
Barbiturates	Increased CNS depression	Increased meperidine metabolites
MAO Inhibitors	Hypertension; hypotension and coma	Not established
Methadone		
Curariform drugs	Increased respiratory depression	Additive
Rifampin	Methadone withdrawal symptoms	Induction of microsomal enzymes
Methyldopa		
Anesthetics, general	Hypotension	Usually additive
Lithium	Increased lithium toxicity	Not established
Sympathomimetic amines	Decreased antihypertensive effect	Pharmacologic antagonism
Tolbutamide	Increased hypoglycemia	Inhibition of microsomal enzymes
Metronidazole		
Alcohol	Increased alcohol toxicity	Inhibition of aldehyde dehydrogenase
Anticoagulants, oral	Increased anticoagulant effect	Inhibition of microsomal enzymes
Miconazole		
Amphotericin B	Decreased anticandidal effect	Not established
Anticoagulants, oral	Increased anticoagulant effect	Not established
Oxytocics		
Ephedrine	Severe hypertension	Additive
Estrogens	Increased uterine contractility	Not established
Sympathomimetic amines	Severe hypertension, vasoconstriction, migraine headache	Additive
Phenothiazines		
Barbiturates	Decreased phenothiazine effect	Induction of microsomal enzymes
Propranolol	Increased effects of chlorpromazine and propranolol	Inhibition of metabolism of both drugs

Drugs	Interaction	Proposed Mechanism
Phenytoin		
Antidepressants, tricyclic	Increased phenytoin toxicity with imipramine	Not established
Contraceptives, oral	Decreased contraceptive effect	Induction of microsomal enzymes
Corticosteroids	Decreased corticosteroid effect	Induction of microsomal enzymes
Doxycycline	Decreased doxycycline effect	Induction of microsomal enzymes
Furosemide	Decreased diuresis	Decreased furosemide absorption
Isoniazid	Increased phenytoin toxicity	Inhibition of microsomal enzymes
Phenylbutazone	Increased phenytoin toxicity	Inhibition of microsomal enzymes
Primidone		
Contraceptives, oral	Decreased contraceptive effect	Induction of microsomal enzymes
Progesterone and Similar Agents		
Antihistamines	Progesterone inhibition	Direct
Phenobarbital	Decreased drug effect	Induction of microsomal enzymes
Phenothiazines	Increased phenothiazine effect	Inhibition of microsomal enzymes
Phenylbutazone	Decreased progestin effects	Induction of microsomal enzymes
Propranolol		
Anesthetics, general	Hypotension	Usually additive
Barbiturates	Decreased β-blocker effect	Induction of microsomal enzymes
Chlorpromazine	Increased effects of both drugs	Inhibition of metabolism of both drugs
Ergots	Headaches, vasoconstriction	Additive
Hypoglycemics, oral	Prolonged hypoglycemia	Decreased glycogenolysis
	Masks tachycardia and tremor	β-receptor blockade
	Hypertension during hypoglycemia	Blocked β effects of epinephrine
Indomethacin	Decreased antihypertensive effect	Possibly by prostaglandin inhibition
Lidocaine	Increased lidocaine effect	Decreased lidocaine clearance
Sympathomimetic amines	Decreased antihypertensive effect	Pharmacologic antagonism
	Hypertension with epinephrine, possibly others	Unopposed α-adrenergic stimulation
Theophylline	Increased theophylline effect with propranolol	Decreased theophylline clearance
Prostaglandin		
Antagonists, including:	Assorted, including:	Inhibition of enzymes in pathway leading to production
Aspirin	Asthma	
Caffeine	Fever	
Indomethacin	Inflammation	
Procaine	Coagulation and platelet function	
Theophylline	Inhibition of uterine stimulation	
Ritodrine		
Anesthetics (general)	Hypotension	Vasodilitation
Corticosteroids	Pulmonary edema	Increased diastolic pressure
Digitalis	Cardiac arrhythmias	Increased conduction velocities
Hypoglycemics	Increased glucose levels	Pharmacologic effect
Propranolol	Antagonism	Pharmacologic antagonism

(*continued*)

Drugs	Interaction	Proposed Mechanism
Salicylates		
Antacids	Decreased salicylate levels	Increased renal clearance
Anticoagulants, oral	Possible increased bleeding risk with aspirin	Inhibition of platelet function
	Increased hypoprothrombinemic effect (more than 2 g/day of salicylates)	Reduction of plasma prothrombin
Heparin	Increased bleeding risk	Inhibition of platelet function
Hypoglycemics	Increased hypoglycemia	Displacement from binding sites; additive
Sulfamethoxazole-Trimethoprim	Same as Sulfonamides	
Sulfonamides		
Anticoagulants, oral	Increased anticoagulant effect	Displacement from binding sites
Hypoglycemics	Increased sulfonylurea hypoglycemia	Not established
Sympathomimetic Amines		
Antihypertensive drugs	Decreased antihypertensive effect	Inhibition of norepinephrine uptake by neuron
β-adrenergic blockers (nonselective)	Hypertension with epinephrine, possibly with others	Unopposed α-adrenergic stimulation
Digitalis drugs	Increased tendency to cardiac arrhythmias	Additive
Tetracyclines		
Antacids, oral	Decreased tetracycline effect	Decreased tetracycline absorption
Barbiturates	Decreased doxycycline effect	Induction of microsomal enzymes
Carbamazepine	Decreased doxycycline effect	Induction of microsomal enzymes
Contraceptives, oral	Decreased contraceptive effect	Not established
Iron, oral	Decreased tetracycline effect	Decreased tetracycline absorption
Phenytoin	Decreased doxycycline effect	Induction of microsomal enzymes
Theophylline		
Cimetidine	Increased theophylline toxicity	Inhibition of microsomal enzymes
Erythromycin	Increased theophylline effect	Inhibition of theophylline metabolism
Influenza vaccine	Increased theophylline effect	Inhibition of theophylline metabolism
Propranolol	Increased theophylline effect	Decreased theophylline clearance
Smoking (tobacco and marijuana)	Decreased theophylline effect	Increased metabolism
Thiazide Diuretics		
Corticosteroids	Increased potassium loss	Additive
Digitalis drugs	Increased digitalis toxicity	Hypokalemia
Indomethacin	Decreased antihypertensive and natriuretic	Possibly by prostaglandin inhibition
Salicylates	Increased CNS toxicity with acetazolamide	Increased plasma nonionized salicylate with increased CNS levels
Thyroid hormones		
Anticoagulants	Increased anticoagulant effect	Increased clotting factor catabolism

Drugs	Interaction	Proposed Mechanism
Tobramycin	See Aminoglycosides	
Vitamin K		
Antibiotics	Decreased clotting factor synthesis	Inhibition of bacterial production of vitamin K due to antibiotic usage
Mineral oil	Decreased clotting factor synthesis	Decreased adsorption of vitamin K

INDEX